In memory of

Gary K. Stewart, MD, MPH
July 26, 1940 – May 31, 1998

Friend, colleague, humanitarian

Preface

You are holding in your hands the seventeenth edition of *Contraceptive Technology*, more than 800 pages of practical information for people who provide and use reproductive health services. This book began in the late 1960s as a stapled sheaf of mimeographed pages prepared for medical students. By 1971, *Contraceptive Technology* was in booklet form, and the section on oral contraceptives was six pages long!

When we look at the long line of editions of *Contraceptive Technology* on the bookshelf (as every one of the authors does), we are struck that over these years the answers change, but the questions remain the same:

- How can we help people have planned and wanted pregnancies?
- How can we help people avoid unwanted pregnancies?
- How can we provide voluntary contraception in a dignified manner?
- How can we help people use contraceptives safely and effectively?
- How can we help people avoid sexually transmitted infections?
- How can we best manage patients with health problems that affect their reproductive lives?
- How can we effectively promote healthy behaviors?
- How can we be clear-eyed advocates for humane and responsible reproductive health policy?

When we answer these questions as truthfully as we can, we honor the goals of reproductive health: every sexual act consensual, pleasurable, and infection-free; every pregnancy intended and safe; and every birth safe and wanted.

The answers do change, that we can count on. Moreover, they have grown more complex. For example, the chronic viral STIs of the 1990s are a greater challenge than the curable bacterial infections that predominated in the 1970s; the explosion of choices for hormonal contraception "overwhelms us with opportunities," as Pogo used to say; and in the span of 17 editions, abortion has been illegal and then legal, though now continuously under pressure—and even under threat of violence.

We have always depended on generous help from our colleagues and patients as contributors to, and reviewers of, chapter drafts. As such, *Contraceptive Technology* distills the thoughts of literally scores of people. With this edition, we have taken the process a step forward and have invited a dozen colleagues to be chapter authors or co-authors. You will notice for the first time that the table of contents and the first page of each chapter include authorship attribution (thereby giving credit for hard work and also exempting our invited authors from responsibility for the words of others).

We invite you to join our contributors and help us refine the answers. Tell us what is helpful, what you need that you do not find here, and what needs to be better. Write to the authors at Contraceptive Technology Communications, P.O. Box 49643, Decatur, GA 30033; or send an e-mail to ctcomm@mindspring.com.

Robert A. Hatcher
Tiger, GA

James Trussell
Princeton, NJ

Felicia H. Stewart
San Carlos, CA

Willard Cates Jr.
Chapel Hill, NC

Gary K. Stewart
Cambridge, MA

Felicia Guest
Atlanta, GA

Deborah Kowal
Decatur, GA

Dedication

We dedicate this edition to nurses, nurses practitioners, and nurse mid-wives—who with unending patience have effectively contributed skills, knowledge, spirit, and leadership toward assuring compassionate, high-quality reproductive health to millions of American women.

Providing clients with comfort, care, and understanding—the primary mission of nursing—is also the essential priority of our field.

Our respect and gratitude are keenly heartfelt. Thank you.

The Authors

Robert A. Hatcher, MD, MPH
Professor of Gynecology and Obstetrics
Emory University School of Medicine

James Trussell, PhD
Professor of Economics and Public Affairs
Director, Office of Population Research
Associate Dean, Woodrow Wilson School of Public and International Affairs
Princeton University

Felicia Stewart, MD
Director of Reproductive Health Programs
The Henry J. Kaiser Family Foundation

Willard Cates Jr., MD, MPH
President, Family Health International
Adjunct Professor of Epidemiology
University of North Carolina School of Public Health
Clinical Professor, Obstetrics and Gynecology
University of North Carolina School of Medicine

Gary K. Stewart, MD, MPH
Consultant, Reproductive Health, Cambridge, MA
Clinical Associate Professor of Obstetrics and Gynecology
University of California-Davis School of Medicine

Felicia Guest, MPH, CHES
Director of Training
Southeast AIDS Training and Education Center
Emory University School of Medicine

Deborah Kowal, MA, PA
President, Contraceptive Technology Communications, Inc.
Consultant, Reproductive Health Communications
Adjunct Assistant Professor
Rollins School of Public Health at Emory University

Invited Chapter Authors

Josefina J. Card, PhD
President, Sociometrics Corporation

Charles S. Carignan, MD
President, Stanwood Associates
Former Medical Director, AVSC International

Charlotte Ellertson, PhD, MPA
Program Associate, The Population Council

Henry L. Gabelnick, PhD
Director, CONRAD Program
Professor of Obstetrics and Gynecology, Eastern Virginia Medical School

John Guillebaud, MA, FRCSE, FRCOG, MFFP
Medical Director, Margaret Pyke Centre
Professor, Family Planning and Reproductive Health, University College, London

Debra W. Haffner, MPH
President, Sexuality Information and Education Council of the U.S. (SIECUS)

Carol J. Rowland Hogue, PhD, MPH
Professor of Epidemiology, Jules and Deen Terry Professor of Maternal and Child
    Health, Rollins School of Public Health at Emory University

Victoria H. Jennings, PhD
Director and Principal Investigator, Institute for Reproductive Health
Associate Professor, Department of Obstetrics and Gynecology, Georgetown
    University Medical Center

Kathy I. Kennedy, DrPH
Director, Regional Institute for Health and Environment Leadership, and Assistant
Clinical Professor of Public Health, University of Denver

Luella Klein, MD
Charles Howard Candler Professor, Emory University School of Medicine
Director, Maternal and Child Health Program, Grady Memorial Hospital

Virginia M. Lamprecht, RN, BSN, MSPH
Clinical Research Specialist, Research Triangle Institute

Anne Brawner Namnoum, MD
Assistant Professor of Gynecology and Obstetrics, Division of Reproductive
    Endocrinology, Emory University School of Medicine

Anita L. Nelson, MD
Associate Professor, Obstetrics and Gynecology, UCLA School of Medicine
Medical Director, Women's Health Care Programs, Harbor-UCLA Medical Center
Chief, Women's Health Care Program, Los Angeles County Coastal Health Centers

Michael S. Policar, MD, MPH
Medical Director, Partnership Health Plan of California
Associate Clinical Professor, Obstetrics, Gynecology and Reproductive Sciences,
    University of California School of Medicine San Francisco

Elizabeth G. Raymond, MD, MPH
Associate Medical Director, Family Health International

William R. Stayton, MDiv, ThD
Adjunct Associate Professor, University of Pennsylvania Graduate School of
    Education
Adjunct Professor, LaSalle University
President, American Association of Sex Educators, Counselors and Therapists

Paul F.A. Van Look, MD, PhD
Associate Director, UNDP/UNFPA/WHO/World Bank Special Programme of
    Research, Development and Research Training in Human Reproduction,
    World Health Organization

D. Lee Warner, MPH
Graduate Student, Rollins School of Public Health at Emory University

Table of Contents

Network

Expanding Perspectives on Reproductive Health

Deborah Kowal, MA, PA

- Evolving market forces and consumer expectations are changing the scope of reproductive health services.
- Many primary care providers are delivering reproductive health services. Conversely, many reproductive health care providers are delivering primary care services.

- Family planning helps not only individuals and families, but also the community at large.

In recent years, reproductive health care in the United States, in parallel with other medical disciplines, has changed to meet the challenges of evolving market forces and broadened consumer expectations. As a result, integrated reproductive health care has expanded in concept. In many cases, shifting management and insurance schemes have placed reproductive health within the domain of primary care. For an increasing number of women, the clinician who provided only family planning now often serves as their health care provider for all primary care. For others, their primary care provider now delivers the family planning services they may previously have received elsewhere.

A broader scope of "family planning" services includes not only fertility but also infertility, not only sexually transmitted infections (STIs) but also reproductive tract infections (RTIs) overall, not only menstruation and fertilization but also the preconceptual and interconceptual periods and menopause, and finally, not only reproductive tract problems but the wide range of risk factors that influence a woman's health in general. As reproductive health care expands in scope, however, two goals are paramount. First, the *planning*, or preventive focus, of family planning must remain a central activity. Second, reproductive health must be recognized for its broader *public health* impact.

PREVENTIVE HEALTH SERVICES

Family planning has always rested on the notion of thoughtful prevention rather than emphasizing the curative orientation practiced in many other medical arenas. This notion of prevention must carry through the entire practice of reproductive health, from providing contraceptives and reducing exposure to STIs to *improving* a woman's general health so she can conceive and deliver a healthy infant and to *minimizing* her risk factors for the diseases and injuries that curtail her life or quality of life.

By knowing which conditions commonly afflict your patient's population group, you can make more efficient use of resources and better assess your patient's risk factors. For example, the most common causes of mortality among women in various age groups provide a starting point (Table 1-1). Simply by screening for the risk factors associated with these problems and counseling about prevention, you can provide a high level of care for a substantial proportion of the patient population. In addition, by knowing what other conditions are uncommon or exceedingly rare, you can limit excessive workups and better identify those cases that truly merit extensive and expensive approaches. Health care provision should be based on more than "Can the patient (or the third-party payor) pay for this?"

Table 1-1 Leading causes of mortality among women

Age	Causes
15–24	Accidents Violence
25–44	Cancer Heart disease Accidents Violence Suicide
45–64	Heart disease Chronic obstructive pulmonary disease Chronic liver disease and cirrhosis Diabetes mellitus Accidents Violence

Source: NCHS (1995).

The U.S. Preventive Services Task Force has designed a recommended schedule of periodic health examinations that cover both general and reproductive health care (Table 1-2). The recommended services reflect only those areas reviewed by the Task Force or those interventions that have documented evidence of value.[23] While many approaches to periodic health screening have been proposed, the Task Force recommendations are considered the blueprint for screening guidelines. These guidelines were developed using an evidence-based methodology. Above all, the Task Force emphasizes that the most cost-effective approach to health is through primary prevention, and primary prevention is most likely met through focused risk assessment and counseling rather than through periodic "one-size-fits-all" laboratory testing and physical examinations. When and how often the preventive services are performed (or other services added) must be based on an individual patient's medical history, physical findings, and risk factors.

Table 1-2 Periodic health examination guidelines, U.S. Preventive Services Task Force

Intervention		Pertinent Chapter in
Ages 11–25	Ages 25–64	*Contraceptive Technology*
Screening		
Measure height and weight	Measure height and weight	
Read blood pressure (≥ 21 years)	Read blood pressure	19. Oral Contraceptives
Perform Papanicolaou test (age 18 or sexual experience)	Perform Papanicolaou test	3. Female Genital Tract Cancer Screening
Screen for chlamydia (sexually active)		8. Reproductive Tract Infections
Take rubella serology or vaccination history	Take rubella serology or vaccination history	
Assess for problem drinking	Assess for problem drinking	
	Measure total blood cholesterol (age 45–64)	
	Order fecal occult blood test or sigmoidoscopy (≥ 50)	3. Female Genital Tract Cancer Screening
	Order mammogram, breast exam (age 50–69)	8. Reproductive Tract Infections
HIGH RISK:	*HIGH RISK:*	
Screen for gonorrhea	Screen for gonorrhea	9. HIV/AIDS and Reproductive Health
Perform HIV test	Perform HIV test	
Injury Prevention (Advise patients to use the following)		
Lap/shoulder belts	Lap/shoulder belts	
Bicycle/ATV helmets*	Bicycle/ATV helmets*	
Smoke detector*	Smoke detector*	

(continued)

Table 1-2 Periodic health examination guidelines, U.S. Preventive Services Task Force *(cont.)*

Intervention		Pertinent Chapter in
Ages 11–25	**Ages 25– 64**	***Contraceptive Technology***

Substance Use (Advise patients of the following)

Avoid tobacco use	Advise tobacco cessation	19. Oral Contraceptives
Avoid underage drinking, illicit drug use*		
Avoid alcohol/ drug use while driving, swimming, boating*	Avoid alcohol/ drug use while driving, swimming, boating*	

Sexual Behavior (Advise patients of the following)

STI prevention: practice abstinence*		13. Abstinence
Avoid high risk behavior*	STI prevention: avoid high-risk behavior*	8. Reproductive Tract Infections
		9. HIV/AIDS
Use condoms*	Use condoms*	16. Male Condoms
Use female barrier with spermicide*	Use female barrier with spermicide*	18. Vaginal Barriers
Unintended pregnancy: use contraception	Unintended pregnancy: use contraception	17. Spermicides and Chapters 12–23

Diet and Exercise (Advise patients of the following)

Limit fat	Limit fat	
Limit cholesterol	Limit cholesterol	
Maintain caloric balance	Maintain caloric balance	
Emphasize grains, fruits, vegetables	Emphasize grains, fruits, vegetables	
Maintain adequate calcium intake	Maintain adequate calcium intake	5. Menopause
Get regular physical activity*	Get regular physical activity*	

Immunizations (Recommended schedule)

Tetanus-diphtheria boosters (11–16 years)	Tetanus-diphtheria boosters	
Rubella (females > 12 years)	Rubella (if not immunized)	25. Preconception
Hepatitis B		
MMR (11–12 years)		
Varicella (11–12 years)		
HIGH RISK:	*HIGH RISK:*	
Hepatitis A	Hepatitis A	
	Hepatitis B	

(continued)

Table 1-2 Periodic health examination guidelines, U.S. Preventive Services Task Force *(cont.)*

Interv	ention	Pertinent Chapter in
Ages 11–25	Ages 25– 64	*Contraceptive Technology*
Chemoprophylaxis		
Prescribe multivitamin with folic acid	Prescribe multivitamin with folic acid	25. Preconception
	Discuss hormone prophy-laxis, peri- and postmeno-pausal	5. Menopause

Source: U.S. Preventive Services Task Force (1996).

*The ability of clinician counseling to influence this behavior is unproven.

RISK FACTORS AFFECTING WOMEN'S HEALTH

Unintended pregnancy. Annually, nearly half of the 6.3 million pregnancies in the United States are unintended.[5,17] About 7.5% of women at risk of pregnancy do not use contraception.[1] Those who do use contraception still face some risk of unintended pregnancy because their use of their chosen method is imperfect. (See Chapter 10 on Essentials of Contraception.) Adequate instruction in how to use a method, provision of a back-up method, and information about emergency contraception could reduce the risk of unintended pregnancy. (See Chapter 12 on Emergency Contraception.)

Exposure to STIs. HIV is fatal, and hepatitis B can be life-threatening; other STIs can cause infertility and pain.[15] A recent report by the Centers for Disease Control and Prevention indicated that STIs accounted for 80% of the top 10 reportable infectious diseases.[11] Younger patients, arguably with the most to lose from a fertility standpoint, account for most STI cases. (See Chapter 8 on Reproductive Tract Infections.) Abstinence, a mutually faithful relationship, and use of condoms merit discussion during each patient encounter.

Cigarette smoking. Just as for men, tobacco smoke is associated with lung cancer and other lung diseases and heart diseases in women smokers. Women smokers in addition have an increased risk of cervical cancer, premature menopause, and impaired fertility. Women who smoke during pregnancy have an increased risk of having an infant of low birthweight, a miscarriage, a stillbirth, or an infant death.[4,9,22] The oral contraceptive user who smokes heavily faces an increased risk of myocardial infarction and thrombotic and hemorrhagic stroke.[16] (See Chapter 19 on Oral Contraceptives.) About one-fourth of women age 18 and older smoke, with smoking concentrated primarily among younger women.[10] Counseling about smoking cessation undoubtedly belongs in the reproductive health office visit.

Substance use. Alcohol use is associated with impaired judgment, increased risk of motor vehicle accidents, use of other addictive substances, cirrhosis, stroke, and hypertension. It is also a leading cause of birth defects.[14] Cocaine may cause sinusitis, allergic rhinitis, upper respiratory tract infections, epistaxis, and weight loss. Marijuana causes fatigue, panic attacks, and anxiety. Sedatives may be associated with headaches, nausea, paranoia, and sleep disturbances.

Violence. Among women age 15 to 24 years, homicide is the second most common cause of death.[21] The warnings of "stranger danger" are misleading—women are 2.5 times more likely to be killed by their husbands than by strangers.[18] Domestic violence is more common than rape or muggings.

Exposure to unintentional injury. The death rate for women occupants in motor vehicle accidents is highest at ages 15 to 24 years and age 75 and older. Three-fourths of female drivers age 20 to 34 years old are killed in night-time, single-vehicle crashes, and one-half of those 35 to 64 years have illegally high blood-alcohol concentrations.[13] Falls in the household (down the stairs or in the shower or tub) are of special concern for the elderly woman who may have problems with balance and muscle tone.

Poor nutrition and exercise patterns. Overnutrition leading to obesity is the primary nutritional problem in the United States. The obese are at increased risk of cardiovascular disease, diabetes, gallbladder disease, some forms of arthritis, and some cancers.[14] Although U.S. women can choose from an abundance of foods, many still have a deficit of vitamins and minerals such as calcium, iron, vitamin B, and folic acid. The fact that folic acid deficiency is associated with neural tube defects implies other nutritional factors may also play heavily in conceptual and pregnancy outcomes.

A lack of exercise is associated with cardiovascular illnesses, musculoskeletal problems, and respiratory insufficiency. Exercise not only reduces the risk of these health problems, but it may also have a favorable effect on mood, depression, anxiety, and self-esteem.[14]

Poverty. The fastest growing segments of people living in poverty are women and children. Over half the poor families in the United States are headed by women with no spouse present.[8] Poverty is not a lifestyle choice; it generally cannot be remedied by changing a lifestyle behavior. However, being poor is a risk factor that must be addressed by clinicians. Poverty is associated with inadequate health care and nutrition, excess stress, and limited alternatives. Having contraceptive services, including thorough education and counseling, is paramount in helping your patient avoid the emotional and financial toll of unintended pregnancy or STI. In many cases, as a contraceptive provider, you may be the indigent woman's *only* health care provider.

PUBLIC HEALTH IMPACT

Effective reproductive health care entails a focused one-on-one encounter between provider and patient. For the average provider, these individual encounters accumulate to a few thousand over a year and many thousand over a career. Though impressive in scope, these direct encounters represent only a fraction of the reproductive health care provider's influence. Although generally considered to affect a woman or a man or a family, reproductive health care potentially has a broader public health effect on a large network of persons.

In the most straightforward and direct example, the woman who receives efficacious contraception will be far less likely to have an unintended pregnancy. She may also influence her friends, relatives, and colleagues to use effective contraception. Some long-time providers anecdotally question whether pregnancy is "contagious." In some sense, peers and role models do shape a cohort's attitudes about intended and unintended pregnancy or the acceptability of given contraceptive methods.

In a parallel example, counseling and treating a man with an STI can break the transmission link so his partner(s) will not be infected. However, treating the man and preventing the infection in his partner(s) could also benefit several others such as the partner's other partner(s) or the pregnancy or offspring of someone involved in the network of spread. Further, by using the most efficacious antibiotic and by counseling the man to use all his medication, you avoid contributing to the growing list of antibiotic-resistant pathogens.

The burden that unintended pregnancies and STIs place on communities is tremendous: each year in the United States, about one and a half million women have an abortion[12] and well over a million persons become infected with an STI.[11] Were it not for the individual providers treating individual patients and indirectly affecting a number of others in the community, the health care burdens could be even greater.

A further, unappreciated, public health influence of reproductive health care, however, lies beyond measurable curative or contraceptive effects. Healthy behavior can be viewed as a continuum of behaviors eventually leading to better health. When you encourage a patient to begin taking steps in the right direction along that continuum, *you and your patient have made progress.* (See Chapter 10 on Education and Counseling.) Moreover, the knowledge and skills you impart can influence many of the patient's other health decisions. The patient may further pass the knowledge and skill to her social network and even to her children.

Just as the health care you provide can influence the community, conversely, the community influences the care you provide:[7]

- At the *individual* level of contraceptive decision making, you and your patient will consider complex factors such as sex partner characteristics; the frequency and timing of intercourse; sex networks; and the safety, cost, and availability of the contraceptive method. At the *community* level, proscriptions or pressures regarding sexual activities, teenage childbearing, and contraceptive choice can aid or limit your influence as a provider.

- At the *individual* level of STI prevention strategies, the goals are to reduce the risk of infection, relieve symptoms, and prevent sequelae of existing STI. At the *community* level, the local prevalence of STIs or the existence of antibiotic-resistant pathogens direct your diagnostic and treatment decisions.[6] Your goal will be to intervene with those *most likely to spread infection* within the community.

Finally, your goal at both the individual and the community levels will be to positively shape the socioeconomic, political, and scientific and biological forces that will characterize reproductive health care at the end of this century.

Table 1-3 U.S. Preventive Services Task Force ratings of interventions

Intervention	Level of Evidence[1]	Strength of Recommendation[2]
Syphilis		
Routine serologic testing		
High-risk persons	II-3	A
Pregnant women	II-3	A
Gonorrhea		
Routine culture or nonculture screen		
High-risk women	II-2, III	B
High-risk pregnant women	II-2	B
Other pregnant women	III	C
High-risk men	II-3, III	C
General population	III	D

(continued)

Table 1-3 U.S. Preventive Services Task Force ratings of interventions *(cont.)*

Intervention	Level of Evidence[1]	Strength of Recommendation[2]
Human Immunodeficiency Virus		
Immunoassay with confirmatory test		
High-risk adolescents and adults	I, II-2	A
High-risk pregnant women	I, II-2	A
Low-risk pregnant women, adolescents and adults	III	C
Chlamydia		
Routine culture or nonculture screen		
Sexually active female adolescents and other high-risk women	I, II-2, III	B
High-risk pregnant women	II-2	B
Other pregnant women	III	C
High-risk men	II-3	C
General population	III	D
Genital Herpes Simplex		
Routine screening		
General population	II-3, III	D
Pregnant women	II-2, II-3, III	D
Examination of pregnant women in labor	II-2, III	C
Clinician counseling of uninfected women who have infected partners to use condoms or abstain	III	C
Asymptomatic Bacteriuria		
Routine urine culture		
Pregnant women 12-16 weeks gestation	I	A
Routine urine dipstick		
Pregnant women	II-2	D
Diabetic women	III	C
School-aged girls	I	E
Sexually Transmitted Infections, including HIV		
Sexual abstinence or mutually faithful relationship	II-2	A
Regular use of condoms	II-2, II-3	A
Regular use of female barriers	I, II-2	B
Clinician counseling to reduce high-risk behavior	I, II-2	C
Unintended Pregnancy		
Sexual abstinence or regular use of contraceptives	II-2	A
Clinician counseling to improve use of contraceptives	II-3	B
Clinician counseling to promote abstinence among adolescents	III	C

(continued)

Table 1-3 U.S. Preventive Services Task Force ratings of interventions *(cont.)*

Intervention	Level of Evidence[1]	Strength of Recommendation[2]
Gynecologic Cancers		
Oral contraceptives to prevent ovarian and endometrial cancer	II-2	B
Avoidance of high-risk sexual activity; use of condoms or female barriers	II-2	A
Clinician counseling about measures to reduce risk of gynecologic cancers	III	C

Source: U.S. Preventive Services Task Force (1996) with permission.

[1]**Quality of Evidence**
I. Evidence obtained from at least one properly randomized controlled trial.
II-1. Evidence obtained from well-designed controlled trials without randomization.
II-2. Evidence obtained from well-designed cohort or case control analytic studies, preferably from more than one center or research group.
II-3. Evidence obtained from multiple time series with or without the intervention.
III. Opinions of respected authorities, based on clinical experience; descriptive studies and case reports; or reports of expert committees.

[2]**Strength of recommendations:**
A. There is *good* evidence to support the recommendation that the condition be specifically considered in a periodic health examination.
B. There is *fair* evidence to support the recommendation that the condition be specifically considered in a periodic health examination.
C. There is *insufficient* evidence to recommend for or against the inclusion of the condition in a periodic health examination, but recommendation may be made on other grounds.
D. There is *fair* evidence to support the recommendation that the condition be *excluded* from consideration in a periodic health examination.
E. There is *good* evidence to support the recommendation that the condition be *excluded* from consideration in a periodic health examination.

REFERENCES

1. Abma JC, Chandra A, Mosher WD, Peterson LS, Piccinino LJ. Fertility, family planning, and women's health: new data from the 1995 National Survey of Family Growth. Vital Health Stat 1997;Series 23, Number 19.
2. American Cancer Society. Cancer facts and figures—1997. Atlanta GA: American Cancer Society, 1997.
3. American College of Obstetricians and Gynecologists. Report of the Task Force on Routine Cancer Screening. ACOG opinion No. 128, October 1993.
4. Blumenthall SJ. Smoking v women's health: the challenge ahead. J Am Med Women's Assoc 1996;51:8.
5. Brown SS, Eisenberg L (eds). The best intentions: unintended pregnancy and the well-being of children and families. Washington D.C.: National Academy Press, 1995.

6. Cates W Jr., Holmes KK. Sexually transmitted diseases. In: Maxcey-Rosenau-Last. Preventive medicine and public health, 14th edition. In press.
7. Cates W Jr., Stone KM. Family planning, sexually transmitted diseases and contraceptive choice. Fam Plann Perspect 1992;24:75-84.
8. Census Bureau. Current population reports, series P60-188. Income, poverty, and valuation of noncash benefits: 1993. Washington D.C.: U.S. Census Bureau, 1994.
9. Centers for Disease Control and Prevention. Reducing the health consequences of smoking: 25 years of progress—a report of the Surgeon General. Atlanta GA: U.S. Department of Health and Human Services, PHS, CDC, 1989.
10. Centers for Disease Control and Prevention. Cigarette smoking among adults—United States, 1994. MMWR 1996;45:588-590.
11. Centers for Disease Control and Prevention. Ten leading nationally notifiable infectious diseases—1995. MMWR 1996:45:.
12. Centers for Disease Control and Prevention. Abortion surveillance: preliminary data—United States, 1994. MMWR 1997;45:1123-1127.
13. Dannenberg AL, Baker SP, Li G. Intentional and unintentional injuries in women. Ann Epidemiol 1994;4:133-139
14. Department of Health and Human Services. Healthy people 2000. National health promotion and disease prevention objectives. Washington D.C.: U.S. Government Printing Office; DHHS Pub. No. (PHS) 91-50213, 1990.
15. Eng TR, Butler WR (eds). The hidden epidemic: confronting sexually transmitted diseases. Washington D.C.: National Academy Press, 1997.
16. Harlap S, Kost K, Forrest JD. Preventing pregnancy, protecting health: a new look at birth control choices in the United States. New York: The Alan Guttmacher Institute, 1991.
17. Henshaw SK, Unintended pregnancy in the United States. Fam Plann Perspect 1998;30:24-29, 46.
18. Kellerman AL, Mercy JA. Men, women, and murder: gender-specific differences in rates of fatal violence and victimization. J Trauma 1992;33:1-5.
19. National Center for Health Statistics. Age-adjusted death rates for selected causes of death, according to sex and race: United States. Hyattsville MD: DHHS Publication No. 97-1232, 1995.
20. Schappert SM. National ambulatory medical care survey: 1992 summary. Advance data from vital and health statistics; no. 253. Hyattsville MD: National Center for Health Statistics, 1994.
21. Sorenson SB, Saftlas AF. Violence and women's health. Ann Epidemiol 1994;4:140-145.
22. Stein Z. Smoking and reproductive health. J Am Med Women's Assoc 1996;51:29-30.
23. U.S. Preventive Services Task Force. Guide to clinical preventive services. 2nd edition. Baltimore MD: Williams & Wilkins, 1996.

Sexuality and Reproductive Health*

Debra W. Haffner, MPH
William R. Stayton, MDiv, ThD

- Sexuality is a natural and healthy part of living.
- Sexuality involves more than sex, and sex involves more than intercourse.
- Sexual feelings and sexual behaviors are integral aspects of reproductive health.
- A client's sexual attitudes, behaviors, and relationships all influence how effective a particular contraceptive method will be.

- Understanding sexual behavior is critical for designing interventions that will reduce unintended pregnancies and sexually transmitted infections (STIs), including infection with the human immunodeficiency virus (HIV).

Sexuality and reproductive health care are interdependent. Reproductive health care providers help people manage their sexual lives. Although contraceptive services have traditionally helped plan the number and spacing of children, most clients seek contraception primarily to separate procreation from the recreational aspects of sexual intercourse.**

---

*Portions of this chapter have been adapted with permission from the following sources: Haffner D (ed). Facing facts: sexual health for America's adolescents. New York: SIECUS, 1995. Stayton W. Sexual and gender identity disorders in a relational perspective. In: Kaslow FW (ed). Handbook of relational diagnosis and dysfunctional family patterns. New York: John Wiley & Sons, 1996.
**While this chapter is directed primarily to heterosexual couples needing contraception, the authors believe sexuality is an important part of most adults' lives: gay men, lesbians, post-reproductive age women, the physically or mentally challenged, and so on.

Sexuality, however, is about much more than sexual intercourse. It encompasses the sexual knowledge, beliefs, attitudes, values, and behaviors of individuals. It includes not only anatomy, physiology, and biochemistry of the sexual response system, but also identity, orientation, roles, personality, thoughts, feelings, and relationships. The expression of sexuality is influenced by ethical, spiritual, cultural, and moral concerns.[3]

Men's and women's sexual attitudes and behaviors influence their choice of contraception and their ability to use the methods effectively. On a very fundamental level, individuals' reproductive health care decisions rest on their ability to make informed and healthy choices about their sexuality. The decision to become sexually involved—whether the relationship is consensual, whether it is monogamous, whether it is protected against unplanned pregnancy and sexually transmitted infections (STIs), or whether sexuality is a pleasurable or painful part of life—are all related to the ability to make responsible sexual choices.

Many reproductive health care clinics have treated an individual's sexuality needs as separate and distinct from contraceptive and other reproductive health needs. Practitioners may not have been trained in addressing sexual health concerns. The pressure to reach the largest number of people in an efficient manner may limit counseling to method instruction and preclude time for helping clients manage their sexual lives in a way consistent with their own values and goals.

The 1994 International Conference on Population and Development (ICPD) directly recognized the relationship of sexuality to reproductive health, acknowledging that sexuality issues must be addressed in reproductive health care settings: "Reproductive health therefore implies that people are able to have a satisfying and safe sex life and that they have the capability to reproduce and the freedom to decide if, when, and how often to do so . . . . Reproductive health . . . also includes sexual health, the purpose of which is the enhancement of life and personal relations, and not merely counseling and care related to reproduction and sexually transmitted diseases."[37] The report was endorsed by more than 200 countries.

Practitioners have a unique opportunity to provide information, education, and counseling to clients who might otherwise have no readily available resource for help. As important, addressing sexual concerns directly with clients as they choose their method may improve how effectively they use contraception.

S EXUAL BEHAVIOR IN THE UNITED STATES

Human sexual interaction is surely the least understood, least investigated behavior in daily life, so reproductive health care practitioners are placed at a serious disadvantage. Solid information on contraceptive use during penile-vaginal intercourse yields knowledge about contraceptive failure and pregnancy risk taking. Solid information on heterosexual and same-gender sexual practices (anal, vaginal, and oral intercourse) and partner networks (who does what with whom and when) yields knowledge about the transmission of STIs, including infection with the human immunodeficiency virus (HIV). Understanding the psychological and social reasons for sexual behaviors is necessary for designing effective interventions to reduce risk taking with regard to pregnancy and infection. Understanding and combating STI transmission can be even more difficult than understanding and combating unintended pregnancy—the sexual behaviors that result in an STI are more varied and the sexual networks extend beyond the present into the past.

Until recently, information about sexual behaviors was limited to questions included in surveys primarily devoted to other topics, such as general social, family, or fertility surveys or non-generalizable surveys of college students or the readers of magazines. In 1994, the National Opinion Research Center (NORC) at the University of Chicago completed the largest, most current study of sexual behaviors in the United States. The study was based on interviews with a national probability household sample of more than 3,400 men and women age 18 to 59 years.[23]

In general, Americans are having less sex than was generally believed. Eighty-three percent of American adults age 18 to 59 had one partner or no partner in the last year of the study, and most people had sexual relations a few times a month. Americans adults were about equally divided among those who have sexual relations with a partner at least twice a week, a few times a month, a few times a year, or not at all (Table 2-1).

Younger Americans behave significantly differently than older Americans. Younger people begin having intercourse earlier, marry later, and have more lifetime partners. One of the surprises of the study is that marriage is a great leveler. Married adults share remarkably similar patterns of sexual behavior, regardless of attitudes, premarital experience, religious

Table 2-1 Survey of sexual behaviors in the United States, 1994

- 83% of Americans had one partner or no partner in the last year.
- Most married couples have sexual intercourse a few times a month.
- The most frequent and most enjoyed sexual behavior for heterosexual adults is penile-vaginal intercourse.
- One-fourth of adults have oral sex regularly.
- 10% of married women and 25% of married men have had an affair.
- More than 4 in 10 adults have had 5 or more sexual partners in their lifetime.
- One in 5 Americans had a new sexual partner in the past 12 months.

Source: Laumann (1994).

or ethnic background, or geography. The vast majority of married people report they are monogamous, engage in sex a few times a month, and focus on penile-vaginal intercourse as their primary sexual behavior.

Gender differences clearly exist when it comes to sexual attitudes and behaviors. Men are much more likely than women to report recreational sex, a greater number of partners, a greater interest in a variety of sexual activities, and less monogamy. Women are much more likely to say their first intercourse was as a result of peer pressure, they do not consistently have orgasms, and they have never masturbated. Men also reported greater access to sexual partners, particularly as they age; although almost 6 in 10 single men age 45 to 59 had a partner last year, only one-third of women did. In fact, 6 in 10 single women in this age group had no partner during the last 12 months of the study.

ADOLESCENT SEXUAL BEHAVIOR

Historically, young women and young men did not reach physical maturity until their middle adolescent years. Marriage and other adult responsibilities followed puberty closely. Today's adolescents are different from young people of generations ago. They reach puberty earlier, have intercourse earlier, and marry later. Women and men who marry today do so 3 to 4 years later than young people did in the 1950s.

A majority of American adolescents date, 85% have had a boyfriend or girlfriend, 85% to 90% have kissed someone romantically, and 79% have engaged in "deep kissing."[9,31] Almost all American adolescents engage in some type of sexual behavior. Although policy debates have tended to focus on sexual intercourse and its negative consequences, young people explore dating, relationships, and intimacy from a much wider framework.[14]

The majority of young people move from kissing to other more intimate sexual behaviors during their adolescent years. More than half of all adolescents have engaged in "petting behaviors." By the age of 14, more than half of all boys have touched a girl's breasts, and a fourth have touched a girl's vulva.[9] By the age of 18, more than three-fourths have engaged in heavy petting.[31] One-fourth to one-half of young people reported experience with fellatio or cunnilingus.[9,29]

Some data suggest the progression from kissing to noncoital behaviors to intercourse varies among different groups of adolescents. While many adolescents move through a progression of intimate behaviors, lower-income adolescents are less likely to follow this progression, moving more rapidly from kissing directly to sexual intercourse.[5]

In the past two decades, there has been a significant change in the numbers of young people who have had intercourse at young ages. At each age of adolescence, higher proportions of adolescent men and women have had sexual intercourse today than had done so 20 years ago.[1]

More than 80% of Americans first have intercourse as adolescents.[1] More than half of women and almost three-fourths of men age 15 to 19 have had sexual intercourse. However, despite the large numbers of young people who experiment with a variety of sexual behaviors, intercourse is generally less widespread and certainly less frequent than many adolescents and adults believe.

Despite the public impression to the contrary, most adolescents who have intercourse do so responsibly. The majority of adolescents use contraceptives as consistently and effectively as most adults. In 1979, less than half of adolescents used a contraceptive at first intercourse.[38] By 1990, that proportion had increased to more than 70%.[26] Recent surveys suggest as many as two-thirds of adolescents now use condoms; these proportions are 2 to 3 times higher than those reported in the 1970s.[7] However, in every survey, less than half of the adolescents who recently used condoms did so all of the time.[6]

SAME-GENDER SEXUAL BEHAVIOR

Reproductive health care practitioners have long understood that presuming heterosexuality can compromise care. Many clinic counselors report they see lesbian clients who prefer the reproductive health care they receive at contraceptive clinics. Many lesbians reluctantly take condoms and foam as a method in exchange for their annual Papanicolaou smears and pelvic exams. However, there are little reliable data on same-gender sexual practices of men and almost none on women who have sex with other women.

In 1948, Alfred Kinsey, in his landmark report on the sexual behaviors of American men, reported that 37% of the total male population had an overt homosexual experience (that did not include orgasm) between adolescence and old age, that 10% of males are more or less exclusively homosexual for at least 3 years between the ages of 16 and 65, and that 4% of white males are exclusively homosexual throughout their lives.[21] Kinsey never published comparable figures for women. These findings about men, which were not based on random samples, led to the widely quoted figure that 10% of American adults are homosexual.

The NORC[23] study used a range of questions to elicit information on same-gender sexual attraction, behavior, and identification. Unfortunately, the small numbers in this study do not reveal a great deal about self-identified gays and lesbians. Respondents were asked, "Do you consider yourself heterosexual, homosexual, bisexual, or something else?" Few women (1.4%) reported themselves as homosexual or bisexual; 2.8%

of men did. This finding was very similar to other recent studies in the United States, England, and France that found 2% to 4% of adults self-identified as gay or lesbian. However, in the NORC study, 10% of the men and 9% of the women reported feeling same-gender sexual attraction, having had sex with someone of the same sex, or self-identifying as gay or lesbian. Forty-four percent of these men and 59% of these women reported desire only.[23]

WHAT DO PEOPLE DO?

The media often give the impression that everybody in America is having more sex, hotter sex, and better sex than they really are. In fact, most Americans are fairly conservative in their sexual practices. When the Kinsey studies were first published, Americans were surprised to find a significant minority of people had visited prostitutes, many people had at least one same-gender sexual experience, and there was a substantial rate of extramarital affairs.[20,21] These data, with all their limitations, suggest changes in sexual behaviors probably began around the turn of the century, and the so-called sexual revolution of the 1960s and 1970s was really just a continuation, and perhaps an acceleration, of these trends.[33]

Several factors have been offered as explanations for these trends. During the mid-1900s, larger numbers of young Americans began to go to college, and the age of marriage was delayed as a result of this education. More women entered the labor force and became financially independent. Marrying later and divorcing more, adults who were single and sexually available increased in number.

In 1948 and 1953, Kinsey found that by the age of 25, three-fourths of men but only one-third of women had had sexual intercourse.[20,21] By 1992, 89% of men and 94% of women age 18 to 24 had had vaginal intercourse. Only 5% of American adults were virgins. The vast majority of Americans first have intercourse by their twentieth birthday, and almost all adults, regardless of marital status, are sexually experienced by their mid-twenties.[23]

The NORC[23] study found that the most frequent, and most enjoyed, sexual behavior for heterosexual adults is penile-vaginal intercourse. About two-thirds of men and 60% of women have had oral sex, although only about a fourth do so regularly. Oral sex is more common in short-term relationships and more likely among whites compared with blacks. Older adults (over age 50) are less likely to engage in oral sex. About one-fourth of men and one-fifth of women report having ever had anal sex, and about 10% of single men and women have had heterosexual anal sex. Rates of anal sex are higher among Hispanics.

Frequency of sexual interactions is a factor of age, relationship duration, and marital status. In general, cohabitating couples have more sex than married couples; married people have more sex than singles. Due to increased age of marriage and the high divorce levels, there are now significantly more heterosexual adults who are not married but are nevertheless sexually involved.[33]

Ten percent of women and 25% of men report they have had an extramarital sexual relationship.[23] Since more men are involved in affairs, presumably without their wives' knowledge, more women may be at risk of STIs than they expect. Research is not available on what proportion of men have same-gender relationships outside of marriage. "These findings suggest not only that the clinician would be wise to ask about behavior rather than sexual orientation, but also that some married persons will perceive themselves to be at no (or low) risk of STIs when in fact their spouse's extramarital sexual activities may place them at risk."[33]

RISK OF HIV AND OTHER STIS

The authors of the NORC study[23] convincingly argue that the 83% of American adults age 18 to 59 years who had either one partner or no partner last year faced little risk of exposure to HIV, unless one or both partners are exposed by sharing injecting-drug equipment. Indeed, they found most American adults have sexual relationships with people very much like themselves; this fact, coupled with the limited infectivity of HIV, is part of the reason that HIV infection has not exploded among heterosexuals in the United States.

However, both the HIV and STI epidemics have clearly affected large numbers of people attending reproductive health clinics. Many people's behaviors place them at risk of infections, and clinics must now address how clients are protecting themselves against these risks. The NORC[23] study found risky behaviors:

- More than 4 in 10 Americans age 18 to 59 years have had 5 or more partners. An estimated 13 million Americans have had 21 or more partners since the age of 18.
- One in 6 Americans report they have had an STI.
- One in 5 Americans have had a new sexual partner in the past 12 months—25% of the men and 15% of the women. Of these, 8.5% had a one-encounter sexual relationship; 12% had a sexual relationship that lasted less than 2 months. The more partners one has had, the less likely they are to be known well, the less likely they are to be from the same social networks, and the less exclusive the relationships are likely to be.

- Condom use is still very low. Only 20% of people who had 3 or more partners in the past 3 years always used condoms with their primary partner. Although knowledge of AIDS is very high, less than half of those surveyed said using a condom is a very effective way to prevent HIV.

Nonvoluntary Sexual Activity

Not all sexual behavior is voluntary, and a history of sexual abuse and sexual assault may severely compromise one's ability to have safe, satisfying sexual relationships. Be sure to ask questions about prior sexual assault and abuse. It is not uncommon for young adolescent women to reveal they are being forced into sexual relationships with older men, some of whom live in the same household.

Almost one-fourth of women report they have been forced to have sexual relations during their adult lives, most often by their committed partner. In the NORC study,[23] 22% of women report they had been forced by their partners to have sexual relations, while only 3% of men report they had ever forced a women. Just under one in 5 men and women report having been sexually abused as children. At least 683,000 adult American women are raped each year.[28] A history of sexual abuse seems to have especially pernicious effects. Women with histories of sexual abuse are more likely than other women to be unhappy, have more than 10 lifetime sex partners, lack interest in sex, be unable to have orgasms, feel sex was not pleasurable in the past year, and report other sexual problems.

Adolescents are particularly vulnerable to sexual abuse, and 6% of boys and 15% of girls are sexually assaulted prior to their sixteenth birthday. In a study of adolescent girls in foster care, 43% reported experiencing some type of sexual abuse. The most prevalent type of abuse was being touched or fondled by an adult against her wishes. One in 6 reported being forced to have intercourse with an adult. One-third of the young women had been sexually abused before their tenth birthday.[30] In fact, nearly one-third of rapes are committed against women 11 to 17 years of age.[28] Nearly three-fourths of young women who had intercourse before age 14 report the experience was involuntary.[1,8]

A disproportionate number of young women who become pregnant during adolescence are victims of childhood sexual abuse. In one study of adolescents who were pregnant or were parents, 70% of whites, 42% of blacks, and 37% of Hispanics had been sexually abused as a child.[4] In another study, 64% of parenting and pregnant adolescents reported they had at least one unwanted sexual experience.[8]

SEXUAL ANATOMY*

MALE SEXUAL ANATOMY

Men tend to be conditioned to focus on genital sexual stimulation rather than whole-body touch arousal. Retraining to be comfortable and to accept and enjoy whole-body stimulation may be a desirable sexual goal for some men. Except for those men who do not respond to nipple caresses and those who deny their sensitivity because of the fear of being unmasculine, the remainder of men are likely to be pleased and excited by nipple stimulation. The sexual sensitivity of male genitalia varies strikingly according to anatomic area. The sites of highly pleasurable sensitivity (in order of decreasing response to touch) are as follows:

- Area of frenular attachment on ventral surface of penis, just behind the glans
- Coronal ridge of glans
- Urethral meatus
- Shaft of the penis
- Penile base located within the perineal area between the area of scrotal attachment and the anus
- Scrotum and testicles
- Perianal skin

FEMALE SEXUAL ANATOMY

Virtually any portion of a woman's skin may give pleasurable and exciting sensations when caressed, providing she is willing and not distracted by extraneous thoughts or events. Women tend to be whole-body oriented for sexual touching rather than genitally oriented as men are trained to be. Breast and nipple sensitivity tends to be high in most women, but some women do not find breast caressing particularly arousing.

For most women, the glans and shaft of the clitoris, the inner surfaces of the labia minora, and the first inch and a half of the vagina are the most sexually sensitive areas of all. Indeed, the clitoral head (glans) may be so exceedingly sensitive that direct touch is sometimes or always

---

*The Sexual Anatomy section is adapted from "Sexuality and Reproductive Health" by M.G. Freeman in the 16th edition of *Contraceptive Technology*.

uncomfortable. Many women enjoy indirect clitoral touch by caressing the clitoral shaft rather than the glans. Women, as men, have (or may acquire) high levels of sexual responsiveness to anal penetration.

The old Freudian argument about clitoral orgasm as being less mature than vaginal orgasm is essentially dead. Neither is more mature than the other. In fact, researchers today suggest women may have three different types of orgasm.[22,35] First is a vulvar or tenting orgasm, where the clitoris or some outside stimuli such as fantasy or breast stimulation is the main focus of the orgasmic experience. Second, a uterine or A-frame orgasm is felt deeper inside the abdomen and may be triggered by stimulation of the Grafenberg spot or G-spot. The G-spot is an area in the front wall of the vagina, an inch or two inside the vagina. Some women report ejaculating a milky-white fluid from the urethra when they reach orgasm through this stimulation. The ejaculate is described as different from urine. It also differs from urine in color, clarity, and odor and does not stain. It should be regarded as a normal variant of female sexual response, not a symptom of urinary incontinence. The third type of orgasm is a blended orgasm, which is a combination of the first two.

It is important to note that none of these orgasmic responses are better than another, and they are definitely not new goals to be reached. Goal-oriented sexual behaviors are seldom as satisfying as pleasure-directed sexual activities, that is, sexual interactions driven by what partners feel is pleasurable.

Many women describe a striking difference in their perception of pleasure in sensation, intensity, and duration of orgasm depending upon how it is achieved (dream, fantasy, kissing, caressing, masturbation, or penile-vaginal intercourse). Women vary greatly in what sort of stimulus produces orgasm. It is common for healthy, normal women to not be orgasmic through penile-vaginal thrusting alone.

S EXUAL RESPONSE

In the past 30 years, the medical and behavioral sciences have yielded information about healthy sexual functioning. Sexual arousal and response are natural to everyone from birth to death. They are not experiences that begin at adolescence and end with menopause, but rather occur to be enjoyed and experienced throughout the life cycle. Reproductive health care providers can incorporate the information that is now available into clinical practice.

There have been three major contributions to the overall understanding and knowledge of adult sexual response.

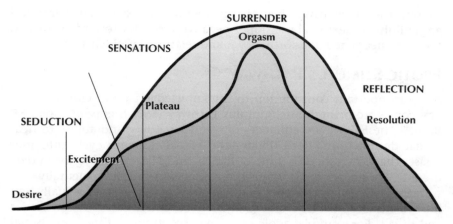

Masters W et al. (1966); Kaplan HS (1979); Stayton WR (1989).

Figure 2-1 Sexual response curve

FOUR PHASES OF RESPONSE

William Masters and Virginia Johnson can be credited with beginning the modern movement toward our understanding of the sexual response cycle. They divided the sexual response cycle into four phases: excitement (or arousal), plateau, orgasm, and resolution. In their seminal book, *Human Sexual Response* (1966),[24] they detail these phases of the response cycle for both men and women (Figure 2-1).

TRIPHASIC MODEL

Another major contribution to our understanding of sexual function comes from Helen Singer Kaplan.[16-19] She described sexual response in a triphasic model consisting of desire, excitement, and orgasm. In discussing her differences with the Masters and Johnson model, she combined their excitement and plateau stages as describing different degrees of her vasodilatory excitement phase. She believed the resolution stage of the Masters and Johnson model merely refers to the absence of sexual arousal.

Kaplan stressed it is natural to have sexual desire.[17] She discussed all the factors that contribute to the inhibition of sexual desire: medication, relational problems, sexual abuse, and the effects of illness and disease.

Among the major psychological contributors to sexual desire disorders are childhood sexual abuse, rape, negative attitudes towards sexuality, low self-esteem, religious orthodoxy, and relational problems.

EROTIC STIMULUS PATHWAY

A most important contribution to the knowledge base in clinical sexology comes from the Erotic Stimulus Pathway (ESP) theory of David M. Reed.[36] The ESP theory enhances our understanding and ability to treat sexual dysfunctions. Reed divides the sexual response cycle into four phases that correspond to those of Kaplan and Masters and Johnson (Figure 2-1). For many people, these phases are learned developmentally.

In the *seduction* phase a person learns how to get aroused sexually and how to attract someone else sexually. Seduction translates into memories and rituals. For example, adolescents may spend much time on personal appearance, choice of clothes, and mannerisms. These can enhance positive self-esteem if the adolescents like the way they feel. If the adolescents feel good about the way they look and feel, then attracting another person will be much easier. As the adolescents get older, these positive feelings are translated into sexual desire and arousal. These seductive techniques are stored in the memory and can be activated later on in life.

In the *sensations* phase, the different senses can enhance sexual excitement and ideally prolong the plateau phase. The early experiences of touch (holding hands, putting arms around a loved one) become very important. The sense of vision (staring at a loved one, holding an image of him or her when absent) is a way of maintaining interest and arousal. Hearing the loved one in intimate conversation or over the telephone becomes very important. Hearing the sounds of a partner responding to sexual stimulation can be titillating. The smell of the loved one, either a particular scent he or she wears or the sexual smell, brings additional excitement. Finally, the taste of a food or drink or the taste of the loved one become important to memory and fantasy. All these senses extend the excitement into a plateau phase, which makes one want to continue the pleasurable moment over a longer period of time. These seduction and sensation experiences are the psychological input to the physiology of sexual response. They are the precursors to sexual climax and orgasm.

In the *surrender* phase, orgasm is a "psycho-physiological surprise." The psycho-dynamic issues surrounding orgasm are power and control. Persons with orgasmic dysfunction may be in a power struggle with themselves or with their partners or with the messages received about sex. Over-control or under-control can affect orgasmic potential and the ability to allow all of the passion to be expressed.

Finally, the *reflection* phase is central to the sexual experience, especially for the person having intercourse for the first time. How does the person feel immediately after the experience? If the person feels it was a positive experience, the reflection will create positive feedback that will affect future desire. If it is negative, it will diminish future desire, at least for that specific partner, if not for sex itself. It is important that the first sexual experience not be traumatic, otherwise it can have a negative effect on future sexual encounters. For example, in a case of sexual abuse or rape, it can take years for the victim to be able to experience sex in a positive way. The effects of early negative sexual experiences can manifest in lack of sexual desire, vaginismus or dyspareunia, orgasmic disorders, sexual orientation confusion, gender dysphoria, low self-esteem, and erotophobia.

CONTRACEPTIVE CHOICE AND SEXUALITY

Attitudes about sexuality and the characteristics of sexual relationships influence choice of a contraceptive method, how effectively the method is used, and satisfaction with the method. Ambivalence about sexuality contributes to unintended pregnancies and STIs. For example, a 1996 study of women found "women who think planning ahead for birth control can spoil the fun of sex are no more or less likely to use contraceptives, but they are less likely to be satisfied with their method, and, if they use the pill, less likely to use it consistently."[12]

There is no perfect, 100% effective, 100% easy-to-use, pleasurable contraceptive. Advise clients to consider comfort with their body, desire to keep contraception independent of intercourse, degree of cooperation they can expect from their partner, and whether they also need protection against STIs (Table 2-2).

FEAR OF INFECTION

Worry about HIV, genital warts, and other incurable viral STIs often clouds the sexual experience for couples. It can be discouraging to realize that assuring protection from unwanted pregnancy is only half the battle for couples with any possible STI risk. Some people give up on sex altogether, some manage excellent safer sex techniques, but many more give up on safety. Your task is to help at-risk patients in their efforts to keep sex pleasurable and infection-free, tailoring advice to fit an individual patient's sexual patterns.

Table 2-2 Sexuality issues and contraceptive selection

	Used at Time of Coitus	Partner Support Required	Affects Sexual Functioning	Can Be Used in Love-making	Okay for Multiple Partners
Pill	No	No	May	No	Yes? With condoms
Diaphragm	Yes	No	No	Yes	Yes? With condoms
Condom	Yes	Yes	Yes	Yes	Yes
IUD	No	No	No	No	No
Abstinence	NA	Yes	Yes	Yes	Yes
Coitus Interruptus	Yes	Yes	Yes	Yes	Yes? With condoms
Fertility Awareness	Yes	Yes	May	Yes	No
Sterilization	No	No	No	No	Yes? With condoms

FEAR OF PREGNANCY AND INFERTILITY

Fear or hope for pregnancy may powerfully affect sexual desire and performance. For men, the subject of pregnancy may cause concerns, but their level of concern tends to be lower than women's. Even among premenarchal, postmenopausal, contracepting, or sterilized women, the fantasy, memory, hope, fear, anticipation, dread, joy, or desperation and despondency of pregnancy have an impact on identity that men generally do not feel. A woman who has more children than she wants may feel she literally risks the further destruction of her life every time she has penile-vaginal intercourse. An infertile woman may put her feminine identity on the line every month she tries to conceive and is likely to feel emotionally intimidated by the typical infertility workup.

Instructions to time intercourse around ovulation can be particularly stressful for both partners. Even among well-adjusted couples, such instructions are likely to precipitate performance anxiety as well as power and control conflicts. After couples begin timed intercourse, the man may experience an inability to achieve or maintain erections and the couple may have major conflicts. The spontaneity and romantic parts of lovemaking disappear, and couples often panic. Couples trying timed intercourse often need counseling and a break from the pressure of trying to conceive.

INFLUENCE OF CONTRACEPTIVE CHOICE

Oral Contraceptives

The primary sexual advantage of oral contraceptive pills is that their use is entirely independent of coitus. Like Depo-Provera and Norplant, the pills do not interrupt lovemaking. Further, women can adopt these methods without the cooperation, or even the knowledge, of their partners. For some couples, assurance of safety from pregnancy leads to increased frequency and satisfaction with sex. There are no timing issues, no stopping to use the method, and virtually no fear of pregnancy. Some women experience increased sexual desire when taking the pill. In addition, some women appreciate being able to use the pill to time their periods so they are not menstruating on weekends, vacations, or other special times.

Conversely, one of the occasional side effects of oral contraceptives is diminution or loss of sexual desire. A woman whose usual sexual response pattern is well established over time is likely to recognize immediately any loss of desire that closely follows the initiation of a new pill as an undesirable effect of the method. Such patients will usually report their symptom. A different pill combination may alleviate the problem. (See Chapter 19 on The Pill: Oral Contraceptives.)

Vaginal Barriers and Spermicides

Diaphragms, cervical caps, films, suppositories, and foam may either increase sexual pleasure or impair sexual functioning. Clients must be comfortable touching and handling their genitals to use these methods successfully. Using these methods often requires women to plan for intercourse in advance or to interrupt love-making. Some couples include inserting the method as part of their sexual play. The extra lubrication is a plus for some couples and a messy interference for others.

For some women, inserting a vaginal barrier method before the beginning of a sexual interaction may increase excitement about the upcoming behavior. For others, carrying the equipment when going out for a date may feel uncomfortable and can alter the negotiation between partners. Inserting the method during precoital play carries the risk of interrupting a tender and romantic interlude with a purely mechanical task. One possible negative sexual outcome of diaphragm use for some women is an increased risk of cystitis infections, thereby making intercourse painful if not impossible. This is particularly true for couples having very frequent or particularly rigorous intercourse. (See Chapter 17 on Vaginal Spermicides and Chapter 18 on Vaginal Barriers.)

The female condom offers particular challenges related to sexual functioning. Although some women users report that it increased their pleasure during intercourse, others report it as awkward to place and use. The external ring requires that oral sex take place before insertion or after removal. Couples have reported the method "squeaks" during intercourse. As one sexologist reports, "This is not a method for a couple without a sense of humor."

Condoms

For many couples, condoms are a sexual boon, while for others, their use dampens sexual experience. Condom use requires that the couple communicate about their decision to have intercourse, which is likely to benefit both the sexual interaction and the relationship as a whole. Condoms can help men maintain their erection longer, perhaps increasing the likelihood that women will achieve orgasm during intercourse.

Yet, everyone knows men who feel using a condom is "like taking a shower with a raincoat on." Couples need careful encouragement on how to integrate putting on the condom as part of foreplay prior to intercourse. Men need to be encouraged to practice condom use when they are not with a partner so they increase their condom skills; women can experiment with erotic techniques for putting condoms on their partners. Some men report they lose their erections when faced with an unrolled condom; practice in private should help alleviate this problem. Speak with young women about how to bring up and negotiate condom use with their male partners. Because so many women have older partners, power issues related to condom use are very real. Role play discussing condom use with her partner and help her develop strategies with a resistant partner. Encourage clients to bring their male partners to the clinic for education and counseling.

Some men lose their erection rapidly after ejaculation whereas others maintain a relatively erect penis for some time, perhaps as long as 15 to 20 minutes. Because even a few minutes of rest and relaxation while the penis is still inside the partner *may result in spillage of semen*, encourage all men to hold the rim of the male condom at the base of the penis as they withdraw. Doing so prevents the condom from slipping off. (See Chapter 16 on Male Condoms.)

Coitus Interruptus

Withdrawal requires the man to pull out and move away from his partner when his desire is to push deeper and hold more firmly. For some heterosexual couples, this contraceptive method may leave the woman in a state of high excitement without orgasmic relief. Couples using withdrawal should make a special effort to reinstitute sexual play after withdrawal to make sure both partners have achieved gratification and relief of sexual tension. The method can encourage attention on performance rather than pleasure.

In adult or X-rated movies the man often withdraws, ejaculates after a few moments of manual stroking, and then rapidly reinserts. It should be noted that this withdrawal is for the purpose of showing the viewer his ejaculation and is not for contraception. Rapid reinsertion when seminal fluid is still in the urethra as well as on the glans and shaft is not a satisfactory technique for contraception. Reinsertion should probably not take place without cleansing the male genitalia (washcloth and warm water with or without soap) and urinating to flush the urethra. (See Chapter 14 on Coitus Interruptus.)

Abstinence

It is likely all adults will go through periods of abstinence. In some cases, single people choose abstinence because of their conviction that sexual intercourse should occur only in marriage. Some single people remain abstinent because they lack a desirable partner. Some couples experience periods of abstinence because of illness, physical separation, or relationship conflicts.

There is no uniformly accepted definition of abstinence. Some people have defined abstinence as no genital contact of any kind outside of a monogamous marriage. Others have defined abstinence as not engaging in penetrative behaviors.

Young people need support for choosing abstinence until they are physically, emotionally, and cognitively ready for a mature sexual relationship. Counsel adolescents that "not everybody is doing it": although many American adolescents have had sexual intercourse, many have not. Adolescents need to understand that sexual intercourse is not a way to achieve adulthood, that adolescents in romantic relationships can express sexual feelings without engaging in intercourse, and that there are many ways to give and receive sexual pleasure without the risks associated with penetrative behaviors.[27] Spend ample time with adolescent clients addressing their decision to be sexually involved.

Adult couples may achieve satisfaction with sexual abstinence providing both select this alternative as the one that most closely meets their individual needs. A relationship can be almost anything so long as both partners agree on what it is to be. When one partner does not agree to abstinence but does not wish to give up the relationship, then a continuing conflict arises that will have emotional consequences for each individual and for the couple. One or both partner(s) may choose abstinence for contraception, for protection from an STI, as part of sexual aversion, or as a symptom of alcoholism or other addiction, depression, or distraction.

The person who feels abandoned because of a partner's decision to abstain may use masturbation as an alternative, may reluctantly accept abstinence also, or may choose to seek another partner outside of the primary relationship. (See Chapter 13 on Abstinence.)

The couple practicing sexual abstinence may lose a major method of nonverbal communication in their relationship and may find it difficult to compensate by communicating in less intimate ways. They must make special efforts to maintain or strengthen other forms of communication.

Fertility Awareness

Couples using fertility awareness methods must carefully assess its impact on their sexual relationship. Both partners must be committed to fertility awareness as the primary contraceptive method for it to be effective. Couples must negotiate in advance what the use of this method will mean during the fertile days: will they abstain from all sexual behaviors, will they abstain only from penile-vaginal intercourse, or will they use a barrier method? How sure are they that they will be able to maintain sexual limits once sexual activity is in progress? It is even possible that abstaining from sexual intercourse may enhance the experience when it does occur.

Intrauterine Devices

The primary advantage of the intrauterine device (IUD) as regards sexual functioning, is that like the pill, its use is completely separate from coitus and it is highly effective. IUD users do not need cooperation from their partner. However, women who experience severe or frequent bleeding with the IUD may find it affects their own and their partner's aesthetic experience during intercourse. (See Chapter 21 on Intrauterine Devices.)

Voluntary Surgical Contraception

Sterilization could improve or hinder sexual functioning. Men considering vasectomy need careful counseling that a vasectomy will not affect or impair their ability to have an erection. As many men are not familiar with their reproductive anatomy, beyond their penis and scrotum, begin with basic anatomy education, including the sexual function of different organs. Help men understand that vasectomy does not affect their erectile or orgasmic potential.

For many women, sterilization removes the fear of pregnancy and leads to an increase in desire and frequency of intercourse. For others, reproductive capacity is intimately connected with sexual desire, and sterilization may have the opposite effect. These issues should be carefully discussed as part of the informed consent process. (See Chapter 22 on Female and Male Sterilization.)

BRIEF INTRODUCTION TO SEXUAL COUNSELING

Few patients who have a sexual problem or dysfunction are beyond help, if they want to change and if you are willing to help. By simply allowing them a place to ventilate or by providing basic information, you can often help patients solve their problems. A brief sexual history is a good place to start (Table 2-3).

The PLISSIT counseling model was developed for providers who are not psychiatrists, psychologists, or sexual therapists but who wish to address the sexual needs and concerns of their patients and make appropriate referrals when necessary.[2] PLISSIT is an acronym for four stages of counseling: *P*ermission giving, *L*imited *I*nformation giving, *S*pecific *S*uggestions, and *I*ntensive *T*herapy.

Permission giving is not the same as telling the patient what to do. Permission is usually for thoughts, feelings, or behaviors and may be expressed as permission to do or not to do. Permission giving from a knowledgeable professional figure is quite powerful. However, you are not required to give permission for thoughts, feelings, or behaviors that violate your own professional value system; however, you are required by professional honesty to indicate to the patient that such is the case and to be frank about differing beliefs and values among professionals. For example, no qualified professionals approve of rape or child sexual abuse. The law requires reporting of all suspect child abuse to the police. This duty supersedes medical confidentiality. Professionals ought not approve

Table 2-3 Taking a sexual history

The following questions may be helpful in encouraging clients to talk about their sexual lives or to choose a contraceptive method:

1. Tell me about your earliest sexual experience.

2. Briefly give me a history of your sexual experiences to date.

3. Did you agree to these experiences?

4. How has contraception fit into your sexual behaviors?

5. Are you willing to use a contraceptive method at the time of intercourse?

6. Does your partner actively support your use of contraception?

7. Are you looking for a method you can integrate into love-making?

8. How likely is it that you will have more than one sexual partner?

9. Do you have any questions or concerns that you would like to discuss about your present sexual response or your relationship?

of behaviors that threaten the physical or psychological health of patients and their partners.

Limited information giving usually involves discussing anatomy and physiology as well as dispelling myths about sex. This task is often easy for health care providers since we know anatomy and physiology. Sexual myths are common, but trained health workers can usually dispel them easily.

Specific suggestions involve skill-building such as changing position for sexual activities, using lubricants (for dyspareunia), or using a squeeze or stop-start technique (for rapid ejaculation).

Intensive therapy will probably prove too time-consuming and involved for all but those who are specially trained and wish to devote considerable time to such work. Intensive therapy may be necessary for body-image problems, relationship problems, identity issues, depression, personality disorders, or psychoses.

Patients are rarely hesitant to provide sexual information if you are professional, concerned, self-confident, and nonjudgmental. Even though the patient may offer no data on the first visit, the experience demonstrates your willingness to deal with these special subjects, and, often on subsequent visits, patients will offer additional significant and useful data.

If the patient has beliefs or practices that may be harmful or dysfunctional (not merely different from yours), then talk about the consequences of those beliefs and practices and discuss alternatives. Refusing to offer care for ethical reasons and then failing to recommend an alternative source of reputable help is not appropriate.

COMMONLY ASKED QUESTIONS

Client's questions about sexuality often indirectly approach personal worries and concerns:

- How often do most couples my age have sex?
- Is it normal to have times in your marriage when you do not want to have sex?
- How often is it okay to masturbate?

The client with these questions is often asking "Am I normal?" Factual information about frequency may help assure the client, but she may also need time to process her own feelings about sexual behavior. Clients can be reassured there is no "right" answer to these questions; people must decide, alone or with their partner, what frequency is acceptable. Assure married clients that sexual drives fluctuate during different periods of life, so communication is essential. The questioner on masturbation needs to know that "once is too much if you don't like it," and that too much is when it interferes with your life, relationship, and work.

- My partner wants to (fill in behavior) and I do not. What can I do?
- My partner wants less sex than I do. What can I do?
- What can I do to improve my sex life?

These clients are seeking assistance with couple issues. For example, they may need permission to discuss this issue with their partner. They may need encouragement to say "no" to sexual behaviors or to ask for more control and input over sexual encounters. These clients and partners may need to be referred for counseling.

- Intercourse is painful for me.
- My partner cannot maintain an erection.
- I have never had an orgasm.

These clients may be helped by simple information. The clinician needs to elicit additional information from the client: how often does this happen? Under what conditions does it happen? The information given in the next section may be helpful.

- How can I tell if my partner has an STI?
- How do I know if my partner is being honest with me?

The reality is that no one can ever know for sure if a partner is being completely honest about past or current sexual history. Unfortunately, some people do lie to their partners, and in some cases, some people may not be aware themselves of their past exposure to STIs and even HIV. To eliminate transmission risk, condoms must be used with each and every act of vaginal, oral, and anal intercourse when a partner's health history is unknown. Of course, if the partner has obvious genital sores, lesions, or secretions, all sexual contact is best avoided until medical advice has been sought and the condition diagnosed and treated.

▌NTRODUCTION TO COMMON SEXUAL DYSFUNCTIONS

Sex therapy in its beginnings was framed in relational terms. In their book, *Human Sexual Inadequacy*, Masters and Johnson said "there is no such thing as an uninvolved partner in any marriage in which there is some form of sexual inadequacy."[25] Even though some sexual dysfunctions, such as female orgasmic disorder, can be treated on an individual basis, it is still important to offer to include her partner so she can become orgasmic with her partner as well as alone.

The effects of a sexual dysfunction on a relationship cannot be overstated. Performance fears, anxiety, and low self-esteem often are direct results of a person feeling like a failure in the bedroom. Depression is common in either or both partners if they cannot get aroused or feel they cannot satisfy their partner. On the other hand, improving sexual functioning can help the entire relationship blossom, just as resolving some of the marital discord can promote a more relaxed and satisfying sexual interaction.

Since 1970, not only has much more been learned about sexual function and dysfunction, but the field of sex therapy has expanded to include a wider range of sexual issues such as sex therapy with persons with a disability, both physical and mental, and gender identity issues.

Most people were not taught to be good lovers. While we are all born sexual and with the capacity for sexual response, we are not born lovers. In America's sexually repressive and sex-negative culture, being a good lover is a matter of learning new attitudes and skills; sex instruction with adults can provide the "how to" of being a lover. Overcoming a sexual dysfunction can be a by-product of learning and practicing the techniques of being a considerate and passionate lover.

While most clinics do not provide sex therapy, it is important to know when to refer a client to a competent sex therapist. Refer clients who require more than information and education to a qualified gynecologist, sex counselor, or therapist. Develop a list of certified practitioners in your area for referrals to a certified sex therapist. Contact the American Association of Sex Educators, Counselors and Therapists (AASECT), PO Box 238, Mount Vernon, Iowa, 52314. In this section are simple suggestions for assessing when to refer a client for sex or relationship therapy.

ETIOLOGY OF SEXUAL DYSFUNCTION

"Human sexual response consists of a complex orchestration of emotional and hormonal influences, via the autonomic nervous system, to trigger basic reflexes. Any agent that alters metabolism, stimulates or depresses the central nervous system, or locally influences anatomy or physiology is likely to affect sexual functioning."[32] Stress, emotional well-being, relational issues, and general health affect attitudes about sexual intimacy and functioning.

Organic factors. Rule out any possibility of organic, physiological, or chemical factors in the sexual dysfunction. Emotional and physiological illness, neurological disorders, use of illicit drugs or medications, or psychotropic drugs can raise or lower sexual desire or function. Perform a complete physical examination when beginning treatment. (See Chapter 6 on Menstrual Problems and Common Gynecologic Concerns.)

Individual psycho-dynamics. When Masters and Johnson[25] first presented their material on sexual inadequacy, it was believed that more than 90% of sexual dysfunction was psychologically caused. Performance anxiety was believed to be the chief culprit. Classically trained analysts believed most sexual dysfunctions were the result of psychological issues such as unresolved Oedipal wishes. Other causes of sexual dysfunction were thought to be borderline personality disorder, obsessive-compulsive personality disorders, anxiety disorders, and depression. While it is true that all of these can effect sexual function, they are not the only factors to be evaluated.

Relationship. It is common for therapists to believe from their own clinical experience and from familiarity with the sex therapy literature that most sexual problems are due to significant relationship problems. Hostility, battles for power and control, poor communications, and excessive dependency are incompatible with sexual intimacy and good functioning. For sex therapy to be successful, problems with the relationship need to be resolved. Otherwise, the behavioral suggestions recommended later in this section will not work and can even increase marital discord. Many clients will need to be referred for couples counseling.

Sociocultural and religious factors. The United States is one of the most sexually repressive cultures in history when compared with both ancient and other contemporary societies. Kaplan as well as Masters and Johnson held that religious orthodoxy has played a major part in the widespread sexual dysfunction of our day. Guilt, fear, and the denial of sex as pleasure have led to sexual inhibition. In recent decades, widely held gender-role stereotypes (males as aggressive, females as passive, and so on) have been challenged. Cultural imprinting or conditioning (males pressured to perform quickly; females conditioned to not stimulate the male directly) can create sexual dysfunctions.

SEXUAL DESIRE DISORDERS

The desire disorders[17] are associated with Reed's seduction phase. In any given case, it must be determined when seduction takes place: in the present or the past? These disorders must create enough distress and interpersonal difficulty for both partners to be motivated to change.

Lack of desire may be lifelong or acquired; that is, desire may have once been there, but then have diminished for some reason. A lack of desire may be generalized, that is, experienced in every situation; or it may be situational, occurring only in certain situations. For example, one may have desire on vacation but not at home in familiar surroundings.

Or one may lack lustful feelings with a long-term partner but feel aroused by others. The dysfunction may be due only to psychological factors or to a combination of psychological and organic disease or chemical factors. Sexual desire disorders should be referred to a trained sex therapist.

In *hypoactive sexual desire disorder*, there is a lack of desire for sexual activity and often an inability to experience sexual fantasies. In a *sexual aversion disorder*, there is an aversion or avoidance to kissing, touching, and genital sexual contact. Using a picture or genital model, discuss the client's feelings about observing or touching the model.

SEXUAL AROUSAL DISORDERS

Female sexual arousal disorder. Women who have difficulty getting aroused will have difficulty lubricating and feeling erotic genital sensations. There is little or no genital swelling. The clinician can recommend lubricants, such as K-Y Jelly or Astroglide, which can be bought over-the-counter. Evaluate the couple's foreplay patterns to assess whether there has been enough attention paid to the woman's arousal. Perimenopausal and menopausal women may benefit from special over-the-counter lubricants like Replens or hormonal creams or treatment, which diminish vaginal dryness. (See Chapter 5 on Menopause.) Sometimes, a psychological component needs to be addressed as well.

Male erectile disorder. If a man has difficulty gaining or maintaining an adequate erection suitable for sexual activity, he suffers from erectile disorder. Obtain a medical evaluation. Even when it is possible to treat the erectile disorder through medical intervention, evaluate the effect of the erectile disorder on the couple's relationship. Currently there are four possibilities of medical intervention:

- Testosterone injections can increase desire and erectile capability for men whose testosterone levels are low.
- Yohimbine helps both desire and erection ability.[10] Yohimbine, a natural ingredient from the bark of the Yohimbe tree, can be obtained from a health food store or by prescription under the name Yocon or Aphrodyne.
- Self-administered penile injections of a combination of Prostaglandin E1, Papaverine. and Phentolomine Regitine are an excellent means for achieving full erections. These injections are considered safe with no long-range scarring or other problems. The injections are painless, but the idea of giving oneself an injection in the penile area may be hard for some men who may prefer a urethral delivery system called Muse.
- The ErecAid System, a device placed over the penis to create a vacuum, draws blood into the penis by the pump. When an erection

is attained, a rubber band is placed over the base of the penis to hold the blood in. The pump can be purchased through mail-order catalogs or sex shops, but it is also a prescription item.

These options should be supplementary to sex therapy, which can help greatly with the relational issues that may occur as a result of the dysfunction. For example, it is common for the non-dysfunctional partner to feel her partner is no longer attracted to her or that he may be interested in someone else. He may have lost his confidence in himself or believe he is no longer attracted to his partner. Both may feel powerless and fearful. Even though he may have regained his erectile capability through a medical intervention, sexual desire may still be affected if the interpersonal issues are not treated.

SENSATE FOCUS FOR MALE AND FEMALE AROUSAL DISORDERS

Simple pleasuring exercises can increase or enhance the arousal process. Masters and Johnson called these exercises sensate focus. First, have the couple sensually touch each other over their entire bodies, except for the genital and breast areas. This is often difficult, because when the couple is experiencing sexual difficulties, one or both often take on spectator roles and try to think about what is going on in their partner's head. They lose the focus on their own pleasure as participants.

Once partners have been able to focus on their own pleasurable experiences, they can explore the breasts and genitals and determine which touches are pleasurable, threatening, or irritating. What many couples do not realize is that different areas on the breasts and genitals can be more erotic and sensitive than other spots. Next the couple caresses the breasts and genitals to produce arousal. If either of the partners experiences arousal, they may go on to non-coital orgasm, unless the dysfunction is directly related to orgasm.

Before trying intercourse when he is able to gain an erection consistently, the man should deliberately lose his erection by having his partner stop stimulating him. Once his erection has gone down, his partner should then restimulate him until he has another erection. The important lesson here is that if there has been no orgasm, he can lose his erection several times and regain it with further erotic stimulation. Too often a man incorrectly believes that if he loses his erection once, the experience is over for him. After the man has accomplished losing and regaining an erection, his partner can stimulate him while he is lying on his back and then mount him and just hold his penis near her labia and clitoris. When she does this and he holds the erection, she can then insert the penis into her vagina without doing any thrusting, so he can experience being contained in her vagina without stimulation. He will then lose his erection and she can restimulate him. When he gets an erection again, she can put his penis into her vagina and begin slowly thrusting. They can continue this exercise until they are having satisfying intercourse.

ORGASMIC DISORDERS

The psychological issues involved in orgasmic disorders usually involve issues of power and control. Other issues include an inability to relax, let go, and let the tension of the sexual response take over. Being vulnerable, fearing failure, or fearing success can affect orgasmic potential.

Female orgasmic disorder.   A woman who has never been orgasmic should begin with self-exploration and stimulation to experience her sexual response cycle without having to perform in front of her partner. The books *For Yourself*,[3] *Sex for One: The Joys of Self-loving*,[11] or *Becoming Orgasmic: A Sexual and Personal Growth Program for Women*[15] are helpful resources for clients to learn about masturbation and orgasm. A vibrator also can be a useful aid in helping the woman experience her orgasmic potential. Once she has become orgasmic, it is easier for her to share with her partner the type of touch that helps her reach an orgasm. As she develops her orgasm response, she can then introduce the experience into intercourse by masturbating or using a vibrator while her partner's penis is inside her. Advise her not to get discouraged if orgasm does not occur during the first few love-making encounters. It takes time, patience, and comfort.

Male orgasmic disorder.   A man who cannot have an orgasm with intercourse is rare and usually has difficulty giving of himself in a relationship. It is most helpful to have him masturbate with his partner so she can experience him having an orgasm. During intercourse, when either partner is ready for orgasm, he should withdraw and masturbate until he feels himself on the brink of orgasm and then again insert his penis in the vagina. The goal is to have him experience having an orgasm. Once this occurs it may be easier for him to get to the point of orgasm through intercourse. A lot of patience and practice are needed for this dysfunction. If he works on his ability to give of himself generally to the relationship, it will help him have an orgasm inside his partner.

Another possibility is that the male orgasm is inhibited because of a fear of an unwanted pregnancy or STI. These men need information about contraception and safer sex methods. Feeling safe can enhance his orgasmic release.

Premature ejaculation.   Premature ejaculation has been successfully treated with both the "stop-start" method and the "squeeze" technique. The "stop-start" method is often the easier and preferred procedure. After the man is aroused, his partner should stimulate (masturbate) him until he is almost ready to ejaculate. He should signal his partner, who then stops any further stimulation until the feeling of ejaculatory inevitability subsides. His partner then resumes stimulation until he again feels he is going to ejaculate, and then the partner stops. After stopping three or four times, he should go ahead and have an ejaculation. This process should be repeated several times a week until the client is able to hold back ejaculation for as long as he likes. Next, he can try intercourse, using the female superior position, going through the same process. When his penis is in her vagina, she should begin moving up and down on the penis, until he feels he is going to ejaculate. She should stop until he loses that feeling, and when he does, start moving up and down again. After repeating this exercise several times, the couple can proceed to have an orgasm. With patience and practice, this method will work.

It is also possible to treat premature ejaculation with a small dose of Prozac or some other antidepressants. Combining the use of one of these medicines with the above exercises can bring about more rapid results.[10]

SEXUAL PAIN DISORDERS

When a client suffers from dyspareunia (painful intercourse), vaginismus (inability to insert the penis into the vagina because of spasms), or vulvodynia (sensitive or painful areas in the vagina), it may be best to refer the client to a certified sex therapist or to a specialist, such as a gynecologist who is trained to help with these dysfunctions. (See Chapter 6 on Menstrual Problems and Common Gynecologic Concerns).

REFERENCES

1. Alan Guttmacher Institute. Sex and America's teenagers. New York: The Alan Guttmacher Institute, 1994.
2. Annon JS. The behavioral treatment of sexual problems. Vol. 1, Brief therapy. Honolulu HI: Mercantile Printing, 1974:100-105.
3. Barbach L. For yourself: the fulfillment of female sexuality. Garden City NY: Doubleday, 1976.
4. Boyer D, Fine D. Sexual abuse as a factor in adolescent pregnancy and child maltreatment. Fam Plann Perspect 1992;24:4-11.
5. Brooks-Gunn J, Furstenberg FF. Coming of age in the era of AIDS. Puberty, sexuality, and contraception. Millbank Quart 1990;68(Suppl 1).
6. Cates W. Teenagers and sexual risk taking: the best of times and the worst of times. JAMA 1991;12:84-94.
7. Centers for Disease Control and Prevention. Selected behaviors that increase risk for HIV infection among high school students. MMWR 1992;41:237.

8. Child Welfare League of America. A survey of 17 Florence Crittenton agencies serving minor mothers. Washington DC: Child Welfare League of America, 1994.

9. Coles R, Stokes F. Sex and the American teenager. New York: Harper and Row, 1995.

10. Crenshaw TL, Goldberg JP. Sexual pharmacology. New York: WW Norton, 1996.

11. Dodson B. Sex for one: the joys of self-loving. New York: Harmony Books, 1987.

12. Forrest JD, Frost JJ. The family planning attitudes and experiences of low-income women. Fam Plann Perspect 1996;28:246-255, 277.

13. Forrest JD, Singh S. The sexual and reproductive behavior of American women, 1982-1988. Fam Plann Perspect 1990;22:206-214.

14. Haffner DW, National Commission on Adolescent Sexual Health. Facing facts: sexual health for America's adolescents. New York: SIECUS, 1995.

15. Heiman J, LoPiccolo J. Becoming orgasmic: a sexual and personal growth program for women. Englewood Cliffs NJ: Prentice-Hall, 1988.

16. Kaplan HS. Active treatment of sexual dysfunctions. New York: Brunner/Mazel, 1981.

17. Kaplan HS. Disorders of sexual desire: and other new concepts and techniques in sex therapy. New York: Brunner/Mazel, 1979.

18. Kaplan HS. Sex aversion, sex phobias and panic disorders. New York: Brunner/Mazel, 1987.

19. Kaplan HS. The evaluation of sexual disorders: psychological and medical aspects. New York: Brunner/Mazel, 1983.

20. Kinsey AC, Pomeroy WB, Martin CE. Sexual behavior in the human female. Philadelphia: WB Saunders, 1953.

21. Kinsey AC, Pomeroy WB, Martin CE. Sexual behavior in the human male. Philadelphia: WB Saunders, 1948.

22. Ladas AK, Whipple B, Perry JD. The G spot: and other recent discoveries about human sexuality. New York: Holt, Rinehart and Winston, 1982.

23. Laumann EO, Gagnon JH, Michael RT, Michaels S. The social organization of sexuality—sexual practices in the United States. Chicago IL: University of Chicago Press, 1994.

24. Masters W, Johnson V. Human sexual response. Boston: Little, Brown & Co., 1966.

25. Masters WH, Johnson VE. Human sexual inadequacy. Boston: Little, Brown & Co., 1970.

26. National Center for Health Statistics. Contraceptive use in the United States: 1982-1990. Advance Data 1995.

27. National Guidelines Task Force. Guidelines for comprehensive sexuality education: kindergarten - 12th grade. Second edition. New York: SIECUS, 1996.

28. National Victims Center. Rape in America: a report to the nation. Arlington VA: National Victims Center, 1992.

29. Newcomer S, Udry J. Oral sex in an adolescent population. Arch Sex Behav 1985;14:41-46.

30. Polit DF, White CM, Morton TD. Child sexual abuse and premarital intercourse among high risk adolescents. JAHC 1990;11:231-234.

31. Roper Starch Worldwide. Teens talk about sex: adolescent sexuality in the 90's. New York: SIECUS, 1994
32. Satterfield S, Stayton W. Understanding sexual function and dysfunction. In: Stayton W (ed). Topics in clinical nursing 1980;1:21-32.
33. Schwartz P, Gillmore M, Civic D. The social context of sexuality. In: Cates W, Hansfield and Holmesk (ed). Sexually transmitted diseases. New York: McGraw Hill, 1996.
34. Sexuality Information and Education Council of the United States. SIECUS position statements. New York: SIECUS, 1995:1.
35. Singer J, Singer I. Types of female orgasm. In: LoPiccolo J, Lopiccolo L (ed). Handbook of sex therapy. New York: Plenum Press, 1978.
36. Stayton WR. A theology of sexual pleasure. American Baptist Quarterly 1989;8:94-108.
37. United Nations. Programme of Action. Reproductive rights and reproductive health. Proceedings of the International Conference on Population and Development, September 5-13, 1994; Cairo, Egypt, 1994; section 7.2:43.
38. Zelnik M. Shah FK. First intercourse among young Americans. Fam Plann Perspect 1983;15:64-68.

Female Genital Tract Cancer Screening

Michael S. Policar, MD, MPH

- Early detection by Papanicolaou (Pap) smear prevents at least 70% of potential cervical cancers. Pap smears should be performed at least every 3 years, depending on the woman's risk factors for cervical cancer.
- Convincing evidence shows that human papilloma virus (HPV atypia) and cervical intraepithelial neoplasia (CIN) I represent the same entity.

- Oral contraceptive use for 10 years or longer reduces the risk of ovarian cancer by as much as 80%.
- Most guidelines recommend mammographic screening every 1 to 2 years for any woman age 50 and older. The value of screening in women younger than age 50 is under debate; however, many experts agree that women with risk factors for breast cancer should initiate regular mammographic screening at age 35 to 40.

A reproductive health care visit represents an ideal opportunity to offer periodic health screening services, including screening for genital tract cancers. As early as the 1920s, the prevalent philosophy of the American medical community was that individuals of all ages should receive an annual physical examination and a battery of routine screening tests to detect early, asymptomatic disease.[2] Over the past decade, however, the wisdom of this practice has been challenged, and research studies and health policy discussions have focused upon the optimal content of periodic health screening: which tests should or should not be performed, how often each screening test should be done, and whether each test should be performed universally or limited to persons of certain age or risk factors.[27,43] While many approaches to periodic health screening have been proposed, the recommendations of the United States Preventive Services Task Force (USPSTF) are considered the blueprint for the screening guidelines developed by most state Departments of Health, professional specialty societies, and health plans.[46] Using an evidence-based methodology, the USPSTF guidelines gauged both the strength of each recommendation and the quality of the research studies used to develop each guideline. The guidelines emphasize that the most cost-effective approach to maximizing health status is by avoiding the development of disease through primary prevention based on focused risk assessment and counseling interventions rather than on periodic physical examination or laboratory testing. (See Chapter 1 on Expanding Perspectives on Reproductive Health.)

Over the years, annual periodic health screening has been linked with the provision of prescription hormonal contraceptives. In many cases, a woman could get a prescription for oral contraceptives (OCs) only when she underwent an annual examination, which necessarily included a breast exam and a Papanicolaou (Pap) smear. In this way, women have been compelled to receive desirable public health screening tests as a by-product of their need for contraception. However, a recent trend among reproductive health programs has been to remove the requirements for genital tract cancer screening from provision of prescription-based contraceptives, based on the philosophy that beneficial screening tests must be supported on their own merits, and any unnecessary barriers to contraceptive services should be removed.[10,44] Regardless of one's attitude on this issue, genital tract cancer screening is a desirable, and in some cases, lifesaving measure, irrespective of a woman's contraceptive method. Furthermore, hormonal methods should never be restricted or withheld from a woman solely because she has an abnormal Pap smear. There is no reason to believe that the use of any contraceptive method will hasten the progression of an existing cervical lesion. All too often, the unfortunate result of withholding contraceptive methods from a woman with cervical dysplasia is unintended pregnancy, which makes diagnosis more difficult and often delays treatment.

SCREENING FOR CERVICAL CANCER

The Pap smear, more than most other screening tests, has proven its cost effectiveness over the years.[23,46] Although negative press reports in the mid-1980s shed doubts upon Pap smear quality, early detection of pre-malignant lesions by Pap smears prevents at least 70% of potential cervical cancers. Of the remaining 30% (16,000 women) who develop new cases of cervical cancer each year:[12,13]

- One-half had not had a Pap smear in the past 3 to 5 years.
- One-half had received a Pap smear within 3 to 5 years that was falsely negative:
  - One half of these falsely negative smears occurred in women whose initial smears were re-read as normal, either because the pre-malignant or malignant lesion had too little exfoliation to be detected, the lesion grew rapidly and so did not exist at the time of the initial Pap smear, or the lesion was a sampling error.
  - The other half occurred in women whose initial smears were re-read as abnormal, suggesting a screening or interpretive error in the cytopathology lab.

In addition, in 1996 the U.S. Food and Drug Administration (FDA) approved a number of new technologies aimed at improving the detection rate of abnormal Pap smears, thereby reducing the rate of false negatives. One approach, the "Thin Prep" sample preparation technique, improves accuracy by increasing the number of cells sampled and by removing blood, mucus, and debris from the background of the smear. Another approach is to evaluate the Pap smear by routine microscopy and then re-screen the negative smears with a computer-based evaluation techniques (PapNet, AutoPap 200) to detect abnormal smears that should be re-evaluated microscopically. Each of these approaches improves Pap smear accuracy by about 30% over current practices; however, evidence is insufficient to determine whether the additional cost associated with these tests justifies their use or, in contrast, if the increased cost of screening actually may lead to fewer Pap smears being performed.[19]

PATHOPHYSIOLOGY

The cervix consists of two types of epithelium:

- Squamous epithelium, which covers the vagina and the portio vaginalis of the cervix
- Columnar epithelium, which covers the endocervical canal, and in younger women, the area around the external cervical os

At menarche, the vaginal pH drops into an acidic range and causes the fragile columnar epithelial cells around the cervical os to be replaced by squamous epithelium, a process referred to as squamous metaplasia. As this process proceeds over decades, the advancing edge of the squamous epithelium (referred to as the squamocolumnar junction) migrates centrally toward the cervical os and ultimately into the endocervical canal. Because squamous cell cancers and their precursors virtually always develop within the field of metaplasia (also called the transformation zone), both cytological and colposcopic evaluation focus upon this area.[37]

There is now widespread agreement that the cause of cervical dysplasia is a DNA mutation in an immature metaplastic cell—a consequence of human papilloma virus (HPV) infection in concert with other carcinogenic co-factors. Although more than 70 DNA-types of HPV have been identified, only a limited number are associated with premalignant and malignant epithelial lesions of the lower genital tract: HPV types 16, 18, 45, and 56 are known to have a high potential for malignancy.[38,42] The high-risk HPV types exert their cancer-causing effects through a series of events leading to the degradation of the p53 tumor suppressor protein in infected cells, reducing the host's ability to reject cells with random DNA mutations. However, HPV infection alone is insufficient to initiate this process. A facilitating agent, or co-factor, appears to be necessary to act in concert with HPV to initiate these premalignant changes. For example, cigarette smoking has been identified as a powerful co-factor, doubling a smoker's risk of cervical cancer.[3,48] HPV types 6 and 11, frequently isolated from cervical condylomata and low-grade lesions, are felt to exhibit low or no malignant potential.

HPV infections are widespread among sexually active adults, costly to characterize virologically, and impossible to eradicate once established. In addition, the role of evaluating and treating the male sexual partner in preventing recurrences of cervical dysplasia in treated women and in preventing spread of the virus to uninfected women is uncertain.[7] From a public health viewpoint, it makes more sense to detect and treat preinvasive lesions, before life-threatening invasive cervical cancers have a chance to develop, rather than to rely on a strategy that focuses on the transmissibility of HPV.

RISK FACTORS FOR CERVICAL CANCER

Epidemiological observations are consistent with the biological mechanism of cervical cancer. The following are primary epidemiological risk factors for the development of cervical cancer:

- Early onset of intercourse (defined as a sexual debut before 20 years old). Metaplasia is most active during adolescence, making a young woman more vulnerable to cell changes.
- Three or more sexual partners in one's lifetime. The greater the number of sexual partners, the greater the risk of acquiring a high-risk type of HPV.

- Male sexual partner who has had other partners, especially if a previous partner had cervical cancer.
- Clinical history of condyloma acuminata. Infection with a low-risk type of HPV is a risk marker for co-infection with a high-risk type.[11]
- Infection with the human immunodeficiency virus (HIV) and other medical conditions associated with immunodeficiency. These illnesses decrease the ability of the immune system to recognize and reject clones of abnormal cells.

Protective factors include virginity, long-term celibacy, life-long mutual monogamy, and long-term use of condoms. Factors that appear to have no effect on cervical cancer risk include history of herpes simplex virus infection, circumcision status of the male partner, religious background, or number of pregnancies. The effect of race and socioeconomic status are controversial. Studies show higher rates of cervical cancer among black women and women of lower socio-economic status; however, it is unclear whether the higher rates are related to poor access to medical care and, consequently, Pap smear services or other undetermined factors.

HIV Infection and Cervical Cancer Risk

Recent studies of cohorts of women with HIV infection have demonstrated disturbing findings regarding cervical neoplasia.[6,30] While the prevalence of dysplasia in reproductive-age women is below 3%, its prevalence is 36% among HIV-positive women and 64% among women with acquired immune deficiency syndrome (AIDS).[22] Although an early uncontrolled study suggested that HIV-positive women had substantially higher rates of falsely negative Pap smears,[32] more recent studies show that the accuracy of Pap smears is the same in HIV-positive as in HIV-negative women.[1,22] When cervical dysplasia occurs in an HIV-infected woman, the lesion may progress more rapidly, especially if she is immunocompromised. It also has been observed that HIV-positive women treated for cervical dysplasia have loop electrosurgical excision (LEEP) failure rates of 40% to 60% (even higher if the women are immunocompromised) compared with failure rates of 10% for HIV-negative women.[31,47] In 1992, the Centers for Disease Control and Prevention changed its surveillance definition of AIDS to include cervical cancer in an HIV-positive woman as an indicator of AIDS.[7] Women with HIV also are more likely to develop multifocal vulvar intraepithelial neoplasia (VIN), as well as pre-invasive and invasive squamous cell cancers of the anus.[21] Three clinical recommendations can be made:

1. Some experts recommend that HIV-positive women undergo a baseline colposcopic evaluation at the time of initial diagnosis of HIV infection. Thereafter, immunocompetent HIV-positive women should receive Pap smears annually; those who are immunocompromised or who have been treated for dysplasia since the time of HIV diagnosis should receive a Pap smear every 6 months.

2. There is no role for expectant management when an HIV-positive woman has an abnormal Pap smear result. Perform a colposcopy after a single reading of atypical squamous cell of undetermined significance (ASCUS) or squamous intraepithelial lesion (SIL).[25] During this examination, check the vagina, vulva, and anus for neoplastic changes.

3. Do not assume that treatment is futile for the woman who has both HIV and premalignant or malignant cervical disease. Aggressive treatment of cervical disease will prolong life in most cases.[29]

TECHNICAL ASPECTS OF CYTOLOGICAL SCREENING

High accuracy in cytological screening depends on a good quality cervical sample, appropriately performed slide preparation, and competent cytopathologic interpretation.

- **Timing.** A Pap smear may be performed whenever heavy menstrual bleeding is not present. However, the optimal timing is at midcycle in a woman who has not has intercourse for 24 hours and has not placed any substances in her vagina for at least 48 hours.

- **Sampling.** Moisten the speculum with warm water. Never use other lubricants because they may cause cell clumping on the slide and interfere with cytological interpretation. Using a large cotton-tipped applicator in a gentle wiping motion, remove excess cervical mucus. The order in which specimens are sampled is critical: since samples most easily contaminated by blood should be obtained early in the sampling sequence, take the Pap smear first. Sampling of the vaginal pool is not helpful in premenopausal women and actually may decrease the quality of the sample by adding degenerating cells and other debris. If additional cervical sampling is necessary for evaluation of infection, collect the sample for gonorrhea testing next and the sample for chlamydia testing last. An exception is the DNA probe test for gonorrhea and chlamydia; these tests are sensitive to blood and should be performed before the Pap smear.

- **Slide preparation.** First sample the exocervix by rotating a wooden or plastic spatula 360 degrees around the exocervix. Immediately place the sample on a glass slide, creating a monolayer covering most of the slide's surface. Second, sample the endocervical canal, preferably using a brush sampling device, or if the brush device is not available, a saline-moistened cotton-tipped applicator. Plate this sample directly over the first sample by gently rolling the brush or swab over the surface of the slide, again attempting to achieve a monolayer of material. Fix the sample immediately in order to avoid air drying. Unless specifically requested by the cytopathology laboratory, separate slides are not needed for each sample, nor is segmenting the slide into a section for the exocervical sample and another for the endocervical sample.

CYTOLOGICAL SCREENING INTERVALS

The issue of Pap smear screening intervals has been a contentious one, mainly because of disagreements over cost effectiveness. In August 1987, a Pap Smear Consensus Statement was issued by a number of medical organizations:[9]

> All women who are or who have been sexually active or who have reached 18 years old (should) have an annual Pap test and pelvic exam. After a woman has had three or more consecutive, satisfactory, normal annual exams, the Pap test may be performed less frequently at the discretion of her physician.

Many clinicians find that this statement provides minimal guidance, because the term "physician discretion" is rather nebulous. The current USPSTF guidelines for cervical cancer screening provide somewhat more specific advice:[46]

- Regular Pap tests are recommended for all women who are or who have been sexually active and who have a cervix.
- Pap smears should be done at least every 3 years, depending upon the woman's risk factors for cervical cancer.
- Discontinue regular testing after age 65 in women who have had regular previous screening in which Pap smears have been consistently normal.
- Women who have had a hysterectomy for benign disease do not need to have further Pap smears.
- Clinicians should consider providing patients with a pamphlet or other written information about the meaning of the abnormal smear to help ensure follow-up and minimize anxiety over possibly false-positive results.

A central concern in determining screening intervals is the roughly 20% risk of a falsely negative Pap smear.[50] The longer the sampling interval, the greater risk that a falsely negative Pap smear will delay the diagnosis of a cervical lesion. For example, if a woman chooses a 3-year sampling interval, a single false-negative smear could result in a delay of up to 6 years in the detection of her lesion.

More useful are guidelines that account for epidemiological risk factors in the design of Pap smear sampling intervals for individual women. Table 3-1 contains the recommendations for Pap smear screening intervals used by Title X Family Planning programs,[45] with modifications based upon the recommendations of the USPSTF.[46]

PAP SMEAR REPORTING SYSTEMS

In the original Pap smear reporting system, premalignant squamous epithelial changes were referred to as dysplasia and lesions with increasing degrees of involvement of the cervical epithelium were graded in severity as mild, moderate, and severe dysplasia; full-thickness epithelial lesions were termed carcinoma-in-situ (CIS). In general, dysplasia was considered of lesser importance than CIS, which in the 1950s was considered equivalent of an early cervical cancer. Since the 1970s, this terminology was replaced with three categories of cervical intraepithelial neoplasia (CIN) nomenclature to stress the fact that premalignant squamous lesions of the lower genital tract represent a continuum of the same process and that the severity of the CIN lesion is irrelevant as long as it is detected and treated before invasion occurs.[38]

The Bethesda Classification System (TBS) for cervical cytological screening[14] (Table 3-2) has become the international standard for cervical cytopathological reporting. One of the most controversial aspects of TBS was the inclusion of "HPV atypia" and CIN I in the same category of low-grade squamous intraepithelial lesions (LG-SIL). Some observers who considered these to be two separate entities feared that placing them in the same category would lead to over-aggressive management of atypia or under-evaluation of potentially high-grade CIN lesions.[15] Convincing evidence, however, shows that HPV atypia and CIN I represent the same entity:[26]

- Virologically, both HPV atypia and CIN I are in most cases associated with the presence of HPV types 6 and 11, although either lesion may demonstrate the presence of high-risk HPV types 16 and 18.
- Morphologically, the two lesions appear colposcopically as acetowhite epithelium with few or no vascular changes.
- Histologically, the nuclear and cytoplasmic characteristics of the lesions are very similar and commonly are indistinguishable under the microscope.

Table 3-1 Pap smear screening intervals

Risk level	Characteristics	Interval
Extremely low-risk	• Virginal • Older than 65 years old with a history of consistently normal Pap smears, including at least one smear at 60 years old or later	Papanicolaou (Pap) smear not necessary
Low-risk	• Onset of sexual activity at >20 years • <3 sexual partners (ever) • User of barrier contraception • No history of HPV or STDs • Non-smoker • Previously normal Pap smears	Yearly for 3 years, then every 2–3 years
High-risk	• Onset of sexual activity at <20 years old • 3 or more sexual partners • History of HPV or STDs • Previously abnormal Pap smear • Cigarette smoker	Yearly
Post-hysterectomy	• Cervical or uterine malignancy • Premalignant cervical lesion • Benign cervix and uterus	• Every 3 months for 2 years, every 6 months for 3 years, then yearly • Every 6 months for 2–3 years, then yearly • Pap smear not necessary
DES-exposed daughters		• First Pap smear at onset of menstruation, 14 years old, or onset of intercourse • Baseline colposcopy after onset of intercourse • Vaginal and cervical Pap smears every 6–12 months until 30 years old Thereafter, yearly cervical and vaginal Pap smears

Finally, and most important, the natural history of two lesions appear to be the same in that 15% to 20% of untreated lesions progress[33] while the remainder either regress or remain unchanged for long periods of time.

Table 3-2 Comparison of The Bethesda Classification, CIN classification, and Papanicolaou reporting

Bethesda System	CIN Classification	Papanicolaou
Low-grade SIL	HPV change	Atypia: koilocytotic, warty, condylomatous
	CIN I	Mild dysplasia
High-grade SIL	CIN II	Moderate dysplasia
	CIN III	Severe dysplasia, carcinoma-in-situ

CIN II and CIN III were combined into the category of high-grade SIL for similar reasons: the lesions are difficult to differentiate histopathologically, and if they are comparable in size, treatment is the same for the two lesions.

MANAGEMENT OF ABNORMAL PAP SMEAR RESULTS

Cervical cytological reports conforming with TBS format will always include a statement of sample adequacy and a general categorization of the sample being normal or abnormal. Abnormalities are grouped into four broad categories: infection, reactive and reparative changes, squamous cell abnormalities, and gland cell abnormalities (Table 3-3).

Normal, Problems with the Adequacy of the Specimen

Satisfactory, but limited by . . . The condition that most often limits interpretation is an inadequate sampling of endocervical cells. Their presence confirms that in the process of sampling the transformation zone, the active squamocolumnar junction was included. If a normal or benign result is reported, take the next Pap smear at a routine interval. A result that describes inadequate or absent endocervical cells but provides no other categorization or diagnosis must be managed as an unsatisfactory smear (see the next subsection).

Even with the best of sampling efforts, however, endocervical cells are absent in as many as 10% of Pap smears obtained from premenopausal women and as many as 50% from postmenopausal women. These cells also are more likely to be absent in smears from women who use oral contraceptives or are pregnant. The proportion of Pap smears with this reading provides an important opportunity to monitor Pap smear technique. If the percentage of Pap smears with no endocervical cells present exceeds 10% to 15%, remedial action is necessary. If clinician education regarding Pap smear technique and a switch to brush sampling devices does not result in improvement, the laboratory's cytopathologist must be

Table 3-3 The Bethesda System reporting categories

Category	Reading
Infection	• Fungus consistent with *Candida sp.* • *Trichomonas vaginalis* • Predominance of coccobacilli consistent with a shift in vaginal flora • Bacteria morphologically consistent with *Actinomyces sp.* • Cellular changes associated with herpes simplex virus
Reactive and reparative changes	• Cellular changes associated with inflammation • Atrophy with inflammation • Miscellaneous: radiation, IUD, DES, etc.
Squamous cell abnormalities	• Atypical squamous cells of undetermined significance (ASCUS) • Low-grade SIL • High-grade SIL • Squamous cell cancer
Gland cell abnormalities	• Endometrial cells, cytologically benign, in a post-menopausal woman • Atypical glandular cells of undetermined significance (AGCUS) • Adenocarcinoma

consulted in order to determine whether the problem lies with the laboratory or the provider and to define further steps necessary to rectify the problem.

Unsatisfactory for evaluation . . . Inadequate sampling, air drying, excessive red or white blood cells, or other factors make interpretation impossible. Repeat the smear, preferably when the woman is at midcycle and has not had intercourse or used vaginal products for at least 24 hours. Do not repeat the Pap smear earlier than 6 weeks from the previous smear; repetitive sampling over short periods of time may increase the risk of falsely negative smears due to decreased exfoliation of abnormal cells and a greater likelihood of reparative changes. Postmenopausal women with one or more unsatisfactory Pap smears due to vaginal atrophy should apply topical vaginal estrogen cream for 4 to 6 weeks, then receive a repeat Pap smear no earlier than 1 week after completing the medication in order to avoid sampling interference caused by the vehicle of the topical medication. Unless a woman has a history of endometrial hyperplasia, progestin withdrawal is not necessary after this short course of estrogen exposure. If the proportion of unsatisfactory smears within a practice is greater than 5%, remedial action in consultation with the cytopathologist is indicated.

ABNORMAL DESCRIPTIVE DIAGNOSES

Infection

Fungus consistent with* Candida *sp. In most cases, *Candida* detected on Pap smear is due to normal vaginal colonization with low levels of *Candida*, rather than frank vaginal candidiasis. *Candida* colonization is not dangerous to the affected woman or her sexual partner. Review the woman's medical record. If she received treatment for vaginal candidiasis at the time the Pap smear was taken or since then, she does not need to be notified. However, if she was not treated for vaginal candidiasis, notify her that *Candida* were present. If she is symptomatic, ask her to return for evaluation and treatment. Repeat the Pap only if the inflammation due to the candidiasis is of sufficient severity that the cytopathologist recommends that the Pap smear be repeated after treatment is complete.

Trichomonas vaginalis. While the Pap smear is a relatively insensitive test for the detection of Trichomonas—it detects trichomonads in only about one-half of infected women—its specificity is as high as 98%.[24] When the Pap report indicates presence of Trichomonas, review the woman's medical record to determine whether the infection was recently treated. If it has been, no further action is required. If it has not been treated, offer treatment to avoid horizontal transmission to a new sexual partner and to prevent conversion of asymptomatic Trichomonas colonization into an uncomfortable case of symptomatic vaginal trichomoniasis. The practice of requiring microscopic saline suspension confirmation of trichomonads is illogical because such a relatively insensitive test (about 60%) should not be used to confirm a test of high specificity. Repeat the Pap smear after the next routine screening interval, unless the narrative report mentions obscuring inflammation and indicates the need to repeat the Pap smear after treatment.

Predominance of coccobacilli consistent with shift in vaginal flora. This reading refers to changes detected in the bacterial flora of the vagina in which the normal *Lactobacillus* are not abundant but coccobacilli are seen in numbers greater than normal. While this description was devised to suggest the possibility of bacterial vaginosis (BV), it is both an insensitive and nonspecific indicator of BV. The clinical diagnosis of BV is made solely on clinical findings (see Chapter 8 on Reproductive Tract Infections), and neither vaginal culture nor Pap smear findings have any role in the diagnosis of this condition. Management is controversial. Many clinicians feel that no further evaluation is necessary and that the next Pap smear should be performed at the routine interval, while others feel that the woman should be informed of that BV is inferred from findings on the smear and be offered clinical evaluation for BV.

***Bacteria morphologically consistent with* Actinomyces spp.** *Act-inomyces israelii* is an anaerobic bacteria capable of causing a severe pelvic infection, especially in long-term IUD users over 35 years of age. A large majority of IUD wearers with *Actinomyces* on Pap smear have asymptomatic cervical colonization (not infection) that does not require antibiotic therapy. Examine IUD users with *Actinomyces* on their Pap smear to determine whether they have evidence of pelvic infection. If symptoms or physical findings suggest pelvic actinomycosis, remove the IUD and initiate intensive antibiotic therapy. Advise the woman to use another method of contraception. While no definitive evidence supports a particular course of action for patients with asymptomatic *Actinomyces* colonization, it is prudent to remove the IUD and insert a replacement IUD only after a repeat Pap smear performed 3 months later shows the absence of *Actinomyces*. (See Chapter 21 on Intrauterine Devices.)

Cellular changes associated with herpes simplex virus (HSV). Although an insensitive indicator of cervical herpes simplex shedding, the Pap smear is a *specific* indicator. A confirmatory HSV culture will be wasteful of resources. Advise the infected woman to tell her obstetrical care provider so that precautions may be taken to minimize the risk of vertical transmission to a newborn. Unless inflammation interferes with the interpretation of the Pap smear, the next Pap smear should be performed at the routine interval.

Reactive and Reparative Changes

Reactive cellular changes associated with inflammation. Nonspecific reactive inflammatory changes may be associated with benign metaplasia, mechanical or chemical irritation, post-traumatic repair, chlamydial or gonococcal endocervicitis, trichomoniasis, viral infection, invasive cervical cancer, or other unknown factors. Of these possibilities, the only infectious conditions amenable to antibiotic therapy are gonococcal and chlamydial endocervicitis and vaginal trichomoniasis. Women who recently have been evaluated for these organisms and found to be uninfected do not require further evaluation or antibiotic therapy. Examine women who have not been evaluated recently. Either provide empirical antibiotic treatment for women diagnosed with mucopurulent cervicitis or perform gonorrhea and chlamydia tests and treat women who test positive. Empirically treating women with inflammatory Pap smears with topical antibiotic sulfa creams is of no value in either the treatment of cervical infection or the resolution of abnormal Pap smears and is to be condemned.[39]

Rarely, the only Pap smear finding in a woman with a preinvasive or an invasive cervical carcinoma is the persistent finding of inflammation or inflammatory atypia. Women who have been treated for a cervical infection or those evaluated and found not to be infected should receive their next two Pap smears at 3- to 6-month intervals. If unexplained inflammation again is found during this surveillance period, colposcopic evaluation is recommended.

Atrophy with inflammation. Atrophy with inflammation is most common in postmenopausal women or those with estrogen-deficiency states. Treatment of the vaginal atrophy is indicated only if the woman has symptomatic atrophic vaginitis; it is not necessary for the asymptomatic woman. Pap smear screening intervals do not need to be modified, and the women does not need to be notified. However, because atrophy may cause a cytological picture similar to dysplasia, a postmenopausal woman with a Pap smear showing ASCUS or low-grade SIL should be treated with a vaginal estrogen cream for 4 to 6 weeks and given a repeat Pap smear.

Intrauterine contraceptive device. Cytological changes associated with the use of an IUD detected on Pap smear are of a benign nature and do not require further investigation.

Squamous Cell Abnormalities

Atypical squamous cell of undetermined significance (ASCUS). The ASCUS reading refers to the finding of cells with nuclear atypia that are not normal yet not consistent with a diagnosis of low-grade SIL. The large majority of ASCUS smears are due to benign HPV infections, although a small percentage of women with this reading have low-grade or high-grade SIL, and very rarely, invasive cancer. Because of confusion regarding the meaning of the ASCUS reading, TBS II permits the cytopathologist to further qualify the reading: "reactive change," "a premalignant/malignant process is favored," or "undifferentiated." While some pathologists have adopted this approach, others believe that it is not technically possible to achieve this degree of differentiation and use a single ASCUS category.

According to the TBS interim guidelines,[25] four acceptable options are available for the management of women with ASCUS results: perform colposcopy, follow with a shorter Pap screening interval, use a second test such as HPV typing to differentiate women who are at low risk or high risk for dysplasia (also called secondary triage), or tailor the management of each individual patient using any of the above approaches based upon the woman's own preference and the likelihood that she will return for follow-up. Recommend colposcopy for women with the following results:

- ASCUS/premalignant change suspected in a woman who is unwilling or unlikely to return for follow-up

- ASCUS with severe inflammation, unexplained by positive gonorrhea or chlamydia tests
- ASCUS in a woman with an immunodeficiency condition

Alternatively, follow-up Pap smears can be performed every 4 to 6 months for three intervals in the following cases:

- ASCUS/premalignant change suspected in a woman willing and likely to return for follow-up
- ASCUS/reactive
- ASCUS/unspecified

If any second Pap smear during the next 12 to 18 months shows ASCUS or SIL, colposcopy should be recommended.

Low-grade SIL. This category encompasses HPV change (koilocytotic atypia, condylomatous atypia) and CIN I. Since only 15% to 20% of women with low-grade SIL lesions will progress to a higher-grade lesion,[34] focus on identifying and treating women whose lesions do not spontaneously regress. In light of the relatively slow temporal progression of SIL lesions, expectant management of women with low-grade SIL on a single Pap smear is acceptable, assuming that the woman is a good candidate for follow-up. In this situation, perform Pap smears every 4 to 6 months for three intervals, and if any subsequent Pap smear report over the next 12 to 18 months shows ASCUS/premalignant change or SIL, recommend colposcopic evaluation. Conversely, if all Pap smears are reported as normal during this period of increased surveillance, the woman may return to a routine screening pattern afterward. Women who may not reliably revisit for follow-up, who request immediate evaluation, or who have immunodeficiency diseases should be advised to receive colposcopic evaluation after a single low-grade SIL Pap smear reading.

High-grade SIL. Refer women with high-grade SIL for colposcopic evaluation, even if the Pap smear was obtained during pregnancy, a benign Pap smear has been obtained since the SIL reading, or no visible cervical lesion is present. A comprehensive list of indications for colposcopy is included in Table 3-4.

Gland Cell Abnormalities
Endometrial cells, cytologically benign, in a postmenopausal woman. Endometrial cells found on Pap smear are an insignificant finding in premenopausal women with normal ovulatory cycling. However, because the endometrium normally is atrophic in postmenopausal women, the finding of endometrial cells may be the result of exfoliation

Table 3-4 Indications for colposcopy

- Papanicolaou (Pap) smear showing high-grade SIL
- Persistent finding of atypical squamous cell of undetermined significance (ASCUS) or low-grade squamous intraepithelial lesion (SIL) on Pap smear (any two abnormal Pap smears performed at 4- to 6-month intervals within a 12- to 18-month observation period) in a patient who will reliably return for repeat smear
- Single Pap smear showing ASCUS or low-grade SIL in woman who is unlikely or unwilling to return for frequent follow-up
- Persistent inflammation after treatment of proven infection or if persistent Pap smear finding with no infection documented
- Pap smear showing atypical glandular cells of undetermined significance (AGCUS)
- Cervical leukoplakia (white lesion visible to the naked eye without the application of acetic acid) or other unexplained cervical lesion, regardless of Pap smear result
- Unexplained or persistent cervical bleeding, regardless of Pap smear result
- Baseline examination of a woman with a history of in-utero DES exposure
- Baseline examination of a woman known to be infected with the human immuno-deficiency virus (HIV)

Refer women with Pap smear results reporting squamous cell or adenocarcinoma of the cervix for immediate expert consultation with a physician experienced in the management of gynecologic cancers.

---

from a focus of endometrial hyperplasia or adenocarcinoma. For this reason, consider the finding of endometrial cells in a postmenopausal woman as a danger sign and sample the endometrium. Because a premenopausal woman with chronic anovulation also is at risk for endometrial hyperplasia, manage the finding of endometrial cells in the same way.

Atypical glandular cells of undetermined significance (AGUS or AGCUS). AGCUS may result from bacterial or HPV infection of glandular cells, adenocarcinoma-in-situ (adenoCIS), or adenocarcinoma. Because adenocarcinomas of the cervix are associated with a rate of false-negative Pap smears as high as 40%,[18] women with AGCUS Pap smears require aggressive evaluation in order to exclude a cancer diagnosis. There is no role for observation (repeat Pap smear) in this situation. Management consists of colposcopic evaluation of the exocervix and a thorough endocervical curettage. If you do not see a lesion, take random biopsies of the anterior and posterior cervix. In cases where only benign epithelium is found, many experts suggest more frequent Pap smear screening intervals for at least 12 months; if AGCUS smears persist, consider performing a cone biopsy to exclude an occult adenocarcinoma.

Squamous cell carcinoma, endocervical adenocarcinoma. Immediately refer women with Pap smear results showing squamous or adenocarcinoma of the cervix for expert consultation with a physician experienced in the management of gynecological cancers.

TREATMENT OF SQUAMOUS INTRAEPITHELIAL LESIONS

Since the early 1990s, management protocols have become much more conservative, due to the recognition that most low-grade SIL lesions will regress rather than progress to higher-grade lesions or cancer. While this conservative trend is likely to continue, both providers and patients should continue to be diligent with follow-up.

Typical papillary condyloma accuminata of the cervix, once histologically proven by cervical biopsy, should be treated rather than observed. This aggressive approach decreases the amount of friable cervical tissue, which will reduce receptivity to HIV infection and may decrease the risk of viral transmission to a partner. Cryotherapy will be the least invasive and most inexpensive treatment modality in most cases, although some situations may require the use of LEEP or laser. The use of trichloroacetic acid and topical 5-fluorouracil (FU) for the treatment of cervical condyloma and SIL is considered investigational and is not recommended.

The optimal treatment of low-grade SIL remains a major focus of controversy. Because the lesion has an indeterminate potential for malignancy, many clinicians assume that progression is a possibility and treat (ablate) the entire "at risk" transformation zone. Alternatively, because risk of progression is only about 20% and the lesion is not dangerous until it does progress, other clinicians follow the patient until there is evidence of high-grade SIL or persistence of low-grade SIL over the period of 1 year. There is universal agreement that high-grade SIL must be treated, because the risk of progression to cervical cancer is both more likely and more immediate.

O VARIAN CANCER SCREENING

Annually in the United States, about 19,000 women develop ovarian cancer, making the cancer the fifth most common among American women. However, because of the low 5-year survival rates with this disease, especially in the later stages when it is more commonly diagnosed, it is the fourth most common cause of female cancer deaths and the leading cause (49%) of gynecologic cancer deaths, accounting for 14,500 deaths in the United States in 1995. The average age at diagnosis is 60 years. A woman's lifetime risk of ovarian cancer is about 1 in 70.

Although some risk factors for ovarian cancer are well known, a majority of women diagnosed with this condition have none.[49] Geographic differences are marked; rates in Sweden and United States are 13 to 15 cases per 100,000 women per year, while the rate in Japan is 3 cases per 100,000 women per year. This difference in part may be related to dietary fat intake, which is higher in the United States and Scandinavia and lower in Japan. A long interval of ovulatory cycles also is associated epidemiologically with ovarian cancer, as low parity, delayed childbearing, and infertility are weak risk factors. Familial predisposition accounts for 5% to 10% of cases, and the risk of ovarian cancer is 5% if one first-degree relative had ovarian cancer and 7% if two or more first-degree relatives had the condition. A site-specific familial ovarian cancer syndrome also has been described that is mediated through a highly penetrant autosomal dominant gene; in these cases, the risk to a first-degree relative is up to 50%. In addition, women with BRCA-1 and BRCA-2 mutations are at greater risk of both ovarian and breast cancer. Because there is no accurate method to detect early ovarian cancer in these high-risk women, some experts recommend prophylactic oophorectomy in women who have two or more first degree relatives with ovarian cancer and who have completed childbearing.[36]

Conversely, oral contraceptive use reduces the risk of ovarian cancer by as much as 80% in women age 40 to 59 years. Not only does longer duration of use provide more protection, but the effect lasts for as long as 15 years after oral contraceptives are discontinued.[41] There is a decreased risk of ovarian cancer in women who are chronic anovulators (also called the polycystic ovary syndrome); protection also is seen with increasing parity and greater duration of lactation. Contraceptive sterilization is associated with a 40% to 50% reduction in the risk of ovarian cancer, and hysterectomy with a 35% reduction.

OVARIAN CANCER SCREENING TECHNIQUES

Early ovarian cancer usually is asymptomatic, and may be detected as a mass found incidentally during pelvic examination or ultrasound. However, ovarian cancer can be associated with pelvic pain, abdominal discomfort and distention, post-prandial bloating, constipation, nausea, urinary frequency, and irregular vaginal bleeding. In advanced-stages, ovarian cancer is often accompanied by non-specific gastrointestinal symptoms, poor appetite and weight loss, increased abdominal girth, or shortness of breath due to pleural effusion.

A number of techniques have been suggested to screen for the early stages of asymptomatic ovarian cancer: periodic bimanual pelvic examination, serum CA-125 level measurement, and transvaginal ultrasound examination. Conducting pelvic examination as part of periodic health examination is inexpensive and safe and may provide valuable information, but it is insensitive and has not been found to be cost-effective when the visit and examination are done for the *sole* purpose of ovarian cancer screening. Screening with the serum tumor marker CA-125 will detect up to 80% of women with advanced non-mucinous ovarian cancers, but the test is only 50% to 70% sensitive for early-stage cancers and has poor specificity (many false positives), which may lead to unnecessary invasive and costly workups. Screening with this test is not cost effective because of the low prevalence of ovarian cancer and the test's moderate sensitivity, poor specificity, and high cost. Vaginal-probe pelvic ultrasound also has been suggested as a screening test because of its high sensitivity (≥98%), but it has poor specificity (high false positives) and the highest cost of any of the screening modalities. While there is general agreement that asymptomatic low-risk women should not be screened routinely with any of these interventions, either alone or in combination, many experts believe that they should offered to women with familial risk factors for ovarian cancer. The current USPSTF guidelines make the following recommendations regarding ovarian cancer screening:[46]

- Screening asymptomatic women for ovarian cancer with ultrasound, tumor markers, or physical exam is not recommended.
- There is insufficient evidence to recommend for or against testing in asymptomatic women at increased risk of ovarian cancer.

B REAST CANCER SCREENING

Breast cancer is the second leading cause of cancer deaths in women in the United States, accounting for one-fourth of all cancer cases and one-fifth of cancer deaths in women (47,000 per year). Incidence rates of breast cancer have increased 1% per year since 1973, although morbidity rates have remained stable. A woman's lifetime risk of breast cancer, assuming she lives to old age, is about 1 in 9.

Risk factors are helpful indicators of risk, but do not predict the development of breast cancer in the majority of cases. Of women with breast cancer, 21% of women age 30 to 54 years have risk factor(s), as do 29% of women between 55 to 84 years old (Table 3-5).[16,17]

BREAST CANCER SCREENING TECHNIQUES

All adult women should learn how to do a *breast self-examination* (BSE). The optimal time for performing BSE is 1 to 7 days after the end of the menses. Performing the exam after a shower, while the skin still is wet, may improve accuracy. After inspecting her breasts while she is sitting or standing in front of a mirror, the woman should palpate each breast; her hand on the side of the breast being examined should be placed behind her head. She should then repeat the exam while lying down. The objective of BSE is to detect a significant change in the breasts from one

Table 3-5 Risk characteristics of breast cancer

Factor	High-Risk Group	Low-Risk Group
Relative risk >4.0		
Age	Old	Young
Country of birth	North America, Northern Europe	Asia, Africa
Two first-degree relatives with breast cancer diagnosed at an early age	Yes	No
History of cancer in one breast	Yes	No
Relative risk = 2.1–4.0		
Nodular densities on mammogram (postmenopausal)	Densities occupy >75% of breast volume	Parenchyma composed entirely of fat
One first-degree relative with breast cancer	Yes	No
Biopsy-confirmed atypical hyperplasia	Yes	No
High-dose radiation to chest	Yes	No
Oophorectomy before age 35	No	Yes
Relative risk = 1.1–2.0		
Socioeconomic status	High	Low
Place of residence	Urban	Rural
Race/ethnicity		
Breast cancer at ≥40 years	Caucasian	Asian
Breast cancer at <40 years	Black	Asian
Religion	Jewish	Adventist, Mormon
Age at first full-term pregnancy	≥30 years	<20 years
Age at menarche	<12 years	>14 years
Age at menopause	≥55 years	<45 years
Obesity (postmenopausal)	Obese	Slender
Breastfeeding	None	Several years
Hormonal contraceptives Breast cancer <45 years	Yes	No
Hormone replacement therapy	Yes	No
Height	Tall	Short
History of primary cancer in endometrium, ovary, or colon	Yes	No
Alcohol consumption	Yes	No

month to the next, not necessarily the finding of a dominant nodule. Although BSE may provide women with a sense of empowerment and may result in earlier detection of a breast mass than might occur by coincidence or at a periodic health examination, studies suggest that breast cancer survival is no greater among those women who perform BSE compared with those who do not,[46] probably because a mass detected through BSE is larger than that detected by other means.

Clinical breast examination (CBE) should be performed routinely at the time of periodic health examinations. Examine the breasts while the woman is sitting with her hands on her hips or behind her head. Repeat the exam while the woman is lying down. Examine each breast in vertical strips or enlarging concentric circles. Palpate with flat portion of your fingers rather than your fingertips. If a woman has very pendulous breasts, place your hand between her breast and chest wall, then palpate tissue between your hands. Be sure to include the axillary tail of the breast in the examination. Lymph node examination of the supraclavicular and axillary nodes is an integral component of the examination. Draw a diagram in the medical record indicating the position and size of abnormalities (dominant nodules have measurable dimensions while fibrocystic change does not).

While most consensus guidelines include breast examination as a component of the periodic health examination in adult women, U.S. Preventive Services Task Force evidence is insufficient to recommend this intervention alone (without mammography), even for women between 50 and 69 years of age. However, it is reasonable to offer all women CBE because it is safe, non-invasive, and adds little extra time to the periodic health examination.

Mammography

When used as a *screening test*, the purpose of mammography is to detect pre-clinical breast cancer between 1 to 10 mm, before a mass can be palpated clinically. Alternatively, when used as a *diagnostic test*, mammography can suggest malignancy at the site of the mass and exclude malignancy elsewhere in the same or opposite breast. *In the presence of a dominant breast nodule, a negative diagnostic mammogram does not exclude the diagnosis of breast cancer.* Tissue sampling, either by fine-needle aspiration cytology or open biopsy, is the only definitive procedure to exclude cancer.

With better technology and improvements in interpretation, the accuracy of mammography as a screening test has improved over the past decade. The false-negative rate is 10% to 15% and the false-positive rate is 15% to 20%. The optimal use of screening, particularly in regard to the age at which routine mammography should be initiated and how frequently it should be performed, has been a subject of ongoing debate in North America and Europe. Large-scale epidemiological studies show screening mammography will reduce breast cancer mortality by 30% to 50% in women age 50 to 69 years, mainly by finding cancers while they still are small and localized. While some consensus statements recommend screening annually, others suggest every 2 years. The USPSTF guidelines state that for women over age 70, the evidence regarding the value of mammography is conflicting and limited. There is no evidence of benefit to women over 75 years old. However, most consensus guidelines do not put an upper age limit on mammographic screening and recommend that it should be performed every 1 to 2 years for any woman age 50 or older.

The area of greatest debate centers on the use of screening mammography in women between 40 and 49 years. Previous guidelines recommended that low-risk women initiate mammograms at age 40 and have them performed every 2 years until age 50. The 1996 USPSTF guidelines made no recommendations because the evidence on costs and benefits was conflicting.[46] In the same year, the National Cancer Institute concluded that a specific recommendation could not be formulated and that the decision whether to have a mammogram should be left to the individual woman.[8] The 1997 American Cancer Society (ACS) guidelines took an opposite position and recommended that mammograms be performed annually in women age 40 to 50 years.[28] This opinion was based upon studies that suggest that breast cancer grows more rapidly among younger women and that, despite its greater cost, annual screening is significantly more likely than biennial screening to detect early cancers and more favorably affect outcomes than is a biennial screening pattern. Given the diversity of opinion, carefully explain to women the pros and cons of screening and refer women who wish to have mammography performed. However, this must be balanced against a lower prevalence of breast cancer among women in their 40s, as well as a higher rate of positive mammograms because of a greater breast density. Most experts agree that women with risk factors for breast cancer should initiate screening at age 35 to 40 and subsequently be screened annually.

REFERENCES

1. Adachi A, Fleming I, Burk RD, Ho GY, Klein RS. Women with human immunodeficiency virus infection and abnormal Papanicolaou smears, a prospective study of colposcopy and clinical outcome. Obstet Gynecol 1993;81:372-377.
2. American Medical Association. Periodic health examination: a manual for physicians. Chicago: American Medical Association, 1940.
3. Brinton LA, Schairer C, Haenszel W, Stolley P, Lehman HF, Levine R, Savitz DA. Cigarette smoking and invasive cervical cancer. JAMA 1986;225(23):3265-3269.

4. Centers for Disease Control. Black-white differences in cervical cancer mortality—United States, 1980-1987. MMWR 1990;39:245-248.
5. Centers for Disease Control. 1993 revised classification system for HIV infection and expanded surveillance case definition for AIDS among adolescents and adults. MMWR 1992;41(RR-17):1-19.
6. Centers for Disease Control. Risk for cervical disease in HIV infected women—New York City. MMWR 1990;39(47):846-849.
7. Centers for Disease Control and Prevention. 1997 sexually transmitted diseases treatment guidelines. MMWR (in press).
8. Eastman P. NCI adopts new mammography screening guidelines for women [news]. J Natl Cancer Inst 1997;89:538-539.
9. Fink DJ. Change in ACS Checkup guidelines for the detection of cervical cancer. CA Cancer J Clin 1988;38:127-128.
10. Grimes DA. Over-the-counter oral contraceptives—an immodest proposal? [editorial]. Am J Public Health 1993;83:1092-1094.
11. Gross G, Ikenberg H, Gissman L, Hagedorn M. Papillomavirus infection of the anogenital region: correlation between histology, clinical picture and virus type. A proposal of a new nomenclature. J Invest Dermatol 1985;85:147-152.
12. Harlan LC, Bernstein AB, Kessler LG. Cervical cancer screening: who is not screened and why? Am J Public Health 1991;81:885-891.
13. Hayward RA, Shapiro MF, Freeman HE, Corey CR. Who gets screened for cervical and breast cancer? Results from a national survey. Arch Intern Med 1988;148:1117-1118.
14. Henry M. The Bethesda System, the pathology of preinvasive lesions, and screening technology. The Bethesda System (TBS) of nomenclature for cervical smears. J Natl Cancer Inst Mongr 1996;13-16.
15. Herbst AL, The Bethesda System for cervical/vaginal cytologic diagnosis: a note of caution [editorial]. Obstet Gynecol 1990;76:4049-4050.
16. Hoskins KF, Stopfer JE, Calzone KA, et.al. Assessment and counseling for women with a family history of breast cancer: a guide for clinicians. JAMA 1995;273:577-585.
17. Hulka, BS, Stark AT. Breast cancer: cause and prevention. Lancet 1995;346:883-887.
18. Hurt WG, Silverberg SG, Frable WJ, Belgrad R, Crooks LD. Adenocarcinoma of the cervix: histopathologic and clinical features. Am J Obstet Gynecol 1977;129:304-315.
19. Hutchinson ML. Assessing the costs and benefits of alternative rescreening strategies [editorial]. Acta Cytol 1996;40-48.
20. Kerlikowske K, Grady D, Barclay J, Sickles E, Ernster V. Effect of age, breast density, and family history on the sensitivity of first screening mammography. JAMA 1996;276:33-38.
21. Korn AP, Autry M, DeRemer PA, Tan W. Sensitivity of the Papanicolaou smear in HIV-infected women. Obstet Gynecol 1994;83:401-404.
22. Korn AP, Landers DV. Gynecologic disease in women infected with human immunodeficiency virus type 1. J Acq Immune Defic Syndr Hum Retrovirol 1995;9:361-370.
23. Koss LG. The Papanicolaou test for cervical cancer detection. A triumph and a tragedy. JAMA 1989;261:737-743.

24. Krieger JN, Tam MR, Stevens CE, Nielsen IO, Hale J, Kiviat NB, Holmes KK. Diagnosis of trichomoniasis: comparison of conventional wet mount examination with cytologic studies, cultures, and monoclonal antibody staining of direct specimens. JAMA 1988;259:1223-1227.
25. Kurman RJ, Henson DE, Herbst AL, Noller KL, Schiffman MH. Interim guidelines for management of abnormal cervical cytology. JAMA 1994;271: 1866-1869.
26. Kurman RJ, Malkasian GD, Sedlis A, Solomon D. From Papanicolaou to Bethesda: the rationale for a new cervical cytologic classification. Obstet Gynecol 1991;77:779-782.
27. Lawrence RS, Mickalide AD. Preventive services in clinical practice: designing the periodic health examination. JAMA 1987;257:2205-2207.
28. Leitch AM, Dodd GD, Costanza, Linver M, Pressman P, McGinnis L, Smith RA. Amercian Cancer Society guidelines for the early detection of breast cancer: update 1997. CA Cancer J Clin 1997;47:150-153.
29. Maiman M, Fruchter RG, Guy L, Cuthill S, Levine P, Serur E. Human immunodeficiency virus infection and invasive cervical carcinoma. Cancer 1993;71:402-406.
30. Maiman M, Fruchter RG, Serur E, Remy JC, Feuer G, Boyce J. Human immunodeficiency virus infection and cervical neoplasia. Gynecol Oncol 1990;38: 377-382.
31. Maiman M, Fruchter RG, Serur E, Levine PA, Arrastia CD, Sedlis A. Recurrent cervical intraepithelial neoplasia in human immunodeficiency virus seropositive women. Obstet Gynecol 1993;82:170-174.
32. Maiman M, Terricone N, Vieira J, Suarez J, Serur E, Boyce JG. Colposcopic evaluation of human immunodeficiency virus-seropositive women. Obstet Gynecol 1991;78:84-88.
33. Montz FJ, Monk BJ, Fowler JM, Nguyen L. Natural history of the minimally abnormal Papanicolaou smear. Obstet Gynecol 1992;80:385-388.
34. Nasiell K, Roger V, Nasiell M. Behavior of mild cervical dysplasia during long term follow-up. Obstet Gynecol 1986; 67:665-669.
35. National Institutes of Health. Rapid communication—The Bethesda System for reporting cervical/vaginal cytologic diagnoses—the report of the 1991 Bethesda workshop. JAMA 1992;267:1892.
36. National Institute of Health Consensus Development Panel on Ovarian Cancer, NIH consensus conference. Ovarian cancer. Screening, treatment, and follow up. JAMA 1995;273:491-497.
37. Reid R. Preinvasive disease. In: Berek JS, Hacker NF (eds). Practical gynecologic oncology (second edition). Baltimore MD: Williams & Wilkins, 1994:210-242.
38. Reid R, Greenberg M, Jenson AB, Husain M, Willett J, Daoud Y, Temple G, Stanhope CR, Sherman AI, Phibbs GD, Lorincz AT. Sexually transmitted papillomaviral infections. I. The anatomic distribution and pathologic grade of neoplastic lesions associated with different viral types. Am J Obstet Gynecol 1987;156:212-222.
39. Reiter RC. Management of initial atypical cervical cytology: a randomized, prospective study. Obstet Gynecol 1986;68:237-240.
40. Richart RM. A modified terminology for cervical intraepithelial neoplasia. Obstet Gynecol 1990;75:131-133.

41. Rosenberg L, Palmer JR, Zauber AG. A case control study of oral contraceptive use and invasive epithelial ovarian cancer. Am J Epidemiol 1994;139: 654-661.

42. Schiffman MH. Recent progress in defining the epidemiology of human papillomavirus infection and cervical neoplasia. J Natl Cancer Inst 1992;84: 394-398.

43. Sox HC, Woolf SH. Evidence-based practice guidelines from the U.S. Preventive Services Task Force [editorial]. JAMA 1993;269:2678.

44. Trussell J, Stewart F, Potts M, Guest F, Ellertson C. Should oral contraceptives be available without prescription? Am J Public Health 1993;83:1094-1099.

45. U.S. Department of Health and Human Services. Improving the quality of clinician Pap smear technique and management, client Pap smear education, and the evaluation of Pap smear laboratory testing: a resource guide for Title X family planning projects. Washington DC: U.S. Department of Health and Human Services, Public Health Service, Office of Population Affairs, Office of Family Planning, 1989:3-4, 59.

46. U.S. Preventive Services Task Force. Guide to clinical preventive services: report of the United States Preventive Services Task Force (2nd edition) Baltimore MD: Williams & Wilkins, 1996.

47. Wright TC, Koulos J, Schnoll F, Swanbeck J, Ellerbrock T, Chaisson M, Richart RM. Cervical intraepithelial neoplasia in women infected with the human immunodeficiency virus: outcome after loop electrosurgical excision. Gynecol Oncol 1994;55:253-258.

48. Winkelstein W, Jr. Smoking and cervical cancer—current status: a review. Am J Epidemiol 1990;131:945-957.

49. Whittemore AS, Harris R, Itnyre J. Characteristics relating to ovarian cancer risk. Collaborative analysis of 12 US case-control studies. II. Invasive epithelial ovarian cancers in white women. Am J Epidemiol 1992;136:1184-1203.

50. Yobs AR, Swanson RA, Lamotte LC Jr. Laboratory reliability of the Papanicolaou smear. Obstet Gynecol 1985;65:235-244.

The Menstrual Cycle

Anne Brawner Namnoum, MD
Robert A. Hatcher, MD, MPH

- Although the idealized 28-day cycle is used as a model for discussion and for some hormonal contraceptive cycling, normal cycles range from 23 to 35 days.
- Normal ovulatory cycles require the integration of hormones and signals from the hypothalamus, pituitary gland, and ovaries.

- The menstrual cycle responds to changing levels of many essential hormones at key moments in time.

A thorough understanding of the menstrual cycle is fundamental to the discussion of contraception. The ovaries are the source of oocytes (eggs) as well as the hormones that regulate female reproduction. In contrast to the male reproductive system where large numbers of gametes are produced continuously, in women only one gamete is released each month from the time of menarche to the time of menopause. During each monthly interval, or menstrual cycle, a series of events occur that culminates in ovulation and the preparation of the endometrium for implantation of an embryo. If pregnancy does not occur, the process of oocyte maturation and endometrial preparation begins anew.

Under complex regulation by the hypothalamus, the pituitary gland, and the ovaries, cyclic changes in gonadotropins and steroid hormones induce the development of a leading follicle, resulting in ovulation and corpus luteum formation.[5] Responding to the cyclic changes in ovarian steroids, the endometrium prepares for implantation should fertilization occur. If pregnancy does not occur, the endometrium sloughs, resulting in menstrual bleeding.

Normal cycles range from 23 to 35 days, and individual women may have considerable variation in their cycles from month to month. Only 15% of women have the idealized 28-day cycle. The cycle can be divided into four functional phases: follicular (pre-ovulatory), ovulatory, luteal, and menstrual.

M ENSTRUAL CYCLE REGULATION
HYPOTHALAMUS AND ANTERIOR PITUITARY

Gonadotropin-releasing hormone (GnRH), a neurohormone synthesized in the hypothalamus, travels via the portal circulation to the anterior pituitary gland. GnRH is secreted in a pulsatile fashion every 60 to 90 minutes, stimulating cells in the anterior pituitary (gonadotropes) to produce follicle-stimulating hormone (FSH) and luteinizing hormone (LH).[3,9] FSH and LH are secreted in a pulsatile manner in response to GnRH pulses. The pulse frequency varies, depending on the phase of the menstrual cycle. FSH plays a dominant role in the promotion of ovarian follicular growth by causing the granulosa cells that line each follicle to proliferate and produce estrogen. LH stimulates androgen production in theca cells adjacent to the granulosa cells. These androgens are the substrates for estrogen production. LH also promotes ovulation and final oocyte maturation and converts estrogen-secreting granulosa cells to progesterone-secreting cells after ovulation.

STEROID PRODUCTION IN THE OVARY

Together, theca cells and granulosa cells synthesize steroid hormones. Theca cells respond to LH by producing the androgens testosterone and androstenedione. These androgens diffuse from the theca cells across the basement membrane of the follicle into granulosa cells, where they are converted to estrogens by the enzyme aromatase. Theca cells have little intrinsic aromatase activity, and granulosa cells are relatively deficient in the enzymes necessary to synthesize androgens; thus the two cell types depend on each other to produce estrogen in the developing follicle. Androgens are critical to follicular development because they are the precursors for estrogens, but if androgens exist in excess amounts, they induce follicular atresia. Androgen production therefore must be delicately balanced to allow for normal ovarian function.

Moderate levels of estrogen produced by the follicles act on both the hypothalamus and the anterior pituitary to inhibit FSH and LH secretion in a classic negative feedback effect.[7] Progesterone and androgens have a negative feedback effect as well, but theirs is not as prominent as that of estrogen. Paradoxically, higher levels of estrogen have a positive feedback effect on gonadotropin secretion during the middle of a cycle, which initiates the preovulatory surge of LH and FSH.[11] When levels of estradiol in the range of 200 to 300 picograms/milliliter (ml) are present for 2 to 3 days, a gonadotropin surge is elicited. Progesterone may amplify this positive feedback effect. The pituitary is the major site of such estradiol action, but there may be a hypothalamic site of action as well. This positive feedback effect of estrogen is critical for ovulation and regular menstrual cycles.

PEPTIDE HORMONES IN THE OVARY

A variety of peptide hormones produced in the ovary help modulate follicular development and steroid production. One of the more important of these substances is inhibin, a protein composed of alpha and beta subunits. Synthesized in granulosa and theca cells, inhibin suppresses FSH secretion.[1] Activin, composed of two of the beta subunits of inhibin, has the opposite effect and enhances FSH secretion. Ovarian follicular fluid contains more inhibin than activin, thus inhibin from the dominant follicle has a negative feedback effect on FSH secretion. Inhibin and activin also act directly within the ovary to regulate androgen and estrogen production. A third peptide, follistatin, also suppresses FSH, probably by binding activin.

Insulin and insulin-like growth factors also seem to play a significant role as regulators within the ovary. Insulin-like growth factor 1 (IGF-1) stimulates cell division and growth in many tissues. The ovary is now known to be a site of IGF-1 production and action. IGF-1 has been shown to amplify LH-stimulated androgen production in theca cells and to amplify FSH action in granulosa cells. It may also serve to communicate messages between granulosa cells and theca cells.

Oocyte maturation inhibitor (OMI), a peptide hormone present in follicular fluid, prevents final maturation of the oocyte until the time of ovulation. OMI suppression ends within hours following the midcycle LH surge just prior to ovulation.

ENDOMETRIUM

The endometrium responds to the cyclic changes in ovarian steroids. Estrogen increases the thickness of the endometrium by increasing the number and size of endometrial cells. Estrogen also stimulates the formation of progesterone receptors on endometrial cells and increases the blood flow (via spiral arterioles) to the endometrium. Progesterone causes the proliferated endometrium to differentiate and secrete proteins that are important in the survival and implantation of an early embryo if pregnancy occurs. Progesterone and exogenous progestins also decrease the proliferative effects of estrogens on the endometrium. Withdrawal of estrogen and progesterone results in the orderly and controlled sloughing of the functional zone of the endometrium. This monthly shedding of the lining of the uterus occurs from 400 to 500 times during a woman's reproductive years.[12]

CERVIX

The cervix and cervical mucus also change in response to estrogen and progesterone. The cervical mucus facilitates selective sperm penetration from the vagina to the fallopian tube during the periovulatory period; at other times, the mucus prevents microorganisms and sperm from entering the uterine cavity. When estradiol levels increase during the mid to late follicular phase, the cervical mucus becomes clear, thin, more profuse, and extrudes from the cervical os into the vagina. The cervix itself swells and softens, and the cervical os dilates. After ovulation, progesterone causes the cervix to become more firm, the cervical os to close, and the cervical mucus to become scant, thick, and turbid. Progesterone and exogenous progestins produce a contraceptive effect by causing a thick cervical mucus that sperm cannot penetrate.

THE INTEGRATED CYCLE

FOLLICULAR PHASE

Pulsatile GnRH release by the hypothalamus results in pulses of FSH and LH. FSH stimulates the proliferation of granulosa cells, which produce estradiol from androgen precursors synthesized in theca cells.[11] In the first half of the follicular phase (days 1 to 5), many follicles are "recruited" and begin to grow. The increasing local estradiol levels induce more FSH receptors on the largest follicle, thus producing greater amounts of estradiol. Estradiol and inhibin begin to provide negative feedback on FSH secretion by the anterior pituitary.

During days 5 to 7 of the cycle, one of the recruited follicles becomes "dominant," producing the most estradiol and developing the most FSH receptors.[5] As FSH levels decline, the dominant follicle survives while the non-dominant follicles undergo atresia. After day 7, the dominant follicle is selected. The dominant follicle continues to mature and produce high levels of estradiol in the latter half of the follicular phase.[2] The length of the follicular phase is variable from individual to individual, but usually ranges from 10 to 17 days.

OVULATORY PHASE

Once the estradiol level has exceeded a critical level for 2 to 3 days, a positive feedback occurs in the pituitary, resulting in a surge of LH and FSH.[6] The estradiol level reaches its peak about 24 hours before ovulation. The LH surge leads to resumption of meiosis I in the dominant oocyte, luteinization of granulosa cells, and resultant progesterone production. Prostaglandins, proteolytic enzymes, and the contraction of smooth muscle cells within the follicle result in a break down of the follicular wall. The oocyte and follicular fluid exude about 32 to 44 hours after the onset of the LH surge. Ovulation predictor kits detect the increasing LH levels.

LUTEAL PHASE

Following the rupture of the follicle, the granulosa and theca cells take up steroids and lutein pigment to give the corpus luteum ("yellow body") a yellow appearance. The hallmark of the luteal phase is the shift from the estrogen-dominated follicular phase to one of progesterone dominance. Progesterone suppresses new follicular growth and causes secretory changes in the endometrium.[8] Peak progesterone production occurs 7 to 8 days after the LH surge, at the approximate time of implantation if fertilization has occurred. The length of the luteal phase tends to be more constant than the follicular phase, approximately 14 days unless pregnancy occurs.

Because progesterone causes an elevation in basal body temperature, daily measurement of basal body temperature can be used to determine whether or not ovulation has occurred. (See Chapter 15 on Fertility Awareness.) Basal body temperatures cannot be used to predict ovulation, as the temperature rise does not occur until after ovulation, but can confirm that ovulation has occurred.

MENSTRUAL PHASE

If pregnancy does not occur, the corpus luteum regresses, resulting in a decline of progesterone and estrogen levels. The withdrawal of these hormones initially shrinks endometrial height, decreases blood flow, and begins vasodilation followed by rhythmic vasoconstriction of the spiral arterioles. Ischemia and stasis are followed by interstitial hemorrhage and tissue disorganization, resulting in menstrual flow.[10]

The normal amount of blood lost during a normal menstrual period is 20 to 80 ml. Seventy percent of the blood will slough by the second day, and 90% by the third day.[12] The average duration of the menstrual phase is 4 to 6 days.

Thrombin-platelet plugs limit blood loss, and rising estrogen levels of the new cycle induce clot formation and regrowth of the endometrium. Delayed, asynchronous, or incomplete shedding of the endometrium, as might occur in anovulatory cycles, can be associated with heavier and longer bleeding.

FERTILIZATION AND IMPLANTATION

A woman is most likely to conceive if fresh sperm are present in the upper reproductive tract when ovulation occurs. The oocyte retains potential for fertilization for 12 to 24 hours, and sperm may remain viable in the reproductive tract for 72 hours or perhaps longer. The several days prior to ovulation are thus the most "fertile" cycle days, or the days that conception is most likely to occur. (See Chapter 27 on Impaired Fertility.) After ovulation and during the very early follicular phase, the likelihood of pregnancy is much lower. If a woman has very regular cycles and is monitoring her cycle closely, it may be feasible to use periodic abstinence during the "fertile" period as a means of contraception. (See Chapter 17 on Fertility Awareness.)

IMPLANTATION

During intercourse, the man deposits into the woman's vagina as many as 300 million spermatozoa suspended in seminal fluid. Because cervical mucus does not mix with semen, the sperm have to pass into the mucus, but this occurs within minutes. Under optimal conditions (in the preovulatory period), the number of sperm that enter the mucus within the first few minutes is often sufficient to accomplish fertilization. Within 30 minutes, several hundred thousand sperm can be found in the cervical canal, and this number remains stable for approximately 24 hours. Because cervical mucus allows easier passage of normal sperm, the sperm population improves over that present in the ejaculate. Sperm pass through the fallopian tubes fairly rapidly, but spermatozoa in the cervical crypts can supply sperm to the upper reproductive tract for several days.

Following extrusion of the oocyte and cumulus complex at the time of ovulation, the oocyte is swept into the lumen of the tube by the fimbria within minutes to hours. Fertilization occurs in the ampullary region of the fallopian tube, and the early embryo is then transported to the uterine cavity within 2 to 3 days. Implantation begins approximately 6 to 7 days after fertilization, when the embryo is at the blastocyst stage.

ANOVULATION

Because normal ovulatory cycles require the integration of hormones and signals from the hypothalamus, pituitary gland, and ovaries, problems at any of these sites may result in anovulation. Inadequate GnRH secretion by the hypothalamus inhibits normal FSH and LH production and results in anovulation. Problems such as weight loss, stress, and anorexia nervosa can interfere with GnRH secretion. Hyperprolactinemia may also result in ovulatory dysfunction or anovulation.

Alterations in the critically balanced factors in the ovary may also lead to anovulation. Excessive concentration of androgens in ovarian follicles may inhibit the emergence of a dominant follicle and result in follicular atresia. As in individuals with polycystic ovarian syndrome, hyperinsulinemia may contribute to the excessive androgen production in the ovaries.

THE MENSTRUAL CYCLE AND AGING

Menstrual cycle length varies as a woman ages. It may be several years after menarche before regular, ovulatory cycles are achieved. Several years prior to menopause, menstrual cycles tend to lengthen and anovulatory cycles become more frequent again.[4]

HORMONAL CONTRACEPTIVE EFFECTS

Hormonal contraceptives prevent fertilization in part by disrupting the menstrual cycle. Combined oral contraceptives contain both estrogen and progestin. Progestin-only contraceptives include Depo-Provera injections, Norplant implants, minipills, and intrauterine devices (IUDs) such as the Progestasert System and the Levonorgestrel IUD. Estrogens and progestins act upon many different organ systems and produce a broad range of effects:[11]

Estrogenic Effects

- Ovulation is inhibited because estrogen suppresses FSH and LH, thus preventing the pituitary gland from releasing ovary-stimulating hormones.
- The endometrial secretions and cellular structured are altered.
- Altered local levels of prostaglandins contribute to the degeneration of the corpus luteum.

Progestational Effects

- Ovulation is inhibited by suppression of the midcycle peak of LH and FSH.
- Thickened cervical mucus decreases sperm penetration.
- The activity of the cilia in the fallopian tubes is reduced.
- The endometrium becomes atrophic and impairs implantation.

REFERENCES

1. Bicsak TA, Tucker EM, Cappel S, Vaughan J, Rivier J, Vale W, Hseuh AJW. Hormonal regulation of granulosa cell inhibin biosynthesis. Endocrinology 1986;119:2711.
2. Clark JR, Dierschke DJ, Wolf RC. Hormonal regulation of ovarian folliculogenesis in rhesus monkey. III. Atresia on the preovulatory follicle induced by exogenous steroids and subsequent follicular development. Biol Reprod 1981;25:332.
3. Filicori M. Santoro N, Merriam GR, Crowley WF Jr. Characterization of the physiological pattern of episodic gonadotropin secretion throughout the human menstrual cycle. J Clin Endocrinol Metab 1986;62:1136.
4. Gosden RG. Follicular status at menopause. Human Reprod 1987;2:617.
5. Henderson KM. Gonadotrophic regulation of ovarian activity. Br Med Bull 1979;35:161.
6. Hoff, JD, Quigley ME, Yen SSC. Hormonal dynamics at midcycle: a reevaluation. J Clin Endocrinol Metab 1983;57:792.
7. Kase NG, Speroff L. The ovary. In: Bondy P, Rosenberg L (eds). Metabolic control and disease. 8th edition. Philadelphia PA: WB Saunders, 1980.
8. Kase NG, Weingold AB, Gershenson DM. Principles and practice of clinical gynecology. 2nd edition. New York: Churchill Livingstone, 1990.
9. Reame N, Sauder SE, Kelch RP, Marshall JC. Pulsatile gonadotropin secretion during the human menstrual cycle: evidence for altered frequency of gonadotropin-releasing hormone secretion. J Clin Endocrinol Metab 1984;59:384.
10. Sixma JJ, Cristiens GCML, Haspels AS. The sequence of hemostasis events in the endometrium during normal menstruation. In: Diczfalusy E, Fraser IS, Webb WTG (eds). WHO symposium on steroid contraception and endometrial bleeding. London: Pittman Press Ltd, 1980.
11. Speroff L, Glass RH, Kasen G. Clinical gynecologic endocrinology and infertility. 5th edition. Baltimore MD: Williams & Wilkins, 1994.
12. Swartz DP, Butler W. Normal and abnormal uterine bleeding. In: Thompson JD, Rock JA (eds). TeLinde's operative gynecology. 7th edition. Philadelphia PA: J.B. Lippincott, 1992.

Menopause

Felicia Stewart, MD

- Women over age 40 have the second highest proportion of unintended pregnancies (77%).
- Perimenopausal and menopausal women generally consume only half to a third of the amount of calcium they need daily. Supplementation may be necessary.
- Annual mammography screening for women age 50 or older reduces breast cancer mortality rates by 20% to 50%.
- Women taking estrogen treatment should be aware of new information about potential risks for cancer of the breast and uterus.

During the decade before menopause, the number of maturing ovarian follicles gradually decreases. The cause of menopause is not known,[57] but when it occurs, the ovaries are no longer able to respond to pituitary stimulating hormones, so estrogen levels are low and production of follicle stimulating hormone (FSH) and luteinizing hormone (LH) increases dramatically. Fertility declines, and menstrual cycles may be erratic with a diminished menstrual flow. This transition of endocrine and somatic changes, called the climacteric, occurs for most women between the ages of 45 and 55.

Menopause, the cessation of menstrual periods, occurs at a median age of 51,[47] but can occur as early as 45 or as late as 55. Menopause before age 45 is defined as premature menopause, and is not rare. Evaluation is therefore reasonable for younger women who are concerned about menopause-like symptoms. Premature ovarian failure before the age of 40 has been estimated to occur in 1% of women,[47] and may follow a hereditary pattern. The likelihood that menopause will occur before age 46 increases from 5% to about 25% for a woman whose family history includes a sister or mother who reached menopause before this age.[13]

Often, the diagnosis of menopause is straightforward: the cessation of menses at an appropriate age accompanied by typical hot flushes. Hot flushes usually begin with a spreading wave of warmth extending from trunk to face. During a flush, the skin may redden and sweating may be evident. Flushes typically last just a few minutes; they may occur a few or many times daily and may awaken the woman at night. The cause of hot flushes is not established, but they were found in a population-based sample of Australian women[26] to occur with most frequency among women who were postmenopausal, had lower estradiol and higher FSH levels, consumed heavier amounts of caffeine, and had a lower body mass index.

Menopausal symptoms may begin months or even years before menopause. Many women have unpredictable, irregular cycles preceding menopause, with intermittent menopause symptoms. If bleeding occurs more frequently than once a month, then evaluate it as abnormal bleeding. (See Chapter 6 on Menstrual Problems and Common Gynecologic Concerns.) FSH levels may be elevated during this interval, but LH is still in the normal range so ovulatory cycles may occasionally occur and contraception is still needed.

If you have any doubt about the diagnosis of menopause, conduct blood tests for FSH and LH. Good evidence that fertility has ended and that a woman can safely stop using contraception is cessation of menstrual periods for 12 months occurring at an appropriate age or elevated FSH and LH levels in the menopause range.

CONTRACEPTION IN THE PERIMENOPAUSAL YEARS

Contraception is an important issue for many women in the perimenopausal years. Although the likelihood is not high, when pregnancy does occur, it is likely to be unintended. Women over age 40 have the second highest proportion of unintended pregnancies, 77%, a proportion exceeded only by the proportion for adolescents 13 to 14 years of age.[22]

Perimenopausal women who are healthy non-smokers with no risk factors for heart disease may want to continue taking oral contraceptives until they reach menopause. Progestin-only minipills also are an option and can be used by some women who are not good candidates for combined oral contraceptives (see Chapter 19 on The Pill: Oral Contraceptives and Chapter 20 on Depo-Provera, Norplant, and Progestin-Only Pills.) Long-acting progestin contraceptives such as Norplant or Depo-Provera can be continued through menopause. However, irregular bleeding patterns sometimes associated with these two methods can create problems for perimenopausal women, because abnormal bleeding that is persistent, even if contraceptive hormone exposure is its most likely cause, will need to be evaluated. Other contraceptive options for women in this age group include condoms, vaginal barriers, and intrauterine devices.

Surgical sterilization is the most prevalent contraceptive method among women in the perimenopausal age range. A decision to undergo tubal ligation during perimenopause, however, deserves a thoughtful evaluation of risks, benefits, and cost. Because her fertility is low, a perimenopausal woman can expect highly effective protection with any of the temporary methods, including vaginal barriers. The advantages of sterilization surgery for perimenopausal women are less compelling than they are for women who make the decision earlier in their reproductive years.

Women using oral contraceptives are unlikely to have signs that indicate when menopause is occurring. Beginning when the woman is age 50, check the serum level of FSH annually to identify menopause so that she can discontinue contraception. Perform the blood test at the end of the pill-free week.

M EDICAL MANAGEMENT ISSUES AT MENOPAUSE

Except for hot flushes, which are extremely common, most women are able to make the climacteric transition without serious difficulty. Problems associated with reduced estrogen levels such as vaginal dryness and diminished bladder control tend to begin later, months or years after menopause, and may persist or worsen; hot flushes usually subside in intensity within the first few years. When a woman reaches menopause, review the personal risks and benefits of postmenopausal hormone treatment (see the section on Estrogen Treatment), information on calcium balance, and routine health screening measures such as mammography, lipid surveillance, and colon cancer screening.

BONE HEALTH

Medical priorities for postmenopausal women include protection against bone loss and home safety precautions to prevent falls and reduce the risk of serious fall-associated injury.[25] Fractures, especially of the hip, cause substantial morbidity and mortality in the elderly.

The minimum daily calcium requirement increases from 1,000 milligrams (mg) daily for perimenopausal adult women to 1,500 mg after menopause for women who do not take estrogen.[54] Dietary sources provide 400 mg to 600 mg of calcium for the average woman, so supplements are likely to be necessary regardless of a woman's decision about hormone treatment. Restriction of dietary calcium has been commonly recommended for individuals who have suffered kidney stones. However, there is no evidence that calcium intake increases the risk for stone formation; moreover, a very large study (involving 45,619 men) found that high dietary calcium intake was associated with a significant decreased risk for kidney stones.[14]

Adequate calcium intake and weight-bearing exercise are helpful, but cannot alone prevent bone loss, especially for women who have one or more risk factors for osteoporosis, such as a family history of osteoporosis, medical problems or medications that adversely affect bone, slenderness and short stature, and nonblack ethnicity. Hormone treatment with estrogen alone, or combined with progestin, improves bone density[51] and also may improve postural balance.[27] Women who do not want to use estrogen, or cannot, should have their bone density assessed at menopause. If the woman's bone density is more than one standard deviation below the median for her age or if other osteoporosis risk factors are present, she should carefully consider the advantages of hormone treatment.[45] Hormone treatment, if not contraindicated, is the simplest approach for preventing osteoporosis or stopping further bone loss. Otherwise, consider alternative treatment options such as alendronate sodium (Fosamax), calcitonin, or etidronate (Didronel). Arrange for continuing surveillance. Pay particular attention to medical problems or medications that might impair balance or attentiveness, and consider whether to conduct further evaluations.

Using hormone treatment to prevent or stop bone loss requires a daily dose of at least 0.625 mg conjugated estrogen or its equivalent, although some evidence suggests that a dose of 0.3 mg accompanied by an aggressive intake of calcium (1,500 to 2,500 mg daily total) can provide a similar benefit.[19] Because there is some evidence that the addition of progestin to a menopausal hormone treatment regimen may increase the positive benefit on bone density, some experts recommend that women who have osteoporosis, or are a high risk for this problem, take progestin along with estrogen whether or not it is needed for protection against uterine cancer.[47] (See the section on Uterine Cancer Risk.) Similarly, initiating hormone treatment for the first time for an elderly woman who has osteoporosis may be reasonable to protect against hip fracture.[44]

MAMMOGRAPHY

Annual mammography screening for women age 50 and older has been shown consistently to reduce breast cancer mortality by 20% to 30%; however, research for younger women is limited and interpreting results to form recommendations has been the subject of continuing controversy.[38] Because breast cancer occurs much less frequently in women age 40 to 50 than in older women, the number of cancers that can potentially be detected at an early stage is much smaller, and the potential years of life saved for the population screened, therefore, is also much smaller. There is conflicting evidence regarding benefits of screening women age 40 to 49; however, a recent review of results from seven clinical trials concluded that screening could reduce mortality in this age group by 24%.[20] (For more detailed discussion of breast cancer screening, see Chapter 3 on Female Genital Tract Cancer Screening.)

In addition to arbitrary age criteria, consider other breast cancer risk factors when helping a woman evaluate her own schedule for mammography. Women who are at increased risk because of one or more risk factors (Table 5-1) should make screening a high priority. At highest risk are women with familial risk because of the BRCA1 or BRCA2 gene mutation. These high-risk families are likely to have multiple relatives (three or more have had breast cancer), often with premenopausal onset and bilateral disease; they also have an increased risk for ovarian and colon

Table 5-1 Breast cancer risk factors

Risk Factor	Relative Risk
Family History	
First-degree relative with breast cancer	1.2–3.0
Premenopausal	3.1
Premenopausal and bilateral	8.5–9.0
Postmenopausal	1.5
Postmenopausal and bilateral	4.0–5.4
Menstrual History	
Age at menarche less than 12 years	1.3
Age at menopause greater than 55 years	1.5–2.0
Pregnancy	
First live birth from ages 25 - 29	1.5
First live birth after age 30	1.9
First live birth after age 35	2.0–3.0
Nulliparous	3.0
Benign Breast Diseases	
Proliferative disease	1.9
Proliferative with atypical hyperplasia	4.4
Lobular carcinoma in situ	6.9–12.0

Source: Bilimoria, et al. (1995) with permission.

cancers. In this situation, refer the woman for genetic counseling so she can plan for needed surveillance and consider the option of prophylactic mastectomy. This hereditary pattern is rare: it accounts for only about 1% of all breast cancer. A non-specific family history, with one or two first degree relatives having breast cancer, is much more common but is associated with only a moderate increase in risk.[8]

ESTROGEN TREATMENT

Hormone treatment is a reasonable option for many women. Reviewing available research, the American College of Obstetrics and Gynecologists concluded that epidemiologic studies "strongly suggest" estrogen treatment reduces the risk of cardiovascular disease for postmenopausal women.[2] There are no large randomized treatment studies to prove cause-and-effect, and heart disease prevention is not an indication that has been approved by the U.S. Food and Drug Administration (FDA) for estrogen use. However, epidemiologic studies suggest the magnitude of benefit from estrogen treatment is large: a 50% reduction in the risk of a coronary event.[5,36] Hormone treatment also prevents osteoporosis and ameliorates symptoms such as hot flushes, vaginal dryness, and sleep disturbance; these are the FDA-approved indications for its use. There is evidence that estrogen can favorably affect memory,[33,45] mood,[41] dental health, and skin thickness and collagen content.[2] It may also significantly reduce the risk for colorectal cancer.[9] Well-being also is likely to be enhanced for women who experience severe flushing or fatigue, irritability, or depression because of chronic sleep disturbance caused by flushes at night. The possible role of estrogen treatment in slowing development of Alzheimer's disease, if this relationship is confirmed, will be especially compelling for many women.[21,40]

Women reluctant to consider hormone treatment commonly cite concerns about the possible role of hormone treatment in the risk of breast and uterine cancer, practical issues such as convenience and cost, and the less serious side effects. Some experts, as well, do not find the cardiovascular disease protection research persuasive and admonish caution because of their concern about the risk of breast cancer.[37] In addition, some women have been advised to avoid estrogen because of a prior history of uterine leiomyomata, endometriosis, endometrial hyperplasia, gallbladder disease, thromboembolic disease, chronic liver disease, or seizure disorder. In a randomly selected sample of women age 40 to 55 who were members of a large health maintenance organization, about 9% had an "absolute" contraindication (breast cancer, 8%; endometrial cancer, 1%), and an additional 33% had one or more "relative" contraindications documented in medical records.[55] New concerns have also been raised about an increased risk (about a three-fold risk among current hormone treatment users) for venous thromboembolism[15,32] and an increased risk for developing asthma (doubled risk after 10 years of hormone use).[52]

Uterine Cancer Risk

The most clearly documented adverse consequence of estrogen treatment after menopause is a fourfold to eightfold increase in risk for endometrial cancer. This consequence can be avoided by providing progestin for at least 10 days each month along with estrogen,[47] although some experts have recommended 12 days or a continuous progestin schedule.[39] Women who use a combined estrogen and progestin regimen after menopause have a lower risk for endometrial cancer than do untreated women. Even if progestin is not provided, overall life-expectancy is greater for estrogen-users than it is for untreated women; this is true even for users who actually develop endometrial cancer.[28]

Breast Cancer Risk

With research results in conflict and the pathophysiology of breast cancer unknown, it is not possible to speculate with confidence about the role that exogenous hormones might play in breast cancer risk. Because breast cancer incidence ranks second only to lung cancer among women, this is a very significant issue. Several carefully executed, large epidemiologic studies have shown no excess risk of breast cancer among menopausal hormone users.[34,48,56] Several other studies, however, have found an increased risk, at least for some users.[7,12] Conclusions from meta-analyses are also conflicting, but the most recent have suggested that current use of hormone treatment, especially prolonged use of high doses, is associated with a modest increase in risk.[12,24,49] One such analysis, based on 16 studies, concluded that breast cancer risk may be increased by 30% after 15 years of estrogen use; no increased risk was apparent until 5 years of use. The risk was greatest for women who had a family history of breast cancer.[49] Another review of 31 studies concluded that current hormone use for 10 years or longer is associated with 20% to 30% increased risk.[12] This analysis did not find an association between increased risk and family history, however, and an increased risk of death has been documented in only one clinical trial. Similarly, clinical research has not found a link between breast cancer and past use of hormone treatment.

Some researchers have suggested a possible protective effect of concomitant progestin administration,[23,48] but others have not found evidence of protection. Analysis of data from the Nurses' Health Study led its researchers to conclude that addition of progestins to estrogen treatment does not reduce breast cancer risk,[11] and a 1989 study of Swedish women found the excess breast cancer risk to be highest for women who took progestin along with estradiol.[7] Unlike estradiol users in this study, women using conjugated estrogen or estriol did not incur increased risk. Until the causes of breast cancer are understood, continuing concern and awareness are appropriate. Breast surveillance with conscientious clinical exams and annual mammography are important for all women in this age group whether or not they are taking hormones.

CAUTIONS AND SIDE EFFECTS

Cautions

Contraindications to menopausal estrogen treatment include the following conditions:[2,42]

- Pregnancy
- Unexplained vaginal bleeding
- Active liver disease; chronic, impaired liver function
- Active thrombophlebitis or thromboembolic disorder
- Carcinoma of the breast
- Known or suspected estrogen-dependent neoplasia

Cautions (relative contraindications) to hormone treatment include seizure disorder, hypertension, familial hyperlipidemia, migraine headache, and gallbladder disease.[2] The risk estrogen may pose for a woman with a past history of thrombosis is unknown. Any woman who has had thrombophlebitis in the past should approach the decision to use estrogen cautiously and be under careful surveillance.

Although a history of breast cancer is a contraindication to estrogen treatment, it is unknown whether estrogen use increases a woman's risk for breast cancer recurrence. One small study of patients who received hormone treatment after previous therapy for breast cancer did not find any evidence of an adverse effect,[18] but further research will be needed to provide a reasonable basis for assessing the overall benefits and risks of this approach.[1] Also unresolved is the balance between benefit and risk for hormone treatment after previous therapy for endometrial cancer. The risk of ovarian cancer and cervical carcinoma recurrence are believed to be unaffected by hormone treatment.[2] Hormone treatment could aggravate endometriosis symptoms or cause growth of uterine leiomyomata, but in practice, these effects are not common.

Side Effects

Breast tenderness, a common initial side effect of treatment, generally subsides after the first few weeks of treatment. Some women have nausea;

taking estrogen at meal time may help. Progestin administration can cause fluid retention and uterine cramps—reasons to reduce the progestin dose or try an alternative progestin such as micronized progesterone. Some women tolerate better the continuous, moderate blood levels of estrogen that occur with use of estradiol patches than they do the daily hormone peaks that occur with oral administration. A night-time peak, however, may be helpful for a woman with sleep disturbance; taking hormone pills in the evening may maximize relief of her symptoms.

PROVIDING HORMONE TREATMENT

A typical hormone treatment regimen provides conjugated estrogen 0.625 mg daily for 25 days each month, with medroxyprogesterone acetate 10 mg daily for the last 10 to 14 days of estrogen treatment in each cycle.[39] Estrogen given continuously, with progestin on the first 10 to 14 days of each month, may be helpful for women who experience menopause symptoms during the non-hormone interval. With these sequential regimens, 80% to 90% of women experience withdrawal bleeding following the progestin phase. Bleeding is much less common (20%) for women using a continuous/combined schedule. Options for this approach include the following:[47]

- Daily estrogen: 0.625 mg conjugated estrogens, *or*
  0.625 mg estrone sulfate, *or*
  1.0 mg micronized estradiol
- Daily progestin: 2.5 mg medroxyprogesterone acetate, *or*
  0.35 mg norethindrone, *or*
  100 mg micronized progesterone

Research to clarify optimal regimens, doses, and choice of drugs for menopause treatment is surprisingly limited. Available products are shown in Table 5-2. Because of the increased risk of endometrial cancer, women who have a uterus and choose to use estrogen alone need an annual endometrial biopsy. Research on endometrial hormone receptors and histologic response to hormone exposure suggests the duration of progestin treatment is important for protection against endometrial cancer. If progestin-related side effects, such as fluid retention, are a problem, reducing the dose of progestin (to 5 mg or 2.5 mg of medroxyprogesterone acetate) is preferable to reducing duration.[39] The effectiveness of continuous or monthly progestin in reducing the risk of uterine cancer has been documented in clinical studies. However, progestin treatment for fewer than 10 days a month has been associated with an increased risk for hyperplasia[10] and endometrial cancer;[6] thus, once-per-3-months progestin treatment regimens have little or no demonstrated

Table 5-2 Menopausal treatment products

Estrogens

Conjugated estrogens	Premarin 0.3 mg (green), 0.625 mg (maroon), 0.9 mg (white), 1.25 mg (yellow), 2.5 mg (purple)
Esterified estrogen	Estratab 0.3 mg (blue), 0.625 mg (yellow), 1.25 mg (orange), 2.5 mg (purple) Menest 0.3 mg (yellow), 0.625 mg (orange), 1.25 mg (green), 2.5 mg (pink)
Estropipate (estrone)	Ogen 0.625 mg, 1.25 mg, 2.5 mg, 5.0 mg Ortho-est "0.625" (0.75 mg), "1.25" (1.5 mg) Estropipate tabs (generic) 0.75 mg, 1.5 mg, 3.0 mg
Estradiol	Estrace 0.5 mg, 1 mg, 2 mg - scored
Micronized	No commercially marketed products: Oral capsules compounded by a pharmacist are available from some pharmacies and through mail order (eg., California Pharmacy & Compounding Center, 307 Placentia Avenue, Newport Beach, CA 92663. Phone: 1-800-279-5709). Prescription required.
Pellets	No commercially marketed products: Implantable pellets containing 25 mg, 50 mg, 75 mg compounded by a pharmacist are available from some pharmacies (see above).

Transdermal	Estraderm 0.05 mg, 0.1 mg - patches
	  (8 in pack) use 2x weekly
	 Climera 0.05 mg/day, 0.1 mg/day - patches
	  (4 in pack) use 1x weekly
	 Vivelle 0.0375, 0.05, 0.075, 0.1 mg/day - patches
	  (8 in pack) use 2x weekly

Vaginal ring	Estring 2 mg, wear continuously for 90 days then remove and replace

Estrogen with Methyl Testosterone (MeT)*

Conjugated estrogen	Premarin 1.25 with MeT 10 mg; Premarin 0.625 with MeT 5 mg
Esterified estrogen (EE)	Estratest 1.25 EE with MeT 2.5 mg (dark green) Estratest H.S. 0.625 EE with MeT 1.25 mg (light green)

Estrogen with Progestin (packaged together)

Conjugated estrogen Medroxyprogesterone acetate	Premphase: Premarin 0.625 mg (days 1-28) with Cycrin 5.0 mg (days 15-28); Two 14-day blister packs to be used consecutively Prempro: Premarin 0.625 mg (daily) with Cycrin 2.5 mg (daily); 14-day blister pack

(continued)

Table 5-2 Menopausal treatment products *(cont.)*

Estrogen Vaginal Creams**

Conjugated estrogen	Premarin Vaginal Cream 0.625 mg/g; 42.5 g tube; 1–4 g applicator
Estropipate	Ogen Vaginal Cream 1.5 mg/g; 42.5 g tube; 1–4 g applicator
Dienestrol	Ortho Dienestrol Cream 0.01% (estrogenic potency unknown) 78 g tube
Estradiol	Estrace Vaginal Cream 0.01% (0.01 mg/g) 42.5 g tube; 1–4 g applicator

Progestins

Medroxprogesterone acetate	Amen 10 mg - scored Cycrin 10 mg - scored Provera 2.5 mg, 5 mg, 10 mg - scored
Norethindrone acetate***	Aygestin 5 mg - scored
Progesterone (micronized)	No commercially marketed products: Capsules containing 100 or 200 mg, compounded by a pharmacist using micronized progesterone powder extracted from plant sources, are available from some pharmacies, and through mail order. (For example, Women's International Pharmacy, Madison, Wisconsin. To order, call 1-800-279-5708). Prescription is required.

Methyltestosterone*

Methlytestosterone	Android 10 mg, 25 mg - scored Oreton 10 mg Testred 10 mg - capsules
Transdermal	Androderm 2.5 mg/day - patches (30 or 60 in pack); Schedule III Controlled Substance Testoderm 4 mg/day; 6 mg/day - patches (30 in pack); Schedule III Controlled Substance

Nonhormonal Products

Clonidine	Clonidine 0.1 mg tablets
Transdermal	Catapres-TTS -1 (0.1 mg/day), Use 1 patch/week Catapres-TTS -2 (0.2 mg/day), Use 1 patch/week Catapres-TTS -3 (0.3 mg/day), Use 1 patch/week
Belladonna 0.2 mg	Bellergal-S - scored
Phenobarbital 40 mg	One tab b.i.d.
Ergotamine 0.6 mg	

(continued)

Table 5-2 Menopausal treatment products *(cont.)*

Nonhormonal Products *(cont.)*	
Bioflavinoids	Hy-C tablets
	Mevanin-C capsules
	Peridin-C tablets

Source: Adapted from Stewart, et al. (1987) with permission.

*Methyltestosterone can cause growth of coarse, dark body hair, scalp hair loss (balding), deepened voice, and unfavorable lipid ratio; risks for developing liver tumor may also be increased.

**Vaginal estrogen absorption results in somewhat lower blood estrogen levels than the same dose given orally. Notice that Estrace and Dienestrol cream contain a smaller amount of estrogen than do the other products available. For a dose equivalent to 0.3 mg conjugated estrogen vaginally, measure 1/8 of an applicator of Premarin, or 1/16 of an applicator of Ogen, or a whole applicator of Estrace or Dienestrol.

***This synthetic progestin may have less desirable blood lipid effects than medroxyprogesterone acetate.

advantage over unopposed estrogen treatment and would require annual endometrial biopsy.

Several small studies indicate that a progestin-releasing intrauterine device (IUD) can protect against endometrial hyperplasia among women using estrogen treatment.[3,4,46] In these studies, women wearing a progestin-releasing IUD became amenorrheic within about 1 year and did not have evidence of endometrial proliferation despite estrogen use. When the 10-year progestin IUD, now widely used in other countries, becomes available in the United States, it may provide an attractive option for many menopausal women using estrogen treatment.

A woman who has had a hysterectomy does not need progestin for protection against endometrial cancer risk. However, use of progestin along with estrogen has been suggested for women with the following characteristics:[47]

- Previously treated Stage I adenocarcinoma of the endometrium or endometrioid tumors of the ovary
- History of pelvic endometriosis (to prevent development of adenocarcinoma in endometriosis tissue)
- Osteoporosis, or at high risk for osteoporosis (to gain the bone-preserving benefit conferred by progestin)
- Elevated triglyceride levels (to attenuate the further estrogen-induced triglyceride increase)

Transdermal estrogen treatment may be advantageous for women with elevated triglyceride levels. Oral estrogen treatment increases triglycerides, but transdermal treatment does not have this effect. Some experts recommend monitoring lipids and changing to the transdermal route if fasting triglyceride levels are 250 mg/deciliter (2.8 nanomoles/liter) or more.[47]

Testosterone treatment has been suggested for women who have problems with diminished libido. Libido increases within a few days after the woman begins oral treatment. Available hormone products include fixed estrogen and methyl testosterone combinations, methyl testosterone oral tablets, and testosterone transdermal patches intended for treatment of men. These patches (classified as a controlled substance because of the potential for steroid abuse), offer the possibility of providing a lower dose by cutting each patch in half or into quarters. Intermittent use of testosterone is an option. Little information is available about long-term effects of testosterone treatment in women, and problems such as acne and increased facial hair have been reported, as have possible adverse effects on plasma lipids (such as suppression of high density lipoprotein [HDL] cholesterol).[16,30,53]

Cyclic hormone treatment is likely to be associated with monthly bleeding after each progestin batch. Bleeding at any other time or any bleeding in a postmenopausal woman not receiving progestin requires prompt evaluation. Irregular bleeding is not uncommon during the first 3 to 6 months of treatment with a continuous regimen of estrogen and progestin. Perform an endometrial biopsy on a woman who has irregular bleeding. Uterine cancer has been reported among women using a continuous regimen.[35]

Alternatives to Estrogen

When estrogen is contraindicated, treatment with progestin such as medroxyprogesterone acetate 10 to 20 mg daily or Depo Provera 150 mg every 3 months may reduce hot flushes. Progestin also provides some protection against bone loss.[47] Estrogen-containing vaginal cream is an option for treating vaginal dryness. Vaginal symptoms respond to local treatment at a much lower dose than is needed systemically. The use of this cream may not be associated with an increased risk of endometrial cancer.[17] Another option is a 3-month, estradiol-releasing silicone vaginal ring (Estring) introduced in 1997. Women wearing the ring have sustained plasma estradiol levels of 20 to 30 pico-moles per liter (pmol/L). This level is not high enough to provide cardiovascular or bone protection, but is lower than the estimated threshold (60 pmol/L) for endometrial proliferation. It is sufficient, however, to reduce symptoms of urogenital atrophy in 90% of wearers. About 20% of women using the ring experience adverse effects including vaginal irritation or ulcers.[29]

Commonly recommended alternatives to hormone treatment for hot flushes include bioflavinoids, Bellergal, and clonidine. Efficacy superior to placebo has been reported only for transdermal clonidine, as a 100 microgram dose applied once weekly.[47] Women who must avoid hormones need to be aware that herbal preparations such as ginseng may not be a wise choice since they, too, have estrogenic effects.[31]

References

1. American College of Obstetricians and Gynecologists. Estrogen replacement therapy in women with previously treated breast cancer. ACOG Technical Bulletin No. 135. Washington DC:ACOG, 1994.
2. American College of Obstetricians and Gynecologists. Hormone replacement therapy. ACOG Technical Bulletin No. 166. Washington DC: ACOG, 1992.
3. Andersson K, Mattsson L-A, Rybo G, Stadberg E. Intrauterine release of levonorgestrel—a new way of adding progestogen in hormone replacement therapy. Obstet Gynecol 1992;79:963-967.
4. Archer DF, Viniegra-Sibal A, Hsiu J-G, Seltman HJ, Muesing R, Ross B. Endometrial histology, uterine bleeding, and metabolic changes in post-menopausal women using a progesterone-releasing intrauterine device and oral conjugated estrogens for hormone replacement therapy. J North Amer Menopause Soc 1994;1:109-116.
5. Barrett-Connor E, Bush TL. Estrogen and coronary heart disease in women. JAMA 1991;265:1861-1867.
6. Beresford SAA, Weiss NS, Voigt LF, McKnight B. Risk of endometrial cancer in relation to use of oestrogen combined with cyclic progestagen therapy in postmenopausal women. Lancet 1997;1:458-461.
7. Bergkvist L, Adami HO, Persoon I, Hoover R, Schaiver C. The risk of breast cancer after estrogen and estrogen-progestin replacement. N Engl J Med 1989;321:293-297.
8. Bilimoria MM, Morrow M. The woman at increased risk for breast cancer: evaluation and management strategies. CA Cancer J Clin 1995;45:263-278.
9. Calle EE, Miracle-McMahill HL, Thun MJ, Heath CW. Estrogen replacement therapy and risk of fatal colon cancer in a prospective cohort of postmeno-pausal women. J Natl Cancer Inst 1995;87:517-523.
10. Cerin A, Heldaas K, Moeller B. (Letters to the editor). Adverse endometrial effects of long- cycle estrogen and progestogen replacement therapy. N Engl J Med 1996;334:668-669.
11. Colditz GA, Hankinson SE, Hunter DJ, Willett WC, Manson JE, Stampfer MJ, Hennekens C, Rosner B, Speizer FE. The use of estrogens and progestins and the risk of breast cancer in postmenopausal women. N Engl J Med 1995;332:1589-1593.
12. Colditz GA, Egan KM, Stampfer MJ. Hormone replacement therapy and risk of breast cancer: results from epidemiologic studies. Am J Obstet Gynecol 1993;168:1473-1480.
13. Cramer DW, XuH, Harlow BL. Family history as a predictor of early meno-pause. Fertil Steril 1995;64:740-745.
14. Curhan GC, Willett WC, Rimm EB, Stampfer MJ. A prospective study of dietary calcium and other nutrients and the risk of symptomatic kidney stones. N Engl J Med 1993;328:833-838.
15. Daly E, Vessey MP, Hawkins MM, Carson JL, Gough P, Marsh S. Risk of venous thromboembolism in users of hormone replacement therapy. Lancet 1996;348:977-980.
16. Davis SR, Burger HG. Clinical review 82: androgens and the postmenopausal woman. J Clin Endocrin Metab 1996;81:2759-2763.

17. Deutsch S, Ossowski R, Benjamin I. Comparison between degree of systemic absorption of vaginally and orally administered estrogens at different dose levels in postmenopausal women. Am J Obstet Gynecol 1981;139:967-968.
18. DiSaia PJ, Grosen EA, Kurosaki T, Gildea M, Cowan B, Anton-Culver H. Hormone replacement therapy in breast cancer survivors: a cohort study. Am J Obstet Gynecol 1996;174:1494-1498.
19. Ettinger B, Genant HK, Cann CE. Postmenopausal bone loss is prevented by treatment with low-dosage estrogen with calcium. Ann Int Med 1987;106:40-45.
20. Feig SA. Estimation of currently attainable benefit from mammographic screening of women aged 40-49 years. Cancer 1995;75:2412-2420.
21. Filley CM. Alzheimer's disease in women. Am J Obstet Gynecol 1997;178:1-7.
22. Forrest JD. Epidemiology of unintended pregnancy and contraceptive use. Am J Obstet Gynecol 1994;170:1485-1489.
23. Gambrell RD Jr. Proposal to decrease the risk and improve the prognosis of breast cancer. Am J Obstet Gynecol 1984;150:119-132.
24. Grady D, Rubin SM, Petitti DB, Fox CS, Black D, Ettinger B, Ernster VL, Cummings SR. Hormone therapy to prevent disease and prolong life in postmenopausal women. Ann Intern Med 1992;117:1016-1041.
25. Greenspan SL, Myers ER, Maitland LA, Resnick NM, Hayes WC. Fall severity and bone mineral density as risk factors for hip fracture in ambulatory elderly. JAMA 1994;271:128-133.
26. Guthrie JR, Dennerstein L, Hopper JL, Burger HG. Hot flushes, menstrual status, and hormone levels in a population-based sample of midlife women. Obstet Gynecol 1996;88:437-442.
27. Hammar ML, LindgrenR, Berg GE, Moller CG, Niklasson MK. Effects of hormonal replacement therapy on the postural balance among postmenopausal women. Obstet Gynecol 1996;88:955-960.
28. Henderson BE, Paganini-Hill A, Ross RK. Decreased mortality in users of estrogen replacement therapy. Arch Intern Med 1991;1511:75-78.
29. Henriksson L, Stjernquist M, Boquist L, Cedergren I, Selinus I. A one-year multicenter study of efficacy and safety of a continuous, low-dose, estradiol-releasing vaginal ring (Estring) in postmenopausal women with symptoms and signs of urogenital aging. Am J Obstet Gynecol 1996;174:85-92.
30. Hickok LR, Toomey C, Speroff L. A comparison of esterified estrogens with and without methyltestosterone: effects on endometrial histology and serum lipoproteins in postmenopausal women. Obstet Gynecol 1993;82:919-924.
31. Hopkins MP, Androff L, Benninghoff AS. Ginseng face cream and unexplained vaginal bleeding. Am J Obstet Gynecol 1988;159:1121-1122.
32. Jick H, Derby LE, Myers MW, Vasilakis C, Newton KM. Risk of hospital admission for idiopathic venous thromboembolism among users of postmenopausal oestrogens. Lancet 1996;348:981-983.
33. Kampen DL, Sherwin BB. Estrogen use and verbal memory in healthy postmenopausal women. Obstet Gynecol 1994;83:979-983.
34. Kaufman DW, Miller DR, Rosenberg L, Helmrich SP, Stolley P, Schottenfeld D, Shapiro S. Noncontraceptive estrogen use and the risk of breast cancer. JAMA 1984;252:63-67.

35. Leather AT, Savvas M, Studd JW. Endometrial histology and bleeding patterns after 8 years of continuous combined estrogen and progestogen therapy in postmenopausal women. Obstet Gynecol 1991;78:1008.

36. Lindsay R, Bush TL, Grady D, Speroff L, Lobo RA. Therapeutic controversy: estrogen replacement in menopause. J Clinical Endocrinol Metab 1996;81:3829-3837.

37. Love S, Lindsey K. Dr. Susan Love's hormone book: making informed choices about menopause. New York: Random House, 1997.

38. Margolese R. Screening mammography in young women: a different perspective. Lancet 1996;347:881-882.

39. Mishell DR Jr, Davajan V, Lobo RA. Infertility, contraception and reproductive endocrinology. 3rd ed. Oradell NJ: Medical Economics Co., 1991.

40. Paganini-Hill A, Oestrogen replacement therapy and Alzheimer's disease. Brit J Obstet and Gynecol 1996;103:80-86.

41. Pearlstein TB. Hormones and depressions: what are the facts about premenstrual syndrome, menopause, and hormone replacement therapy? Am J Obstet Gynecol 1995;173:646-653.

42. Physicians' desk reference. 51st edition. Oradell NJ: Medical Economics Co., 1997.

43. Riggs BL, Melton LJ. The prevention and treatment of osteoporosis. N Engl J Med 1992;327:620-627.

44. Schneider DL, Barrett-Conner EL, Morton DJ. Timing of postmenopausal estrogen for optimal bone mineral density. JAMA 1997;543-547.

45. Sherwin BB, Tulandi T. "Add-back" estrogen reverses cognitive deficits induced by a gonadotropin-releasing hormone agonist in women with leiomyomata uteri. J Clin Endocrinol Metab 1996;81:2545-2549.

46. Shoupe D, Meme D, Mezrow G, Lobo RA. (Letters to the Editor) Prevention of endometrial hyperplasia in postmenopausal women with intrauterine progesterone. N Engl J Med 1991;325:1811-1812.

47. Speroff L, Glass RH, Kase NG. Clinical gynecologic endocrinology and infertility. 5th ed. Baltimore: Williams & Wilkins Co., 1994.

48. Stanford JL, Weiss NS, Voigt LF, Daling JR, Habel LA, Rossing MA. Combined estrogen and progestin hormone replacement therapy in relation to risk of breast cancer in middle-aged women. JAMA 1995;274:178-179.

49. Steinberg KK, Thacker SB, Smith SJ, Stroup DF, Zack MM, Flanders WD, Berkelman RL. A meta-analysis of the effect of estrogen replacement therapy on the risk of breast cancer. JAMA 1991;265:1985-1992.

50. Stewart F, Guest F, Stewart G, Hatcher RH. Understanding your body: every woman's guide to gynecology and health. New York: Bantam Books, 1987.

51. The Writing Group for the PEPI Trial. Effects of hormone therapy on bone mineral density: results from the postmenopausal estrogen/progestin interventions (PEPI) trial. JAMA 1996;276:1389-1396.

52. Troisi RJ, Speizer FE, Willett WC, Trichopoulos D, Rosner B. Menopause, postmenopausal estrogen preparations, and the risk of adult-onset asthma: a prospective cohort study. Am J Respir Crit Care Med 1995;152:1183-1188.

53. Urman B, Pride SM, Yuen BH. Elevated serum testosterone, hirsutism, and virilism associated with combined androgen-estrogen hormone replacement therapy. Obstet Gynecol 1991;77:595-598.

54. Utian WH, Avioli L, Bonnick SL, Ettinger B, Miller PD, Voda AM (eds). A consensus opinion: calcium supplementation for the prevention and treatment of osteoporosis. Menopause Management 1994;III(Suppl):4-15.

55. Whitlock EP, Valanis B, Ernst D, Smith L. Prevalence of contraindications to hormone replacement therapy in middle-aged women in a managed care setting. J Women's Health 1995;4:293-302.

56. Wingo PA, Layde PM, Lee NC, Rubin G, Ory HW. The risk of breast cancer in postmenopausal women who have used estrogen replacement therapy. JAMA 1987;257:209-215.

57. Wise PM, Krajnak KM, Kashon ML. Menopause: the aging of multiple pacemakers. Science 1996;273:67-70.

Menstrual Problems and Common Gynecologic Concerns

Anita L. Nelson, MD

- Take a systems approach when evaluating menstrual problems:
  - for primary amenorrhea, determine the status of uterine and breast development;
  - for secondary amenorrhea, assess (1) the uterus and lower genital tract, (2) the ovaries, and (3) the pituitary and hypothalamus;
  - for dysfunctional uterine bleeding, conduct your workup based on whether the DUB is ovulatory or anovulatory.

- About 3% to 10% of reproductive-age women in the United States have endometriosis. Nearly 25% to 35% of infertile women have endometriosis.
- Pelvic masses are fairly common; the relative frequencies of different types of masses change with a woman's age. Rule out ectopic pregnancy immediately.
- As many as 50% of married couples experience some sexual dissatisfaction, but few women present sexually related complaints to their health care provider.

Reproductive health care providers deal with a wide range of gynecologic complaints in conjunction with counseling and providing contraceptive methods to women. Many of these problems, including sexually transmitted infections (STIs) and vulvovaginitis, are addressed in other chapters. This chapter focuses on problems women have with menstrual cycle disorders and some of the more common gynecologic problems such as vulvar lesions, pelvic masses, endometriosis, and sexual dysfunction.

MENSTRUAL PROBLEMS

During their reproductive years, women frequently experience disorders in menstrual cycling such as excessive bleeding, infrequent bleeding, or painful menses. In addition, even normal menstrual cycling can be associated with other problems such as premenstrual syndrome (PMS), menstrual migraine headaches, and increased seizure activity.

DYSMENORRHEA

Dysmenorrhea, Greek for painful menstruation, is classified as *primary* (intrinsic and usually lifelong) or *secondary* (due to some physical cause and usually of later onset). In a study of young women attending a family planning clinic, 72% of those surveyed experienced dysmenorrhea; for 15% it was severe enough to interfere with their normal activities.[5]

In addition to painful uterine cramping with menses, women with dysmenorrhea may also experience nausea, vomiting, diarrhea, headaches, or symptoms of vasomotor instability such as weakness or fainting. Symptoms may vary in severity from cycle to cycle but generally continue through the reproductive years. Dysmenorrhea can be an incapacitating problem, causing significant disruption each month. Young women lose days at school, and older women are unable to function at home or in the workplace.

Primary Dysmenorrhea

Primary dysmenorrhea has mainly physiologic, not psychological, causes. Early investigators held that dysmenorrhea occurred in "maladjusted women who were intensely rejecting their feminine role and suffered from deep hostility."[13] Today, it is understood that the problem is not in the woman's head but in her uterus. Measurements with intrauterine catheters demonstrate that women with primary dysmenorrhea generate intrauterine pressures similar to those generated during the second stage of labor.[109,122,128] Women with primary dysmenorrhea are generally ovulatory and produce progesterone in the luteal phase. Progesterone stimulates the production of a balanced mixture of prostaglandins in the base of the endometrium. When the endometrium sloughs, women with primary dysmenorrhea have been found to produce excessive amounts of prostaglandins,[86] which increase the force of myometrial contractions. These contractions reduce uterine blood flow, causing ischemia and intensifying pain. In addition, intermediates in the production of prostaglandins (cyclic endoperoxides) in the presence of high prostaglandin levels can directly cause pain. When injected into the general circulation by uterine contractions, prostaglandins can also precipitate systemic symptoms such as headache, nausea, vomiting, and diarrhea.

Symptomatic therapies include rest, applying a heating pad, or taking teas or medications to treat the discomfort (such as aspirin or over-the-counter nonsteroidal anti-inflammatory agents [NSAIDs]). Strong pain relievers, such as narcotics, may be required to treat severe pain. Usually, however, women seeking medical care have already tried these measures without success and are in need of treatment targeted to treat the pathophysiology underlying their complaints. Two complementary strategies target the underlying problem: reducing the thickness of the endometrial lining and reducing prostaglandin production.

Endometrial thinning. Hormonal therapies control the thickness of the endometrium, the amount of blood loss, and the production of prostaglandins.[26] Combination oral contraceptives (OCs) generally reduce menstrual blood flow at least 40% within 3 months when used in cyclic fashion.[7] Within 3 to 4 months of beginning oral contraceptive therapy, 90% of women experience marked decreases in the severity of pain.[26,73,95] Oral contraceptive formulations with a higher ratio of progestin to estrogen are more effective in thinning the endometrium than are formulations with a high estrogen ratio.[73] Women can achieve additional relief by reducing their number of withdrawal bleeds, thereby reducing the number of days of discomfort. Continuous use of active pills for 6 weeks (eliminating the placebo pills in one of the two packages) or for 9 weeks (eliminating the placebo pills in two sequential packages) can be very helpful.[117] These approaches, referred to as "bicycling" and "tricycling," use only monophasic pill formulations. (See Chapter 19 on The Pill: Oral Contraceptives.) Depot-medroxyprogesterone acetate (DMPA) is also helpful in treating dysmenorrhea. After their third injection, nearly half of DMPA users become amenorrheic and avoid dysmenorrhea.

Other hormonal manipulations are also available to achieve amenorrhea, but their use is limited due to side effects and cost. Danazol, an androgen used to treat endometriosis, effectively induces amenorrhea but can be used for only 4 to 6 months due to unpleasant androgenic side effects including acne, hirsutism, oily skin, clitoral enlargement, and voice deepening. Gonadotropin releasing hormone (GnRH) agonists, FDA-approved for treatment of endometriosis, induce amenorrhea and therefore eliminate dysmenorrhea. However, GnRH agonists can be used only for a short course of therapy because they cause hypoestrogenic side effects such as vasomotor symptoms (hot flashes), vaginal dryness, and osteoporosis.

Prostaglandin inhibition. Prostaglandin synthetase inhibitors such as NSAIDs are more effective than placebo.[29] Taken at the onset of menses or just prior to menses, NSAIDS reduce prostaglandin release into the menstrual fluid and significantly reduce dysmenorrhea as well as blood loss.[29] Aspirin is no more effective than placebo.[19]

Rule out other causes of pain in women who fail to respond to these therapies. Some women who have primary dysmenorrhea early in life may subsequently develop other problems, such as endometriosis, which then result in *secondary* dysmenorrhea. Women with persistent complaints often benefit from a psychological evaluation and treatments for chronic pain. Some investigators report that a transcutaneous electrical nerve stimulation (TENS) unit reduces dysmenorrhea. Some investigators have suggested that dietary manipulations such as supplementing omega-3 polyunsaturated fatty acids may decrease dysmenorrhea in adolescents.[55] Surgical interventions including a presacral nerve ablation, endometrial ablation, and hysterectomy are treatments of last resort, reserved for patients who do not benefit from medical and other approaches.

Secondary Dysmenorrhea

Women with secondary dysmenorrhea also complain of painful uterine cramping with menses but may have other accompanying complaints, such as dyspareunia or non-menstrual pelvic pain. The pain women with secondary dysmenorrhea experience is, by definition, due to uterine or pelvic pathology. The most common causes are adenomyosis, endometriosis, and adhesions. Adenomyosis often develops in parous women after endometrial glands and stroma embed in the myometrium (the muscular lining of the uterus) during labor. The monthly hormonal swings cause this ectopically located endometrium to slough, irritating the uterus. An implantation of endometrial tissue in other parts of the pelvis is called endometriosis (see the section on Endometriosis). Women with endometriosis experience painful menses in part due to the sloughing of tissue, but also due to internal scarring. Pelvic adhesions from previous pelvic inflammatory disease (salpingitis or tubo-ovarian abscesses), appendicitis, and pelvic or abdominal surgery can also cause dysmenorrhea. Other pelvic pathology, including as uterine fibroids, cervical stenosis, and some types of pelvic masses may also cause painful menses. Often diagnostic laparoscopy is needed to fully evaluate the causes of the patient's pain. Copper intrauterine devices (IUDs) sometimes are associated with heavier or more uncomfortable menses but are an unusual cause of clinically significant secondary dysmenorrhea.

The treatment of secondary dysmenorrhea depends upon its etiology, as well as other factors, including the patient's desire for fertility. In the absence of problems requiring surgical intervention, the treatments outlined for primary dysmenorrhea are often at least partially successful for treatment of symptoms of secondary dysmenorrhea. If these interventions are not sufficiently effective, more definitive surgical treatments may be needed. For example, secondary dysmenorrhea caused by pelvic scarring may benefit from surgical lysis of adhesions. For women with fibroids, a myomectomy might more effectively reduce menstrual flow and discomfort. Consider more significant therapies such as endometrial ablation and hysterectomy to treat only incapacitating, intractable dysmenorrhea unresponsive to more conservative measures.

AMENORRHEA

Amenorrhea, the absence of menses, is also classified as primary or secondary. *Primary* amenorrhea is the lack of menarche or any secondary sexual characteristics by age 14, the lack of menses by age 16 1/2, or no menses in the 2 years after the breasts develop (thelarche) or pubic and axillary hair appear (pubarche or adrenarche). *Secondary* amenorrhea occurs only in women who have previously menstruated. Technically, secondary amenorrhea is the absence of menses for at least 3 months in a the woman who previously has had regular monthly menses and for at least 6 to 12 months in a woman who normally experiences irregular menses. The absence of menses for a shorter period of time is referred to as "delayed menses."

Begin the evaluation of amenorrhea in a sexually active reproductive-age woman with a pregnancy test. History may be helpful in identifying women at risk for pregnancy, but it is not always reliable. The woman need not have had vaginal intercourse to become pregnant; genital exposure to semen is sometimes sufficient. Once you have ruled out pregnancy as a cause of the patient's amenorrhea, evaluating amenorrhea further depends upon its classification. Both primary and secondary amenorrhea have a multitude of causes, so take a systematic approach to find answers in a cost-effective manner.

Primary Amenorrhea

Usually the evaluation of primary amenorrhea involves consultation with experts, but a fundamental understanding of the possible etiologies can be helpful to advise the patient and her often anxious family. An efficient evaluation of primary amenorrhea relies on two physical findings: the uterus and breast development (Figure 6-1).[75]

Uterus present, no breast development. If the patient has a uterus but no breast development, it can be assumed that she is genetically female but that she is not producing estrogen. The problem may reside in her hypothalamus, pituitary, or ovary. A helpful test to distinguish among the causes is her serum level of follicle stimulating hormone (FSH).

- **Low FSH level.** If her FSH is low, her ovaries have not been stimulated and the problem lies in the functioning of her pituitary or

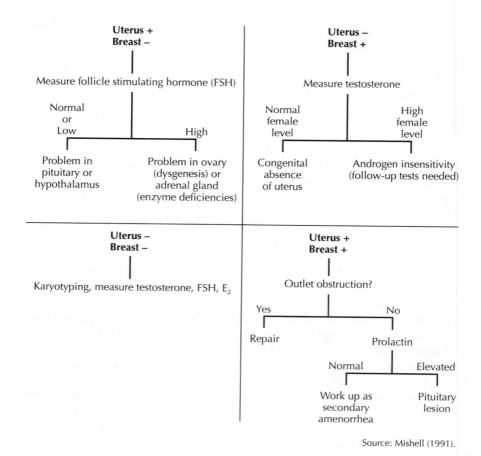

Source: Mishell (1991).

Figure 6-1 Diagnostic evaluation for primary amenorrhea

hypothalamus. Isolated pituitary failure is extremely rare. Hypo-thalamic failure can be demonstrated by administering a GnRH stimulation test. If the patient responds to GnRH stimulation by making FSH and luteinizing hormone (LH), her problem is at the hypothalamic level. Give her long-term pulsatile GnRH agonists or try hormonal cycling using postmenopausal regimens or oral contraceptives.

- **Elevated FSH level.** If her FSH is elevated, she has gonadal fail-ure. Genetic causes often underlie gonadal failure: Turner's syn-drome, mosaicism, pure gonadal dysgenesis, or life-threatening 17x-hydroxylase deficiency or autoimmune disease. Occasionally, chemotherapy or radiation treatments for carcinoma destroy ovarian function. Whatever the cause, once you have confirmed the diagnosis of ovarian failure and counseled the patient about infertility, give her estrogen and progestin therapy to establish female secondary sexual characteristics and to mitigate the effects of hypoestrogenism on her bone and the cardiovascular system. Additional therapy may be needed to control other aspects of her disorder.

Uterus absent, breast development. If a woman has breasts but no uterus, check her serum testosterone levels. If her testosterone levels are within the range for a normal woman, her diagnosis is a congenital absence of the uterus. If her levels are in the range for a man, she has androgen-resistance syndrome (testicular feminization). Further tests will be needed to confirm that she is genetically 46 XY. However, since she is phenotypically a woman and has been raised as a woman, her sexual identity should not be altered. She needs counseling about her infertility, since she has no uterus and her ovaries are abnormal. Her gonads have a high potential for malignancy; after puberty, she should undergo a gonadectomy and receive life-long hormone replacement therapy.[31]

Uterus absent, no breast development. Women without breasts or uterus need to undergo genetic testing since many of these women have male karyotypes.

Uterus present, breast development. Thirty percent of women with primary amenorrhea have both breasts and uterus. Consider an outlet obstruction such as imperforate hymen, transverse vaginal septa, pituitary adenoma without galactorrhea, and other causes commonly found in women with secondary amenorrhea. Evaluate these other women as per "secondary amenorrhea."

A special case of primary amenorrhea occurs in young athletes or women with profound eating disorders who experience a delay in puberty.[46,47] These young women have a uterus with or without breast development. The delay in puberty may result in bone loss at a time when a young woman should be accumulating bone.[7]

Another unusual condition in this category is a true hermaphrodite, but often these hermaphrodites will also have elements of male genitalia. Also since there is often a mixture of tissue in the gonads, the ovotestes need to be removed early to reduce the risk of carcinoma.

Secondary Amenorrhea

The absence of menses is an important symptom because it can indicate a serious systemic medical problem or represent a problem confined to the reproductive system. Even if a woman does not desire fertility, she must be evaluated because the underlying problem or its consequences may require prompt therapy.

Conduct a thorough history and physical examination. Take a careful menstrual history, emphasizing ovulatory symptoms (mittelschmerz), moliminal complaints (bloating, cramping, skin changes heralding the onset of menses), and any vasomotor symptoms she may be experiencing. Question her about recent changes in weight, dietary habits, complexion, hair growth, cold or heat intolerance, galactorrhea, medications, recent pregnancy, genital tract procedures, medical problems, stress, and exercise patterns. On examination, pay close attention to signs of androgen excess (hirsutism), hypoestrogenism (dry, flattened vaginal mucosa), prolactin excess (galactorrhea), or thyroid dysfunction (skin, pulse, and reflex changes). A complete drug history is helpful because many classes of medications can induce amenorrhea or oligomenorrhea.

If an obvious reason for the woman's amenorrhea emerges from this initial screening, order specifically targeted diagnostic tests to confirm the diagnosis. For example, if the patient has spontaneous galactorrhea, measure her prolactin and thyroid stimulating hormone (TSH) levels. A 50-year-old woman who complains of hot flashes and has had no menses for a few months may only need her FSH levels measured to confirm the diagnosis of menopause. A 20-year-old woman with a recent onset of hirsutism and amenorrhea will need to have her androgen status evaluated. On the other hand, a woman using DMPA needs no further workup when she develops amenorrhea in the absence of other symptoms.

More frequently, however, no single cause is discovered on the basis of history and physical examination. Several systematic approaches have been developed by experts in the field, but one particularly cost-effective protocol[112] divides the reproductive system into four components: uterus and lower genital tract, ovaries, pituitary and hypothalamus (Figure 6-2).

Uterus and lower genital tract. Evaluation begins with the uterus and lower genital tract. A physical examination will have already ruled out functional blockage of menstrual flow from the vagina such as an imperforate hymen or transverse septum. (These commonly cause primary, but not secondary, amenorrhea.) First test the functional capacity of the uterus and lower genital tract with a progestin challenge test. Give the patient medroxyprogesterone acetate 5 to 10 milligrams (mg) for 7 to 10 days or progesterone in oil 100 to 150 mg intramuscularly.

- If she experiences a withdrawal bleed, then it is established that her cervix is patent, she is producing estrogen, and her endometrium is functional. She will need an evaluation of her ovaries (see the next section).

Step 1: **Evaluate Uterus and Lower Genital Tract**
Perform progestin challenge test

Medroxyprogesterone acetate 5-10 mg orally once a day
for 7-10 days or 150 mg progesterone in oil (intramuscularly)

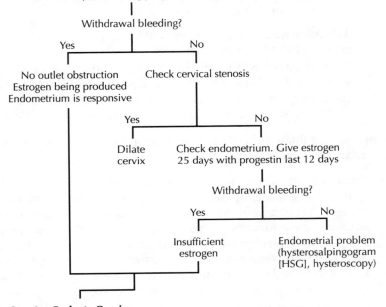

Withdrawal bleeding?

Yes — No outlet obstruction / Estrogen being produced / Endometrium is responsive

No — Check cervical stenosis

Yes — Dilate cervix

No — Check endometrium. Give estrogen 25 days with progestin last 12 days

Withdrawal bleeding?

Yes — Insufficient estrogen

No — Endometrial problem (hysterosalpingogram [HSG], hysteroscopy)

Step 2: **Evaluate Ovaries**
**Measure serum levels of follicle stimulating hormone (FSH),
luteinizing hormone (LH), estradiol (E$_2$)**

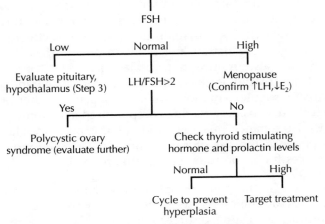

FSH

Low — Evaluate pituitary, hypothalamus (Step 3)

Normal — LH/FSH>2

High — Menopause (Confirm ↑LH,↓E$_2$)

Yes — Polycystic ovary syndrome (evaluate further)

No — Check thyroid stimulating hormone and prolactin levels

Normal — Cycle to prevent hyperplasia

High — Target treatment

Step 3: **Evaluate Function of Pituitary Gland and Hypothalamus**
Consider imaging. Consider GnRH challenge test

Source: Modified from Speroff et al. (1994).

Figure 6-2 Systematic diagnostic evaluation for secondary amenorrhea

- If she does not experience a withdrawal bleed, she needs a detailed evaluation of her uterus and cervix. Check for cervical stenosis by passing a uterine sound. Assess the responsiveness of the endometrium by priming her uterus with estrogen for 25 days, adding progestin the last 10 to 12 days.

  — **Withdrawal bleed.** Her endometrium is functional. She will need an evaluation of her ovaries.

  — **No withdrawal bleed.** She may have Asherman's syndrome, tuberculosis, schistosomiasis or some other disorder in her uterine lining. She will benefit from direct endometrial evaluation by hysteroscopy or perhaps by hysterosalpingogram (HSG).

Ovaries. Evaluate the ovaries by measuring serum levels of FSH, LH, and, perhaps, estradiol (E_2).

- If the patient's gonadotropins (FSH and LH) are elevated and her E_2 is low, she is menopausal. If she is younger than 35 to 40 years of age, conduct a more detailed evaluation of other possible autoimmune endocrinopathies. In any event, offer physiological sex steroid replacement or combination oral contraceptives to reduce the long-term effects of hypoestrogenism, such as osteoporosis and increased risk of cardiovascular disease.
- If the patient's gonadotropins are not abnormally elevated, evaluate the patient for polycystic ovarian syndrome (see the section on Polycystic Ovaries). Often the LH/FSH ratio is greater than or equal 2.

Pituitary. If the patient's gonadotropins are low or within normal limits, her pituitary warrants evaluation. Initial tests include TSH and prolactin tests because both hypothyroidism and hyperprolactinemia can interfere with estrogen production and result in amenorrhea. Primary hypothyroidism can also induce hyperprolactinemia. If you detect abnormalities of the thyroid, evaluate the patient for related endocrine problems; thyroxine supplementation will be therapeutic. If her prolactin levels are elevated, consider ordering computerized axial tomography (CT) or magnetic resonance imaging (MRI) of the pituitary gland to determine the presence and size of a prolactinoma. Bromocriptine therapy is usually successful in controlling prolactin production.

Hypothalamus. If the gonadotropins are low or normal and no other abnormalities are identified, the patient's hypothalamus may be implicated. Consider an eating disorder even in a woman of normal weight. One study found that 55% of amenorrheic women had an eating disorder.[126] For young women with hypothalamic amenorrhea, low-dose oral contraceptives are very helpful. Newer therapies, such as with Naltrexone, have also been suggested to treat women with weight-loss-related amenorrhea.[49] If you suspect an intracranial neoplasia, obtain appropriate imaging studies. A woman who has stress due to extreme exercise, eating disorders, or situational factors should have her underlying problems addressed; she also needs hormonal modulation to induce regular bleeding and maintain adequate estrogen levels to prevent osteoporosis.[106] Recent work has shown that young women with hypothalamic amenorrhea will have improved bone mineralization when given oral contraceptives but not when given medroxyprogesterone or placebo.[59]

OLIGOMENORRHEA

When the interval between a woman's menses exceeds 35 days but is not long enough to qualify as being amenorrhea, she by definition has oligomenorrhea. Most women with oligomenorrhea have anovulatory cycles. Often this menstrual pattern is lifelong; many women with polycystic ovary syndrome (PCO) have consistently irregular and infrequent menses (see the next section). Sometimes oligomenorrhea develops as a result of excessive weight gain or after significant weight loss. It is important to identify the etiology of the oligomenorrhea to reduce other consequences of an underlying endocrinopathy and to help improve fertility potential when she is ready to conceive.

Oligomenorrhea is appropriately viewed as a symptom on a continuum between normal ovulatory cycling and secondary amenorrhea. Many of the causes of amenorrhea can, in milder forms, present as oligomenorrhea. Medical problems such as hypothyroidism, hyperprolactinemia, and liver dysfunction can cause oligomenorrhea, as can certain medications. Women with stress and those who engage in extreme exercise or excessive dieting often develop oligomenorrhea, which can progress to amenorrhea. Cheerleaders and women engaging in seasonal sports may have irregular menses for the months they are involved in those activities. In these women, oligomenorrhea results from suppressed estrogen production. Adequate sex steroid levels can be maintained with oral contraceptives. On the other hand, women with other causes of oligomenorrhea, such as extreme increases in weight and PCO usually have excessive amounts of unopposed estrogen. Unopposed estrogen leads to uninterrupted endometrial stimulation and increases the risk for endometrial hyperplasia and carcinoma. These women need a cyclic source of progesterone to offset the estrogen stimulation and induce a periodic endometrial sloughing. Cyclic administration of progestin or oral contraceptives, or endometrial suppression with DMPA or continuous administration of oral contraceptives, are reasonable alternatives.

Polycystic ovary syndrome (PCO). Previously called Stein-Leventhal syndrome, PCO is a common cause of oligomenorrhea. In textbook descriptions, women with PCO are obese, hirsute, oligomenorrheic, and subfertile. In reality, many women with PCO are not overweight and many do not have hirsutism.[39] Even its name is not defining; many women with polycystic ovaries do not have PCO.[50] A common theme in women with PCO, however, is hyperandrogenism and chronic anovulation, which has caused many leaders in the field to rename the syndrome *hyperandrogenic chronic anovulation* (HCA).

The central problem in PCO is aberrant GnRH release and gonadotropin response, which is associated with high serum levels of LH.[89] LH stimulates ovarian androgen production.[20] This testosterone adds to the high levels of adrenally produced androgens (dehydroepiandrosterone) and causes hyperandrogenism, responsible for the classical PCO problems such as hirsutism and acne. The excessive *androgen* levels, paradoxically, also induce a *hyperestrogenic* state. Androgens circulate to the adipose cells where they are converted to estrone (E_1). The E_1 recirculates and stimulates endometrial proliferation and simultaneously suppresses pituitary production of FSH. In the absence of the initial FSH rise, ovarian cycling and luteal progesterone production cease. Endometrial proliferation continues unchecked, resulting in irregular, uncoordinated endometrial sloughing and a long-term increased risk of endometrial cancer. With anovulatory cycles, fertility is compromised. However, women with PCO can have unpredictable ovulatory cycles on an intermittent basis and should not be considered to be protected against unintended pregnancy by their condition.

There are other associated health risks for which women with PCO should be monitored. Many overweight women (body mass index greater than 27) with PCO have insulin resistance, which increases the risk for overt diabetes.[32] Insulin-like growth factors are produced by the ovary in PCO, which can contribute to coronary artery disease.[70] Many women with PCO have unhealthy lipid profiles with high ratio of total cholesterol/high density lipoprotein (HDL); androgenized women with polycystic ovaries have lipid profiles similar to male profiles.[53,127] Both the lipid and insulin abnormalities are independent risk factors for cardiovascular disease. Women with PCO often also have elevated levels of prolactin. Several authors have suggested a genetic component to PCO and recommend screening relatives for insulin resistance.[64]

Therapy is designed to reduce long-term adverse health consequences and to address the patient's immediate complaints. Initiate weight reduction, exercise, and sensible diets (low in fat and high in complex carbohydrates) to reduce cardiovascular disease risks. Both hyperinsulinemia and hyperandrogenemia in obese women with PCO can be reduced with a weight loss of at least 5% of their initial weight.[85] Weight distribution is also important. Women with PCO tend to have more android obesity when the waist-to-hip ratio is greater than 0.85 (which is associated with a higher risk for myocardial infarction than is gynecoid obesity (waist-to-hip ratio less than 0.75]).[63] Oral contraceptives with low androgenicity can moderate hirsutism, prevent unopposed endometrial proliferation, and provide contraceptive protection. DMPA can prevent endometrial proliferation and reduce pregnancy risks. Cyclic progestin with 10 mg medroxyprogesterone acetate each month can reduce the risk of endometrial hyperplasia.

If the patient desires fertility, give her a trial of clomiphene citrate to block the negative feedback estrone has on pituitary reproduction of FSH. Failing that, add dexamethasone, betamethazone, GnRH agonists, or human menopausal gonadotropins either to block the production of LH or to override it.

Treatment of PCO-associated hirsutism. Women with hirsutism may be offered estrogenic oral contraceptives to suppress ovarian production of androgens and increase sex human binding globulin (SHBG). This increase in SHBG will reduce serum levels of biologically active unbound androgens to reduce further hair growth. When the woman also suffers from acne, these mechanisms will decrease stimulation of the pilo-sebaceous unit and help reduce her outbreaks. Continuous oral contraceptive administration is superior to cyclic oral contraceptive use in controlling LH and testosterone levels.[100] Other indicated therapies to slow the progression of new hair growth include spironolactone or corticosteroids (if adrenal androgen overproduction is implicated by levels of dehydroepiandrosterone [DHEAS] greater than 75 mg/ml). Cyproterone acetate-estrogen regimens have been reported to be as effective as spironolactone.[33] Anti-androgens such as flutamide and finasteride, which directly inhibit hair growth without serious side effects, represent a new approach to the treatment of hirsutism in women with PCO.[69,121] Gonadotropin-releasing agonists with estrogen add-back therapies have also been used to block new hair growth, but this approach is still considered experimental. Newer agents are being investigated. Overall, the clinical response is usually slow, and removal of existing hair by electrolysis is also often necessary.

ABNORMAL UTERINE BLEEDING

Menorrhagia and *hypermenorrhea* refer to prolonged bleeding (>7 days) or excessive blood loss (>80 cc) occurring at regular intervals. *Metrorrhagia* refers to irregular but frequent uterine bleeding of variable amounts. *Menometrorrhagia* refers to prolonged uterine bleeding occurring with completely irregular frequency. *Polymenorrhea* describes uterine bleeding occurring at short intervals (<21 days). *Intermenstrual bleeding* is bleeding of variable amounts occurring between regular menses. *Postcoital bleeding* occurs after sexual intercourse.

The "normal" values for the frequency and duration of menses as well as the amount of blood loss vary widely (Table 6-1). A woman's history of her menses may not be accurate. Common pitfalls are that women may

Table 6-1 Range of normal values for menses

	Range	Average
Frequency	21–35 days	28 days
Duration	2–6 days	4 days
Blood Loss	20–80 cubic centimeters (cc)	30–35 cc

report bleeding-free days rather than cycle length measured from first day of bleeding in one cycle to the next. Some women report that their menses occur on exactly the same date each month and are concerned if they have 2 periods in one month even if one starts on the first of the month and the second on the last day. Quantifying actual blood loss may also be quite challenging.[22,41,58] Estimates derived from numbers of pads or tampons are complicated by variations in fastidiousness among women. By the time excessive menstrual bleeding causes anemia, a woman has endured very significant bleeding. At least as important as the absolute numbers of days or amounts of blood loss is any *change* the patient may perceive from what has been established as normal for her. A woman who has historically bled 3 days per cycle and now notices that she bleeds for 6 to 7 days may still be within an arbitrary range for "normal," but she merits an evaluation since she is experiencing a significant change from her baseline pattern.

Causes of abnormal uterine bleeding may be classified into several categories to facilitate evaluation (Table 6-2). *Organic gynecologic disease* is the first concern when women present with abnormal bleeding. Pregnancy and its complications (e.g., threatened abortion or ectopic pregnancy) and infection of the cervix, endometrium, or fallopian tubes are primary differential diagnoses for sexually active women. Endometrial and cervical

Table 6-2 Excessive uterine bleeding

Assess clinic stability

- Vital signs
- Hemoglobin/hematocrit
- Urine pregnancy test

Consider causes

- Obstetrical: pregnancy or pregnancy complications
- Medication (e.g., phenytoin, anticoagulants, digitalis, estrogen)
- Systemic diseases: coagulation disorders, endocrinopathies (e.g., thyroid or adrenal disorders); hepatic or renal failure
- Cervical abnormalities: infection, polyp, cancer
- Uterine abnormality: fibroids, infection, hyperplasia, polyp, cancer
- Dysfunctional uterine bleeding (DUB) = diagnosis of exclusion

polyps and uterine leiomyoma and adenomyosis can cause menorrhagia. Endometrial hyperplasia and carcinoma are often associated with heavy and prolonged menses as well as intermenstrual bleeding. Cervical infection or carcinoma more classically present with postcoital bleeding.

Systemic diseases such as thyroid dysfunction, liver cirrhosis, active hepatitis, adrenal hyperplasia, incipient renal failure, and hypersplenism can cause prolonged or heavy menses by altering estrogen metabolism or coagulation factor production. Similarly, women with intrinsic blood dyscrasias such as Von Willebrand's disease, idiopathic thrombocytopenia purpura (ITP), aplastic anemia, or platelet dysfunction often have chronic menorrhagia. Acute problems such as leukemia, severe sepsis, or disseminated intravascular coagulation (DIC) may also induce menorrhagia. Medications such as digitalis, phenytoin, anticoagulants, and plastic and copper IUDs are associated with increased menstrual flow. Occasionally, heavy menstrual bleeding can result from trauma such as sexual abuse or the presence of a foreign body in the vagina.

Evaluation of Abnormal Uterine Bleeding

Take a complete menstrual history, emphasizing the last several months. The age of the patient and the pattern of her bleeding guides the evaluation. Perform pregnancy tests for all reproductive-age women who have abnormal bleeding. If anemia is a concern, determine the patient's hemoglobin or hematocrit. Rule out vaginal and cervical abnormalities (infection, carcinoma, or polyps) by screening for gonorrhea and chlamydia and taking a Papanicolaou (Pap) smear. Perform a bimanual examination to determine the size and shape of the uterus and to detect any ovarian or adnexal masses. Check for rebound tenderness. Perform thyroid function tests for women with suspicious signs or symptoms. If a menarcheal woman has bleeding severe enough to require transfusion, evaluate her for blood dyscrasias.[24] Women with a life-long history of heavy and prolonged menses should be evaluated for Von Willebrand's disease, especially if her female relatives have had the same menstrual pattern. Endometrial biopsy to rule out endometrial hyperplasia or carcinoma in women with abnormal uterine bleeding is appropriate for those with risk factors such as advanced reproductive age (over 35), obesity, or unopposed estrogen exposure from either iatrogenic (medications) or intrinsic (PCO) sources. Some practitioners use hysteroscopically directed biopsy to evaluate vaginal bleeding initially, but the technique is more frequently used to evaluate women whose bleeding persists after endometrial sampling fails to provide a diagnosis.

Women with unexplained bleeding may have dysfunctional uterine bleeding (DUB). There are two types of DUB—anovulatory DUB and ovulatory DUB (Table 6-3).

Table 6-3 Characteristics and types of dysfunctional uterine bleeding

Type of DUB	Characteristics	Treatment

Anovulatory (90% of DUB)	• Occurs at extremes of reproductive ages
	• No moliminal symptoms
	• Irregular, unpredictable bleeding, sometimes excessive
	• Underlying problems:
	  — Unopposed estrogen stimulation
	  — Lack of progesterone priming of prostaglandins
	  — Excessive vasodilating prostaglandins
		• Cycle endometrium
		  — Oral contraceptives monthly
		  — Cyclic progestin (last 12 days of cycle)
		• Suppress endometrium
		  — DMPA
		  — Oral contraceptives (bicycling/tricycling)
		  — Danazol
		  — GnRH agonists
		  — Progestin IUD
		• Provide vasoconstrictive prostaglandins
		  — NSAIDS starting first day of menses x 3 days

Ovulatory (10% of DUB)	• Occurs in peak reproductive years
	• Bleeding predictable but excessive and prolonged
	• Bleeding due to imbalance in prostaglandins
	  — Inadequate vasoconstrictive prostaglandins
		• Suppress endometrium
		  — Oral contraceptives monthly, bicycling/tricycling
		  — DMPA
		  — Danazol
		  — GnRH agonists
		  — Progestin IUD
		• Correct prostaglandin imbalances
		  — NSAIDS starting first day of menses x 3 days

- **Anovulatory DUB.** Anovulatory DUB usually develops during the extremes of reproductive life—adolescence and perimenopause.[79] Within the first year of menarche, approximately 55% of cycles are anovulatory.[60] Anovulation results in unopposed estrogen stimulation of the endometrium, which produces a thick lining. Without progesterone, there is an uncoordinated endometrial sloughing, an imbalance in prostaglandins, and a relative excess of PGE—the vasodilating prostaglandin. Under these influences, women develop heavy and prolonged bleeding.

- **Ovulatory DUB.** Ovulatory DUB occurs in reproductive-age women and accounts for 10% of all DUB. The underlying problem many of the women with ovulatory DUB experience is that their endometria fail to produce adequate amounts of the vasoconstricting prostaglandin $PGF_{2\alpha}$.

Treatment of Abnormal Uterine Bleeding

Treat any identified problem causing vaginal bleeding, such as infection, polyps, miscarriage, etc. The treatment for dysfunctional uterine bleeding depends on the severity and acuteness of the problem.

Acute, severe bleeding. Women with significant acute bleeding that causes anemia may require hospitalization. Perform a diagnostic endometrial sampling or a dilation and curettage (D&C) in any woman who is hypovolemic or has a risk factor for endometrial hyperplasia or carcinoma. For acute bleeding the goal is to promptly heal the denuded areas of the endometrium. The drug of choice is estrogen, because it will cause endometrial proliferation and seal over the actively bleeding sites within the uterus. Administer estrogen orally using either high-dose estrogen replacement preparations such as 2.5 mg conjugated equine estrogen or high-dose oral contraceptive preparations with 50 µg ethinyl estradiol four times a day. Success rates for these preparations are comparable in the 80% to 85% range.[68,107] Alternatively, the estrogen may be given intravenously at higher and more frequent doses, but this regimen is usually associated with more pronounced gastrointestinal side effects.[30]

NSAIDS are useful as adjunctive therapeutic agents in the acute phase. Bleeding generally stops or dramatically slows after 12 to 24 hours of estrogen therapy. At that time, support endometrial growth by adding progestin (typically, medroxyprogesterone acetate 10 mg per day). Maintain high-dose hormonal therapy for a few days after the initial response and then lower the dose to the minimal amount necessary to forestall bleeding; continue the regimen for at least 1 to 2 weeks. When the hormonal support is withdrawn, the patient should undergo a coordinated (and therefore limited) endometrial sloughing. If the patient does not respond promptly to initial estrogen therapy, she should have a diagnostic dilation and curettage.

Acute, prolonged but less significant bleeding. For women with significantly less bleeding, outpatient therapy with lower-dose hormones or NSAIDs can be sufficient.[17] Methergine has no demonstrated efficacy in controlling uterine bleeding in nonpregnant women.[80]

Long-term medical therapies. After an acute bleeding event, the goal is to prevent future bleeding episodes. Therapy depends on the etiology of the woman's dysfunctional uterine bleeding (Table 6-3).

- *Anovulatory bleeding.* For women with an ongoing problem with anovulatory dysfunctional uterine bleeding, prevent a recurrence by pharmacologically inducing cyclic withdrawal bleeding with oral contraceptives or progestins or by suppressing her cycles altogether with DMPA and other agents.[11] If a woman does not desire to use oral contraceptives, offer her medroxyprogesterone acetate 5 to 10 mg a day for 12 to 14 days in the second half of the month to produce withdrawal bleeding. In women with oligomenorrhea, many protocols delay initiation of progestin therapy until cycle day 35 to permit spontaneous menses, if possible.

Other medical therapies have been successful for short-term use. Danazol (400 to 600 mg/day) is an androgenic hormone that blocks gonadotropins and suppresses ovarian and endometrial activity. Danazol's androgenic side effects limit its use to only 6 to 9 months. GnRH agonists effectively suppress gonadotropin and ovarian estrogen production to thin the endometrium and induce amenorrhea. GnRH agonists also result in hypoestrogenism, which can lead to osteoporosis if used for any significant period of time. Newer regimens combining GnRH agonists and cyclic hormonal therapy may hold promise for the future but currently are costly and experimental.[119]

The Levonorgestrel-20 IUD has been used in Europe for treatment of abnormal uterine bleeding, including DUB, and has been extremely effective.

- *Ovulatory dysfunctional bleeding.* Women with ovulatory dysfunctional uterine bleeding have consistently heavy menses that can last for more than 8 days per cycle. These women have an underlying imbalance between prostaglandins E_2 and $F_{2\alpha}$[110] which can be effectively treated by administering NSAIDS starting at the beginning of menses and continuing through the heavy flow days. Hormonal therapies with oral contraceptives or DMPA can also be effective.[40,80] Oral contraceptives reduce blood loss by more than 50% in women with chronic menorrhagia.[80] The Levonorgestrel IUD holds promise for these women, too.

Surgical therapies.   Many women with significant bleeding undergo a D&C for the immediate control of bleeding as well as for diagnosis. However, the effects of a D&C are only temporary. Initiate medical care to avoid the recurrence of the problem. Other surgical interventions such as endometrial ablation with laser, resectoscope or roller ball,[84] and hysterectomy are reserved for women who have other pelvic pathology and for those who fail to improve with conservative therapy.

MENSTRUALLY INDUCED EXACERBATIONS OF OTHER MEDICAL PROBLEMS

Migraine headaches are quite common, especially in reproductive-age women; approximately 17.6% of women have a history of migraine. Hormones have been implicated because over two-thirds of adults with migraines are women, and oral contraceptives may worsen the symptoms or frequency of migraine headaches in 15% to 50% of women. In general, women who have common migraines should use combined oral contraceptive pills with caution and those who have classic migraines (preceded by an aura) should avoid oral contraceptive pills altogether.

However, there is one type of migraine that may be treated with appropriately timed hormonal contraception. Menstrual migraines are a special subset of migraines that may start 2 to 3 days before menses and continue into the menses but occur at no other time. Pure menstrual migraines comprise 7% to 9% of all migraines. In addition, another 35% of women suffer a worsening of migraine symptoms during menses. An intriguing set of experiments linked the onset of menstrual migraine headaches to downward swings in estrogen levels. Administering estrogens premenstrually delayed the headaches but did not alter menses; in contrast, administering progesterone delayed menses but did not affect headaches.[111] Some investigators have suggested that suppressing ovulation with oral contraceptives may be helpful in blocking estrogen-withdrawal headaches.[72,118] Continuous use of active oral contraceptives for two to three cycles may eliminate withdrawal headaches for long stretches of time.[54,112] If the patient desires to have monthly menses, make every cycle a first-day start to minimize the menstrual hypoestrogenism. Alternatively, severe menstrual migraines have been shown to respond well to treatment with GnRH agonist and add-back therapy.[76]

Nonhormonal treatments for menstrual migraine include NSAIDS or judicious use of narcotics and injectable agents such as dihydroergotamine or sumatriptan. If those fail to treat the pain adequately and the pain keeps a woman from her usual productivity at least 2 days a month, most physicians would recommend preventive therapy. Prophylactic agents include beta blockers (Inderol), calcium channel blockers, and selective anti-depressants. Other important self-help measures include regular physical exercise and avoidance of headache triggers (food and other sensory stimuli). Some women report that incipient menstrual migraines can be curtailed by sexual activity and orgasm. The National Headache Foundation maintains a 24-hour headache hotline at 1-800-843-2250.

Other diseases that worsen with menstrual cycling, such as some seizure disorders, asthma, and Behcet's disease (oral and genital ulcers as well as ophthalmia), may similarly respond to hormonal manipulations.[14] Between 10% and 70% of women with seizure disorders suffer catamenial seizures exacerbated by or occurring only during menses. Some authors have suggested that treatment with progestogenic oral contraceptives might be helpful,[16] but few clinical data support these ideas. Sequential oral contraceptives alleviate the symptoms of Behcet's disease in some resistant cases.

Hormonal methods to suppress menstrual blood loss can also aid women with medical problems associated with anemia, such as sickle cell disease, renal failure, and coagulopathies (such as hemophilia or Von Willebrand's disease). Other women taking medications that increase menstrual blood loss, such as anticoagulants, long-term NSAIDS, and some anticonvulsants, may distinctly benefit from oral contraceptives or DMPA to reduce or eliminate monthly drains on their hemoglobin reserves. Women who have blood dyscrasias also benefit from ovulation suppression, which removes the threat of internal hemorrhage posed by monthly follicle extrusion.[16,78]

PREMENSTRUAL TENSION SYNDROME (PMS)

Premenstrual syndrome (PMS) is a heterogeneous collection of signs and symptoms that share one common characteristic: a temporal relationship to the menstrual cycle. By definition, PMS is the cyclic appearance of at least one symptom prior to menses followed by an entirely symptom-free time starting with the first day of menses. To be considered clinically significant, the problem must be of a magnitude sufficient to affect a woman's work, lifestyle, or interpersonal relationships.[91] The most common symptoms of PMS include abdominal bloating, anxiety, breast tenderness, crying spells, depression, fatigue, irritability, thirst, appetite changes, and edema. Women with PMS rarely have only physical complaints; they also have behavioral and psychological complaints. A related syndrome called *premenstrual dysphoric disorder* has been defined by the American Psychiatry Association (Table 6-4) that focuses more on affective disorders than on emotional or behavioral problems often seen with PMS.[3]

About 20% to 30% of women have moderate to severe PMS, and another 1% to 10% have debilitating symptoms.[108] Premenstrual dysphoria affects 3% to 8% of North American women during their reproductive years.[57,61,94] PMS can increase marital strain, sexual dysfunction, social isolation, work absenteeism, suicide, and psychotic behavior. Some law courts around the world have accepted PMS as a mitigating factor for criminal behavior and, in some cases, a grounds for a plea of temporary insanity. Many PMS symptoms can persist even after hysterectomy. Women with functioning residual ovaries can experience symptoms, as can women using cyclic post-menopausal hormone replacement therapy.

After a thorough history and a complete examination have ruled out other causes, the key to diagnosing PMS is a *prospective* charting of symptoms for at least 2 to 3 cycles. A woman who is overwhelmed by a series of complaints should chart only the 3 to 5 complaints that most profoundly bother her. This chart should also include her weight and, if pos-

Table 6-4 DSM-IV criteria for premenstrual dysphoric disorder

- Need at least five symptoms including:
  At least one of the following:
  — Affective lability
  — Persistent and marked anger or irritability
  — Marked anxiety and tension
  — Markedly depressed mood, feeling of hopelessness
- With 1–4 of the rest from the following:
  — Decreased interest in usual activities
  — Easy fatigability or marked lack of energy
  — Subjective sense or difficulty in concentration
  — Marked change in appetite
  — Sleep disorders
  — Physical symptoms—breast tenderness, headache, edema, joint or muscle pain, weight gain

Source: American Psychiatric Association (1994).

sible, a record of her basal body temperatures. (See Chapter 15 on Fertility Awareness Methods.) No laboratory tests are needed to diagnose PMS although, if clinically indicated, hypothyroidism or other endocrinopathies may need to be ruled out. Panels to measure sex steroid hormonal levels are unnecessary,[21] and their use reflects a basic misunderstanding of the underlying pathophysiology.

Carefully study the patterns of the patient's symptoms. Symptoms do not need to reappear with equal intensity in each cycle; different symptoms may occur during different cycles. It is the timing that is critical. PMS symptoms peak in the luteal phase and completely disappear with the onset of menses. For many women, clinical depression and other serious problems worsen premenstrually, but this is not PMS, because those women never have a symptom-free interval.[99] As many as half the women with self-diagnosed PMS have other problems, which require careful evaluation and therapies different from those for PMS.[56] Even women with PMS-like symptoms verified by daily charting frequently may have underlying or concomitant psychiatric problems. In one study, 59% of women with PMS also had clinical depression or an anxiety disorder.[35]

The cause of PMS is unknown. Early investigators suggested that PMS was due to a lack of progesterone, and many therapies were developed to provide progesterone supplements to women with PMS.[28,38] Subsequent investigations failed to find a difference in any significant hormone levels (FSH, LH, estradiol, progestin, prolactin, SHBG, testosterone) between PMS sufferers and controls.[98] Similarly, in controlled studies, women using progesterone supplements did no better than controls.[44] However, women whose symptoms vary from cycle to cycle appear to have variation in the *ratio* of their ovarian hormones. More recently, researchers have suggested that some women with PMS have a central opioid abnormality resulting in lower beta endorphin levels,[23] although other studies have challenged this hypothesis.[103] PMS sufferers have no deficiencies in magnesium, zinc, vitamin A, vitamin E, thiamine, or vitamin B_6, refuting nutritional deficiencies as a cause of PMS.[74] One investigator found low adrenocorticotropin levels in women with PMS.[90] Other hypotheses include the suggestion that women with PMS have abnormal prostaglandin production, endogenous hormone allergies, or psychosomatic influences.

Increasing evidence suggests that serotonin dysregulation may be important in the pathogenesis of many of the psychological elements in PMS such as tension, irritability, and dysphoria.[34,65,88,97,114,129,130] In clinical trials, half of women with premenstrual dysphoria improved with treatment to selectively inhibit the reuptake of serotonin.[115] However, many women did not improve, so serotonin disorders are not an etiology for all PMS sufferers. It is likely that several mechanisms are involved in PMS. Therapy needs to be individualized for each woman's specific problems.

Treatment for PMS

PMS treatment is a strongly influenced by a placebo effect. In a wide range of studies, researchers report that 40% to 94% of patients will improve in the short term regardless of the treatment used. This reinforces the need for relying on controlled studies rather than case reports of and private testimonials for the efficacy of a particular drug or treatment for PMS.

Overall, a comprehensive approach to treatment is needed. Reassure the woman with physiologic moliminal changes. Give her emotional support, education, reassurance, and perhaps, dietary manipulation. Both the patient and her family benefit from discussion of hormonal changes and PMS. Charting the symptoms can help the patient gain more insight into her problem and more control over the situation, even if she decides not to take medication. Cognitive behavioral therapy may be helpful for some women. Self-help groups formed within a clinic or private practice can help women learn coping skills from experts and from each other. Although exogenous stress does not cause PMS, women with PMS have less tolerance for stress and may benefit from stress-reduction strategies. Relaxation, exercise, biofeedback, and acupuncture have all been reported to be helpful.[52,81,124] Regular exercise can reduce stress and physical complaints, but it does not alter the emotional components of PMS.[87] There has been some suggestion that aerobic exercise may be more helpful than body-building exercise.[113] When recommending exercise, set a realistic achievable program to avoid additionally burdening a woman with a sense of failure.

Diet.   Dietary manipulations have been recommended for years in the treatment of PMS. Traditionally, women have been advised to resist carbohydrate cravings premenstrually. Newer evidence suggests that carbohydrate-rich, low-protein foods consumed during the luteal phase may improve mood swings.[102] Caffeine may worsen PMS symptoms—increasing nervous tension, heart rate, and a general body awareness. Avoiding caffeine and related compounds from all sources (coffee, tea, chocolates, over-the-counter medications, and so on) may be helpful. Be sure to advise the patient to abstain from caffeine throughout her cycle to avoid monthly symptoms of caffeine withdrawal.

Vitamins.   Vitamin therapy has been recommended to reduce PMS symptoms. Pyridoxin (vitamin B_6) is important in the biosynthesis of neurotransmitters. One prospective controlled study found significant improvement of PMS symptoms among women taking vitamin B_6.[1] However, several subsequent studies failed to detect any differences.[66] Some companies market multivitamin PMS supplements with daily doses of high levels of vitamins B_6, A, and E in addition to magnesium and calcium. Neuropathy can occur when vitamin B_6 is taken at doses of 200 mg or more a day. Both vitamin E and primrose oil are prostaglandin precursors used routinely in other countries, based primarily on the results of uncontrolled studies. Primrose oil can be expensive but otherwise poses no known dangers. If a patient is interested in vitamin therapy, recommend she take a daily multivitamin supplemented calcium and 50 mg or less of vitamin B_6.[42,120]

Medical therapy.   Medical therapy is useful for women whose symptoms are severe or do not respond to education, counseling, or stress-reduction and related techniques. The mainstay of medical treatment today is selective serotonin reuptake inhibitors (SSRIs). About 60% of women with PMS, especially those with emotional or behavioral changes, improve on SSRIs.[44] Even some women with physical complaints improve. SSRIs differ, so carefully select the agent. For example, fluoxetine may be more appropriate for women with complaints of depression and fatigue, because it has activating properties, whereas sertraline may be a better choice for women who suffer from insomnia, irritability, or anxiety.[44] If one agent is not successful, try another before abandoning SSRIs as a class.

SSRIs at doses used to treat depression on a chronic basis may be relatively expensive and may be associated with higher incidence of side effects, such as decreased libido, anorgasmia, and weight gain. Many women with PMS improve on lower doses,[115] and some do not require daily dosing despite the known delay in onset of action. Several options for administration are outlined Figure 6-3.

For women whose symptoms do not respond to SSRIs, consider prescribing anxiolytics. For PMS sufferers, the preferred agent is alprazolam.[44]

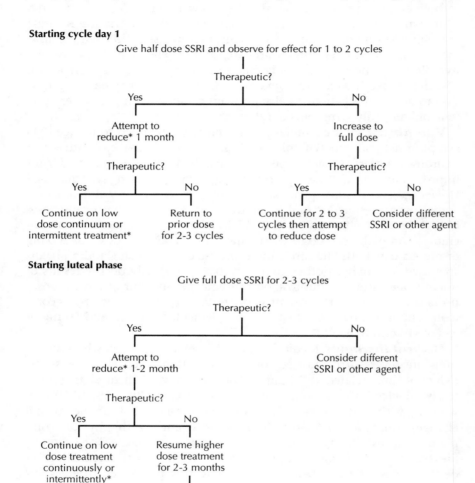

Starting cycle day 1

Give half dose SSRI and observe for effect for 1 to 2 cycles

Therapeutic?

Yes — No

Attempt to reduce* 1 month — Increase to full dose

Therapeutic? — Therapeutic?

Yes — No — Yes — No

Continue on low dose continuum or intermittent treatment* — Return to prior dose for 2-3 cycles — Continue for 2 to 3 cycles then attempt to reduce dose — Consider different SSRI or other agent

Starting luteal phase

Give full dose SSRI for 2-3 cycles

Therapeutic?

Yes — No

Attempt to reduce* 1-2 month — Consider different SSRI or other agent

Therapeutic?

Yes — No

Continue on low dose treatment continuously or intermittently* — Resume higher dose treatment for 2-3 months

Consider intermittent therapy*

* Intermittent therapy options:
  • Administer SSRI only during luteal phase or
  • Administer low-dose SSRI during follicular phase, increase to therapeutic dose during luteal phase

Source: Freeman EW (1995).

Figure 6-3 Flexibility in SSRI use for premenstrual syndrome (PMS)

Begin therapy at low doses (e.g., 0.25 mg three times a day) and progressively increase the dose (e.g., 1 mg to 2.5 mg a day) until the patient improves. Alternatively, try increasing the morning and evening doses while holding the mid-day dose low or dividing the dose into a four-times-a-day regimen. The most effective pattern of use for alprazolam in the treatment of PMS is still controversial. Some studies have found therapeutic response with intermittent use (e.g., 4 to 5 days preceding menses) while other studies have found such protocols no better than placebo. It is likely that individualizing therapies will be the key. To avoid withdrawal symptoms, taper the alprazolam doses each time it is discontinued. Be careful when prescribing these agents, which have potential for abuse; women with histories or current problems with alcoholism or other substance abuse are not appropriate candidates. Buspirone HCl, 10 mg three times a day, may be an effective alternative.[93]

Ovulation suppressants may also be helpful in the treatment of PMS. Oral contraceptives are beneficial for women with complaints of dysmenorrhea, irritability, and anger. For some oral contraceptive users, PMS symptoms are milder and shorter, but others have an increase in depression, breast tenderness, and bloating. Carefully select patients who may benefit, and monitor the results. Similarly, Danazol and GnRH agonists may provide relief,[77] but side effects limit their use to 4 to 6 months. Symptoms return once these agents are discontinued.

The 150 symptoms associated with PMS have been grouped into five categories to help target therapy. Some therapies have been shown to be effective in subsets of symptoms:

- **Anxiety.** Nervous tension, mood swings, irritability, restlessness, and impatience. If the patient's symptoms are debilitating, complement counseling and supportive measures with other efforts to reduce stress, including tips on organization. Unfortunately, studies have failed to demonstrate the efficacy of physical exercise. Serotonergic antidepressants and benzodiazepines have proven effective. Premenstrual use of prostaglandins inhibitors may also be helpful.

- **Depression.** Crying, confusion, social withdrawal, and insomnia must be carefully evaluated to rule out an underlying depressive or thyroid disorder. Antidepressants administered on a daily basis with prostaglandin inhibitors are most successful as short-term therapy.

- **Pain.** Severe uterine cramping, backache, and breast pain. Problems with cramping and backache respond well to the therapies outlined under the discussion of dysmenorrhea. Breast tenderness can be eased with a fitted support bra (sized for the luteal phase, when breast volume may increase 20%). Avoidance of methylxanthines found in coffee, tea, chocolate, and many prepared foods may be helpful. Bromocriptine has not been found to be a useful agent in any of the reported studies. Danazol is effective with mastalgia but can be taken for only a few months.

- **Water retention.** Weight gain, swelling, breast tenderness, and abdominal bloating. Many women experience no absolute increase in weight, but have fluid shifts. Spironolactone 25 mg taken orally two to four times a day for 14 days has efficacy in some studies. Other diuretics, most notably hydrochlorothiazide, are inappropriate for this problem.

- **Hypoglycemia.** Headaches, cravings for sweets, increased appetite, fatigue, and reduced coordination can be treated by eliminating sex steroid cycling or by dietary manipulations such as avoiding simple sugars and fats, eating several small meals of complex carbohydrates, and consuming fresh foods.

GYNECOLOGIC PROBLEMS
VULVAR LESIONS

Vulvar lesions present both diagnostic and therapeutic challenges. Since the vulva is composed of squamous epithelium with a full range of underlying glandular structures, virtually any pathology found anywhere on the skin can also be found on the vulva.[45] Psoriasis, eczema, vitiligo, moles, freckles, basal cell carcinoma, and squamous cell carcinoma can occur on the vulva. Often because of moisture and other local influences, common lesions on the vulva look different than they do when they appear elsewhere on the body. Psoriasis on the vulva often has a more velvet appearance with less scaling. Melanomas of the vulva occur at a rate nearly three times higher than would be expected based on the surface area of the vulva, because there are three times as many melanocytes in the vulvar skin. Sexually transmitted lesions such as condyloma lata and condyloma acuminata and molluscum contagiosum are predominately located in the vulva and other genital areas. Similarly, lesions such as Paget's disease of the vulva, hydradenitis suppurativa, and Bartholin's cysts involve the vulva exclusively or primarily due to the relatively unique glandular structures underlying the vulva. The epidermis of the vulva is subjected to a variety of local conditions that put it at risk for developing unique changes such as dystrophy, hyperplasia and lichen sclerosis. The vulva can also be a site for metastasis and spread of diseases from other areas. For example, the vulva can be a site of fistula for Crohn disease and for metastasis of choriocarcinoma.

The patient can play a pivotal role in diagnosing and detecting vulvar disease. If she does serial self-vulvar examinations, she may be able to draw a clinician's attention to a new lesion or to reassure the clinician that a lesion has had no growth for years. Every woman should be encouraged to do self-examination as a part of a comprehensive program of preventive health care. The clinician can help her learn more about this traditionally taboo area of her body by providing her a mirror during her routine pelvic exams.

The key to successful treatment of vulvar lesions is early detection. Carefully examine all the surfaces of the vulva under adequate illumination. Use a hand-held magnifying lens. To reveal suspicious areas for biopsy, prepare the vulvar tissue for at least 5 minutes with a gauze pad soaked in acetic acid. Colposcopy can occasionally be helpful in detecting microtrauma induced by rape and in identifying epithelial changes, but it is not useful for grading the severity of the changes (as it can on the cervix) because the vulva epithelium is too thick to permit an appreciation of vascular changes.

Vulvar lesions are categorized by the color of the underlying lesion: white, red, or pigmented.

White Lesions

White lesions often represent structural changes in the epidermis and dermis. *Lichen sclerosis et atrophicus* is a generalized thinning of the epidermis with loss of the dermal papilla. It can occur in females of any age, including young girls. Patients complain of pruritus, which can at times be intense. Over time as more of the vulva becomes involved, the skin loses elasticity and can split painfully and bleed during intercourse or a pelvic examination. In contrast, *hyperplasia,* which involves a profound thickening of the epidermis with no nuclear changes, also appears as a white lesion but often with a brighter color and a coarser texture without the linear crinkling characteristic of lichen. The differences between the two lesions may not be obvious on inspection and it is possible to have a mixture of hyperplasia and lichen. Base the diagnosis on biopsy results from a number of the lesions. *Dystrophy* can induce a chronic burning sensation of the vulva. Lesions may not be immediately obvious on inspection, but after a 5 minute application of 5% acetic acid-soaked gauze, characteristic sharp-bordered, bright, white lesions appear. On the other hand, the whitened areas of *vitiligo* are quite evident and often parallel changes occurring elsewhere on the body.

In sexually active women condyloma are more common than epithelial changes. *Condyloma acuminata*, caused by HPV, first appear as sessile, fleshy lesions. At this stage, they are easily treated with topical chemotherapeutic agents such as podophyllin, bichloracetic acid (BCA), or trichloracetic acid (TCA). (See Chapter 8 on Reproductive Tract Infections.) Mature lesions with thicker epithelia may be more resistant to topical therapies. Local destruction with cryotherapy, laser, LEEP, or surgical excision may be necessary. Interferon applied topically or injected locally may be helpful in treating recurrent lesions. Injectable interferon is very expensive. Biopsy is required only if the diagnosis is questionable or if the lesion fails to respond to conventional treatments. Recurrences are common, especially as the so-called "ring-around-the-lesion." Newer topical interferon agents sometimes reduce wart reoccurrence. Women with vulvar condyloma acuminata may have warts on other exposed surfaces, including the vagina, cervix, anus, urethra and buccal mucosa. They are also at higher risk for cervical dysplasia and require Pap smears annually or more frequently. *Condylomata lata* are vulvar warts that develop in secondary syphilis, when the blood tests for syphilis will be positive. The lesions teem with spirochetes and are very contagious. Systemic antibiotic therapy is needed. *Molluscum contagiosum* appears as dome-shaped papules with central umbilication. Over time they may resolve on their own and form skin tag-like lesions; however, some experts recommend removing the central core and touching the base of each lesion with ferric subsulfate (Monsel's) solution to control oozing.[62] (See Chapter 8 on Reproductive Tract Infections.)

Red Lesions

Red lesions are usually characteristic of infection but also may be associated with general skin changes and with neoplasms. The first lesion of *primary syphilis* is a painless clean, shining, indurated chancre. Painful inguinal adenopathy can develop days to weeks after the chancre. Serology tests will be negative, but darkfield microscopy can demonstrate corkscrew-shaped spirochetes. In the absence of darkfield microscopy, treatment can be initiated on the basis of the lesion's classical appearance. *Lymphogranuloma venereum* (LGV) also first presents as a painless, raised lesion that the patient may not notice. It has a more injected, necrotic appearance compared with the glistening surface of the chancre. If LGV is untreated, painful inguinal adenopathy can develop in 1 to 3 weeks. The adenopathy is usually unilateral and can have a characteristic "double groove" sign in women. (See Chapter 8 on Reproductive Tract Infections.)

In contrast to these relatively painless ulcers, herpes simplex and chancroid can produce extremely painful lesions. *Herpetic* lesions start as vesicles that rupture and leave clearly defined, isolated ulcers. *Chancroid* may start as isolated annular lesions but rapidly spreads by autoinoculation to form serpiginous (snake-like) bilateral lesions. If a chancroid is untreated, a tender inguinal bubo can form and rupture, leaving an open, weeping ulcer in the groin. *Granuloma inguinale* starts as a relatively painless nodule that ruptures and creates an open, fleshy, oozing lesion that slowly fibroses, eventually constricting the surrounding tissue. While some of these lesions are relatively uncommon in the United States, their incidence is increasing and may contribute to the spread of AIDS. For more information on treating these lesions, see Chapter 8 on Reproductive Tract Infections.

Candida vulvovaginitis presents with erythema, edema, and often, excoriation. Characteristic satellite lesions dot the periphery of the lesion. Similarly *tinea* ("jock itch") can infect the labia. Today many women use a wide range of feminine hygiene products that incite painful or pruritic allergic reactions that can mimic fungal infections. If the offending agent is on a pad, the vulvar erythema may have a classic hour-glass shape reflecting the areas of contact. The lack of satellite lesions helps distinguish delayed allergic reactions from candidal infections. *Other infections* such as trichomoniasis, nits, Bartholin's abscesses, hidradenitis suppurativa, and folliculitis tend to present with more localized erythema and purulence. *Non-infectious* problems such as eczema and psoriasis generally appear as red lesions on the vulva. *Trauma* to the vulva also presents with red lesions. *Paget's disease* of the vulva usually has a red, velvety appearance. Deep biopsies of the lesion are needed because an underlying adenocarcinoma occurs in about 10% of cases.

Pigmented Lesions

Pigmented lesions range from benign lentigo (freckles) to invasive squamous cell carcinoma of the vulva. These lesions present the greatest diagnostic challenges. Lesions may have distinctly different and more subtle presentations in women with darker pigmentation. Even in women with lighter-colored skin, it is often difficult to be confident that a compound nevus is not an early melanoma. Carefully examine the lesion with a hand-held magnifying lens to ensure the nevus has clear borders, smooth surface contours, and no variegation in color. If any of these features is present, biopsy is mandatory. *Basal cell carcinoma* has a characteristic round, cored out "rat-bite" lesion with raised pearly edges. *Vulvar intraepithelial neoplasia* (VIN) is usually multicentric in premenopausal women and may appear as darkened areas with a rougher surface. It is usually not possible to distinguish VIN from early *squamous cell carcinoma* by inspection alone. Determining the full extent of the disease is crucial, so multiple biopsies are often necessary.

Although not associated with a visible lesion, many women suffer from vulvodynia (burning vulvar syndrome), a term used when women complain of vulvar pain not adequately explained by physical findings.[67] Occasionally vulvodynia may result from nerve irritations due to previous laser therapy or from topical treatments such as corticosteroids or antibiotics. Pudendal neuralgia can result from previous damage to the pudendal nerve such as diabetes, infection with the herpes simplex virus, degenerative disc disease or tumor, and obstetrical, surgical, or other trauma. Vulvar vestibulitis may present as vulvodynia or dyspareunia.

ENDOMETRIOSIS

Endometriosis is the condition that occurs when endometrial glands and stroma from the lining of the uterus become seeded in locations outside the uterus. Endometriosis has many different appearances. The classical implant is nodular and brown, black, or reddish in color with a puckering of the surrounding tissue in a "powder burn" pattern. Papular implants that are whitish, yellow, or nonpigmented are common, as are implants buried deep within pelvic adhesions. *Endometriomas* are cystic masses of endometriosis contained within the ovary and filled with thick brownish fluid, which give the lesions their popular name—"chocolate cysts."

Endometriosis most frequently involves the peritoneal surfaces of pelvic organs—the cul de sac, ovaries, fallopian tube, uterus, broad ligament, ureters, rectovaginal system, and uterosacral ligaments. The bowel, including the appendix, is often involved both superficially and intrinsically. Other more unusual sites include surgical scars, the bladder, the vulva, and the lungs.

Endometriotic implants are transported out of the uterus primarily by retrograde menstruation. As the uterus contracts to expel the sloughed endometrial lining, some of the material is compressed out the fimbria and into the pelvic cavity. Other mechanisms such as hematogenous and lymphatic spread create more distal implants. Once the material implants, it usually forms a small cyst. The initial red endometriotic implants respond to monthly sex steroid stimuli the same way the endometrial lining does—by proliferating, hypertrophying, and ultimately sloughing at the end of the cycle. With the escape of the "local menstrual blood," the cysts generally perforate. The extruded material incites an inflammatory response creating adhesions to adjacent structures. Ultimately, the inflammatory reaction leads to fibrosis characterized by black and white lesions.[18] If the cyst on the ovary does not perforate early, large endometriomas can form. On the uterosacral ligament or within the sigmoid, the same process leads to creation of the deep nodules.

Endometriosis is a fairly common problem: about 3% to 10% of reproductive-age women in the United States have endometriosis. Women
undergoing laparotomy for gynecologic diseases have higher rates: 14%
to 21%. Nearly 25% to 35% of infertile women have endometriosis.[25,82]
Rates may be twice as high in Asian women, women who delay childbearing, and women with a family history of endometriosis.

Symptoms of Endometriosis

The symptoms associated with endometriosis are variable. Over 50% of
affected women complain of secondary dysmenorrhea; the pain often
precedes the onset of vaginal bleeding each month. Dyspareunia is quite
common; dyschezia (painful defecation) may also occur. There is no constant relationship between the extent of endometriosis and a woman's
symptoms. On physical examination, a fixed retroverted uterus and tender nodular uterosacral ligaments, with or without an adnexal mass, are
consistent with advanced endometriosis. However, a definitive diagnosis
requires direct visualization, usually via laparoscopy. Biopsies help confirm the visual impression. A formal classification system has been developed by the American Society for Reproductive Medicine to help stage
the extent of disease and guide therapy and counseling.[4]

Treatment of Endometriosis

Treatment is guided by the nature and severity of the patient's symptoms
and disease as well as the couple's desire for fertility. Women with clinically apparent endometriomas require surgical cystectomy because
endometriomas are not amenable to medical therapy and do have a potential for rupture, causing chemical peritonitis. Surgery is also appropriate for
women whose endometriosis is resistant to medical management.

Severe endometriosis with dense adhesions throughout the pelvis com-
promises fertility and requires surgical and medical therapies. However,
the relationship between mild endometriosis and infertility is unclear. A
90% 5-year cumulative pregnancy rate has been reported for women
with untreated minimal to mild endometriosis.[9] Treatment of women with
mild endometriosis does not increase fertility rates.[36,48]

Women with symptoms of dysmenorrhea can be given trials of medical
therapy. Dysmenorrhea may be reduced by NSAIDS or oral contraceptives.
Bicycling or tricycling oral contraceptives is particularly helpful. (See
Chapter 19 on The Pill: Oral Contraceptives.) Progestins have long been a
mainstay of therapy. A recent study demonstrated significant symptomatic relief from DMPA use.[125] Other agents with proven efficacy include
danazol and GNRH agonists. These medications are particularly helpful in
shrinking and softening the implants to make them more amenable to
surgical excision or ablation. They are also useful after surgery to treat

residual disease and to prevent re-seeding. As stand-alone therapy, however, their use is limited. Danazol can be used at most for 6 to 9 months because it causes side effects: acne, hirsutism, and virilization. GNRH agonists induce hypoestrogenic states causing vasomotor symptoms and osteoporosis. Coupling GNRH agents with low-dose estrogen and progestin may be possible but is still considered experimental and is costly.

PELVIC MASS

Pelvic masses are fairly common, but the evaluation may be somewhat challenging. The differential diagnoses of a pelvic mass include not only gynecologic causes (ovarian, tubal, and uterine masses) but also non-gynecological sources (a kidney in the pelvis and masses arising from the kidney, bladder, rectum, intestine, peritoneum, omentum, and rarely the blood vessels and nerves of the pelvis).[101] Although pelvic masses may cause symptoms, they are generally an incidental finding in asymptomatic women. The relative frequencies of different types of pelvic masses change with a woman's age:[12]

- **Girls.** A pelvic mass usually presents with pain and is frequently related to gastrointestinal problems (volvulus or appendicitis) or urinary pathology (bladder distension, Wilms' tumor, or neuroblastoma). The most common gynecological cause for a pelvic mass in young girls is a germ cell tumor of the ovary, followed closely by a simple ovarian cyst.

- **Reproductive-age women.** Consider pregnancy (intrauterine and ectopic) and infection (pyosalpinges or hydrosalpinges) as well as hormonally related cysts and the full range of benign and malignant neoplasms of the ovary, fallopian tube, and uterus. Uterine malformations such as bicornuate uterus, as well as paratubal and paraovarian cysts, can present as masses. Non-gynecological causes other than appendiceal abscess and surgical adhesions are relatively rare.

- **Post-menopausal women.** The most common non-gynecological causes are diverticular abscesses and colon cancer. Colon cancer occurs more frequently than ovarian or endometrial cancer. Gynecological causes are more likely to be malignant in this age group; 40% of palpated ovarian masses are malignant.[12]

Pregnancy-Related Masses

Promptly rule out pregnancy when a reproductive-age woman appears with an adnexal mass. Ectopic pregnancy may be suggested by a history of irregular vaginal spotting or bleeding, pelvic pain, and symptoms of pregnancy. The cervix may be cyanotic, and the uterus will be slightly enlarged and globular. Cervical motion tenderness may localize the lesion to one side, where an adnexal mass may be palpable. However, the pelvic mass that is palpated often is not the pregnancy itself but the corpus luteum cyst. Perform a pregnancy test. The rest of the evaluation depends on her clinical status. Acutely ill women require surgical evaluation and treatment. A stable, minimally symptomatic patient may be evaluated with serial ß-hCG titers and transvaginal ultrasound study of the uterus. A dilation and curettage (D&C) that fails to yield products of conception can also point to an ectopic pregnancy. Treatment for small, nonacute ectopic pregnancies may be surgical or medical. (See Chapter 26 on Pregnancy Testing and Management of Early Pregnancy.)

Other masses related to pregnancy include the corpus luteum cyst or a luteoma of pregnancy. The latter may cause significant androgenic changes. Fibroids tend to grow rapidly in pregnancy to form palpable masses and may cause extreme pelvic pain as they undergo necrosis.

Infection

If a woman is sexually active, consider the possibility of an infection, especially if she has a history of fever, vaginal discharge, and pelvic pain. The classic presentation of gonorrhea-associated pelvic inflammatory disease (PID) is high fever, gastrointestinal problems, and severe lower abdominal pain appearing near the end of menses. The affected woman stoops and walks with a slow gait (the "PID shuffle") and has both abdominal tenderness and bilateral rebound in the pelvis. Her cervix is edematous and has a purulent discharge. On bimanual exam she has marked cervical motion tenderness and, if she is able to tolerate abdominal pressure, may be found to have bilateral masses—pyosalpinges.

Today the most common cause of salpingitis is chlamydia, which has a more subtle presentation. Its onset can be anytime in the menstrual cycle. The cervix is friable and has a purulent discharge, cervical motion tenderness is present, but adnexal masses may not be palpable. Other infectious causes of salpingitis are less common but include actinomycosis (rarely found except in current IUD users) and tuberculosis.

Cysts

A symptomatic ovarian masses in reproductive-age women are most likely to be physiological (follicular or luteal) cysts. Women who use hormonal methods that suppress ovulation should not form corpora lutea. Moderately sized asymptomatic physiological cysts may be permitted to resolve spontaneously. The most common ovarian neoplasm in young women is a cystic teratoma (dermoid), a mobile mass floating near the anterior abdominal wall and characterized on ultrasound by internal echoes representing fat, hair and teeth inside. Other common neoplasms include endometrioma, mucinous cystadenoma, and serous cystadenoma. Carcinoma, including borderline lesions, is a rare but ever-present possibility.

Surgical therapy is usually necessary for diagnosis as well as for therapy for any mass that persists or is greater than 8 to 10 cm. Laparoscopic removal of adnexal masses has decreased the costs, physical discomfort, and recovery time of abdominal surgery. Ovarian preservation is the goal for women in their reproductive years; cystectomy, therefore, is the standard procedure unless malignancy is discovered, surgical difficulties present, or bleeding is not otherwise controllable.

A woman who has a pelvic mass accompanied by intermittent pain, fever, and gastrointestinal complaints may have torsion of an ovarian mass (e.g., dermoid or physiologic cyst) or of tubal mass (e.g., paratubal cyst or distal portion of previously transected tube). The diagnosis of torsion often may require diagnostic laparoscopy for confirmation and treatment. Other causes of acutely symptomatic pelvic masses include rupture of an endometrioma or a ruptured hemorrhagic corpus luteal cyst.

Benign Uterine Tumors

Uterine tumors such as fibroids (leiomyoma) also present as pelvic masses, especially during the reproductive years. About 20% of women in their late 30s to 40s have fibroids.

- When a fibroid is submucosal and protrudes into the uterine cavity, it may cause heavy menses but only a normal sized or minimally enlarged uterus.
- When a fibroid is intramural, the uterus will be more enlarged and asymmetrical.
- When the fibroid is subserosal, it may cause no bleeding changes but will result in a markedly irregular contour to the uterus ("lumpy, bumpy, sack of potatoes").
- When a fibroid is pedunculated and attached to the outer surface of the uterus by only a stalk, it causes no change in bleeding but may be felt as an adnexal mass.

It is sometimes difficult to distinguish uterine masses from ovarian masses. If the ovary can be felt to be distinct from the pelvic mass, then the mass is less likely to be ovarian. If, during a bimanual exam, the mass can be moved without moving the uterus, it is more consistent with an adnexal mass. Ultrasound is helpful but not mandatory to characterize and measure the fibroids; it can also document the normalcy of the ovaries and permit conservative management in almost all asymptomatic women. If women have abnormal bleeding, it may still be necessary to perform endometrial biopsies to rule out hyperplasia or carcinoma. Surgery such as myomectomy or hysterectomy is generally reserved for women who are symptomatic and refractory to medical therapy or who have rapidly growing masses.

Adenomyosis

Another cause of uterine enlargement is adenomyosis. The endometrial glands and stroma embed in the muscular layer of the uterus and cause a generalized enlargement and tenderness of the uterus. Women with adenomyosis usually experience heavy and often painful menses.

Ovarian Cancer

Ovarian cancer strikes over 26,000 women each year in the United States, and nearly half of that number die each year. Survival rates, stage for stage, are equivalent to other gynecologic cancers, but ovarian carcinoma is the leading cause of death due to gynecologic cancer because the most cases are diagnosed only in advanced stages. The bimanual exam is the standard screening test for asymptomatic, low-risk women. Women with family histories suggesting a high risk or genetic predispositions to breast/ovarian carcinoma (BRCA1 mutation) may be more appropriately screened by transvaginal ultrasonography and serum tumor markers, such as CA 125.[105]

Postmenopausal Masses

Two or 3 years after menopause, a woman's ovaries should be significantly atrophied and difficult to detect on pelvic exam. A palpable postmenopausal ovary merits evaluation.[10] Perform transvaginal ultrasound to characterize and measure the size of the mass[96] and draw serum to measure tumor markers such as CA 125 if you suspect an organic mass. Color-flow Doppler may be of assistance. If the ultrasound image shows that the mass is a small simple cyst and the patient's CA 125 levels are low, conservatively manage the condition through repeated testing or explore the pelvis by laparoscopy.[83] If the ultrasound image demonstrates any complexity within the mass or if the patient's CA 125 levels are elevated, more extensive surgery is usually required to rule out carcinoma.[27] These new non-invasive testing modalities have reduced the need for surgery to diagnose ovarian cancer.[51]

SEXUAL DYSFUNCTION

Sexuality serves many purposes in human interaction. It is necessary for routine reproduction; it can form a bond between people; it can relieve tension and promote relaxation. Severe sexual dysfunction can deprive couples of many of its benefits. Women's health care providers are in a pivotal position to identify women with sexuality problems, to develop diagnoses and to guide the couple to more complete sexual functioning or to refer them to appropriate resources to help them.

Sexual dysfunction is a relatively common problem. As many as 50% of all married couples experience some sexual dissatisfaction or dysfunction.[116] Despite the widespread prevalence of sexual problems, women often hesitate to volunteer their complaints to health care providers. In one study, only 3% of women seen in a typical gynecological practice presented with sexually related complaints, but another 16% acknowledged problems during a comprehensive review of systems.[8] The most common complaint was dyspareunia (48%), followed by decreased sexual desire (21%), partner problems or dysfunction (8%), vaginismus (6%), anorgasmia (4%), and other problems (13%).

Once a sexual problem has been identified, it has to be more completely characterized and placed within the context of the woman's complete sexual history. Make no assumptions about the patient's sexual orientation. Be aware of your own comfort, and ask open-ended questions in a non-judgmental manner to reduce the patient's embarrassment.[71]

DYSPAREUNIA

Dyspareunia accounts for nearly half of all women's sexual complaints. The causes are widespread but can be generally grouped into three categories:

Pain on intromission. Some vulvar problems can be easily identified on careful inspection: the small exquisitely tender "red dot" characteristic of vestibulitis; the shallow ulcer of Bechet's disease; herpetic lesions; vulvovaginal candidiasis with its red swollen excoriated appearance; the smooth, reddened areas of allergic reactions; the white cigarette paper changes of lichen sclerosus; and an imperforate hymen. Vulvodynia, most likely due to chronic peripheral nerve irritation, is less obvious but may also cause pain on initiation of intercourse. Severe, prolonged hypoestrogenism and lichen sclerosis can result in inelastic tissue that does not expand to accommodate penile penetration. Therapy in each of these cases targets the underlying pathology and attempts to break the pain-aversion cycle once the acute problem has been resolved.

A special cause of pain on intromission is vaginismus. Although vaginismus is a relatively infrequent problem in the general population, it comprises a disproportionately large proportion of women with sexual problems. Women with extreme vaginismus may not be able to tolerate touch of their genitalia either during sexual encounters or physical examination. A desensitizing program of progressive vaginal dilatation may be helpful but it often needs to be complemented with counseling to deal with the women's fears.[2,123] (See Chapter 2 on Sexuality and Reproductive Health.)

Pain in mid-vagina. Pain that starts immediately after intromission can be due to problems in the vagina or in any of the adjacent structures. An episiotomy scar may be sensitive due to tender granulation tissue or may have entrapped nerve endings that trigger pain when touched. An overly corrected colporrhaphy may create too constricted an orifice to permit comfortable intercourse. Intrinsic anatomical defects such as a congenital septum may be painful during thrusting against its leading edge. Infections may cause dyspareunia, so test for urethral or bladder tenderness to help rule out urethritis and cystitis as causes of mid-vaginal dyspareunia. Lack of adequate lubrication can cause pain during early thrusting. Lack of lubrication can be due to sexual practices (such as inadequate foreplay) or to hypoestrogenism in menopause or to breastfeeding.

Pain with deep thrusting. Dyspareunia that occurs during deep thrusting usually involves upper tract pelvic organs or other intraperitoneal structures. Intercourse during active salpingitis can be quite uncomfortable, but usually the longer-term consequences of infection are responsible for chronic deep-thrust dyspareunia. Adhesions formed by PID, endometriosis, and previous pelvic or abdominal surgery fix the pelvic organs and do not allow for movement to accommodate the pressure exerted against them during intercourse. The stretch placed on the adhesions can cause a tearing or ripping sensation, which can be quite painful. Interestingly, there is no observable relationship between the amount of adhesions and the severity of a woman's symptoms. Gossamer adhesions cause profound pain while dense adhesions may not cause any noticeable discomfort. Women who have undergone hysterectomy occasionally have an ovary adherent to the vaginal cuff; this condition is quite sensitive to forceful contact during intercourse. Piriformis sensitivity has been reported to cause pain than can be reproduced by pressing against the lateral vaginal fornix. For acute infections, a history and physical exam supported by limited laboratory testing is generally sufficient for making a diagnosis. In more chronic conditions, a thorough digital exam of the entire vault can help define the problem: a fixed uterus suggests adhesions while nodules along the uterosacral ligament suggest endometriosis. Adjunctive testing with ultrasound and, often, diagnostic laparoscopy may be needed to make a definite diagnosis. Suggest using different coital positions to direct the penis away from sensitive areas and provide some degree of pain avoidance. Chronic constipation can also cause dyspareunia.

Some women suffer pain with orgasm due to painful uterine or abdominal muscle contractions. Others develop severe headaches.

Prophylactic administration of nonsteroidal agents 1 hour prior to intercourse can reduce or eliminate these problems. Postcoitally, if a woman has been unable to achieve orgasm to release the venous pressure built up during the arousal phase, she may experience a dull aching or throbbing sensation in her pelvis. This is referred to as pelvic congestion syndrome. Some women with this problem will benefit from couples counseling on coital timing; others may benefit from instructions about masturbation.

SEXUAL DISINTEREST

Complaints about decreased libido have only recently achieved attention as medical concerns. They were not even addressed in the Masters and Johnson work in the 1970s. But sexual disinterest is apparently widespread. In one survey, 2 out of every 10 women reported difficulty being sexually aroused; one-third said they had difficulty maintaining excitement and another one-third expressed a complete disinterest in sex.[37] However, 83% of these couples rated their marriages as happy or very happy. While perfect sexual function is not a necessary prerequisite for marital happiness, sexual disinterest can create stresses with the relationship. And the obverse is also true; relationship stresses frequently first manifest themselves in the bedroom.

Medical problems and medications can affect libido.[104] Chronic diseases such as diabetes are often associated with decreased sexual activity. Persons recovering from myocardial infarction may be extremely apprehensive about engaging in strenuous activities. Women who have had mastectomy, colostomy, or vulvectomy may feel unattractive and have diminished libido. Pain from arthritis and other diseases that limit motion may discourage sexual activity. Psychological problems, such as pronounced depression, may first manifest as decreased libido. A history of sexual abuse can leave deep psychological scars and can transform pleasurable sexuality into repeated reminders of former nightmares. Pregnancy can introduce difficulties with sexual relations. Patients can benefit from reassurance as well as explicit advice about safer coital positioning.[15] (See Chapter 2 on Sexuality and Reproductive Health.)

Medications such as sedatives, narcotics, hypnotics, anticonvulsants, centrally acting antihypertensives, tranquilizers, anorectics, and some antidepressants may interfere with sexual desire and/or sexual function.[6] Estrogen has a more complex set of effects; while it increases vaginal lubrication, it also increases sex hormone binding globulin, which may decrease free serum androgen levels and thus may decrease libido. In small amounts, alcohol may decrease inhibition, but, primarily, it is a depressant and decreases a woman's arousal.

Lifestyle issues are pivotal to a woman's sexuality.[92] Fatigue and stress over finances or other issues rob her of libido as profoundly as medications. Distraction by daily tasks or lack of privacy can subdue passion. Over time, predictability combined with a limited sexual menu can replace anticipation and excitement with sheer routine and boredom and result in diminished desire. Stresses within the relationship are also strong determinants of libido. At a practical level, a partner's sexual techniques can profoundly affect a woman's libido; rapid, self-centered, or rough sexual practices may leave the woman unaroused. In retrospect, these influences are obvious but in a clinical setting they may not be as clear. Using open-ended questions, carefully and sensitively inquire about the couple's sexual dynamics.

References

1. Abraham GE, Hargrove JT. Effect of vitamin B_6 on premenstrual symptomatology in women with premenstrual tension syndrome: a double-blind crossover study. Infertility 1980;3:155-165.
2. American College of Obstetricians and Gynecologists. Sexual dysfunction. ACOG technical bulletin, no. 211, 1995.
3. American Psychiatric Association. Diagnostic and statistical manual of mental disorders, fourth edition (DSM-IV). Washington DC: American Psychiatric Association, 1994.
4. American Society for Reproductive Medicine. Revised American Society for Reproductive Medicine classification of endometriosis. Fertil Steril 1985;43:351-352.
5. Andersch B, Milsom I. An epidemiologic study of young women with dysmenorrhea. Am J Obstet Gynecol 1982;144:655-660.
6. Anonymous. Drugs that cause sexual dysfunction: an update. Med Lett Drugs Ther 1992;34:73.
7. Ayers JWT, Gidwana GP, Schmidt IMV, Gross M. Osteopenia in hypoestrogenic young women with anorexia nervosa. Fertil Steril 1984;41:224-228.
8. Bachmann GA, Leiblum SR, Grill J. Brief sexual inquiry in gynecological practice. Obstet Gynecol 1989;73:425.
9. Badway SZA, Elbarkry MM, Samuel F, Dizer M. Cumulative pregnancy rates in infertile women with endometriosis. J Reprod Med 1988;33:757-760.
10. Barber H, Graber E. The PMPO syndrome (postmenopausal palpable ovary syndrome). Obstet Gynecol 1971;38:921-923.
11. Bayer SR, DeCherney AH. Clinical manifestations and treatment of dysfunctional uterine bleeding. JAMA 1993;269:1823-1828.
12. Bennington JL, Fergusen BR, Haber SL. Incidence of relative frequency of benign and malignant ovarian neoplasms. Obstet Gynecol 1968;32:627-632.
13. Berry C, McGuire F. Menstrual distress and acceptance of sexual role. Am J Obstet Gynecol 1972;114:83-87.
14. Beynon HLS, Harbet NE, Barnes PJ. Severe premenstrual exacerbations of asthma: effect of intramuscular progesterone. Lancet 1988;2:370-372.

15. Bing E, Colman L. Making love during pregnancy. New York: Bantam Books, 1977.
16. Boggess KA, Williamson HO, Homm RJ. Influence of the menstrual cycle on systemic diseases. Obstet Gynecol Clin North Amer 1990;17:321-342.
17. Bonnar J, Sheppard BL. Treatment of menorrhagia during menstruation: randomized controlled trial of ethamsylate, mefenamic acid, and tranexamic acid. BMJ 1996;313:579-582.
18. Brosens IA. Endometriosis—a disease because it is characterized by bleeding. Am J Obstet Gynecol 1997;176:263-267.
19. Chan WY. Prostaglandin inhibitors and antagonists in dysmenorrhea therapy. In: Dawood MY (ed). Dysmenorrhea. Baltimore: Williams & Wilkins, 1981.
20. Chang RJ, Mandel FP, Lu JK, Judd JL. Enhanced disparity of gonadotropin secretion by estrone in women with polycystic ovarian disease. J Clin Endocrinol Metab 1982;54:490-494.
21. Chihal HJ. Premenstrual syndrome: an update for clinicians. Obstet Gynecol Clinics North Amer 1990;17:457-481.
22. Chimbira TH, Anderson ABM, Turnbull AC. Relation between measured menstrual blood loss and patient's subjective assessment of loss, duration of bleeding, number of sanitary towels used, uterine weight and endometrial surface area. Br J Obstet Gynaecol 1980;87:603-609.
23. Chuong CH, Coulam CB, Kao PC, Bergstrahl EJ, Go VI. Neuropeptide levels in premenstrual syndrome. Fertil Steril 1985;44:760-765.
24. Claessens EA, Cowell CA. Dysfunctional uterine bleeding in the adolescent. Pediatr Clin North Am 1981;28:369-371.
25. Cramer DW. Epidemiology of endometriosis. In: Wilson EA (ed). Endometriosis. New York: Alan R. Liss, 1987:5-22.
26. Creatsas G, Deligeoroglou E, Zachari A, Loutradis D, Papadimitriou T, Miras K, Aravantino D. Prostaglandins $PGF_{2\alpha}$, PGE_2, 6-Keto-$PGF_{1\alpha}$, TXA_2 and TXB_2 serum levels in dysmenorrheic adolescents before, during and after treatment with oral contraceptives. European J Obstet Gynecol and Repro Biol 1990;36:292-298.
27. Curtin JP. Management of the adnexal mass. Gynecol Oncol 1994;55:S42-S46.
28. Dalton K. The premenstrual syndrome and progesterone therapy. London: William Heimann, 1984.
29. Dawood MY. Nonsteroidal anti-inflammatory drugs and reproduction. Am J Obstet Gynecol 1993;169:1255-1265.
30. Devore GR, Owens O, Kase N. Use of intravenous Premarin in the treatment of dysfunctional uterine bleeding: a double-blind, randomized control study. Obstet Gynecol 1982;59:285-291.
31. Doody KM, Carr BR. Menstrual cycle disorders. Obstetrics and gynecology clinics of North America. Philadelphia: W.B. Saunders Co., 1990;17:361-387.
32. Dunaif A, Green G, Phelps RG, Lebwohl M, Futterweit W, Lewy L. Acanthosis nigricans, insulin action, and hyperandrogenism: clinical, histological, and biochemical findings. J Clin Endocrinol Metab 1991;73:590-595.
33. Erenus M, Yucelten D, Gurbuz, O, Durmusoglu F, Pekin S. Comparison of spironolactone-oral contraceptive versus cyproterone acetate-estrogen regimens in the treatment of hirsutism. Fertil Steril 1996;66:216-219.

34. Eriksson E, Hedberg MA, Andersch B, Sunblad C. The serotonin reuptake inhibitor paroxetin is superior to the noradrenaline reuptake inhibitor maprotiline in the treatment of premenstrual syndrome: a placebo-controlled trial. Neuropsychopharmacology 1995;12:167-176.
35. Fava M, Pedrazzi F, Guaraldi GP, Romano G, Genazzani AR, Facchinetti F. Comorbid anxiety and depression among patients with late luteal phase dysphoric disorder. J Anx Disorders 1992;6:325-335.
36. Fedele L, Parzzini F, Radici E, Bocciolone L, Bianchi S, Bianchi C, Canadiani GB. Buserelin acetate versus expectant management in the treatment of infertility associated with minimal or mild endometriosis: a randomized clinical trial. Am J Obstet Gynecol 1992;166:1345-1350.
37. Frank E, Anderson C, Rubinstein P. Frequency of sexual dysfunction in "normal" couples. N Engl J Med 1978;299:111.
38. Frank RT. The hormonal causes of premenstrual tension. Arch Mem Psychiatry 1931;26:1053-1057.
39. Franks S. Polycystic ovary syndrome: a changing perspective. Clin Endocrinol 1989;31:87-120.
40. Frasier IS. Menorrhagia—a pragmatic approach to the understanding of the causes and the need for investigations. Br J Obstet Gynaecol 1994;101 (Suppl 11):3-7.
41. Fraser IS, McCarron G, Markham R. Blood and total fluid content of menstrual discharge. Obstet Gynecol 1985;65:194-198.
42. Freeman EW, Kielich AM, Sondheimer SJ. PMS: new treatments that really work. Cont Ob/Gyn 1996;25:44.
43. Freeman E, Rickels K, Sondheimer SJ, Polansky M. Ineffectiveness of progesterone suppository treatment for premenstrual syndrome. JAMA 1990;264:349-358.
44. Freeman EW, Rickels K, Sondheimer SJ, Polansky M. A double-blind trial of oral progesterone, alprazolam, and placebo in treatment of severe premenstrual syndrome. JAMA 1995;274:51-57.
45. Friedrich Jr EG. Major problems in obstetrics and gynecology. Vol. 9. Philadelphia: W.B. Saunders 1983:35-60.
46. Frisch R, Wyshak G, Vincent L. Delayed menarche and amenorrhea in ballet dancers. N Engl J Med 1980;303:17-19.
47. Frisch RE, Gotz-Welbergn AV, McArthur JW, Albirght T, Witschi J, Bullen B, Birnholz J, Reed RB, Hermann H. Delayed menarche and amenorrhea of college athletes in relation to age of onset of training. JAMA 1981;246:1559-1563.
48. Garcia CF, Davis SS. Pelvic endometriosis: infertility and pelvic pain. Am J Obstet Gynecol 1977;129:740-747.
49. Genazzani AD, Petraglia F, Gastaldi M, Volpogni C, Gamba O, Genazzani AR. Naltrexone treatment restores menstrual cycles in patients with weight loss-related amenorrhea. Fertil Steril 1995;64:951-956.
50. Givens JR. Polycystic ovaries—a sign, not a diagnosis. Semin Reprod Endocrinol 1984;2:271-280.
51. Goldstein SR. Postmenopausal adnexal cysts: how clinical management has evolved. Am J Obstet Gynecol 1996;175:1498-1501.
52. Goodale IL, Domar AD, Benson H. Alleviation of premenstrual syndrome with the relaxation response. Obstet Gynecol 1990;75:649-655.

53. Graf MJ, Richards CJ, Brown V, Meissner L, Dunaif A. The independent effects of hyperandrogenemia, hyperinsulinaemia, and obesity on lipid and lipoprotein profiles in women. Clin Endocrinol 1990;33:119-131.
54. Guillebaud J. The pill and other hormones for contraception. 4th edition. Oxford, England: Oxford University Press, 1991.
55. Harel Z, Biro FM, Kottenhahn RK, Rosenthal SL. Supplementation with omega-3 polyunsaturated fatty acids in the management of dysmenorrhea in adolescents. Am J Obstet Gynecol 1996;174:1335-1338.
56. Harrison WM, Robkin JH, Endicott J. Psychiatric evaluation of premenstrual changes. Psychosomatics 1985;26:789.
57. Haskett RF, DeLongis A, Kessler RC. Premenstrual dysphoria: a community survey [abstract]. Presented at the 140th annual meeting of the American Psychiatric Association, May 9-15, 1987, Chicago, IL.
58. Haynes PJ, Hodgson H, Anderson ABM, Turnbull AC. Measurement of menstrual blood loss in patients complaining of menorrhagia. Br J Obstet Gynaecol 1977;84:763-768.
59. Hergenroeder AC, Smith EO, Shypailo R, Jones LA, Klish WJ, Ellis K. Bone mineral changes in young women with hypothalamic amenorrhea treated with oral contraceptives, changes in young women with hypothalamic amenorrhea treated with oral contraceptives, medroxyprogesterone or placebo over 12 months. Am J Obstet Gynecol 1997;176:1017-1025.
60. Hillard PA. Heavy uterine bleeding in adolescents. Contemporary Ob/Gyn 1995;40:21-32.
61. Johnson SR, McChesney C, Bean JA. Epidemiology of premenstrual symptoms in a nonclinical sample. I. Prevalence, natural history and help-seeking behavior. J Reprod Med 1988;33:340-346.
62. Kaufman RH, Faro S, Friedrich Jr EG, Gardner HL. Benign diseases of the vulva and vagina. St. Louis: Mosby 1994.
63. Lapidus L, Bengtsson C, Larsson B, Pennert K, Rybo E, Sjostrom L. Distribution of adipose tissue and risk of cardiovascular disease and death: a 12-year follow up of participants in the population study of women in Gothenburn, Sweden. Br Med J 1984;289:1257-1261.
64. Legro RS. Is polycystic ovary syndrome a genetic disease? Contemporary Ob/Gyn 1996;9:43-57.
65. Lepage P, Steiner M. Gender and serotonergic dysregulation: implications for late luteal phase dysphoric disorder. In: Cassano GB, Akiskal HS (eds). Serotonin-related psychiatric syndromes: clinical and therapeutic links. London: Royal Society of Medical Services, 1991:131-143.
66. London RS, Bradley L, Chiamore NY. Effect of a nutritional supplement on premenstrual symptomatology in women with premenstrual syndrome: a double-blind longitudinal study. J Am Coll Nutr 1991;10:494.
67. Lynch PJ, Edwards L. Genital dermatology. New York: Churchill Livingstone, 1994:237-249.
68. Magos AL. Management of menorrhagia. Br J Med 1990;300;1537-1538.
69. Marcondes JAM, Minnani SL, Luthold WW, Wajchenberg BL, Samojilk E, Kirschner MA. Treatment of hirsutism in women with flutamide. Fertil Steril 1992;57:543-547.
70. Mason HD, Margara R, Winston RL, Seppala M, Koistinen R, Franks S. Insulin-like growth factory-I (IGF-I) inhibits production of IGF-binding protein-1

while stimulating estradiol secretion in granulosa cells from normal and polycystic human ovaries. J Clin Endocrinol Metab 1993;76:1275-1279.

71. Masters WH, Johnson VE. Human sexual response. Boston: Little Brown & Co., 1996:141-168.
72. Mattson RH, Rebar RW. Contraceptive methods for women with neurologic disorders. Am J Obstet Gynecol 1993;168:2027-2032.
73. Milsom I, Sundell G, Andersch B. The influence of different combined oral contraceptives on the prevalence and severity of dysmenorrhea. Contraception 1990;42:497-506.
74. Mira M, Stewart PM, Abraham SF. Vitamin and trace element status in premenstrual syndrome. Am J Clin Nutr 1988;47:636-641.
75. Mishell DR. Infertility, contraception and reproductive endocrinology. Boston: Blackwell Scientific Publications, 1991.
76. Murray SC, Muse KN. Effective treatment of severe menstrual migraine headaches with gonadotropin-releasing hormone agonist and add-back therapy. Fertil Steril 1997;67:390-393.
77. Muse KN, Futterman LA, Yen SSC. The premenstrual syndrome: effects of "medical ovariectomy." N Engl J Med 1984:1345-1346.
78. Neinstein LS. Issues in reproductive management. New York: Theime Medical Publishers, 1994.
79. Neinstein LS. Menstrual problems in adolescents. Med Clin North Am 1990;74;1181-1203.
80. Nilsson L, Rybo G. Treatment of menorrhagia. Am J Obstet Gynecol 1971;110:713-720.
81. Oleson T, Flocco W. Randomized controlled study of premenstrual symptoms treated with ear, hand and foot reflexology. Obstet Gynecol 1993;82:906-911.
82. Olive DL, Schwartz LB. Endometriosis. N Engl J Med 1993;328:1759.
83. Parker WH. The case for laparoscopic management of the adnexal mass. Clin Obstet Gynecol 1995;38:362-369.
84. Paskowitz RA. "Rollerball" ablation of the uterus. J Reprod Med 1995;40:333-336.
85. Pasquali R. Antenucci D, Casimirri F, Venturoli S, Paradisi R, Fabbri R, Balestra V, Melchiondra N, Barbara L. Clinical and hormonal characteristics of obese amenorrheic hyperandrogenic women before and after weight loss. J Clin Endocrinol Metab 1989;68:173-179.
86. Pickles VR, Hall WJ, Best FA, Smith GN. Prostaglandins in endometrium and menstrual fluid from normal and dysmenorrheic subjects. J Obstet Gynaecol Br Comm 1965;72:185-192.
87. Prior JC, Vigna Y, Sciarreta D, Alojado N Schulzer M. Conditioning exercise decreases premenstrual symptoms: a prospective controlled 6 month trial. Fertil Steril 1987;47:402-408.
88. Rapkin AJ. The role of serotonin in premenstrual syndrome. Clin Obstet Gynecol 1992;35:629-636.
89. Rebar RW. Gonadotropin secretion in polycystic ovary disease. Seminars Reprod Endocrinol 1984;2:223-230.
90. Redei E, Freeman EW. Preliminary evidence for plasma adrenocorticotropin levels as biological correlates of premenstrual syndrome. Acta Endocrinol 1992;128:536.

91. Reid RL. Premenstrual syndrome. Curr Probl Gynecol Fertil 1985;8:1-57.
92. Renshaw DC. When the patient's chief complaint is sexual disinterest. Prim Care Update Ob/Gyns 1994;1:194-198.
93. Rickels K, Freeman EW, Sondheimer SJ, Albert J. Fluoxetine in the treatment of premenstrual syndrome. Curr Ther Res 1990;48:161-166.
94. Rivera-Tovar AD, Frank E. Late luteal phase dysphoric disorder in young women. Am J Psychiatry 1990;147:1634-1636.
95. Robinson JC, Plichta S, Weisman CS, Nathanson CA, Ensminger M. Dysmenorrhea and use of oral contraceptives in adolescent women attending a family planning clinic. Am J Obstet Gynecol 1992;166:478-483.
96. Rodriguez MH, Platt LD, Medearis AL, Lacarra M, Lobo RA. The use of transvaginal sonography for evaluation of postmenopausal ovarian size and morphology. Am J Obstet Gynecol 1988;159:810-814.
97. Rojansky N, Halbreich U, Zander K, Barkai A, Goldstein S. Imipramine receptor binding and serotonin uptake in platelets of women with premenstrual changes. Gynecol Obstet Invest 1991;31:146-152.
98. Rubinow DR, Hoban C, Grover G, Galloway DS, Roy-Byrne P, Andersen R, Merriam GR. Changes in plasma hormones across the menstrual cycle in patients with menstrually related mood disorders and in control subjects. Am J Obstet Gynecol 1988;158:5-11.
99. Rubinow DR, Roy-Bryne P, Hoban MC, Gold PW, Post RM. Prospective assessment of menstrually related mood disorders. Am J Psychiatry 1984;141:684-686.
100. Ruchhoft EA, Elkind-Hirsh KE, Malinak R. Pituitary function is altered during the same cycle in women with polycystic ovary syndrome treated with continuous or cyclic oral contraceptives on a gonadotropin-releasing hormone agonist. Fertil Steril 1996;66:54-60.
101. Russell DJ. The female pelvic mass: diagnosis and management. Med Clin N Amer 1995;79:1481-1493.
102. Sayegh R, Schiff I, Wurtman J, Spiers P, McDermott J, Wurtman R. The effect of a carbohydrate-rich beverage on mood, appetite, and cognitive function in women with premenstrual syndrome. Obstet Gynecol 1995;86:520-528.
103. Schmidt PJ, Nieman LK, Grover GN, Muller KL, Meriam GR, Rubinow DR. Lack of effect of induced menses on symptoms in women with premenstrual syndrome. New Engl J Med 1991;324:1174-1179.
104. Schover LR, Jensen SB. Sexuality and chronic illness. New York: Guilford Press, 1988.
105. Seltzer V. Screening for ovarian cancer: an overview of the screening recommendations of the 1994 NIH consensus conference. Prim Care Update Ob/Gyn 1995;2:132-134.
106. Shangold M, Rebar RW, Colston Wentz A, Schiff I. Evaluation and management of menstrual dysfunction in athletes. JAMA 1990;263:1665-1669.
107. Shaw RW. Assessment of medical treatments of menorrhagia. Br J Obstet Gynaecol 1994;101 (Suppl 11):15-18.
108. Shoupe D. Premenstrual syndrome: diagnosis and management. In: Mishell DR Jr, Brenner PF (eds). Management of common problems in obstetrics and gynecology. Boston: Blackwell Scientific Publications, 1994.
109. Smith RP. Cyclic pelvic pain and dysmenorrhea. Obstet Gynecol Clin North America 1993;20:753-764.

110. Smith SK, Abel MH, Kelly RW, Baird DT. Prostaglandin synthesis in the endometrium of women with ovular dysfunctional uterine bleeding. Br J Obstet Gynaecol 1981;88:434-442.
111. Somerville BW. The role of estradiol withdrawal in the etiology of menstrual migraine. Neurology 1972;22:355-365.
112. Speroff L, Glass RH, Kase NG. Clinical gynecologic endocrinology and infertility. 5th edition. Baltimore: Williams & Wilkins, 1994.
113. Steege JF, Blumenthal JA. The effects of aerobic exercise on premenstrual symptoms in middle-aged women: a preliminary study. J Psychosom Res 1992;37:127-133.
114. Steiner M. Female-specific mood disorders. Clin Obstet Gynecol 1992;35:599-611.
115. Steiner M, Steinberg S, Stewart D, Carter D, Berger C, Reid R, Grover D, Streiner D. Fluoxetine in the treatment of premenstrual dysphoria. N Engl J Med 1995;332:1529-1534.
116. Stenchever MA. Counseling the patient. Comprehensive gynecology. St. Louis MO: Mosby Yearbook, 1992;192.
117. Sulak PJ, Cressman BE, Waldrop E, Holleman S, Kuehl TJ. Extending the duration of active oral contraceptive pills to manage hormone withdrawal symptoms. Obstet Gynecol 1997;89:179-183.
118. Szigethy A, Dienes L. The relationship between atypical migraine and multiphasic oral contraceptives. Therapia Hungarica 1991;40:185-188.
119. Thomas EJ, Okuda KJ, Thomas NM. The combination of depot gonadotropin releasing hormone agonist and cyclical hormone replacement therapy for dysfunctional uterine bleeding. Br J Obstet Gynecol 1991;98:1155-1159.
120. Thys-Jacobs S, Ceccarelli S, Bierman A, Weisman H, Cohen MA, Alvir J. Calcium supplementation in premenstrual syndrome: a randomized crossover trial. J Gen Intern Med 1989;4:183-189.
121. Tolino A, Petrone A, Sarnacchiaro F, Cirillo D, Ronsini S, Lombardi G, Nappi C. Finasteride in the treatment of hirsutism: new therapeutic perspectives. Fertil Steril 1996;66:61-65.
122. Tolman EL, Partridge R. Multiple sites of interaction between prostaglandins and nonsteroidal anti-inflammatory agents. Prostaglandins 1975;9:349-359.
123. Valens L. When a woman's body says no to sex. New York: Penguin Books, 1988.
124. Van Zak DB. Biofeedback treatments for premenstrual and premenstrual affective syndromes. Int J Psychosom 1994;41:53-60.
125. Vercellini P, DeGiorgi O, Oldani S, Cortesi I, Panazza S, Crosignani PG. Depot medroxyprogesterone acetate versus an oral contraceptive combined with very-low-dose danazol for long-term treatment of pelvic pain associated with endometriosis. Am J Obstet Gynecol 1996;175:396-401.
126. Warren MP, Holderness CC, Lesobre V, Tzen R. Hypothalamic amenorrhea and hidden nutritional insults. J Soc Gynecol Invest 1994;1:84-88.
127. Wild RA, Painter PC, Coulson PB, Carruth KB, Ranney GB. Lipoprotein lipid concentrations and cardiovascular risk in women with polycystic ovary syndrome. J Clin Endocrinol Metab 1985;61:946-951.
128. Wilson L, Kurzrok R. Uterine contractility in functional dysmenorrhea. Endocrinology 1940;27:23-28.

129. Yatham LN. Is 5HT$_{1A}$ receptor subsensitivity a trait marker for late luteal phase dysphoric disorder? A pilot study. Can J Psychiatry 1993;38:662-664.
130. Yonkers KA, Halbreich U, Freeman EW. Efficacy of sertraline for treatment of premenstrual dysphoric disorder [abstract #NR278]. New research program and abstracts of the American Psychiatric Association 148th annual meeting, May 20-25, 1995, Miami, FL.

HIV/AIDS and Reproductive Health

Felicia Guest, MPH, CHES

7

- Women age 15 to 44 years constitute the fastest-growing segment of the U.S. epidemic of human immunodeficiency virus (HIV). Many are not aware of their infection.
- Every patient merits skill-building for HIV prevention. Ask each person, "What do you do to protect yourself from AIDS?"
- Reproductive health care settings are a critical conduit to HIV testing. The standard of care is to offer counseling and voluntary testing to each patient.

- The standard of prenatal care is to counsel and to strongly recommend voluntary HIV testing for all pregnant women. Offer infected women drug regimens that can reduce the likelihood of perinatal transmission.
- Ensure infected women have access to primary and reproductive health care, either by direct treatment or careful referral.
- Preventing unintended pregnancy in infected women is a more humane and more cost-effective approach to preventing perinatal transmission than are antiretroviral drug regimens.

TRENDS IN WOMEN OF REPRODUCTIVE AGE

Infection with the human immunodeficiency virus (HIV) is a global pandemic, with 90% of cases occurring in developing countries, where a small percentage of the world's HIV prevention resources are deployed. Some 31 million people have been infected as of late 1997, including perhaps 12 million women. On almost every continent, acquired immunodeficiency syndrome (AIDS) is a leading cause of death among young women. Most have been infected via sexual exposure to infected men.[43,77]

Between 115,000 to 155,000 U.S. women are already infected with HIV.[44] They are demographically similar to women who seek reproductive health care in family planning, prenatal, abortion, and STI service sites. Several other characteristics describe the epidemic in women:

Young women. Women with HIV are young. About 22% of women are 20 to 29 years old when their AIDS is reported, suggesting many were infected in their teen years. All states report cases of AIDS, and 28 states report cases of HIV infection. Through 1996, 80% of women with AIDS and 90% of women with HIV were 13 to 44 years old.[16] Another disturbing trend is that younger groups have higher proportions of infected females than do older groups. Among AIDS cases reported in 1996, 19% of those age 25 and older were women, compared with 37% of 20 to 24-year-olds and 46% of teenagers.[16]

Women of color. Black and Hispanic women are disproportionately represented by reported AIDS cases, particularly in urban areas of the Northeast and the rural South. About 84% of children with perinatally acquired AIDS are black or Hispanic.[16]

Heterosexual women. Heterosexually acquired HIV is increasing rapidly in women. Sex with an HIV-infected male accounts for 40% of all AIDS cases in U.S. women in recent years. Heterosexual exposure is a major risk factor among younger women, accounting for 53% of cumulative cases among 20- to 24-year-olds and 54% among teenagers.[16] The number of women with heterosexually acquired HIV may be higher than what is officially reported. Women are twice as likely as men to have their AIDS reported without an established risk factor for transmission, and many of these "no identified risk" cases may have been transmitted heterosexually.[22]

Women who have sex with women can also be at risk. Although the frequency of woman-to-woman sexual HIV transmission is rare, these women may be at risk for HIV from injecting drug use, heterosexual sex, and other risk factors. In San Francisco, for example, 40% of lesbian and bisexual women reported unsafe heterosexual sex practices and 10% of the group reported injecting drug use. The HIV prevalence rate among these women was 1.2%.[51]

Injecting drug users. Injecting drug use played a huge role in the first decade of AIDS in U.S. women. About 45% of all AIDS cases are among women who injected drugs with shared and uncleaned injection equipment. Thousands more women were infected by male sex partners who were injecting-drug users.[16]

Geographic clustering. States in the Northeast and South have a higher incidence of women with HIV than other states, and urban areas have a higher incidence than small towns and rural areas, except in rural areas of the South where prevalence is high, particularly among childbearing women.[74]

HIV PREVENTION IN THE REPRODUCTIVE HEALTH CARE SETTING

All reproductive health care patients merit some sort of HIV prevention intervention. Even the patient in a long-term mutually faithful relationship is theoretically one risky choice away from HIV, whether that choice is made by her or by her partner. Many patients are not in long-term mutually faithful relationships. Others want and need new HIV prevention skills to help others, including their own children.

Prevention takes place on multiple levels. *Primary* prevention: Uninfected women remain uninfected by using condoms and other safer sex techniques, and by avoiding IV drug use, especially with shared equipment. *Secondary* prevention: Infected women who do not want a pregnancy choose the best possible contraceptive and practice safer sex techniques to protect uninfected sex partners. *Tertiary* prevention: Infected pregnant women reduce their likelihood of perinatal transmission by taking antiretroviral drug regimens.

HIV RISK ASSESSMENT

Ask each and every patient, *"What do you do to protect yourself from AIDS?"*[5] You can always encourage your patient, even during a brief discussion, to take one step further in skill mastery. You may even be able to determine readiness for behavior change by assessing the answer given to your question. The patient who answers, "I thought I would get some condoms while I'm here today" is more ready to try new behavior than is the patient who answers, "Who, me?" (See Chapter 10 on Education and Counseling.)

With new patients, and with all patients in areas of high HIV prevalence, use a more explicit HIV risk assessment checklist (Table 7-1) whenever time allows. These questions provide a springboard to assess each patient's personal experiences. Although reproductive health physicians are more likely than other primary care physicians to ask about sex and drug behavior,[46] many are reluctant to risk offending patients. It may be helpful to begin with, "I'm going to ask you some personal questions that we ask everyone because we think it is so important to your health. Is that all right with you?"

Simply ask questions or give patients a questionnaire to complete. Understand your client population's literacy skills and cultural feelings about open sexual discussion. Always provide a private setting. Document only what is critical to good patient care, and rigorously protect the written record under lock and key. Once the questionnaire has been discussed, some health care providers return it to the patient with the assurance that only minimal information will be recorded.

Table 7-1 Assessing HIV risk behaviors

Answer these questions for all the time in your life from 1977 to now.

Sex

Had an oral, vaginal, or anal sexual experience with another person?

With how many different people? One? Two or three? Four to 10? More than 10?

Have your partners been men, women, or both? What about your partner's partners?

Ever felt that a sex partner put you at risk for AIDS? (injecting drug user, bisexual)

Ever had a sexually transmitted infection, such as herpes, gonorrhea, genital warts, or chlamydia?

Ever had sex against your will?

What do you do to protect yourself from AIDS?

Do you use male condoms? Female condoms? Other barriers? Please describe how you use them.

Drugs

Used injecting drugs with shared equipment, including street drugs, steroids?

Had sex with a person who uses and shares?

Had sex while stoned, high, or drunk, so that you can't remember details?

Exchanged sex for drugs, money, shelter?

Blood

Had a blood transfusion?

Had sex with a person who had a blood transfusion?

Have hemophilia?

Had sex with a person with hemophilia?

Received donor semen, egg, transplanted organ or tissue?

Shared equipment for tattoo, body piercing?

Other

Ever had a test for HIV?

Ever worried about AIDS, and would like to talk to someone about it?

Avoid making an "ophthalmic" assessment, that is, deciding a patient's sexual and other behaviors based on appearances:

- Single people have many partners and risky practices.
- Older people have few partners and infrequent sex.
- Sexually experienced people know how to use safer sex techniques.
- Married people are heterosexual.
- People with good jobs don't use drugs.

Remember that terminology can sometimes get in the way of clarity with this type of risk assessment. For example, teens may not know the word "monogamous." Lay people may think "sexually active" means vigorous sex, or lots of partners. Many people who engage in same-gender sexual practices do not think of themselves as "homosexual."

SUBSTANCE ABUSE ASSESSMENT

Assess substance use. A survey of high-school-age students found one-third of boys and one-sixth of girls used alcohol or drugs the last time they had intercourse.[14] Abuse of alcohol and drugs increases HIV risk because of potentially self-destructive risk taking, such as sex with someone just met or exchanging sex for drugs, money, food, or shelter. The riskiest substance-using behavior of all is using uncleaned injection equipment. Having sex with an injecting-drug user is also extremely risky, and because injecting-drug use in the present or past is often a carefully hidden practice, some patients will not be aware that a sex partner uses injecting drugs.

Ask behavior-based screening questions such as, "How many drinks of beer, wine, spritzers, and hard liquor have you had in the last 7 days?" "Do you ever have sex when you are so stoned or drunk or high that you don't remember the details?" "Do you think alcohol or drugs ever got you into trouble?"

EXPLICIT SAFER SEX SKILLS

Teach explicit safer sex skills, including correct use of male and female condoms and other latex and plastic barriers, to all at-risk patients (Table 7-2). Be sure to discuss prevention skill for oral sex, because HIV transmission through oral sex appears possible (perhaps especially during the weeks of primary HIV infection).[68]

Advise all patients that a crucial time for diligent safer sex practices is the first 3 months of a new relationship. Delaying intercourse allows for a deeper relationship, a fuller assessment of partner trustworthiness, and an opportunity to get an HIV test. Using male or female latex or plastic condoms consistently during the more infectious early HIV infection interval protects against what might be a legacy from a recent past relationship.[66]

Use audiovisual, print, and electronic teaching aids appropriate to the patient's comfort, pleasure, age, and learning style.

PARTNER ASSESSMENT SKILLS

Teach patients to ask about and look for genital tract infections in sexual partners. Genital tract shedding of HIV increases in the presence of other

Table 7-2 Safer sex options for physical intimacy

Safe

Sexual fantasies
Massage
Hugging
Body rubbing
Dry kissing
Masturbation without contact with partner's semen or vaginal secretions
Erotic conversation, books, movies, videos
Erotic bathing, showering
Eroticizing feet, fingers, buttocks, abdomen, ears, other body parts
All sexual activities, when both partners are monogamous, trustworthy, and known by testing to be free of HIV

Possibly Safe

Wet kissing with no broken skin, cracked lips, or damaged mouth tissue
Hand-to-genital touching (hand job) or mutual masturbation on healthy, intact skin or with a latex or plastic barrier
Vaginal or anal intercourse using latex or plastic condom correctly with adequate lubrication
Oral sex on a man using a latex or plastic condom
Oral sex on a woman using a latex or plastic barrier such as a female condom, dental dam, or modified male condom (especially if she does not have her period or a vaginal infection with discharge)
All sexual activities, when both partners agree to a monogamous relationship and trust each other

Unsafe in the absence of HIV testing and trust and monogamy

Blood contact of any kind, including menstrual blood
Any vaginal or anal intercourse without a latex or plastic condom
Oral sex on a woman without a latex or plastic barrier such as a female condom, dental dam or modified male condom (especially if she is having her period or has a vaginal infection with discharge)
Semen in the mouth
Oral-anal contact
Shared sex toys or douching equipment
Any sex (fisting, rough vaginal or anal intercourse, rape) that causes tissue damage or bleeding

untreated infections,[72] so advise patients to avoid sex or at least use condoms until a health care provider can answer any questions about HIV and other infections.

SKILL-BUILDING

Teach skills, not just facts. Most Americans know what AIDS is, know it is lethal, and know it is transmitted through sexual fluids and blood. However, sexual decisions are not generally based on reason. Human beings tend to act not out of what they know, but out of what they *feel* and *see* and *want*. Patients need our help, therefore, with skills for forging relationships with trustworthy low-risk people, sexual negotiating in relationships, and operating from an internal value system rather than from external pressures.

POSTEXPOSURE PROPHYLAXIS

In cases of isolated high-risk exposures to HIV—unprotected vaginal or anal intercourse, rape, receptive oral sex with ejaculation, or sharing injection equipment when the partner is known or suspected to be infected—postexposure chemoprophylaxis may be considered. Begin treatment as soon as possible, up to 72 hours after exposure, using a 4-week regimen of zidovudine (200 milligrams [mg] three times a day) and lamivudine (150 mg twice a day). Add a protease inhibitor such as indinavir (800 mg three times a day) if the infected partner has advanced disease, a high viral load, or has been treated with antiretroviral medications.[45]

FACTORS AFFECTING HIV PREVENTION

At least 75% to 85% of the 31 million HIV infections worldwide have been sexually transmitted.[43,77] Likelihood of sexual HIV transmission is variable, and is influenced by characteristics in both the infected partner and the uninfected partner.[66] Risk of sexual transmission may be *increased*:

- During early HIV infection, the first months of illness when infectiousness is high
- During late HIV infection, when infectiousness often increases as the immune system becomes less effective in controlling the virus
- When the infected partner has a concurrent reproductive tract infection (RTI)
- When the uninfected partner has cervical ectopy

Risk of transmission may be *decreased*:

- If the infected partner follows an effective antiretroviral drug regimen
- If the uninfected partner has a specific mutation in an HIV receptor gene
- If either the infected or the uninfected partner is circumcised

Contraceptive Choice

Contraceptive method also influences the likelihood of sexual transmission. One powerful reason women of all ages like oral contraceptives, other hormonal methods, intrauterine devices (IUDs), and surgical sterilization is that nothing mechanical or intrusive gets in the way of lovemaking. Therefore, special effort may be needed to encourage these patients to add male or female condoms for HIV protection. An inverse relationship exists between the use of more effective noncoital contraceptives and concurrent condom use.[8,15] In Baltimore, for example, more than three-fourths of sterilized women never used a condom, compared with 46% of nonsterilized women.[15] Among 12,000 U.S. high school students, 19% of pill users also used condoms at last intercourse, compared with 54% of other sexually active students; pill use was the single strongest predictor of failure to use condoms, even stronger than alcohol or drug use or multiple partners.[24] Pills-plus-condoms is by no means the norm for sexual protection. This behavior is rarely modeled in the media, and pregnancy often feels more like a genuine personal threat than does HIV. Almost everyone knows someone involved in an unplanned pregnancy, while many people have never (to their knowledge) known anyone with HIV.

Male condoms. The take-home message for all patients is that always using male condoms and always using them correctly works as HIV prevention. Halfway measures do not work.[38,65] The counseling goal is to teach this message without causing patients to conclude, "Nobody's perfect every time, so why bother using them at all?" Help patients clarify their personal barriers to condom use, and support their efforts to come as close to consistent, correct use as they possibly can.

Latex and plastic condoms are the best way to reduce HIV risk during intercourse and fellatio. In a study of HIV-discordant heterosexual partners, no HIV infections occurred among couples who always used condoms, versus a 10% infection rate in couples who used condoms intermittently.[31] Three other studies of HIV-discordant couples have demonstrated a protective effect from condoms.[38]

Giving patients precise answers about how much protection they can count on remains difficult. One problem is that we do not know how to factor in slippage and breakage effects. (See Chapter 16 on Male Condoms.) Further, other behavioral and biological factors play a role in HIV transmission. Most HIV-infected men shed HIV in semen intermittently, regardless of disease stage or antiretroviral treatment. An infected man can never safely omit condoms and other safer sex behaviors.[47] Help patients understand that male condoms prevent sexual HIV transmission, but more precise quantifying of condom efficacy depends on personal circumstances and behaviors.

Timing when to put on a male condom is a practical issue. Some men leak seminal fluid from the urethral meatus once the penis is fully erect. This clear pre-ejaculatory fluid can contain HIV and other pathogens (although not motile sperm capable of causing pregnancy).[39,62] When a condom is used for safer sex, it must be rolled on the penis well before the penis has any contact with the partner's mouth, vagina, anus, or any broken skin.

Spermicides. For decades, nonoxynol-9-based spermicide products have been the "chicken soup" of reproductive health care, as providers have generally advised users of other contraceptive methods to add a spermicide for improved contraceptive efficacy and for STI protection. In the late 1990s this advice is being re-evaluated in the context of HIV risk, in part because spermicide can cause vulvovaginal microabrasions and altered vaginal flora, which could theoretically increase susceptibility to HIV. Evidence is conflicting, with the best evidence demonstrating no protective effect against HIV for nonoxynol-9.[64] Also, how HIV-negative partners might be affected by vulvovaginal microabrasions in an HIV-infected woman is unclear.

Epithelial disruption could be affected by spermicide dose, delivery system, or frequency of use,[38] so it may be prudent to caution patients who use spermicides routinely.

Although the Public Health Service recommends latex condoms with *or* without spermicide for HIV prevention,[21] patients concerned about vaginal or penile irritation may want to avoid spermicidally lubricated brands. (See Chapter 16 on Male Condoms and Chapter 17 on Vaginal Spermicides.)

Oral contraceptives. The combined oral contraceptive pill may increase the vascularity of the cervical epithelium, extend the area of cervical ectopy, and alter certain immune parameters.[7,38] Whether combined pill use increases susceptibility to HIV in any way, for women or for their male partners, remains unclear. Advise pill users to use male or female latex or plastic condoms unless they are confident both partners are free of HIV and other STIs.

Progestin pills, implants, and injections. In rhesus monkeys, female animals given progesterone implants were more likely to be infected by a vaginal exposure to SIV (a virus similar to HIV) than were animals without progesterone.[53] One possible explanation for the higher risk in monkeys is progesterone-mediated thinning of their vaginal epithelium. However, human studies of Depo-Provera users do not show an HIV prevalence pattern consistent with increased susceptibility.[32] Moreover, vaginal biopsies of Norplant users do not show increased epithelial thinning. On the basis of the inconsistency of these findings, encourage users of these methods to add male or female latex or plastic condoms unless they are certain both partners are free of HIV.

IUDs. Reproductive health clinicians routinely advise against the IUD for the patient at high risk for RTIs, including HIV. However, current data support wider IUD use by women at moderate-to-low risk of RTI. A past history of STI, if cured, does not rule out IUD use for women desiring this method. Factors that might increase the risk of HIV transmission by women using IUDs are longer, heavier periods and disrupted endometrial or cervical epithelium.[38]

Female condoms. In vitro studies show that this condom is an effective barrier against HIV transmission, but no human studies of transmission effects exist.[38]

Diaphragms and cervical caps. No data exist on the efficacy of diaphragms or caps for HIV protection. HIV can be heterosexually transmitted to a woman via vaginal exposure alone, so diaphragms and caps that cover the cervix and a small portion of the vagina may not offer adequate protection.[38] (See Chapter 18 on Vaginal Barriers.)

Sterilization. Tubal sterilization has no known effect on HIV transmission risk. HIV persists in semen after vasectomy.[38,59]

Male Circumcision

Lack of circumcision increases the risk of sexual HIV acquisition for both women and men. The foreskin may cause vaginal microabrasions during intercourse,[38] and it may hold HIV, as it does other pathogens, in a moist environment that facilitates transmission to the male.[56,73]

Advice for Contraceptive Patients

Until further data are available, it seems prudent to advise all patients as follows:

- Use male or female latex or plastic condoms each time you suspect even the slightest risk of HIV but choose to have vaginal or anal intercourse anyway.

- Use latex or plastic condoms for men and latex or plastic vulvar barriers for women any time you suspect any risk of HIV but choose to have oral sex anyway.

- If you cannot use condoms, vaginal spermicides are a weaker option to prevent bacterial infections such as gonorrhea and chlamydia.[7] Vaginal spermicides are not recommended to protect against HIV.[21]

- Any tissue damage to the vulva or vagina or penis could increase susceptibility to HIV and other RTIs. Avoid intercourse until you are healed. See your care provider for help with healing.

- These directions can be modified for gay male, lesbian, and bisexual patients.

SPECIAL CONSIDERATIONS IN HIV PREVENTION

Romance. It is difficult to hold simultaneously the two thoughts, "I am in love with you," and "You might pose an infection risk to me." Romantic (germ-free) fantasy is a hallmark of midadolescence,[42] and many people never manage to be clear-eyed about romance even when realism pervades other aspects of the adult world view. Therefore, the reproductive health care provider is frequently in the unenviable position of bubble-burster, attempting to foster self-protective health behavior where there is only desire, emotional need, and single-minded devotion to the idealized romantic relationship.

Effective HIV prevention counseling with patients who are in love does not set up the beloved as a bad person, but stresses that all people can and do harm other people even when they do not mean to, and that people who love each other would certainly try to help each other maintain good health!

Power. Sometimes women make a personal commitment to HIV prevention but have little hope of enlisting the cooperation of the male partner. They say, for example, "You might as well not give me any condoms, because I know he won't use them." In all U.S. cultural groups, women typically lack economic, social, and personal power equal to that of men. Even when couples negotiate and achieve a relationship with equal decision-making power, they are likely to have begun the relationship with a power imbalance.

One direct way to address this issue is to invite women to bring in their partners and to offer prevention skill-building for these men, either together with the female partner or alone. When men cannot or will not come in, offer telephone counseling with a male counselor. When no way exists to speak directly with the patient's partner, give patients audiotape or print messages to give to men. Remember that community and cultural norms vary substantially in how sexual decisions are made and by whom, so be sure counseling is grounded in the reality of your patient's life. For example, assess her risk of abuse, battering, rape, or abandonment should she insist on condom use.

A woman-controlled vaginal microbicide is a high research priority for HIV prevention,[70] but it may be a decade away. Meanwhile, women at risk must be encouraged to use male and female latex or plastic condoms and other safer sex techniques as consistently as they possibly can, even when they are unaccustomed to such expressions of personal power.

Special needs of adolescents. The critical challenge is to implement effective HIV prevention strategies for adolescents who are entering into sexual and perhaps drug-use experimentation. Interventions in the first 15 years of the HIV epidemic have increased knowledge (86.3% of high schoolers have been taught about HIV in school[14]) and sometimes led to modest behavior change. However, in general, adolescents still take too many risks. More than half of all high school students have had intercourse, and about half of them report using a condom the last time they had sex.[14] Among a cohort of urban adolescents moving into young adulthood, risk-taking behaviors remained about the same over a 5-year period, regardless of their knowledge about HIV, number of sources of information, acquaintance with infected people, perception of personal risk, or experience with HIV test counseling.[71] Most of these young people disliked condoms, did not use them on a regular basis, and did not trust condoms to be protective.

A bold six-step plan for improving HIV-prevention efforts with adolescents is essential:[36]

- Use teenagers as spokespersons, and not as irresponsible stereotypes, in prevention campaigns.
- Replace abstinence-only campaigns with a more balanced approach aimed at delaying first intercourse and other risky sexual experimentation.
- Saturate the adolescent environment with appropriate and explicit risk-reduction messages.
- Link prevention programs with easy access to testing and medical services.
- Help adults learn to deal with sexuality and HIV, including parents, teachers, youth workers, and health care workers.
- Link on-site condom availability with HIV prevention programs in schools and youth agencies.

Deciding to be safe. Deciding to protect oneself (and others) from HIV is not one choice, like flipping a switch, but rather a series of hundreds of choices made day after day in the arenas of sex and drug use. When patients tell their stories, point out to them all their decision points, the places where they made safe and unsafe decisions, and whether they made them actively or passively. An important take-home message for patients is that HIV prevention decisions are made *every single day*, and we can always learn from our past experiences.

HIV TESTING AND COUNSELING

About one-third of U.S. women age 18 to 44 have had an HIV test, excluding those tested as blood donors.[17] An increasing number of reproductive health care facilities now offer HIV testing as a standard component of their services.

WHEN TO OFFER TESTING

No more important conduit to HIV testing services exists for women than the reproductive health care provider. *Offer routine counseling and voluntary HIV testing with informed consent to all women.* With tools to help uninfected women remain uninfected, to help control the advance of HIV-related immunodeficiency and illness, and to markedly reduce the likelihood of perinatal transmission, providers can do no less. This policy is the standard of care in the United States, endorsed by the American College of Obstetricians and Gynecologists (ACOG),[2] the American College of Nurse-Midwives,[1] and the Centers for Disease Control and Prevention.[13] Routine counseling and voluntary HIV testing for all *pregnant* women are further endorsed by the American Academy of Pediatrics and ACOG in a joint statement.[3]

Even with a policy of routine counseling and voluntary testing, certain situations require extra effort to assure that patients have access to HIV counseling and testing services:

- Any time the patient requests testing
- Any time history reveals a present or past sex or drug-use risk behavior (Table 7-1)
- Any time the patient is pregnant or planning a pregnancy
- Any time you diagnose gynecological or other infections or constitutional signs consistent with HIV infection (see the section on Medical Care and Psychosocial Support for Infected Women)
- Any time the patient has had an STI
- Any time history reveals consensual or coerced sex with a person whose health history and HIV status are unknown
- Any time the patient had a blood transfusion before March 1985 or has had multiple transfusions of blood or blood products at any time
- Any time the patient has lived in a geographic area where HIV is endemic
- Any time the patient has a workplace or other injury or accident that could result in HIV exposure

TEST COUNSELING

The decision to be tested for HIV belongs to the patient. Your role is to explain how the test is done, what the routine screening procedure will and will not reveal, characteristics of anonymous and confidential testing, and instructions on learning test results. Some patients do not return for test results, so use the pre-test session to teach personalized and explicit risk-reduction skills. A counselor checklist (Table 7-3) for the pretest session (and for devising an informed consent document) and checklists for giving negative and positive test results to patients may be helpful (Tables 7-4 and 7-5). All providers who give positive HIV-antibody test results to patients will need training to master the particular skills of breaking bad news.[61] This special encounter must help support the patient, while it accomplishes at least one or two educational goals. Many patients report that they remember little or nothing the care provider said after hearing the word, "positive."

Table 7-3 Components of pre-test counseling

Reason for considering test

- Elicit patient's reason(s) so counselor can be as helpful as possible

About the HIV antibody test

- What kind of sample is used for testing: blood, oral mucosal transudate, urine
- What antibodies are
- How soon the test is accurate
- Why this is not a test for AIDS

How people get infected with HIV

- Through unprotected oral, vaginal, or anal intercourse with an infected person
- Through bloodstream-to-bloodstream contact with an infected person
    - Sharing equipment for injectable drugs, steroids, tattoos, skin piercing
    - Transfusion of blood product before March 1985
- From infected woman to child during pregnancy, labor and delivery, or breastfeeding. Risk depends on amount of virus in woman's body; usual risk 15-30%, but can be reduced with medication

Deciding whether to have the test

- Your right to decide whether to be tested
- Unforced informed consent
- Anonymous versus confidential testing
- Who will see the results if test is done here, including state law
- Other sites for testing; home collection kit

(continued)

Table 7-3 Components of pre-test counseling *(cont.)*

Benefits of being tested

- Peace of mind; knowing, one way or the other
- If infected:
  - — Begin treatments for slowing HIV, managing related problems
  - — Prevent transmission to others
  - — Make informed childbearing decisions
  - — Diagnose illness or symptoms
  - — Access assistance programs

Difficulties with being tested

- Anxiety, waiting for results
- If infected:
  - — Learning you have a very serious illness
  - — Telling sex or injecting-drug-equipment-sharing partners
  - — Possible relationship difficulties with partner, family, friends
  - — Possible threat to job
  - — Possible difficulty getting or keeping insurance
  - — Few experienced care providers in some locales

What your results will mean

- If antibody positive:
  - — You are infected
  - — You can pass the virus on to other people
- If antibody negative or indeterminate:
  - — You are not infected

    or
  - — You are infected, but your body has not yet made enough antibodies for test to be positive

Reducing risk for HIV

- Develop a personalized risk reduction plan today with counselor (using Tables 7-1 and 7-2 as starting points)

For more information

- National AIDS Hotline 800/342-AIDS
- Local and regional hotlines
- Resources to meet personal needs

Source: Modified from Southeast AIDS Training and Education Center (1997) with permission.

Table 7-4 Post-test counseling for negative results

Give results promptly. Do not expect people to digest much advice once they have their results. Allow time for supportive counseling about relief, other personal feelings and concerns, then move to education and skill-building. Information can be reinforced in print. Make return appointment for more skill-building if warranted and reasonable.

What the HIV antibody screening test looked for

- Antibodies to HIV, not the virus itself (additional tests can look for the virus itself)
- Evidence of infection acquired longer ago than 1–6 months

What negative results mean

- You may not have been exposed

  or

- You may have been exposed, but did not become infected; you cannot count on this good fortune in the future

  or

- You were infected recently, and it is too soon for the test to be positive; if you have had a possible exposure in the past 6 months, consider getting another test 2-3 months from now, and use safer sex and other prevention measures in the meantime

Reducing risk for HIV

- Develop a personalized risk reduction plan today with counselor (using Tables 7-1 and 7-2 as starting points)

How this office can help

- Condoms and other safer sex supplies
- Help with a risk reduction plan
- Referral for drug, alcohol treatment

For more information

- National AIDS Hotline 800/342-AIDS
- Local and regional hotlines
- Resources to meet personal needs

Source: Modified from Southeast AIDS Training and Education Center (1997) with permission.

Table 7-5 Post-test counseling for positive results

Give results promptly. Do not expect people to take in much new information after they hear that they are infected. Allow plenty of time for supportive counseling about feelings, following patient's lead. Give information in print to read later on, and make a return appointment or referral for ongoing counseling and care. Be sure patients have a reasonable plan of action (where to go when they leave you, whom to tell, etc.) before leaving your office.

What the positive HIV antibody screening test result means

- You have antibodies for HIV in your blood (oral transudate, urine or other tested body fluid)
- You are infected with the virus that causes AIDS
- You can pass the virus on to other people

What the test result does NOT tell you

- How long you have been infected
- Whether you already have AIDS
- The present status of your immune system

Could the test be wrong?

- On rare occasions, a negative person's test result comes back positive
- The chance of this happening is less than 1 in 1000
- Consider being retested by a different testing laboratory if you believe your test result is wrong

What next?

- Learn about HIV; for many people, knowledge is emotional and physical power
- Visit a care provider experienced with HIV for a workup, including
  — T-cell count (CD4 count)
  — Viral load test
  — TB test
  — Any needed medicines

- Start now to keep your body as healthy as you can
  — Eat well, get plenty of rest, moderate exercise
  — Limit or stop drugs that you drink, inhale, inject, or swallow
  — Avoid new STIs (sexually transmissible infections) and treat any infections you have (these infections can increase the amount of HIV in your body)

How this office can help

- Assist with or refer for immediate needs (housing, financial)
- Help you tell others about your HIV
- Answer your questions, and questions from friends and family
- Assist with finding a care provider experienced with HIV
- Supply condoms and other safer sex equipment
- Supply contraception for you, partner
- Help you develop a plan of action
- Assist with or refer for emotional support resources
- Other, based on resources available

(continued)

Table 7-5 Post-test counseling for positive results *(cont.)*

Whom you should tell

- Medical and dental care providers, so proper care can be offered
- Past and present sex partners and people with whom you shared injecting drug equipment
- Learn about HIV before you talk to him/her/them
  — Talk in private
  — Avoid casting blame
  — Think ahead of time how to react if the person gets upset
  — Strongly suggest testing as soon as possible
    • For peace of mind, if negative
    • For early access to medicine to control HIV
    • For taking steps to avoid giving HIV to others
    • For informed childbearing decisions

How to avoid giving HIV to others

- Tear up any donor cards
- Do not donate blood, tissue, eggs, semen, organs
- Do not share razors, toothbrushes (in case any blood is on them)
- Clean up spilled blood or bloody body fluids promptly, using bleach and water
- Inform sex partner, and negotiate a safer sex plan ahead of time
- Do not share injection drug, tattoo, or body piercing equipment
- Limit or stop any drug use that impairs your judgment (alcohol, crack, cocaine)
- Avoid pregnancy, or use medicine during pregnancy to reduce risk of HIV for child
- Avoid breastfeeding

For more information

- National AIDS Hotline 800/342-AIDS
- Local support resources for HIV-infected persons
- Resources to meet personal needs, e.g. drug treatment

Source: Modified from Southeast AIDS Training and Education Center (1997) with permission.

Counselors who are experienced at HIV test counseling generally allow 15 to 30 minutes for a pre-test session, 10 to 15 minutes for a negative post-test session, and 30 to 45 minutes or longer for a positive post-test session.

We naturally dread telling a young woman she has a grave illness. Test counseling is time-consuming. It also requires training and mastery of new referral sources. Be careful to provide sensitive staff training and support both before and after your work setting initiates testing and counseling.

COUNSELING AND TESTING ISSUES

Anonymous vs. confidential testing. Anonymous testing never links a name to the sample presented for evaluation (although age, county of residence, sex, and other general demographic characteristics are often recorded). The anonymous patient is given a number code to bring back or telephone in after a specific time interval for getting test results. Confidential testing is name-linked, and information is protected to a degree determined by state law and the formal policies and staff commitment to confidentiality at the testing site.

Allow patients to choose the approach they prefer, and be prepared to make a careful referral for anonymous testing if you do not provide it on-site. Most laboratories are willing to work out a coding system for anonymous samples. Patients not offered anonymous testing and reluctant to have an HIV test on record are likely to go to a test site where they are not known and to use a false name. Another alternative for anonymous testing is home collection of a test sample using an over-the-counter kit, discussed below.

Discourage patients who have recently practiced risky behaviors from donating blood as a way to learn HIV status; they could possibly donate falsely negative blood early in HIV infection.

Options for testing. Reliance on hospital-, office-, and clinic-based collection of blood for HIV testing has given way to new technologies and expanded choices.[4]

- Patients reluctant to visit a care provider can purchase a drugstore kit, collect their own finger-prick blood sample, mail off the sample to a lab, and call for anonymous results and telephone counseling a few days later.[33] One brand, Home Access, is available for about $35 to $50 per test, as of early 1997.

  Concerns about moving HIV testing out of the traditional health care setting will be familiar to reproductive health care providers who remember the advent of home pregnancy testing. What about tester error? How will people find any follow-up care they need? Will telephone counseling be supportive and skilled enough to make appropriate referrals? Early reports are reassuring. One study of home blood collection found that 98% of the time subjects were able to obtain a testable blood specimen and they correctly answered 96% of the HIV risk questions after pre-test counseling by telephone. Study subjects could elect to use interactive automated information recordings or live telephone counselors;

only one-third of subjects chose a live counselor during the pre-test or post-test call.[33]

- Patients who fear needles can search out a care provider who collects oral mucosal transudate samples for testing.[34] This test collects IgG-rich transudate onto a swab placed for 2 minutes between the lower gum and cheek. Orasure brand is sold only to health care professionals at about $99 for three tests. (Call Epitope, Inc. at 1-888-ORASURE, ext. 302 for details.)

- Providers in need of a rapid initial screening test can consider the Single-Use Diagnostic System (SUDS) from Murex for a 10-minute serum enzyme immunoassay (EIA) result, with no return visit required for negative results. Positive results require a Western blot or other confirmatory test. A 30-test kit was $283 in early 1997.[4]

- Another option for routine screening that avoids needles and blood is a urine EIA using the Sentinel kit from Seradyn, at about $816 for 192 tests. This test is slightly less sensitive (98.7%) than other EIAs.[4]

Without doubt, more technological refinements will follow, perhaps even home HIV test kits that supply rapid results without requiring a needle stick, blood, or even a live or automated telephone counselor. Be prepared to encounter patients whose first conversation with a health professional about HIV comes weeks, months, or years after learning positive test results on their own at home, in the dorm, or anywhere at all.

Test accuracy. Both the serum HIV ELISA test and the Western blot confirmatory test are very sensitive and specific.[60] Yet neither test is perfect, so an HIV test is reported as positive only after at least two ELISA tests and one Western blot or other confirmatory test are all positive. Known causes of incorrect ELISA test results are given in Table 7-6. As with any screening test, population prevalence is the single biggest factor in determining a test's predictive value; the higher the prevalence, the greater the likelihood that a positive test result means that the person is truly infected.[60] Always regard HIV test results in the context of the total patient history and clinical picture, and re-evaluate when the two are not in accord. The 23-year-old injecting-drug-using woman with thrush who tests negative merits further evaluation, as does the healthy 30-year-old lesbian woman with no drug use or transfusion history who tests positive.

Prenatal testing. Many women learn they have HIV when testing is done as part of routine prenatal care, and acceptance of HIV testing in this setting is fairly high.[40] Of women who refused prenatal testing, the most common reasons were prior HIV testing, absence of apparent exposure risk, and fear of testing.[40,75] Counseling about pregnancy options becomes an important component of post-test counseling if the HIV diagnosis is learned early in pregnancy; the patient may be overwhelmed

Table 7-6 False results with HIV antibody ELISA testing

False Negatives

Test performed too early, <3–6 months after infection
Test performed during advanced disease when ability to form antibodies is impaired
History of replacement transfusion
Bone marrow transplant
Use of test kit for antibody only to p24 antigen
Tester error

False Positives

Cross-reacting antibodies such as those against class II human leukocyte antigens (HLA),
  most often seen in multiparous women, persons with multiple transfusions
Cross-reacting antibodies against smooth muscle or parietal cells, anti-mitochondrial antibodies, antinuclear antibodies, anti-T-cell antibodies
Tester error

Source: Modified from Saag (1995).

by the large amount of highly emotional information to absorb at once. Pregnant infected women make the same sorts of reproductive decisions as uninfected women, with similar percentages of terminated pregnancies and live births. For the infected woman who chooses to continue the pregnancy, follow post-test counseling with guidance about her immune status, medicines to help control the advance of her HIV, medicines to reduce the likelihood of perinatal transmission, and the potential impact of all these medicines on her developing fetus. (See the following section for more on the care of pregnant women.)

Charting. Charting HIV test results is clearly important for ongoing medical care, although problems with confidentiality may result. This dilemma can be addressed by maintaining HIV-related information in a separate chart, by using a code for HIV test results, or by removing HIV-related information before releasing the chart. This latter practice is required by law in some states. State and local professional associations may offer guidance for appropriate charting that does not compromise patient, care provider, or health care.

MEDICAL CARE AND PSYCHOSOCIAL SUPPORT FOR INFECTED WOMEN

CHARACTERISTICS OF HIV IN WOMEN

The course of HIV infection in women is similar to the illness in men. Early symptoms, laboratory findings, opportunistic infections, treatment responses, and duration of illness are consistent with findings in men once access to care and immune status at diagnosis are taken into account.[23] Women also have a whole constellation of gynecologic problems related to HIV.

During the primary infection, most people experience a month-long flu-like or mononucleosis-like syndrome characterized by fever, skin rash, headache, diarrhea, malaise, and lethargy.[6,68] Few people recognize this syndrome as HIV, and this lack of awareness could lead to unsafe behaviors in a time of relatively high infectiousness.

After the primary infection period, adults with HIV typically feel well for months or years, then progress (especially in the absence of antiretroviral treatment) from minor skin and constitutional symptoms, to discrete opportunistic illness, to a cascade of illnesses, then to end-stage disease. Specific patterns of immune response to HIV in the first few weeks after infection may predict what pattern of progression the illness will follow. The typical duration, characteristics, CD4 cell count, viral load, and reproductive health concerns differ according to the stage of HIV infection in women (Table 7-7). Whether all people with HIV ultimately progress along this course is not clear.

Beginning in the 1980s, HIV was treated with single-drug antiretroviral medications such as zidovudine (AZT or ZDV), didanosine (DDI), lamivudine (3TC), and other nucleoside analog reverse transcriptase inhibitors. In the 1990s, non-nucleoside reverse transcriptase inhibitors, such as nevirapine, and protease inhibitors, such as indinavir and ritonavir, were added to the drug arsenal and combination therapy began to replace single-drug therapy.

Protease inhibitors are a class of antiretroviral drugs that act on an entirely different phase of the HIV life cycle than do other anti-HIV formulations. Some patients have used protease inhibitors in combination with two or more older drugs to lower viral load to undetectable levels. The combination works by making it extremely difficult for HIV to mutate into a form that is not vulnerable to the drugs. However, the daily pill-taking schedule is demanding, and HIV mutation and resistance can occur quickly if the regimen is not followed carefully. The success of this combination drug approach varies from patient to patient and long-term effects are not yet known. Moreover, combination regimens are expensive, and some patients cannot tolerate the drugs.

Combination therapy with protease inhibitors and viral load testing have made it possible to attack HIV with greater success than ever before. Viral load testing uses branched-DNA signal amplification assays to measure the actual amount of HIV in plasma, permitting an accurate determination of real-time viral activity and a rapid assessment of antiretroviral drug efficacy. For example, you can now assess baseline viral load, start one or more antiretroviral drugs, look at viral load again in 2 to 4 weeks, and quickly abandon an ineffective regimen that is not lowering viral load. Before this technology became available, care providers could only assess antiretroviral drug efficacy by watching symptoms and CD4 counts—which decline slowly as the immune system fails—over many months. Formerly the clinician had only an odometer, a record of how much damage the virus had *already done*, and now has a speedometer as well, a record of what the virus is *doing today*.

The advent of viral load testing and protease inhibitors makes it possible to demonstrate the value of a "hit it early and hit it hard" approach to HIV management, and most patients are offered some form of antiretroviral therapy as soon as they are diagnosed. Much remains to be learned about treating HIV, and many infected people have little or no access to these new technologies. Nonetheless, there is renewed hope that HIV can be a truly manageable disease.

Infected women need high-quality primary care from a clinician experienced with and comfortable with HIV management. Reproductive health care would ideally be managed in the primary health care setting also, but in some cases the primary care provider and reproductive health care provider are two different people in two different sites, so careful attention to shared information, shared decision making, and collaboration is essential.

A natural role for all staff in the care setting is to assist patients with health promotion practices that will engender optimism and contribute to well-being. Provide guidance on normal nutrition, stress management, exercise, rest, and reduction or elimination of tobacco, alcohol, and drugs.[41]

GYNECOLOGIC MANAGEMENT

The keys to successful management of gynecologic infections in women with HIV are high index of suspicion, prompt diagnosis, aggressive treatment, and secondary prophylaxis when appropriate.

Vulvovaginal candidiasis. Candidiasis is common in HIV, and recurrences may appear when immune status weakens.[23] First-line treatment is one of the topical antifungals and is usually successful. If topical treatment proves unsatisfactory, consider oral fluconazole.[9]

Human papilloma virus. Genital warts caused by human papilloma virus (HPV) are common in HIV-infected women and may progress more rapidly in the presence of a declining immune status. Consider baseline colposcopy or cervicography, 6-month Pap smear intervals, and prompt colposcopy and loop excision of any abnormal findings. Cervical intraepithelial neoplasia occurs in 25% to 50% of women with HIV, and treatment of abnormal or neoplastic cervical disease should be prompt and aggressive.[52]

Table 7-7 Stages of HIV infection and reproductive health concerns

	Primary HIV Infection/ Seroconversion	Symptom-Free	Early Symptoms	Discrete Illness/Cascade of Illness/Endstage
Duration	Average 1–8 weeks	Few months to many years	Few months to several years	Few months to several years
CD4 Cell Count/ L Normal = 500–1600	Normal or slightly low	Typically >500	Typically <500	AIDS diagnosis automatic at 200 or less
Viral Load/ml	High	Variable	Rising (without antiretroviral therapy)	High (without antiretroviral therapy)
Characteristics	Some notice a flu-like illness and rash that resolves on its own	Likely to test positive 6–12 weeks after infection	Fevers, night sweats, zoster, candida, hairy leukoplakia, skin problems, weight loss, fatigue, loss of appetite	Mild or severe multiple opportunistic bacterial, viral, fungal, parasitic infections
	Would test negative for HIV antibody in "window period" that typically lasts 6–12 weeks post-infection	Without test, may have no reason to suspect infection	Symptoms may cue testing and diagnosis	Neoplastic diseases: Kaposi's sarcoma (uncommon in women), lymphoma, cervical cancer
	Might test positive for p24 antigen or HIV RNA	With test, difficult to resolve feeling well with grave diagnosis	Should begin antiretroviral therapy	Neurologic: dementia, memory loss, peripheral neuropathy, affect, gait may be affected
		With test, loss of sense of health, and loss of uncomplicated sex	Loss of strength, stamina	Many medications daily, side effects likely. Multiple prophylaxes added to antiretroviral regimen.
		Not sure how long feeling well will last		Loss of looks, ability to work or care for self, ability to interact with others
		May begin antiretroviral therapy, especially if high viral load		Saying goodbye

(continued)

Table 7-7 Stages of HIV infection and reproductive health concerns *(cont.)*

	Primary HIV Infection/ Seroconversion	Symptom-Free	Early Symptoms	Discrete Illness/Cascade of Illness/Endstage
Reproductive Health Concerns	No screening test available for early diagnosis and so sex partner(s) and offspring may be placed at risk Assess contraception, safer sex	May not know diagnosis, so may not protect sex partner(s) and offspring May be tested as part of routine prenatal screening Offer anticipatory guidance on future pregnancy planning Pap every 6 months, aggressive management of abnormal findings Pregnancy likely to be normal except for transmission risk for offspring Assess contraception, safer sex	Pregnancy likely to be normal except for transmission risk for offspring Pap every 6 months, aggressive management of abnormal findings Aggressive management of gynecologic infections Assess contraception, safer sex	Aggressive management of reproductive tract infections (RTIs) Prophylaxis drugs may interfere with hormonal contraception; assess drug interactions Assist with short-range and long-range child care plans Pregnancy may result in prematurity, low birth weight, premature rupture of membranes, other complications Pap every 6 months, aggressive management of abnormal findings Assess contraception, safer sex
Risk of Transmission to Offspring	15–50% each pregnancy without treatment. Decreased to one-third with treatment.	15–30% each pregnancy without treatment. Decreased to one-third with treatment.	15–30% each pregnancy without treatment. Decreased to one-third with treatment.	15–30% each pregnancy without treatment. Risk may rise as disease advances.

Source: Modified from McKusick (1992).

Pelvic inflammatory disease (PID). Most HIV specialists recommend inpatient management of PID using standard CDC treatment regimens for all women.[23] With proper treatment, the course of PID in HIV-infected women is similar to PID in other women.

Herpes. Herpes lesions may be more extensive, more painful, and slower to heal in the presence of immune dysfunction. Consider suppressive doses of acyclovir, although acyclovir resistance can develop.[9]

Menstrual problems. Two cross-sectional studies did not find significant menstrual changes in women with CD4 counts above 200. It may be that studies of more profoundly immunosuppressed women will increase our understanding of HIV-related menstrual abnormalities.[27] Infected women, like other women, cope with menopause and may need hormonal replacement therapy.[28] Hormonal intervention also may be offered for heavy bleeding and anemia and to ease discomfort. All menstrual irregularities merit a full evaluation; do not assume HIV is always the culprit.

PSYCHOLOGICAL CARE AND SUPPORT

Women with HIV are likely to be caregivers themselves, accustomed to attending to the needs of children, spouse, parents, and others; they may resist moving into a self-care mode. Women may make sure their children's clinic appointments are kept, for example, but be less diligent about keeping their own appointments. Gently remind the patient that she deserves care as well. Collaborate in establishing family-centered HIV clinics where all family members are cared for at the same time.

Often the infected woman is not the only infected person in her household; her spouse or partner and one or more children may also have HIV, so the disruption of daily life may be profound.

When infected women discuss their biggest worries and concerns, several fundamental needs are often mentioned:

- Having housing
- Earning an income
- Having a caregiver for children when mother is not feeling well
- Worrying about the health of children
- Feeling dread about disclosing illness to loved ones, especially children
- Fearing loss of the ability to care for oneself
- Worrying about the relationship with a partner
- Coping with addiction

Any guidance, support, and referral you can offer to assist with these fundamental concerns is likely to be welcome and helpful. Remember that for some women—an addicted woman, perhaps, or a woman in poverty—HIV may not be at the top of her list of problems to worry about.

REPRODUCTIVE HEALTH CARE

Women with HIV in their reproductive years may make many active or passive decisions about their reproductive lives, including contraceptive practice, desire for pregnancy, outcome of an unintended pregnancy, and prenatal practices to reduce perinatal transmission of HIV. Infected women are free to make reproductive choices for themselves just as other women do. Support them with information and time to reflect on decisions in an unpressured environment.

Reproductive decision making for infected women is similar to uninfected women, and desire for a child is often profound. Counseling for the infected woman who is pregnant or contemplating pregnancy includes important medical issues:

- Impact of HIV on pregnancy
- Impact of pregnancy on HIV
- Effect of medicines on woman and developing fetus
- Risk of woman-to-offspring transmission
- Options for reducing woman-to-offspring transmission
- Risk of breastfeeding for HIV transmission
- Course of HIV in perinatally infected infants

Counseling for pregnancy optimally includes a full understanding of the patient's personal goals, her support network, an understanding of stressors in her life, and her overall physical and emotional status. Once this groundwork is in place, guide the patient through specific questions to help her predict how she would feel, how others would feel, and what would happen:[30]

- Are you able and willing to love and care for a baby, whether or not he or she is infected?
- Do you have the support of a partner, family members, or friends who can help you care for a child?
- Who will care for your child—teach your child about his or her culture, remember you, and raise your child according to your values—if you become sick or die?
- In what ways (good or bad) will having a baby change your life?

- What are the reasons that you want (or do not want) to have a child?
- Do you feel pressured by others to have (or not have) a child?
- Do you have enough information to make an informed decision?

Clearly, this is difficult counseling work, best carried out by counselors with experience, compassion, and the ability to help with the feelings of grief and loss that these scenarios will likely generate. The goal is to guide each patient to an uncoerced, thoughtful decision.

HIV-infected women who do not wish to become pregnant, like other women, are more likely to succeed with a contraceptive method they have chosen for themselves and feel comfortable using (Table 7-8). The goal is high contraceptive efficacy, low risk of woman-to-partner HIV transmission (if applicable), and low risk of partner-to-woman STI transmission. This goal is met by choices such as oral contraceptives plus male latex or plastic condoms. In reality, infected women often choose a contraceptive without regard to disease transmission factors, just as uninfected women often do.

Thousands of U.S. women with HIV give birth each year. Generally, HIV-infected women who are immunocompetent have uneventful pregnancies with normal labor and delivery. Just as with any women with serious systemic illness, immunocompromised women may have complicated pregnancies, including prematurity, low birth weight, and premature rupture of membranes. However, the effects of HIV on pregnancy are hard to differentiate from the effects of poverty, poor health care, or addiction. Pregnancy does not appear to speed HIV progression.[23]

Antiretroviral drugs and nonteratogenic antibiotics are usually continued in pregnancy, especially for women with <200 CD4 cells or a relatively high viral load. When the woman has reasonable immune status and a relatively low viral load, her own judgment is crucial as she evaluates the benefit of treatment for herself versus any possible adverse effects of medication on the developing fetus.

Without antiretroviral therapy, each offspring of an infected woman faces a 15% to 30% risk (range 13% to 40%) of being infected in utero, during birth, or while breastfeeding.[13] Infants will all test positive for HIV antibody at birth because of the presence of maternal antibodies in infant blood. The HIV screening test becomes accurate for the infant's true status at 15 to 18 months. Polymerase chain reaction (PCR) testing will reveal the infant's true infection status by about age 6 months.

Reducing perinatal transmission risk. More than 6,500 U.S. children have become infected with HIV because they were born to infected women.[14] A 1994 multicenter controlled trial of 477 HIV-infected pregnant women (called AIDS Clinical Trial Group 076 or ACTG 076)

Table 7-8 Contraception for the HIV-infected woman

Method	Possible Benefits	Possible Drawbacks
Oral Contraceptives	Good effectiveness with consistent use	Unclear interaction of steroids and immune function
	Less blood loss to avoid anemia	Interaction with certain antibiotics, antiretrovirals, other drugs
		Possible increased shedding of virus from cervix
		No RTI protection
		No HIV protection for partner
Norplant Depo-Provera	Good low-maintenance effectiveness	Unclear interaction of steroids and immune function
		Possible increased shedding of virus from cervix
		No RTI protection
		No HIV protection for partner
IUD	Good low-maintenance effectiveness	Risk of uterine infection secondary to insertion
		No RTI protection
		No HIV protection for partner
		Increased days of bleeding, possible anemia
Diaphragm, Cap, Spermicides	Some RTI protection	Vulvovaginal irritation increases vulnerability to UTIs for some users
		Requires good technique
Male, Female Condom	Good RTI protection	Male condom requires partner co-operation; partner cooperation helpful with female condom
	HIV protection for partner	
		Requires good technique
Surgical Sterilization	Good low-maintenance efficacy for women who desire no more children	No RTI protection
		No HIV protection for partner

Source: Denenberg (1993a) and (1993b), Kurth (1995).

demonstrated that zidovudine (AZT) lowered perinatal transmission from 26% to 8% when given to women during pregnancy and to their newborn children during the first 6 weeks of life.[25] No worrisome short-term maternal or infant effects were noted. Similar results were found in a cohort of mother-infant pairs studied before and after ACTG 076 results were published, with transmission rates declining from 19% to 8%.[26]

On the basis of ACTG 076, it is now the *standard of care to offer this zidovudine regimen to all HIV-infected pregnant women.*[11] This regimen is the basic tool of tertiary HIV prevention for women, using one or more anti-retroviral drugs to reduce HIV infection risk for their offspring. Many urgent questions are now under investigation to further clarify strategies for reducing perinatal transmission:

- Will there be long-term effects in the exposed children?
- Will the regimen work as well in women whose HIV is advanced?
- What should women do whose HIV strain is resistant to zidovudine?
- Can more convenient, less expensive regimens effectively and safely reduce the likelihood of perinatal transmission?

Transplacental zidovudine in mice produced liver, lung, and reproductive tract tumors in offspring exposed to very high doses or to a lifelong regimen. However, National Institutes of Health experts concluded that the known benefits of zidovudine for preventing perinatal transmission appear to far outweigh the hypothetical concerns of transplacental carcinogenesis. The panel recommended that this issue be routinely discussed when women are counseled about the benefits and risks of zidovudine treatment.[57]

As with HIV testing, the decision to accept or refuse zidovudine belongs to the woman. The care provider's role is to teach the facts clearly, neutrally, and thoroughly, and to assure that access to care and quality of care will not be influenced by the patient's decision. In North Carolina and New York City, 25% of women declined the therapy.[49]

Decisions about anti-HIV therapy during pregnancy are likely to become more complex as new drugs appear. Many clinicians offer combination drug regimens, ensuring that one of the drugs is zidovudine. Steps to provide optimal care for infected women should not be compromised during pregnancy, and optimal care is likely to reduce viral load, thereby protecting offspring as well.[55]

Labor and delivery. An estimated 50% of perinatal transmissions occur around the time of labor and delivery,[13] and a number of strategies can reduce exposure of the neonate to maternal blood and secretions. Suggested approaches include vaginal disinfection, RTI treatment during pregnancy to lower viral shedding at term, avoidance of intrapartum invasive procedures, and cesarean delivery. However, current data do not justify routine cesarean delivery for HIV-infected women.[58] Avoid delays in delivery once membranes have ruptured. The risk of perinatal HIV transmission increases when fetal membranes rupture more than 4 hours before delivery, 25% versus 14%.[50]

Breastfeeding. Advise infected women in the United States to bottle feed infants in order to reduce the risk of postnatal HIV transmission via breast milk.[10] In developing countries, where the risk of infant mortality from bottle feeding is high, women are advised to breastfeed regardless of HIV status.[76] The precise risk of HIV transmission via breast milk is difficult to quantify, and may be influenced by the woman's HIV status (with high viral loads during primary infection and late stage disease), her use of antiretroviral drugs, breastfeeding patterns, and other factors. (See Chapter 23 on Postpartum Contraception and Lactation.) Little is known about the impact of breastfeeding on the HIV-infected woman's nutritional status and overall health, or about the immunoprotective qualities of the breast milk produced by immunocompromised women.[37]

WORKPLACE SAFETY

Persistent concern with personal safety is normal when providing care for HIV-infected patients. When agency policies and staff training are managed appropriately, worker safety can be maintained at high levels. Workplace safety procedures regarding HIV and other blood-borne pathogens have these essential components:

- Universal precautions or another infection control system for protecting the worker (and patient) from body fluid exposure
- Hepatitis B vaccination for all workers with any risk of exposure to blood or bloody body fluid
- A post-exposure plan for appropriate management of needle sticks and other accidental exposures (see below)
- Appropriate procedures for prompt evaluation and respiratory isolation for known or suspected tuberculosis

INFECTION CONTROL

In the ambulatory reproductive health care setting, most care providers use universal precautions. This means they treat as potentially infectious all blood; bloody body fluids; semen, vaginal and cervical secretions; and amniotic, cerebrospinal, pleural, peritoneal, and pericardial fluids. The following precautions are recommended:[18]

- Wash hands before and after every patient contact.
- Dispose of needles and sharps in puncture-resistant containers, and *never* recap needles.
- Wear latex or vinyl gloves when likely to touch body fluids, mucous membranes, or broken skin.

- Wear protective eye wear and mask when eyes and mucous membranes may be splashed.
- Wear a water-repellent gown when clothing could be soiled with body fluids.
- Cover any broken skin that could come into contact with body fluids.

OCCUPATIONALLY ACQUIRED HIV

Several cases of occupationally acquired HIV are reported annually to the Centers for Disease Control and Prevention (CDC). Needlesticks and other percutaneous exposures have accounted for 86% of cases.[18] Almost all exposures have been to blood or to concentrated virus in a laboratory setting. No infections have been observed from blood exposure to intact skin, from airborne droplets, or from environmental surfaces.[18] What proportion of occupationally acquired infections are actually reported to the CDC is unknown.

The rate of occupational HIV infection following a single needlestick or other percutaneous exposure is about 0.3% in 6,498 reported accidental exposures in the U.S. and other countries.[35] Not all exposures are equally likely to transmit HIV, however. Deep injuries, visibly bloody instruments, instruments previously placed in the source patient's artery or vein, and exposure to source patients who died within 60 days (and presumably had a high viral load) appear to increase risk.[12,18]

POSTEXPOSURE MANAGEMENT

The current recommendations for postexposure management acknowledge the limited data available on this subject:

- *Recommend* chemoprophylaxis to workers with highest-risk exposures, such as a deep injury with a bloody hollow-bore needle. *Offer* chemoprophylaxis for lower-risk exposures, such as injury with a solid suture needle from a source patient with asymptomatic HIV or a blood splash to mucous membranes. *Do not offer* chemoprophylaxis for negligible-risk exposures such as a non-bloody urine splash.
- Use a regimen of zidovudine 200 mg three times a day *and* lamivudine 150 mg two times a day for 4 weeks. Consider *adding* indinavir 800 mg three times a day for highest risk exposures or when zidovudine-resistant HIV strains are present or suspected. Try to begin the regimen within 1 or 2 hours after exposure.

For more precise guidance about a wide range of accidental exposure variables, consult the Centers for Disease Control and Prevention published recommendations.[18]

Some care providers may wish to keep a dose of the chemoprophylaxis drugs on hand at the worksite. They can initiate treatment immediately in the event of accidental exposure, and then decide later on whether to continue treatment, based on source patient characteristics, personal pregnancy status, and other factors.

INFECTED HEALTH CARE PROVIDERS

Many thousands of health care providers have acquired HIV through sex and the other typical transmission routes. Whether HIV-infected health care workers place patients at risk is an important question. Retrospective studies using voluntary HIV testing of patients cared for by 51 infected physicians, surgeons, and dentists found no evidence of transmitted infection in any of the more than 22,000 patients evaluated.[63] Infected dentists, physicians, and other care providers are usually advised to make practice decisions in consultation with the personal physician, supervisor, and other professional groups as appropriate.

PERSONAL PERSPECTIVE ON WORKPLACE SAFETY

The health care workplace is not, and has never been, 100% safe. Ultimately, each care provider is responsible for her or his own safety and must insist on sound workplace policies and procedures, appropriate safety devices,[19,20] high-quality barriers, and adequate staff training. In emergency situations, take the extra seconds to protect yourself and your coworkers with barriers and careful disposal of sharps. Most important, find a way to maintain compassionate touching, even when a latex barrier must sometimes come between care provider and patient.

REFERENCES

1. American College of Nurse-Midwives. Statement on HIV/AIDS. Washington DC, March 1996.
2. American College of Obstetricians and Gynecologists. Human immunodeficiency virus infection: physicians' responsibilities. ACOG Committee Opinion No. 130. Washington DC, November 1993.
3. American College of Pediatrics, American College of Obstetricians and Gynecologists. Joint statement on human immunodeficiency virus screening. August 1995.
4. Brodie S, Sax P. Novel approaches to HIV antibody testing. AIDS Clinical Care 1997;9:1-5;10.

5. Bush DM. Personal communication to F. Guest, November 10, 1991.
6. Carr A, Cooper DA. Primary HIV infection. In: Sande MA, Volberding PA (eds). The medical management of AIDS (5th edition). Philadelphia PA: W.B. Saunders, 1997.
7. Cates Jr. W, Stone KM. Family planning, sexually transmitted diseases and contraceptive choice: a literature update—part 1. Fam Plann Perspect 1992;24:75-84.
8. Cates Jr. W. Contraception, unintended pregnancies, and sexually transmitted diseases: why isn't a simple solution possible? Am J Epidemiol 1996;143:311-318.
9. Celum C. Diagnosis and treatment of STDs in HIV-infected women. In: Cotton D, Watts DH (eds). The medical management of AIDS in women. New York: Wiley-Liss, 1997.
10. Centers for Disease Control and Prevention. Recommendations for assisting in the prevention of perinatal transmission of human T-lymphotropic virus type III/lymphadenopathy-associated virus and acquired immunodeficiency syndrome. MMWR 1985;34:721,731-732.
11. Centers for Disease Control and Prevention. Recommendations for the use of zidovudine to reduce perinatal transmission of human immunodeficiency virus. MMWR 1994;43:1-20.
12. Centers for Disease Control and Prevention. Case-control study of HIV seroconversion in health-care workers after percutaneous exposure to HIV-infected blood—France, United Kingdom, and United States, January 1988-August 1994. MMWR 1995(a);44:929-933.
13. Centers for Disease Control and Prevention. U.S. Public Health Service recommendations for human immunodeficiency virus counseling and voluntary testing for pregnant women. MMWR 1995(b);44:1-15.
14. Centers for Disease Control and Prevention. CDC Surveillance Summaries, September 27, 1996. MMWR 1996(a);45:16-19.
15. Centers for Disease Control and Prevention. Contraceptive method and condom use among women at risk for HIV infection and other sexually transmitted diseases—selected U.S. sites, 1993-1994. MMWR 1996(b)45:820-823.
16. Centers for Disease Control and Prevention. HIV/AIDS surveillance report. 1996(c);8(2):1-39.
17. Centers for Disease Control and Prevention. HIV testing among women aged 18-44 years—United States, 1991 and 1993. MMWR 1996(d);45:733-737.
18. Centers for Disease Control and Prevention. Update: provisional public health service recommendations for chemoprophylaxis after occupational exposure to HIV. MMWR 1996(e);45:468-472.
19. Centers for Disease Control and Prevention. Evaluation of blunt suture needles in preventing percutaneous injuries among health-care workers during gynecologic surgical procedures—New York City, March 1993-June 1994. MMWR 1997(a);46:25-29.
20. Centers for Disease Control and Prevention. Evaluation of safety devices for preventing percutaneous injuries among health-care workers during phlebotomy procedures—Minneapolis-St. Paul, New York City, and San Francisco, 1993-1995. MMWR 1997(b);46:21-25.
21. Centers for Disease Control and Prevention. 1998 Guidelines for treatment of sexually transmitted diseases. MMWR 1998;47(SS-4):1-132.

22. Chu SY, Wortley PM. Epidemiology of HIV/AIDS in women. In: Minkoff HL, DeHovitz JA, Duerr A (eds). HIV infection in women. New York: Raven Press, 1995.
23. Clark R. Clinical manifestations and the natural history of human immuno-deficiency virus infection in women. In: Cotton D, Watts DH (eds). The medical management of AIDS in women. New York: Wiley-Liss, 1997.
24. Collins J, Holtzman D, Kann L, Kolbe L. Predictors of condom use among U.S. high school students, 1991. Abstract #WSC134. Presented at the Ninth International Conference on AIDS, June 6-ll, 1993, Berlin, Germany.
25. Connor EM, Sperling RS, Gelber R, Kiselev P, Scott G, O'Sullivan MJ, VanDyke R, Bey M, Shearer W, Jacobson RL, Jimenez E, O'Neill E, Bazin B, Delfraissy J-F, Culnane M, Coombs R, Elkins M, Moye J, Stratton P, Balsley J, for the Pediatric AIDS CTG Protocol 076 Study Group. Reduction of maternal-infant transmission of human immunodeficiency virus type 1 with zidovudine treatment. N Engl J Med 1994;331:1173-1180.
26. Cooper ER, Nugent RP, Diaz C, Pitt J, Hanson C, Kalish LA, Mendez H, Zor-rilla C, Hershow R, Moye J, Smeriglio V, Fowler MG, for the Women and Infants Transmission Study Group. J Infectious Dis 1996;174:1207-1211.
27. DeHovitz JA. Natural history of HIV infection in women. In: Minkoff HL, DeHovitz JA, Duerr A (eds). HIV infection in women. New York: Raven Press, 1995.
28. Denenberg R. Female sex hormones and HIV. Aids Clinical Care 1993(a); 5:69-71;76.
29. Denenberg R. Gynecological care manual for HIV positive women. Durant OK: Essential Medical Information Systems, 1993(b).
30. Denison R. Update: AZT and pregnant women. WORLD 1994;April:4.
31. deVincenzi I. A longitudinal study of human immunodeficiency virus trans-mission by heterosexual partners. N Engl J Med 1994;331:341-346.
32. Duerr A, Warren D, Smith D, Nagachinta T, Marx PA. Contraceptives and HIV transmission [letter]. Nature Medicine 1997;3:124.
33. Frank AP, Wandell MG, Headings MD, Conant MA, Woody GE, Michel C. Anonymous HIV testing using home collection and telemedicine counseling. Arch Intern Med 1997;157:309-314.
34. Gallo D, George JR, Fitchen JH, Goldstein AS, Hindahl MS. Evaluation of a system using oral mucosal transudate for HIV-l antibody screening and con-firmatory test. JAMA 1997;277:254-258.
35. Gerberding JL. Prophylaxis for occupational exposure to HIV. Ann Intern Med 1996;125:497-501.
36. Hein K. "Getting real" about HIV in adolescents. Am J Public Health 1993;83:492-494.
37. Heymann J, Brubaker J. Breast feeding and HIV infection. In: Cotton D, Watts DH (eds). The medical management of AIDS in women. New York: Wiley-Liss, 1997.
38. Howe JE, Minkoff HL, Duerr AC. Contraceptives and HIV. AIDS 1994;8: 861-871.
39. Ilaria G, Jacobs JL, Polsky B, Koll B, Baron P, MacLow C, Armstrong D, Schle-gel PN. Detection of HIV-1 DNA sequences in pre-ejaculatory fluid. Lancet 1992;340:1469.

40. Irwin KL, Valdiserri RO, Holmberg SD. The acceptability of voluntary HIV antibody testing in the United States: a decade of lessons learned. AIDS 1996;10:1707-1717.

41. Jewett JF, Hecht FM. Preventive health care for adults with HIV infection. JAMA 1993;269:1144-1153.

42. Johnson R. Adolescent growth and development. In: Hofmann A, Greydanus D (eds). Adolescent medicine, 2nd ed. Norwalk CT: Appleton & Lange, 1989.

43. Joint United Nations Programme on HIV/AIDS. The HIV/AIDS situation in mid-1996: global and regional highlights. UNAIDS Fact Sheet, July 1, 1996.

44. Karon JM, Rosenberg PS, McQuillan G, Khare M, Gwinn M, Petersen LR. Prevalence of HIV infection in the United States, 1984-1992. JAMA 1996;276:126-131.

45. Katz MH, Gerberding JL. Postexposure treatment of people exposed to the human immunodeficiency virus through sexual contact or injection-drug use. New Engl J Med 1997;336:1097-1100.

46. Kerr SH, Valdiserri RO, Loft J, Bresolin L, Holtgrave D, Moore M, MacGowan R, Marder W, Rinaldi R. Primary care physicians and their HIV prevention practices. AIDS Patient Care and STDs 1996;10:227-235.

47. Krieger JN, Coombs RW, Collier AC, Ho DD, Ross SO, Zeh JE, Corey L. Intermittent shedding of human immunodeficiency virus in semen: implications for sexual transmission. J Urology 1995;154:1035-1040.

48. Kurth A, Minkoff HL. Pregnancy and reproductive concerns of women with HIV infection. In: Kelly P, Holman S, Rothenberg R, Holzemer SP (eds). Primary care of women and children with HIV infection: a multidisciplinary approach. Boston: Jones and Bartlett, 1995.

49. Landers DV, Sweet RL. Reducing mother-to-infant transmission of HIV—the door remains open. N Engl J Med 1996;334:1664-1665.

50. Landesman SH, Kalish LA, Burns DN, Minkoff H, Fox HE, Zorrilla C, Garcia P, Fowler MG, Mofenson L, Tuomala R, for the Women and Infants Transmission Study. Obstetrical factors and the transmission of human immunodeficiency virus type 1 from mother to child. N Engl J Med 1996;334:1617-1623.

51. Lemp GF, Jones M, Kellogg TA, Nieri GN, Anderson L, Withum D, Katz M. HIV seroprevalence and risk behaviors among lesbians and bisexual women in San Francisco and Berkeley, California. Am J Public Health 1995;85:1549-1552.

52. Maiman M. Management of cervical neoplasia in HIV-positive women. In: Cotton D, Watts DH (eds). The medical management of AIDS in women. New York: Wiley-Liss, 1997.

53. Marx PA, Spira AI, Gettie A, Dailey PJ, Veazey RS, Lackner AA, Mahoney CJ, Miller CJ, Claypool LE, Ho DD, Alexander NJ. Progesterone implants enhance SIV vaginal transmission and early virus load. Nature Medicine 1996; 2:1084-1089.

54. McKusick L. Counseling across the HIV spectrum. HIV Frontline 1992; No. 8, June 1992:1-8.

55. Minkoff H, Augenbraum M. Antiretroviral therapy for pregnant women. Am J Obstet Gynecol 1997;176:478-489.

56. Moses S, Plummer FA, Bradley JE, Ndinya-Achola JO, Nagelkerke NJD, Ronald AR. The association between lack of circumcision and risk for HIV infection:

a review of the epidemiological data. Sexually Transmitted Diseases 1994;21:201-210.

57. National Institute of Allergy and Infectious Diseases, National Institutes of Health. Summary of a meeting of a panel to review studies of transplacental toxicity of AZT. January 14, 1997.

58. Peckham C, Gibb D. Mother-to-child transmission of the human immunodeficiency virus. N Engl J Med 1995;333:298-302.

59. Peterson G, Akridge RE, Gibson J, Nikolaeva I, Ross S, Lee W, Dragavon J, Nirapathpongporn A, Krieger J, Coombs RW. Detection of HIV-l in semen and blood by nucleic acid amplification: effect of vasectomy on the recovery of HIV-1 RNA from seminal plasma. Abstract #I017. Presented at the 36th Interscience Conference on Antimicrobial Agents and Chemotherapeutics, 1996.

60. Pins MR, Teruya J, Stowell CP. Human immunodeficiency virus testing and case detection: pragmatic and technical issues: In: Cotton D, Watts DH (eds). The medical management of AIDS in women. New York: Wiley-Liss, 1997.

61. Ptacek JT, Eberhardt TL. Breaking bad news: a review of the literature. JAMA 1996;276:496-502.

62. Pudney J, Oneta M, Mayer K, Seage G, Anderson D. Pre-ejaculatory fluid as a potential vector for sexual transmission of HIV-1. Lancet 1992;340:1470.

63. Robert LM, Chamberland ME, Cleveland JL, Marcus R, Gooch BF, Srivastava PU, Culver DH, Jaffe HW, Marianos DW, Panlilio AL, Bell DM. Investigations of patients of health care workers infected with HIV. Ann Intern Med 1995;122:653-657.

64. Roddy RE, Zekeng L, Ryan K, Tamoufé U, Weir SS, Din E. A randomized controlled trial of the effect of nonoxynol-9 use on male-to-female transmission of HIV-l. Presented in Bethesda, Maryland, April 9, 1997.

65. Roper WL, Peterson HB, Curran JW. Commentary: condoms and HIV/STD prevention—clarifying the message. Am J Pub Health 1993;83:501-503.

66. Royce RA, Seña A, Cates Jr. W, Cohen MS. Sexual transmission of HIV. N Engl J Med 1997;336:1072-1078.

67. Saag MS. AIDS testing now and in the future. In: Sande MA, Volberding PA (eds). The medical management of AIDS (4th edition). Philadelphia PA: W.B. Saunders, 1995.

68. Schacker T, Collier AC, Hughes J, Shea T, Corey L. Clinical and epidemiologic features of primary HIV infection. Ann Intern Med 1996;125:257-264.

69. Southeast AIDS Training and Education Center. HIV Antibody Testing Counseling Checklists, 1997. Unpublished.

70. Stein Z. Editorial: more on women and the prevention of HIV infection. Am J Public Health 1995;85:1485-1488.

71. Stiffman AR, Earls F, Dore P, Cunningham R. Changes in acquired immunodeficiency syndrome-related risk behavior after adolescence: relationships to knowledge and experience concerning human immunodeficiency virus infection. Pediatrics 1992;89:950-956.

72. St. Louis ME, Wasserheit JN, Gayle HD. Editorial: Janus considers the HIV pandemic—harnessing recent advances to enhance AIDS prevention. Am J Pub Health 1997;87:10-12.

73. Stratton P, Alexander NJ. Heterosexual spread of HIV infection. In: Cotton D, Watts DH (eds). The medical management of AIDS in women. New York: Wiley-Liss, 1997.
74. Ward JW, Petersen LR, Jaffe HW. Current trends in the epidemiology of HIV/AIDS. In: Sande MA, Volberding PA (eds). The medical management of AIDS (5th edition). Philadelphia: W.B. Saunders, 1997.
75. Wong VK, Silebi M. HIV testing of pregnant women: risk factors for refusal. Abstract #I044. Presented at the 36th Interscience Conference on Antimicrobial Agents and Chemotherapeutics, 1996.
76. World Health Organization/UNICEF. Consensus statement from the consultation on HIV transmission and breastfeeding. J Hum Lact 1992;8:173-174.

LATE REFERENCE

77. UNAIDS/WHO Working Group on Global HIV/AIDS and STD surveillance. Report on the global HIVAIDS epidemic. December 1977.

Reproductive Tract Infections

Willard Cates Jr., MD, MPH

- Reproductive tract infections (RTIs) are frequently encountered by reproductive health professionals. RTIs include both the traditional sexually transmitted infections (STIs) and also other common infections of the genital tract.
- RTIs have four serious health consequences:
  - Tubal occlusion leading to infertility and ectopic pregnancy
  - Pregnancy loss and neonatal morbidity caused by transmission of the infection to the infant during pregnancy and childbirth
  - Genital cancers
  - Enhanced transmission of the human immunodeficiency virus (HIV)
- Preventing RTIs and their consequences requires persons to adopt preventive behaviors and clinicians to diagnose and treat existing infections effectively.
- Assessing a client's risks for RTI can help the client better select appropriate contraceptive methods and help clinician better diagnose and treat the client.

Healthy sexual relations and reproductive events should be free of infection.[25] However, preventing, diagnosing, and treating RTIs are growing more challenging, since an increasing number of people are infected with more severe infections:[17]

- Persistent viral infections, including the human immunodeficiency virus (HIV), herpes simplex virus (HSV), hepatitis B virus (HBV), and human papilloma virus (HPV), have afflicted millions of people with incurable diseases.

- Trichomonal and chlamydial infections are at high levels worldwide.
- Long-term consequences of pelvic inflammatory disease (PID) such as infertility, ectopic pregnancy, and chronic pain have increased.
- Neoplastic sequelae such as cervical cancer and hepatocellular carcinoma have been closely linked to some RTIs such as HPV and HBV.

In *Contraceptive Technology*, the generic term RTI covers three types of infection: (1) sexually transmitted infections (STIs), (2) endogenous vaginal infections including bacterial vaginosis and candidiasis, and (3) iatrogenic infections associated with insertion of an intrauterine device (IUD) or induced abortion.

Preventing an infection is the most effective way to reduce the adverse consequences of RTIs. Diagnosing and treating a current infection in a timely manner can also prevent complications in the individual and interrupt transmission in the community. This chapter provides general background about RTI management in the reproductive health care setting.

M AGNITUDE AND RISKS OF RTIs

The number of people infected with RTIs or affected by their consequences is a major problem for our society.[17] The estimated total number of people newly infected each year with curable STIs is 330 million worldwide. In the United States, the annual cost of pelvic inflammatory disease (PID) and its consequences was estimated to be $4.2 billion. Infertility caused by PID accounts for over $1 billion of health care costs and much emotional misery. Although deaths due to RTIs (primarily syphilis and PID) have declined over the past four decades, RTIs still cause almost one-third of reproductive mortality in the United States.

Individuals under age 25 account for a majority of RTI cases. Two-thirds of reported cases of gonorrhea and chlamydia occur in persons 24 years of age or younger.[6] Rates of syphilis, gonorrhea, vaginitis, and PID are highest in adolescents and decline steadily as adults age. Cases are concentrated in socio-geographic clusters, the so-called "core-populations." For example, persons of lower socioeconomic status are more likely to have RTIs than are persons of higher socioeconomic status.

Most RTIs show a "biological sexism." Compared with men, women suffer more severe long-term consequences, including PID, infertility, ectopic pregnancy, chronic pelvic pain, and cervical cancer. They are less likely to seek health care for infection because a higher proportion of their RTIs are asymptomatic or unrecognized as being serious.[25] In addition, most RTIs are more difficult to diagnose in women than in men.

Finally, due to the transmission dynamics of intercourse, women are more likely than men to acquire an STI from any single sexual encounter.

The probability that unprotected sexual intercourse will lead to an RTI or its consequences differs from the probability of unintended pregnancy (Table 8-1). The risk of pregnancy varies throughout the menstrual cycle. The risk of acquiring an RTI depends on (1) having intercourse with an infected person, (2) the transmissibility of the particular RTI, and (3) the gender of the infected person. For example, the risk of acquiring gonorrhea from a single sex act (where one partner is infectious) is approximately 25% for men and 50% for women.[19,27] The probability of suffering consequences from an RTI depends on whether or not the person received proper diagnosis and treatment.

One of the fundamental concepts underlying RTI risk is the "epidemiological synergy" between HIV and other RTIs.[33] Organisms that cause genital ulcers (HSV, syphilis, and chancroid) are most strongly correlated with the transmission and acquisition of HIV. Moreover, because immune dysfunction caused by HIV disease makes the ulcerative symptoms persist, the infections have a potentiating influence on each other. RTIs that produce vaginal or urethral discharge (such as gonorrhea, chlamydia, and trichomoniasis) have also been associated with higher levels of HIV infection. Because vaginal and urethral discharge are more common than genital ulcers, they account for more transmission of HIV. Always suspect HIV may be present in persons diagnosed with another RTI.

Table 8-1 Comparative risk of adverse consequences from coitus—RTI and unintended pregnancy

---

Unintended pregnancy/coital act[32]

17%-30% midcycle
<1% during menses

Gonococcal transmission/coital act[19]

50% infected male, uninfected female
25% infected female, uninfected male

PID per woman infected with cervical gonorrhea[27]

40% if not treated
0% if promptly and adequately treated

Tubal infertility per PID episode[35]

8% after first episode
20% after second episode
40% after third or more episodes

R TI PREVENTION AND PERSONAL BEHAVIORS

Different individuals accept different levels of risk to satisfy personal needs. Not everyone will follow every safer sex recommendation but, with the proper knowledge, each person can make his or her own informed choices about reducing sexual risks. Just as with many other daily health decisions, each person will assess differently the factors affecting sexual choices. Thus, simplistic messages urging absolutist policies are ineffective.

Preventive measures for avoiding transmission of all RTIs are generally consistent with guidelines for reducing the risk of HIV infection. (See Chapter 7 on HIV/AIDS and Reproductive Health.) Risk-free options include having a mutually faithful relationship with an uninfected partner or completely abstaining from sexual activities that involve semen, blood, or other body fluids, or that allow for skin-to-skin contact. Examining a partner for lesions, discussing each new partner's previous sexual history, and avoiding partners who have had many previous sexual partners can augment other measures to prevent the transmission of RTIs.

Genital self-examination (GSE), a simple exercise that should be performed by sexually active persons, can help educate clients about the symptoms and signs of RTIs and how to look for them. Persons who detect a potential problem during GSE can receive diagnosis and treatment earlier than those who wait for an annual check-up to detect the problem or for severe symptoms to develop. Early treatment is more effective than later treatment, decreases the risk of serious consequences, and prevents the transmission of the disease. Educating patients about their bodies and teaching them to be active participants in their health care gives them more control over their reproductive health.

CONTRACEPTIVE CHOICE

Choice of contraception directly affects the risk of RTI (Table 8-2). Condoms protect against both bacterial and viral RTIs. Spermicides provide some measurable protection, albeit small, against chlamydia and gonorrhea, but no data support their ability to prevent viral infections, including HIV.[9] Diaphragms used with spermicides provide a barrier against cervical infection, but they have been associated with vaginal and bladder infections. Although oral contraceptives are usually associated with an increase in chlamydia detected in the cervix, they protect against symptomatic PID, but not unrecognized endometritis.[26] IUDs are associated with an increased risk of PID, especially in the first month after insertion.

Table 8-2 Effects of contraceptives on bacterial and viral RTI

Contraceptive Methods	Bacterial RTI	Viral RTI
Condoms	Protective	Protective
Spermicides	Modestly protective against cervical gonorrhea and chlamydia	No evidence of protection *in vivo*
Diaphragms	Protective against cervical infection, Associated with vaginal anaerobic overgrowth	Protective against cervical neoplasia
Hormonal	Associated with increased cervical chlamydia, Protective against symptomatic PID, but not unrecognized endometritis	Not protective
IUD	Associated with PID in first month after insertion	Not protective
Fertility Awareness	Not protective	Not protective

Source: Adapted from Cates (1996).

OTHER RISK BEHAVIORS

In addition to sexual activities, other practices have been linked to a risk of RTI. Routine douching for hygiene purposes has been associated with an increased risk of PID and ectopic pregnancy.[14,36] Postcoital washing or urination have been poorly studied, but appear to have little effect, if any, on reducing the risk of acquiring an RTI. Because postcoital urination could wash away bacteria that could cause cystitis, it was generally recommended for women susceptible to cystitis. However, recent data have not supported this routine practice.[16]

Drug use influences the transmission of RTIs. Besides the risks associated with needle-sharing (hepatitis B, HIV infection), using drugs such as crack cocaine has been associated with sexual behaviors that increase a person's risk of acquiring and transmitting many RTIs. Outbreaks of syphilis, antibiotic-resistant gonorrhea, and chancroid have been linked to crack-related sexual behaviors.[22] Use of other drugs, especially alcohol, also have been associated with risky sexual practices.

ASSESSMENT, DIAGNOSIS AND TREATMENT IN THE REPRODUCTIVE HEALTH CARE SETTING

Professionals in the fields of family planning and RTI have common reproductive health goals:[7]

- Educating all patients about RTIs
- Providing diagnostic services that include risk assessment, RTI screening, and voluntary HIV testing
- Ensuring all persons diagnosed with an RTI get appropriate treatment, preferably before leaving the facility
- Counseling individuals about the need for simultaneous treatment for their sex partner(s)
- Assisting patients in choosing a contraceptive that will reduce their risk of acquiring an RTI

Risk assessment can help clinicians provide better contraceptive counseling and more cost-efficient RTI management. Risk assessment balances a variety of demographic, behavioral, and clinical information (other than laboratory test results) to assess the likelihood that persons are infected with an RTI or are at high risk of future infection and to counsel clients in selecting appropriate contraceptive methods. For example, an RTI risk assessment scale can help identify women who may be good candidates for barrier methods or inappropriate candidates for IUDs.[5]

With the emergence of HIV infection and its endpoint, acquired immunodeficiency syndrome (AIDS), clients need to be educated about using condoms for infection prevention, even in conjunction with other contraceptive methods for pregnancy prevention. In some populations, as many as 50% of people supplement their contraceptive with condoms to prevent RTIs.[4]

Laboratory diagnosis of most RTIs can be performed in nearly every reproductive health care setting.[34] For example, over the past 4 years, routine screening for chlamydia has been associated with a decreased incidence of the infection among clients attending family planning clinics in the Pacific Northwest.[24] In addition, some family planning clinics have extended their range of services to male clients, including RTI diagnosis, treatment, and counseling. Finally, family planning staff have become more familiar with their local STI programs to help provide appropriate referrals.

The sensitive area of STI partner notification is not part of the usual menu of services in reproductive health care clinics. However, an increasing number of counselors are being trained in this essential public health strategy. Going into the community to notify partners is probably most easily handled by the STI program.[29] Confidentiality is crucial, just as it is in all aspects of family planning and RTI care.

RTI Diagnosis and Treatment

Counseling patients with RTI requires an approach different than that generally used in family planning settings. For couples trying to prevent unplanned pregnancies, non-directive counseling allows maximal opportunity for them to choose the best contraceptive method. However, for patients who have RTIs, *directive counseling* is important to (1) prevent new infections; (2) increase compliance with treatment and follow-up; and (3) offer guidance on talking to partners about their RTI exposure. Patients must be made aware of both the potential serious consequences of RTIs and the behaviors that increase the likelihood of reinfection.

Education about disease and treatment. Make sure patients understand what disease they have, how it is transmitted, why it must be treated, and exactly when and how to take prescribed medication. Because unpleasant side effects from many medications may discourage patients from continuing treatment, discuss ways to minimize side effects. For example, doxycycline taken on an empty stomach may cause nausea that prompts the patient to stop taking the medication early. Advise a snack with medication.

Completion of treatment. Urge patients to finish their entire supply of medication even though their symptoms may diminish or disappear in a few days. Discontinuing antibiotics before the infection is completely cured can lead to recurrent infection and increase the likelihood that hard-to-cure strains of the pathogen may flourish. Advise patients to avoid intercourse until they complete the full course of therapy. After the infection is cured, urge the patient to use condoms to prevent repeated infection, especially if a woman wishes to have children in the future or continues to have intercourse with new partners.

Comfort. Provide patients with somatic and emotional comfort to enhance compliance with treatment. Treat nausea, pain, itching, or other physiologic discomforts symptomatically, if possible. Overcoming the psychosocial component of genital discomfort can be exceedingly important in RTI treatment. Remember, patients may be afraid or ashamed to ask a partner to seek treatment, embarrassed to admit their sexual practices, or concerned about confidentiality. Telling patients they have a sexually transmissible *infection* rather than *disease* may prevent some people from feeling stigmatized.

Partner notification. Notify and treat sex partner(s) to prevent both reinfection of the patient and spread of disease through the community.

Assist patients in notifying their partners by coaching them in partner notification techniques (patient referral) and using STI caseworkers (provider referral) to contact partners. An increasing number of family planning professionals are being trained in partner notification skills.

Managing RTI requires clinicians have a high index of suspicion. Often a patient will have two or more RTIs concurrently. Be alert for symptoms different from those normally associated with the primary RTI infection. Treat all presumptive RTIs. For example, when gonorrhea is diagnosed, provide dual therapy for both gonorrhea and chlamydia—an approach that is epidemiologically indicated, cost-effective, and safe for the patient.

All states require the traditional "venereal diseases" (e.g., syphilis, gonorrhea, and chancroid) be reported to public health officials; many states have instituted reporting systems for specific STIs such as chlamydial infections and genital herpes. Nearly all states require HIV infection and AIDS be reported. Reporting of STI to public health authorities is not a breach of confidentiality; in fact, statutory protection of patients' names is a crucial part of STI control strategies. Accurate reporting of STI helps (1) identify trends in disease, (2) gain resources for high-prevalence communities, and (3) evaluate STI intervention efforts. Confer with STI control officials to ensure prompt and accurate reporting of the notifiable STIs.

RTI DURING PREGNANCY

Question pregnant women and their sex partners about their risk of RTIs; counsel them about the possibility of transmitting an infection to their infant.[3] Because of the severe effects RTIs may have on both the pregnancy and the developing fetus, assess whether the pregnant woman should be screened for infections with HIV, syphilis, hepatitis B, chlamydia, gonorrhea, bacterial vaginosis, and trichomoniasis (Tables 8-3 and 8-4). Encourage voluntary screening for HIV to detect infected women who could benefit from prophylactic zidovudine to reduce maternal-to-infant transmission. Routine screening for HPV and HSV is *not* recommended.

Management of specific RTIs is discussed in the Alphabetical Catalog of RTIs in this chapter. HIV and pregnancy is discussed in Chapter 7. For more complete information on RTIs in pregnant women, refer to *Guidelines for Perinatal Care*, jointly published by the American College of Obstetricians and Gynecologists and the American Academy of Pediatrics.[1]

RTI AND SEXUAL ASSAULT

In cases of sexual assault and abuse, clinicians must attend not only to physical and psychological trauma, but also the possibility of pregnancy or RTI. Any of the sexually transmissible infections, including HIV, can

Table 8-3 Risks of sexually transmitted bacterial organisms and syndromes in pregnancy and childbirth

Organism/Syndrome	Maternal Infection Rate (%)[1]	Infant Effects	Transmission Risk from Infected Mother	Prevention	Treatment of Mother, Neonate
Neisseria gonorrhoeae	1–30	Conjunctivitis, sepsis, meningitis	Approximately 30%	Screening: culture mother; apply ocular prophylaxis	Ceftriaxone
Chlamydia trachomatis	2–25	Conjunctivitis, pneumonia, bronchiolitis, otitis media	25%–50% conjunctivitis 5%–15% pneumonia	Screening in third trimester: culture mother, apply ocular prophylaxis prophylaxis	Amoxicillin, Erythromycin
Treponema pallidum	0.01–15	Congenital syphilis, neonatal death	50%	Serologic screening in early and late pregnancy	Penicillin
Trichomonas vaginalis	10–35	Low birthweight, preterm delivery	N/A	Screening	Metronidazole
Bacterial vaginosis	10–35	Low birthweight, preterm delivery	N/A	Screening	Metronidazole

Source: Adapted from Cates (1995).

[1]Percentage of pregnant women with evidence of infection

Table 8-4 Risks of sexually transmitted viral organisms and syndromes in pregnancy and childbirth

Organism/Syndrome	Maternal Infection Rate (%)[1]	Infant Effects	Transmission Risk from Infected Mother	Prevention	Treatment of Mother, Neonate
Hepatitis B Virus	1–10	Hepatitis, cirrhosis	10%–90%	Active HBV immunization	Post-exposure passive HBV immunization
Herpes Simplex Virus	1–30	Disseminated, central nervous system, localized lesions	Recurrent: 3% at delivery primary: 30% at delivery	Cesarean delivery if lesions present at delivery	Vidarabine, Acyclovir
Human Papilloma Virus	10–35	Laryngeal papillomatosis	Rare	None	Surgical
Human Immunodeficiency Virus	0.01–20	Pediatric AIDS	27% without ZDV 7% with ZDV	Pregnancy prevention; ZDV during pregnancy	Zidovudine

Source: Adapted from Cates (1995).

[1]Percentage of pregnant women with evidence of infection

CONTRACEPTIVE TECHNOLOGY

be acquired during a sexual assault.[13] Some RTIs, such as gonorrhea or syphilis, are almost exclusively sexually transmitted and are therefore useful markers of assault in persons not previously sexually active.

To reduce the risk of pregnancy, emergency contraception can be used. (See Chapter 12 on Emergency Contraception.) To reduce the risk of RTI, the Centers for Disease Control and Prevention (CDC) recommends the following approach:[11]

Adult evaluation. If possible, initially evaluate the patient within 24 hours of the assault and take specimens to culture for *N. gonorrhoeae* and *C. trachomatis*. Examine microscopically for *T. vaginalis* and bacterial vaginosis (BV). Perform a pregnancy test, and keep a frozen serum sample for possible future testing. If treatment is not administered, schedule a repeat evaluation for 2 weeks later.

Treatment. Presumptive treatment remains controversial. While no regimen provides coverage against all potential pathogens, the following should be effective against the most frequent RTIs:

- Ceftriaxone 125 milligrams (mg) given intramuscularly (IM)
- Metronidazole 2 grams (g) given orally
- Azithromycin 1 g given orally
- Hepatitis B vaccination, first dose
- Post-exposure prophylaxis against HIV may also be considered (See Chapter 7 on HIV/AIDS and Reproductive Health) and
- Advise clients to use condoms until test results are reported.

Child

In general, identification of an STI in a child beyond the neonatal period suggests sexual abuse. However, unlike gonorrhea or syphilis, specific infections such as bacterial vaginosis (BV), genital mycoplasmas, and genital warts are not conclusive evidence of sexual abuse. Evaluation is essentially the same as described for adult victims, except culture specimens should be collected from the pharynx and rectum as well as from the vagina or urethra because the child's report of assault may not be complete. Presumptive treatment may be given at the family's request.

For more complete information regarding laboratory procedures, diagnosis, and treatment for sexual assault and abuse victims, refer to the *1998 Guidelines for Treatment of Sexually Transmitted Diseases.*

A LPHABETICAL CATALOG OF REPRODUCTIVE TRACT INFECTIONS

Acquired immunodeficiency syndrome (AIDS) and **HIV** (human immunodeficiency virus) **infections** are covered in Chapter 7.

Acute urethral syndrome (dysuria-pyuria syndrome) can be caused by *E. coli, C. trachomatis, N. gonorrhoeae,* or other gram-negative bacteria.[31] Bacterial cystitis itself is not sexually transmitted per se; however, it is sexually-associated. "Honeymoon" cystitis is believed to be caused by friction against the urethra during sexual intercourse. The underlying etiology is mechanical, and coital movements help vaginal organisms ascend into the bladder. Use of the diaphragm with spermicides and spermicidally coated condoms have been associated with higher levels of acute urethral syndrome.

Prevalence.   Urinary tract infections are second in prevalence only to upper respiratory infections. Depending on the population studied, as many as 10% to 25% of reproductive-age women report dysuria during the previous year.

Symptoms.   Painful, urgent, and frequent urination, as well as dyspareunia, characterizes this syndrome. Occasionally hematuria is the precipitating event for seeking clinical evaluation. Consider pyelonephritis if a patient's temperature exceeds 101° F or if costovertebral angle pain or tenderness are present.

Diagnosis.   Women with >10^5 organisms (coliform bacteria or other uropathogens) per milliliter (ml) of urine have *bacterial cystitis*; however, smaller number of organisms may also cause symptoms. Women with dysuria, frequency, pyuria (10 white blood cells [WBCs] per 400x field on microscopic examination of urinary sediment), and a negative Gram stain of unspun urine have the *acute urethral syndrome*. A definitive diagnosis of the etiologic organism requires cultures of the urethra or urine. Dysuria may also be caused by vaginitis or genital herpes simplex virus infection.

Treatment.   Acute urethral syndrome can be treated with a variety of antibiotics that achieve a high concentration in urine. Fluoroquinolones (e.g., ciprofloxacin 250 mg twice a day, OR ofloxacin 200 mg twice a day) can be effective. The length of therapy is dictated by clinical response, but 3 days is the usual course. Initial episodes of bacterial cystitis can be treated with appropriate single-dose therapy such as sulfamethoxazole 1.6 g plus trimethoprim 320 mg (Bactrim or Septra). However, higher cure rates are achieved with longer courses of therapy.

Potential complications. Left untreated, infections of the lower genito-urinary tract can ascend to the upper tract, leading to acute pyelonephritis, chronic pyelonephritis, and eventual kidney failure.

Behavioral messages to emphasize. Understand how to take any prescribed oral medications. Drink copious fluids to flush the genitourinary system. If *C. trachomatis* or *N. gonorrhoeae* organisms are isolated, refer sex partner(s) for examination. Return for evaluation 4 to 7 days after initiation of therapy.

Bacterial vaginosis (BV) is a clinical syndrome in which several species of vaginal bacteria (including *Gardnerella vaginalis, Mycoplasma hominis,* and various anaerobes) replace the normal H_2O_2-producing lactobacillus species and cause vulvovaginitis symptoms. Bacterial vaginosis is a sexually associated condition, but is not usually considered a specific STI. Treatment of the male partner has not been found to be effective in preventing the recurrence of BV.

Symptoms. Excessive or malodorous discharge is a common finding. Other signs or symptoms include erythema, edema, and pruritis of the external genitalia.

Diagnosis. The presumptive clinical criteria are typical clinical symptoms of vulvovaginitis, elevated vaginal pH (greater than 4.7), and identification of clue cells (small coccobacillary organisms associated with epithelial cells) in a saline wet mount or Gram stain of vaginal discharge. The diagnosis is further supported when a mixture of the vaginal discharge and 10% KOH liberates a fishy odor of volatile amines (Whiff test). Alternatively, a Gram stain of the vaginal discharge can reveal the relative absence of lactobacilli with replacement by numerous other anaerobic organisms. Cultures for *G. vaginalis*, *M. hominis*, or *Mobiluncus* are *not* useful and are not recommended for diagnosing this syndrome.

Treatment. Only patients with symptomatic disease require treatment. The three recommended regimens are metronidazole, 500 mg orally twice daily for 7 days; OR clindamycin cream, 2%, one applicator full (5 g) intravaginally at bed time for 7 days; OR metronidazole gel, 0.75%, an applicator full (5 g) intravaginally two times a day for 5 days. Two alternatives are metronidazole 2 g orally in a single dose OR oral clindamycin 300 mg two times a day for 7 days. During the second and third trimester of pregnancy, oral metronidazole 250 mg three times a day for 7 days is the preferred treatment. Lower doses of medication are recommended during pregnancy because of the general desire to limit fetal exposure. Treatment is not recommended for asymptomatic carriers of *G. vaginalis* or male partners of women with this syndrome.

Potential complications. Secondary excoriation may occur. Recurrent infections are common. Bacterial vaginosis is associated with an increased risk of adverse pregnancy outcomes, including preterm delivery and low birthweight.

Behavioral messages to emphasize. Understand how to take or use any prescribed medications. Return if the problem is not cured or recurs. Use condoms to prevent future infections. Avoid drinking alcohol until 24 hours after completing metronidazole therapy.

Candidiasis is caused by *Candida albicans* (and other *Candida* species), which are dimorphic fungi that grow as oval, budding yeast cells and as chains of cells (hyphae). *Candida* are normal flora of the skin and vagina and are *not* considered to be STIs. Treatment with antibiotics predisposes women to develop vulvovaginal candidiasis.

Symptoms. Clinical presentation varies from no signs or symptoms to erythema, edema, and pruritis of the external genitalia. Symptoms or signs alone do *not* distinguish the microbial etiology. Male sex partners may develop balanitis or cutaneous lesions on the penis.

Diagnosis. The presumptive criteria are typical clinical symptoms of vulvovaginitis and microscopic identification of yeast forms (budding cells) or hyphae in Gram stain or KOH wet-mount preparations of vaginal discharge. Candidiasis is definitively diagnosed when a vaginal culture is positive for *C. albicans* or other *Candida* species in a symptomatic woman. However, cultures are not recommended. Yeasts are part of the resident microflora of the vagina and anogenital skin. Cultures for *Candida* species may detect clinically insignificant infections, which should not be treated.

Treatment. Single dose oral fluconazole, 150 mg is a convenient therapy. In addition, many topical formulations provide effective candidiasis treatment. Examples include miconazole vaginal suppositories 200 mg intravaginally at bedtime for 3 days; OR miconazole 2% vaginal cream, one full applicator (5 g) intravaginally at bedtime for 3 days (and applied externally for vulvitis); OR clotrimazole vaginal tablets 100 mg intravaginally daily for 3 days; OR butoconazole cream, 2%, 5 g intravaginally for 3 days. A variety of other effective treatment regimens exist. In general, 3- to 7-day regimens are preferred for more severe infections. Over-the-counter preparations for intravaginal administration of miconazole, clotrimazole, and butaconazole are available.

Potential complications. Secondary excoriation may occur. Recurrent infections are common, particularly with antibiotic use or diabetes. Persistent candidiasis may indicate HIV infection.

Behavioral messages to emphasize. Understand how to take or use any prescribed medications. Return if the problem is not cured or recurs. Wear a sanitary pad to protect clothing. Change pads frequently. To reduce moisture in the area, avoid panty hose and non-cotton panties to reduce moisture. Store suppositories in a refrigerator. Continue taking medicine even during your menstrual period.

Chancroid is caused by *Hemophilus ducreyi*, a gram-negative bacillus with rounded ends commonly observed in small clusters along strands of mucus. On culture, the organism tends to form straight or tangled chains. Chancroid is well-established as potentiating HIV transmission.

Prevalence. Chancroid occurs more frequently in the developing than in the developed world. However, chancroid is endemic in selected areas of the United States, and specific chancroid outbreaks have occurred in settings where sex is exchanged for drugs or money.

Symptoms. Women are frequently asymptomatic. Usually a single painful ulcer, surrounded by erythematous edges, appears in men. Ulcers may be necrotic or severely erosive with a ragged serpiginous border. Painful inguinal lymphadenopathy presents in about half the cases and may rupture in 25% to 60% of cases. Ulcers usually occur on the coronal sulcus, glans, or shaft of the penis.

Diagnosis. A painful ulcer, particularly if accompanied by a unilateral bubo, suggests chancroid. Because other RTIs cause genital ulcers (principally syphilis and herpes), all ulcers should be examined with darkfield microscopy when adequate facilities exist. Serologic tests for syphilis and HIV should be performed. When the only organisms seen in a bubo aspirate or ulcer smear are arranged in chains or clumps along strands of mucus and they are morphologically similar to *H. ducreyi*, the diagnosis of chancroid is highly likely. The diagnosis is definitive when *H. ducreyi* is recovered by culture or appropriate selective media. Biopsy may be diagnostic but is not usually performed. PCR testing for *H. ducreyi* may soon be available.

Treatment. Azithromycin 1 g orally in a single dose OR ceftriaxone 250 mg IM in a single dose OR ciprofloxacin 500 mg orally twice a day for 3 days OR erythromycin base 500 mg orally four times a day for 7 days. Persons infected with HIV have higher rates of treatment failure with single-dose therapy. The susceptibility of *H. ducreyi* to this combination of antimicrobial agents varies throughout the world. Evaluate the results of therapy after a maximum of 7 days, and continue therapy until ulcers or lymph nodes have healed. Fluctuant lymph nodes should be aspirated through healthy, adjacent, normal skin. Incision and drainage or excision of nodes will delay healing and are contraindicated. Apply compresses to ulcers to remove necrotic material. All sex partners should be simultaneously treated.

Potential complications. Systemic spread is not known to occur. Lesions may become secondarily infected and necrotic. Buboes may rupture and suppurate, resulting in fistulae. Ulcers on the prepuce may cause paraphimosis or phimosis.

Behavioral messages to emphasize. Because genital ulcers can be a risk for HIV infection, get an HIV test at baseline treatment and again in 3 months. Refer sex partner(s) for examination as soon as possible. Return for evaluation 3 to 5 days after therapy begins and thereafter return weekly for evaluation until the infection is entirely healed. The prepuce should remain retracted during therapy, except in the presence of preputial edema. Use condoms to prevent future infections.

Chlamydia is the common name for infections caused by *Chlamydia trachomatis*. Genital chlamydial infection is the leading cause of preventable infertility and ectopic pregnancy. Chlamydia is now the most commonly reported infectious disease in the United States. An estimated 2 to 4 million new cases occur annually. Like viruses, chlamydiae are obligate intracellular parasites and can be isolated in the laboratory only by cell culture. Unlike viruses, *C. trachomatis* is susceptible to antibiotics. Because many chlamydial infections are asymptomatic and probably chronic, widespread screening is necessary to control this infection and its sequelae.[12,30] For further information about the syndromes caused by *C. trachomatis*, see the sections on Mucopurulent Cervicitis, Nongonococcal Urethritis, and Pelvic Inflammatory Disease (PID) in this chapter. The recommended regimens for all sites of uncomplicated chlamydial infection are azithromycin 1 g taken orally in a single dose OR doxycycline 100 mg orally twice a day for 7 days. Alternatives are ofloxacin 300 mg orally two times a day for 7 days OR erythromycin base 500 mg orally four times a day for 7 days OR erythromycin ethylsuccinate 800 mg orally four times a day for 7 days. During pregnancy, the recommended regimens are amoxicillin 500 mg orally three times daily for 7 days OR erythromycin base 500 mg orally four times daily for 7 days.

Genital herpes is caused by herpes simplex virus (HSV) types 1 and 2 DNA viruses that cannot be distinguished clinically. HSV type 2 (HSV-2) is more common in genital disease.

Prevalence. Symptomatic primary (or initial) HSV infections affect an estimated 200,000 persons each year. Recurrent HSV infections are much more common. An estimated 40 million Americans are infected with genital HSV, though most infections are asymptomatic.[18] Persons without symptoms transmit most of the HSV infections.[23]

Symptoms. Single or multiple vesicles, which are usually pruritic, can appear anywhere on the genitalia. Vesicles spontaneously rupture to form shallow ulcers that may be very painful. Lesions resolve spontaneously with minimal scarring. The first clinical occurrence is termed first episode infection (mean duration 12 days). Subsequent, usually milder, occurrences are termed recurrent infections (mean duration 4.5 days). The interval between clinical episodes is termed latency. Viral shedding from the cervix, vulva or penile skin occurs intermittently without clinical symptoms during latency. HSV-2 genital infections are more likely to recur than is HSV type 1 (HSV-1), thus identification of the type of infecting strain has prognostic value.

Diagnosis. When typical genital lesions are present or a pattern of recurrence has developed, suspect herpes infection. A presumptive diagnosis is further supported by direct identification of multinucleated giant cells with intranuclear inclusions in a clinical specimen (Tzanck smear) prepared by a Pap smear or other histochemical stain OR by increased serologic titer in convalescent serum. An HSV tissue culture demonstrates the characteristic cytopathic effect following inoculation of a specimen from the cervix, the urethra, or the base of a genital lesion. Nonculture tests, although not as sensitive as culture, may be used.

Treatment. No cure for HSV has been found; however, antiviral drugs have been helpful in reducing or suppressing symptoms. Oral administration is more clinically useful than topical, both in treating clinically symptomatic episodes and in suppressing or reducing recurrent outbreaks. For clinical illness, oral acyclovir can be given in 400 mg doses three times a day OR in 200 mg capsules five times a day for 7 days (or until clinical resolution occurs). In addition, famciclovir 250 mg orally five times a day OR valacyclovir 1.0 g orally two times a day are recommended for first episode clinical illness. To prevent recurrences, acyclovir 400 mg orally twice a day, OR famciclovir 125 mg orally twice a day, OR valacyclovir 500 mg orally once a day have been used as daily suppressive therapy. Topical therapy with acyclovir is substantially less effective. Intravenous acyclovir is used to treat uncommon disseminated forms of herpes infection requiring hospitalization. The new therapeutic agents offer more convenient dosing but are not more effective clinically than acyclovir.

The safety of systemic acyclovir in pregnant women has not been established. In pregnant women without life-threatening disease, systemic treatment should not be used to treat recurrent genital herpes episodes or, as suppressive therapy, to prevent reactivation near term.

Potential complications. *Men and women*: HSV infection can cause neuralgia, meningitis, ascending myelitis, urethral strictures, and lymphatic suppuration. *Women*: Pregnancy loss and preterm delivery have been associated with HIV infections, usually in primary stages. *Neonates*: During vaginal delivery, virus from an active genital infection can cause neonatal herpes. Neonatal herpes ranges in severity from clinically inapparent infections to local infections of the eyes, skin, or mucous membranes or to severely disseminated infection that may involve the central nervous system. The full-blown infection has a high fatality rate, and survivors often have ocular or neurologic sequelae.

Behavioral messages to emphasize. Because both initial and recurrent lesions shed high concentrations of the virus, abstain from sexual activity while ulcers are present. The risk of HSV transmission also exists during asymptomatic intervals. Because of the large number of persons with asymptomatic HSV infections, most HSV is transmitted by this group. Condoms offer some protection.

The risk of transmission to the neonate from an infected mother is highest among women with primary herpes infection (the first time they have been infected with either HSV-1 or HSV-2) at the time of delivery, less with women with nonprimary first episode of the disease and lower among women with recurrent herpes. At the onset of labor, describe any symptoms and get examined for lesions. If you have no signs or symptoms, your infant may be delivered vaginally. Infants delivered through an infected birth canal should be cultured and followed carefully.

Genital herpes (and other diseases causing genital ulcers) has been associated with an increased risk of acquiring HIV infections. Evaluating asymptomatic partners has little value for preventing transmission of HSV.

Genital warts (Condyloma acuminata) are caused by several of the many types of human papilloma virus (HPV), a small, slowly growing DNA virus belonging to the papovavirus group. Types 6 and 11 usually cause the visible genital warts. Other HPV types in the genital region (16, 18, 31, 33, 35) are associated with vaginal, anal, and cervical dysplasia.

Prevalence. Genital warts account for more than 1 million physician office visits annually, making condyloma the most common symptomatic viral RTI in the United States. The most sensitive measures of HPV indicate up to half of all sexually active young women are infected with this virus.[2] Cases of condyloma have been correlated with earlier onset of sexual activity, multiple sex partners, and a higher frequency of casual relationships than in controls.

Symptoms. Single or multiple soft, fleshy, papillary or sessile, painless keratinized growths appear around the vulvovaginal area, penis, anus, urethra, or perineum. Women infected with condyloma may exhibit typical growths on the walls of the vagina or cervix and may be unaware of their existence. Regular genital self-examinations may be helpful in detecting such growths on the external genitalia of both women and men. From 60% to 90% of male partners of women with condyloma have HPV infection on the penis, although infection may not be visible to the naked eye.

Diagnosis. No evidence supports the use of HPV DNA tests in the routine diagnosis or management of visible genital warts. Therapeutic decisions should *not* be made on the basis of this test. A diagnosis may be made on the basis of either typical clinical signs on the external genitalia or koilocytosis on Papanicolaou (Pap) smear specimens. Colposcopy is valuable for diagnosing flat warts, which are difficult to see. Exclude the possible diagnosis of condylomata lata by obtaining a serologic test for syphilis. A biopsy is usually unnecessary but would be required to make a definitive diagnosis. When neoplasia is a possibility, take a biopsy of any atypical lesions, or persistent warts before initiating therapy.

Treatment. Several different treatment regimens can be used, depending on client preference, available resources, and the experience of the health care provider. None of the currently available treatments is superior to others or are ideal for all patients or all warts. The currently available treatments for visible genital warts consists of two types: (1) patient-applied therapies and (2) provider-administered therapies.

Patient-applied therapies:

- *Podofilox* 0.5% solution or gel. Patients apply podofilox solution with a cotton swab, or a podofilox gel with a finger, to visible genital warts twice daily for 3 days, followed by 4 days of no therapy. This process may be repeated up to a total of four times. Podofilox should not be used during pregnancy.

- *Imiquimod* 5% cream. Patients should apply imiquimod cream with a finger, at bed time, 3 times a week, for up to 16 weeks. They should wash with mild soap and water after 6 to 10 hours. Imiquimod should not be used during pregnancy.

Provider-administered therapies:

- *Cryotherapy* with liquid nitrogen or cryoprobe. Repeat applications every 1 to 2 weeks.

- *Podophyllin resin* 10% to 25% in tincture of benzoin. A small amount of podophyllin should be applied to each wart and allowed to air dry. Avoid normal tissue. Wash off thoroughly in 1 to 4 hours to reduce local irritation. Podophyllin should not be used during pregnancy.

- *Trichloroacetic acid (TCA) or bichloroacetic acid (BCA)* 80% to 90%. Apply a small amount only to the warts and allow to dry, at which time a white "frosting" develops. Repeat weekly as needed.

- *Surgical removal.* Scissor or shaving excision, curette, or electrosurgery are possible.

HPV infection is a chronic condition even when asymptomatic. No therapy has been shown to eradicate the virus. In 80% of cases, HPV recurs.

HPV has been demonstrated in adjacent tissue even after attempts to eliminate subclinical HPV by extensive laser vaporization of the anogenital area. The effect of genital wart treatment on HPV transmission and the natural history of HPV is unknown. Therefore, the goal of treatment is the temporary removal of visible genital warts and the amelioration of symptoms and signs, not the eradication of HPV.

Potential complications. Lesions may enlarge and destroy tissue. Giant condyloma, while histologically benign, may simulate carcinoma. In pregnancy, warts enlarge, are extremely vascular, and may obstruct the birth canal to necessitate a cesarean delivery. Neither routine HPV screening tests nor cesarean delivery for prevention of the transmission of HPV to the newborn is indicated. The perinatal transmission rate is unknown, although it is thought to be low. Persons with HIV disease can have rapidly growing genital warts. Women infected with HIV have an increased risk of progressive HPV-cervical disease.

Behavioral messages to emphasize. Return for regular treatment until lesions have resolved. Once warts have responded to therapy, no special follow-up is necessary. If you have anogenital warts, you are contagious to uninfected sex partners. The majority of partners are probably already infected. Examination of sex partners is not necessary. Use of condoms may help reduce transmission to those who are uninfected. To reduce risks of sequelae from cervical cancer, annual Pap smears are *crucial* for all women with documented HPV infection. Smoking cessation will reduce the risk of HPV and neoplasia.

Gonorrhea is caused by *Neisseria gonorrhoeae*, a gram-negative diplococcus.

Prevalence. About 600,000 new cases of gonorrhea occur each year, making it the second most commonly reported infectious disease in the United States.

Symptoms. Symptomatic men usually have dysuria, increased frequency of urination, and purulent urethral discharge. An estimated one-fourth of infected men can be asymptomatic. Women may have abnormal vaginal discharge, abnormal menses, dysuria, or most commonly are asymptomatic. Pharyngeal gonorrhea can produce symptoms of pharyngitis.

Diagnosis. Presumptive diagnosis relies on microscopically identifying typical gram-negative intracellular diplococci on smear of urethral exudate (men) or endocervical material (women). Definitive diagnosis, especially in women, requires recovery of bacteria with typical colonial morphology, positive oxidase reaction, and typical Gram-stain morphology, grown on a selective culture medium. Ideally, all gonorrhea cases should be diagnosed by culture to facilitate antimicrobial susceptibility testing. However, increasing use of nonculture tests has increased the number of women tested. A definitive diagnosis by culture is required if the specimen is extragenital, from a child, or medico-legally important.

Treatment. In many areas of the United States about one-fourth of men and two-fifths of women with gonococcal infections also have a coexisting chlamydial infection. For this reason, use *both* a single-dose anti-gonococcal drug AND an anti-chlamydial regimen unless screening tests are negative. The recommended therapies for gonorrhea include ceftriaxone 125 mg IM once; OR ciprofloxacin 500 mg orally once; OR cefixime 400 mg orally once; OR ofloxacin 400 mg orally once. For chlamydia, the recommended therapies are azithromycin 1 g orally in a single dose OR doxycycline 100 mg orally two times a day for 7 days. Treat patients with a history of oral-genital sex with a regimen effective against pharyngeal gonorrhea.

Potential complications. Up to 40% of untreated women with cervical gonorrhea develop PID and are at risk for its sequelae (see the section on PID), including involuntary sterility and pelvic abscesses. Men are at risk for epididymitis, urethral stricture, and sterility. Newborns are at risk for ophthalmia neonatorum, scalp abscess at the site of fetal monitors, rhinitis, or anorectal infection. All infected untreated persons are at risk for disseminated gonococcal infection.

Behavioral messages to emphasize. Understand how to take any prescribed oral medications. Refer sex partner(s) for examination and treatment. Avoid sex until patient and partner(s) have been treated. Use condoms to prevent future infections.

Granuloma inguinale (Donovanosis) is caused by *Calymmatobacterium granulomatis* (formerly known as *Donovania granulomatis*), a bipolar, gram-negative bacterium (Donovan body) that in a crush preparation, appears in vacuolar compartments within histiocytes, white blood cells, or plasma cells.

Prevalence. Although one of the traditional venereal diseases, granuloma inguinale is rare in the United States. However, it is endemic in certain less developed countries including the Caribbean, India, Central Australia, and Southern Africa.

Symptoms. Initially, single or multiple subcutaneous nodules appear at the site of inoculation. Nodules erode to form granulomatous, heaped ulcers that are painless, bleed on contact, and enlarge slowly. Spread by autoinoculation is common.

Diagnosis. The typical clinical presentation is sufficient to suggest the diagnosis. Resolution of the lesions following specific antibiotic therapy supports the diagnosis. The patient's or partner's history of travel to endemic areas helps substantiate the clinical impression. A microscopic examination of biopsy specimens from the ulcer margin reveals the pathognomonic Donovan bodies. Tissue culture of *C. granulomatis* is not feasible.

Treatment. Recommended initial regimens are trimethoprim-sulfamethoxazole, 1 double-strength tablet twice a day OR doxycycline 100 mg orally twice a day until all lesions have completely healed (usually a minimum of 3 weeks). Alternatives are ciprofloxacin 750 mg orally twice a day OR erythromycin 500 mg orally four times a day.

Potential complications. Lesions may become secondarily infected. Fibrous, keloid-like formations may deform the genitalia. Pseudo-elephantoid enlargement of the labia, penis, or scrotum occurs. Necrosis and destruction of the genitalia may result.

Behavioral messages to emphasize. Understand how to take prescribed oral medications. Return for evaluation 3 to 5 days after therapy begins. Assure examination of sex partner(s) as soon as possible. Return weekly or biweekly for evaluation until the infection is entirely healed.

Hepatitis B is caused by hepatitis B virus (HBV), a DNA virus with multiple antigenic components.

Prevalence. In the United States, about 5% of the general population show evidence of past HBV infections. An estimated 70,000 to 120,000 new cases of HBV infection are transmitted sexually each year. Heterosexual intercourse is now the predominant mode of HBV transmission.

Symptoms. Most HBV infections are not clinically apparent. When present, symptoms include a serum sickness-like prodrome (skin eruptions, urticaria, arthralgias, arthritis), lassitude, anorexia, nausea, vomiting, headache, fever, dark urine, jaundice, and moderate liver enlargement with tenderness.

Diagnosis. HBV infection is clinically indistinguishable from other forms of viral and other hepatitis. A patient with the typical clinical symptoms and exposure to a patient with definitive or presumed HBV infection may be presumed to have HBV infection. Serodiagnosis of HBV infection is the best method for clinicians to reach a definitive diagnosis. Positive results of the following tests are reliable:

- Hepatitis B surface antigen (HBsAg): Acute HBV infection or, with no acute disease exposure, the chronic carrier state (infectious)
- HBe antigen: More infectious than if just HBsAg-positive, because the virus is actively replicating
- Anti-HBsAg: Past infection with present immunity
- Anti-HB core antigen: Past or current infection

Treatment. No specific therapy exists. Provide supportive and symptomatic care. HBV is the only STI for which we have a vaccine. Vaccines made from recombinant genetic material are available. Specific vaccination and post-exposure prophylaxis strategies are of proven efficacy in preventing hepatitis B. Vaccinating all newborn infants and adolescents against hepatitis B is currently recommended.[1] In addition, the Advisory Committee on Immunization Practices recommends HBV vaccination for all persons with recent STI and those who have a history of sexual activity with more than one partner in the previous 6 months. Subsidized HBV vaccine programs are available in many states through the hepatitis B coordinator.

Potential complications. Long-term sequelae include chronic, persistent, active hepatitis, cirrhosis, hepatocellular carcinoma, hepatic failure, and death. Rarely, the course may be fulminant with hepatic failure.

Behavioral messages to emphasize. HBV vaccination is strongly encouraged for all young, sexually active clients. The full three-vaccination regimen is necessary for maximum protection. Follow patients with hepatitis to see if they become HBsAg carriers and are capable of infecting others.

Human papilloma virus (HPV) See Genital Warts.

Lymphogranuloma venereum (LGV) is caused by immunotypes L1, L2, or L3 of *C. trachomatis*.

Prevalence. LGV infections are more common than ordinarily believed. They are endemic in Asia and Africa but are rare in the United States.

Symptoms. The primary lesion of LGV is a 2 to 3 mm painless vesicle or nonindurated ulcer at the site of inoculation. Patients commonly fail to notice this primary lesion. Regional adenopathy follows a week to a month later and is the most common clinical symptom. A sensation of stiffness and aching in the groin, followed by swelling of the inguinal region, may be the first indications of infections for most patients. Adenopathy may subside spontaneously or proceed to the formation of abscesses that rupture to produce draining sinuses or fistulae.

Diagnosis. LGV is often diagnosed clinically and may be confused with chancroid because of the painful adenopathy. The LGV complement fixation test is sensitive; 80% of patients have a titer of 1:16 or higher. Levels of 1:64 are considered diagnostic. Because the sequelae of LGV are serious and preventable, do not withhold treatment pending laboratory confirmation. A definitive diagnosis requires isolating *C. trachomatis* from an appropriate specimen and confirming the isolate as an LGV immuno-type. However, these laboratory diagnostic capabilities are not widely available.

Treatment. Give doxycycline 100 mg orally two times a day for 21 days OR erythromycin 500 mg orally four times a day for 21 days. Aspirate fluctuant lymph nodes as needed. Incision and drainage or excision of nodes will delay healing and are contraindicated.

Potential complications. Dissemination may occur with nephropathy, hepatomegaly, or phlebitis. Large polypoid swelling of the vulva (esthiomene), anal margin, or rectal mucosa may occur. The most common severe morbidity results from rectal involvement: perianal abscess and rectovaginal or other fistulae are early consequences, and rectal stricture may develop 1 to 10 years after infection.

Behavioral messages to emphasize. Understand how to take prescribed oral medications. Return for evaluation 3 to 5 days after therapy begins. Assure examination of sex partner(s) as soon as possible.

Molluscum contagiosum is caused by molluscum contagiosum virus, the largest DNA virus of the poxvirus group.

Prevalence. As an RTI, molluscum contagiosum occurs infrequently, about 1 case for every 100 cases of gonorrhea. Outbreaks have been reported among groups at high risk for other RTIs.

Symptoms. Lesions are 1 to 5 mm, smooth, rounded, firm, shiny flesh-colored to pearly-white papules with characteristically umbilicated centers. They are most commonly seen on the trunk and anogenital region and are generally asymptomatic.

Diagnosis. Infection is usually diagnosed on the basis of the typical clinical presentation. Microscopic examination of lesions or lesion material reveals the pathognomonic molluscum inclusion bodies.

Treatment. Lesions may resolve spontaneously without scarring. However, they may be removed by curettage after cryoanesthesia. Treatment with caustic chemicals (podophyllin, trichloroacetic acid, silver nitrate) and cryotherapy (liquid nitrogen) have been successful. If every lesion is not extirpated, the condition may recur.

Potential complications. Secondary infection, usually with staphylococcus, may occur. Lesions rarely attain a size greater than 10 mm in diameter.

Behavioral messages to emphasize. Return for reexamination 1 month after treatment so any new lesions can be removed. Sex partner(s) should be examined.

Mucopurulent cervicitis (MPC) can be caused by *C. trachomatis, N. gonorrhoeae (rarely)*, or possibly mycoplasmas.

Prevalence. Based on extrapolation from local studies, mucopurulent cervicitis probably occurs more frequently than male urethritis. Up to 3 million cases per year may occur annually.

Symptoms. The mucopurulent discharge is exuded from the cervix. Often the patient does not recognize the discharge or may perceive it as normal vaginal discharge.

Diagnosis. Diagnosis is made by finding either mucopus on a swab of the endocervical secretions or friability (bleeding) on the first swabbing. Some clinicians diagnose MPC by finding 30 or more polymorphonuclear leukocytes per microscopic field at a magnification of 1000X, but this criterion suffers from a low positive predictive value. A definitive etiologic diagnosis is made when either gonorrhea or chlamydia is diagnosed.

Treatment. Chlamydia is treated with azithromycin 1 g orally in a single dose OR doxycycline 100 mg orally twice a day for 7 days. (See the section on Gonorrhea.)

Potential complications. PID (with subsequent infertility) and pelvic abscesses may complicate infection. In addition, neonatal chlamydial infections, such as ophthalmia or pneumonia, may be acquired during delivery if the mother has an infected endocervix. If a pregnant woman is infected, she may be at risk for postpartum endometritis.

Behavioral messages to emphasize. Understand how to take prescribed oral medications. If your infection involves *C. trachomatis* or *N. gonorrhoeae*, refer your sex partner(s) for examination and treatment. Avoid sex until you and your partner(s) are cured. Return early if symptoms persist or recur. Use condoms to prevent future infections.

Nongonococcal urethritis (NGU) is caused by *Chlamydia trachomatis* about 30% of the time. Other sexually transmissible agents, which cause 10% to 45% of NGU, include *Ureaplasma urealyticum*, *Trichomonas vaginalis*, and herpes simplex virus. The etiology of the remaining cases is unknown.

Prevalence. NGU appears more frequently than gonorrhea in both public STI clinics and private practices. More than 1 million cases annually are estimated to occur in men.

Symptoms. Men usually have dysuria, urinary frequency, and mucoid to purulent urethral discharge. Many men have asymptomatic infections.

Diagnosis. Men with typical clinical symptoms are presumed to have NGU when their gonorrhea tests are negative and they have either white blood cells (WBCs) on Gram stain of urethral discharge or sexual exposure to an agent known to cause NGU. Asymptomatic men with negative gonorrhea tests are also presumed to have NGU if >5 WBCs per oil immersion field appear on an intraurethral smear. Chlamydia testing is strongly recommended for a specific diagnosis. Gonococcal and non-gonococcal urethritis may coexist in the same patient.

Treatment. When the etiology is *C. trachomatis, U. urealyticum,* or unknown, the following treatment is recommended: azithromycin 1 g orally in a single dose OR doxycycline 100 mg orally twice daily for 7 days. Alternatives for patients who fail their first trial are erythromycin 500 mg orally four times a day for at least 7 days OR ofloxacin 300 mg orally twice a day for 7 days. For *T. vaginalis* or herpes simplex infections, see the sections of this chapter that deal specifically with these agents.

Potential complications. Urethral strictures or epididymitis may occur. If *C. trachomatis* is transmitted to female sex partners, the condition may result in mucopurulent cervicitis and PID. If *C. trachomatis* is transmitted to a pregnant woman, complications may include neonatal infections such as ophthalmia or pneumonia.

Behavioral messages to emphasize. Understand how to take any prescribed oral medications. Refer sex partner(s) for examination and treatment. Avoid sex until your and your partner(s) are cured. Use condoms to prevent future infections.

Pelvic inflammatory Disease (PID) can be caused by varying combinations of *N. gonorrhoeae, C. trachomatis,* anaerobic bacteria, facultative gram-negative rods (such as *E. coli*), *Mycoplasma hominis,* and a variety of other microbial agents. Clinical PID is usually of polymicrobial etiology. *N. gonorrhoeae* and *C. trachomatis* may cause antecedent inflammation, which makes the tubes susceptible to invasion by anaerobic organisms.[8]

Prevalence. PID accounts for nearly 180,000 hospitalizations every year in the United States. More than 1 million episodes occur annually. Among American women of reproductive age, 1 in 7 reports having received treatment for PID.

Symptoms. Based on retrospective reports, many women with PID have atypical or no symptoms. Women may have pain and tenderness involving the lower abdomen, cervix, uterus, and adnexae, possibly combined with fever, chills, and elevated white blood cell (WBC) count and erythrocyte sedimentation rate (ESR). The condition is more likely if the patient has multiple sex partners, a history of PID, has recently had an IUD inserted, or is in the first 5 to 10 days of her menstrual cycle.

Diagnosis. Women who have the typical clinical symptoms are presumed to have PID if other serious conditions, such as acute appendicitis or ectopic pregnancy, can be excluded. The diagnosis of PID is often based on imprecise clinical findings.[20] Maintain a low threshold for diagnosing PID, because even mild or moderate PID have the potential for reproductive sequelae. Clinicians should use objective criteria to monitor response to antibiotics, especially if ambulatory treatment is given. Direct visualization of inflamed (edema, hyperemia, or tubal exudate) fallopian tube(s) during laparoscopy or laparotomy makes the diagnosis of PID definitive. Cultures of tubal exudate may help establish the microbiologic etiology.

Treatment. Because the causative organism is usually unknown at the time of the initial therapy, use treatment regimens that are active against the broadest possible range of pathogens. Antimicrobial coverage should include *N. gonorrhoeae*, *C. trachomatis*, anaerobes, Gram-negative facultative bacteria, and streptococci.

Hospitalization and inpatient care: Strongly consider hospitalizing patients with acute PID when (1) surgical emergencies, such as appendicitis and ectopic pregnancy, are not definitely excluded; (2) severe illness precludes outpatient management; (3) the woman is pregnant; (4) the woman is unable to follow or tolerate an outpatient regimen; or (5) the woman has failed to respond to outpatient therapy. Special consideration may be given to adolescents both to preserve their fertility and improve their compliance.

Combined drug therapy is recommended in all cases since the full bacterial etiology of PID is not clear and is generally polymicrobial.

Parenteral treatment: Two parenteral regimens are recommended for both inpatient and outpatient care:

- *Regimen A*: Doxycycline 100 mg intravenously (IV) twice daily PLUS either cefoxitin 2.0 g IV four times a day, OR cefotetan 2.0 g IV twice daily for at least 2 days *after* the patient clinically improves. Continue doxycycline 100 mg orally twice daily after discharge to complete at least 14 days of therapy. This regimen provides optimal coverage for all strains of *N. gonorrhoeae* and *C. trachomatis*. It may not provide optimal treatment for anaerobes, pelvic mass, or an IUD-associated PID.
- *Regimen B*: Clindamycin 900 mg, IV three times a day, PLUS gentamicin 2 mg per kilogram (kg) IV loading dose and maintenance 1.5 mg/kg IV three times daily. Continue oral therapy as above.

Oral treatment: Either of two oral regimens are recommended:

- *Regimen A*: Cefoxitin 2.0 g IM along with probenecid 1.0 g orally; OR ceftriaxone 250 mg IM PLUS doxycycline 100 mg taken orally twice daily for 14 days.
- *Regimen B*: Ofloxacin 400 mg twice daily PLUS metronidazole 500 mg two times a day for 14 days.

Potential complications. Potentially life-threatening complications include ectopic pregnancy and pelvic abscess. Other sequelae are involuntary infertility, recurrent or chronic PID, chronic abdominal pain, pelvic adhesions, premature hysterectomy, and depression.

Behavioral messages to emphasize. For outpatient therapy, return for evaluation 2 to 3 days after initiation of therapy. Return for further evaluation 4 days after completing therapy. Refer sex partner(s) for evaluation and treatment (up to half of sex partners of women with PID are infected but asymptomatic). Avoid sexual activity until the patient and her partner(s) are cured. If she used an IUD, consult with a family planning physician. Use condoms to prevent future infections. Understand how to take prescribed oral medications.

Syphilis is caused by *Treponema pallidum*, a spirochete with 6 to 14 regular spirals and characteristic motility.

Prevalence. Primary and secondary syphilis currently affect approximately 20,000 persons each year in the United States.[28] Congenital syphilis occurs in about 1 in 10,000 pregnancies. Southeastern states have the highest rates of both syphilis and congenital syphilis.

Symptoms.

Primary: The classical chancre is a painless, indurated ulcer, located at the site of exposure. The differential diagnosis for all genital lesions should include syphilis.

Secondary: Patients may have a highly variable skin rash, mucous patches, condylomata lata (fleshy, moist tissue growths), lymphadenopathy, alopecia, or other signs.

Latent: Patients are without clinical signs of infection.

Diagnosis.

Primary: Patients have typical lesion(s) and either a positive darkfield exam; a fluorescent antibody techniques in material from a chancre, regional lymph node, or other lesion; or their present serologic test for syphilis (STS) titer is at least fourfold greater than the last; or they have been exposed to syphilis within 90 days of lesion onset.

Secondary: Patients have the typical clinical presentation and a strongly reactive STS; condyloma lata will be darkfield positive.

Latent: Patients have serologic evidence of untreated syphilis without clinical signs.

Primary and secondary syphilis are definitively diagnosed by demonstrating *T. pallidum* with darkfield microscopy or fluorescent antibody technique. A definitive diagnosis of latent syphilis cannot be made under usual circumstances.

Treatment.

Primary, secondary, or early syphilis of less than 1 year duration: benzathine penicillin G 2.4 million units IM in a single dose.

Syphilis of indeterminate length or of more than 1 year duration: benzathine penicillin G 7.2 million units total; 2.4 million units IM, weekly, for 3 successive weeks.

Patients allergic to penicillin: Doxycycline 100 mg orally two times a day. [Note: Duration of therapy depends on the estimated duration of infection. If duration has been less than 1 year, treat the infection for 14 days; otherwise, treat for 28 days.]

Penicillin-allergic pregnant women or for doxycycline-intolerant patients only: Consult the *1998 Guidelines for Treatment of Sexually Transmitted Diseases*.

Congenital syphilis or if the patient is simultaneously infected with syphilis and HIV: Refer to the *1998 Guidelines for Treatment of Sexually Transmitted Diseases*.[11]

Potential complications. Late syphilis and congenital syphilis, both complications of early syphilis, are preventable with prompt diagnosis and treatment. Sequelae of late syphilis include neurosyphilis (general paresis, tabes dorsalis, and focal neurologic signs), cardiovascular syphilis (thoracic aortic aneurism, aortic insufficiency), and localized gumma formation.

Behavioral messages to emphasize. Because genital ulcers may be associated with HIV infection, get an HIV test. Return for follow-up syphilis serologies at 3 and 6 months for early syphilis, and at 6 and 12 months for late latent disease. HIV-positive patients should return 1, 2, 3, 6, 9, and 12 months after therapy; pregnant partners should be followed monthly. Understand how to take any prescribed oral medications. Refer sex partner(s) for evaluation and treatment. Avoid sexual activity until you and your partner(s) are cured. Use condoms to prevent future infections.

Trichomoniasis is caused by *Trichomonas vaginalis*, a motile protozoan with an undulating membrane and four flagella.

Prevalence. Trichomoniasis is the most common curable STI, in the United States and worldwide. Each year an estimated 3 million U.S. women become infected.

Symptoms. Excessive, frothy, diffuse, yellow-green vaginal discharge is common, although clinical presentation varies from no signs or symptoms to erythema, edema, and pruritis of the external genitalia. Dysuria and dyspareunia are also frequent. The type of symptoms or signs alone does *not* distinguish the microbial etiology. Male sex partners may develop urethritis, balanitis, or cutaneous lesions on the penis; however, the majority of males infected with *T. vaginalis* are asymptomatic.

Diagnosis. Trichomoniasis is diagnosed when a vaginal culture or fluorescent antibody is positive for *T. vaginalis* OR typical motile trichomonads are identified in a saline wet mount of vaginal discharge. Trichomonads found by Pap smear should be verified by examination of vaginal secretions.

Treatment. Metronidazole 2.0 g orally at one time. An alternative regimen is metronidazole 500 mg orally twice daily for 7 days. Metronidazole-resistant *T. vaginalis*, although uncommon, can occur. Most treatment failures respond to higher doses of therapy. Sex partners should be simultaneously treated with the same regimen as the index client.

Potential complications. Secondary excoriation may occur. Recurrent infections are common. Trichomoniasis has been associated with an increased risk of salpingitis, low birthweight, prematurity, and acquisition of HIV.

Behavioral messages to emphasize. Understand how to take or use prescribed medications. Return if the problem is not cured or recurs. Make sure sex partner(s) are treated. Use condoms to prevent future infections. Avoid drinking alcohol until 24 hours after completing metronidazole therapy.

REFERENCES

1. American College of Obstetrics and Gynecology and American Academy of Pediatrics. Guidelines for Perinatal Care, 4th edition. Washington DC: American College of Obstetrics and Gynecology, and American Academy of Pediatrics, 1996.
2. Bauer HM, Ting Y, Greer CE, Chambers JC, Tashiro CJ, Chimera J, Reingold A, Manos MM. Genital human papillomavirus infection in female university students as determined by a PCR-based method. JAMA 1991;265:472-477.
3. Cates W Jr. Sexually transmitted diseases. In: Sachs BP, Beard R, Papiernik E, Russell C (eds). Reproductive health care for women and babies: analysis of medical, economic, ethical and political issues. New York: Oxford University Press, 1995:57-84.
4. Cates W Jr. Contraception, unintended pregnancies, and sexually transmitted diseases: why isn't a simple solution possible? Am J Epidemiol 1996;143:311-318.
5. Cates W Jr. A risk assessment tool for integrated reproductive health services. Fam Plann Perspect 1997;29:41-43.
6. Cates W Jr, Berman SM, Darroch JE, Berkley SF. Epidemiology of STDs and STD sequelae. In: Hitchcock PJ, Berkley SF, Boruch R, Flay B, Darroch JE, Barouse D, Whitley R (eds). Adolescents and sexually transmitted diseases. New York: Oxford University Press (in press).
7. Cates W Jr, Stone KM. Family planning, sexually transmitted diseases, and contraceptive choice: a literature update—Part I. Fam Plann Perspect 1992;24(2):75-84.
8. Cates W Jr, Rolfs RT Jr, Aral SO. Sexually transmitted diseases, pelvic inflammatory disease, and infertility: an epidemiologic update. Epidemiol Rev 1990;12:199-220.

9. Cates W Jr, Stewart FH, Trussell J. The quest for women's prophylactic methods: hopes vs. science. Am J Public Health 1992;82:1479-1482.
10. Celum CL, Wilch E, Fennell C, Stamm WE. The management of sexually transmitted diseases. Second edition. Seattle, WA: University of Washington, Health Sciences Center for Educational Resources, 1994.
11. Centers for Disease Control and Prevention. 1998 Guidelines for treatment of sexually transmitted diseases. MMWR 1998;47(ss-4):1-132.
12. Centers for Disease Control and Prevention . Recommendations for the prevention and management of Chlamydia trachomatis infections. MMWR 1993;43(RR-12):1-39.
13. Davies AG, Clay JC. Prevalence of sexually transmitted disease infection in women alleging rape. Sex Transm Dis 1992;19:298-300.
14. Forrest KA, Washington AE, Daling JR, and Sweet RL. Vaginal douching as a possible risk factor for pelvic inflammatory disease. J Natl Med Assoc 1989;81:159-165.
15. Holmes KK, Mardh PA, Sparling PF, Lemon SM, Stamm WE, Piot P, Wasserheit JN (eds). Sexually transmitted diseases, third edition. New York: McGraw-Hill, 1998.
16. Hooton TM, Scholes D, Hughes JP, et al. A prospective study of risk factors for symptomatic urinary tract infection in young women. N Engl J Med 1996;335:468-474.
17. Institute of Medicine, Eng TR, Butler WT (eds). The hidden epidemic: confronting sexually transmitted diseases. Washington DC: National Academy Press, 1997.
18. Johnson RE, Nahmias AJ, Magder LS, Lee FK, Brooks CA, Snowden CB. A seroepidemiological survey of the prevalence of herpes simplex virus type 2 in the United States. N Engl J Med 1989;321:7-12.
19. Judson FN. Gonorrhea. Med Clin N Amer 1990;74:1353-1366.
20. Kahn JG, Walker CK, Washington AE, Landers DV, Sweet RL. Diagnosing pelvic inflammatory disease. JAMA 1991;266:2594-2604.
21. Lande RE. Controlling sexually transmitted diseases. Popul Rep 1993;Series L: No 9.
22. Marx R, Aral SO, Rolfs RT, Sterk CE, Kahn JG. Crack, sex and STD. Sex Transm Dis 1991;18:92-101.
23. Mertz GJ, Benedetti J, Ashley R, Selke SA, Corey L. Risk factors for the sexual transmission of genital herpes. Ann Intern Med 1992;116:197-202.
24. Mosure DJ, Berman S, Fine D, DeLisle S, Cates W Jr, Boring JR. Genital chlamydial infections in sexually active female adolescents: do we really need to screen everyone? J Adolesc Health Care 1997;20:6-13.
25. National Academy of Sciences, Tsui AO, Wasserheit JN, Haaga JG (eds). Reproductive health in developing countries: expanding dimensions, building solutions. Washington DC: National Academy Press, 1997.
26. Ness RB, Keder LM, Soper DE, Amortequi AJ, Gluck J, Weisenfield H, Sweet RL, Rice PA, Peipert JF, Donegan SP, Kanbour-Shakir A. Oral contraception and the recognition of endometritis. Am J Obstet Gynecol 1997;17:580-585.
27. Platt R, Rice PA, McCormack WM. Risk of acquiring gonorrhea and prevalence of abnormal adnexal findings among women recently exposed to gonorrhea. JAMA 1983;250:3205-3209.

28. Rolfs RT, Nakashima AK. Epidemiology of primary and secondary syphilis in the United States, 1981 through 1989. JAMA 1990;264:1432-1437.
29. Rothenberg RB, Potterat JJ. Strategies for management of sex partners. In: Holmes KK, Mardh P-A, Sparling PF, Wiesner PJ, Cates W Jr, Lemon SM, Stamm WE (eds). Sexually transmitted diseases, 2nd edition. New York: McGraw-Hill, 1990:1081-1086.
30. Scholes D, Stergachis A, Heidrich FE, Andrilla H, Holmes KK, Stamm WE. Prevention of pelvic inflammatory disease by screening for cervical chlamydial infection. N Engl J Med 1996;334:1362-1366.
31. Stamm WE, Hooton TM. Management of urinary tract infections in adults. N Engl J Med 1993;329:3128-3134.
32. Trussell J, Kost K. Contraceptive failure in the United States: a critical review of the literature. Stud Fam Plann 1987;18:237-283.
33. Wasserheit JN. Epidemiological synergy. Interrelationships between human immunodeficiency virus infection and other sexually transmitted diseases. Sex Transm Dis 1992;19:61-77.
34. Wentworth BB, Judson FN, Gilchrist MJR, eds. Laboratory methods for the diagnosis of sexually transmitted diseases, second edition. Washington DC: American Public Health Association, 1991.
35. Westrom L, Joesoef R, Reynolds G, Hadgu A, Thompson SE. Pelvic inflammatory disease and fertility. A cohort study of 1,844 women with laparoscopically verified and 657 control women with normal laparoscopic results. Sex Transm Dis 1992;19:185-192.
36. Zhang J, Thomas AG, Lebovich E. Vaginal douching and adverse health effects: a meta analysis. Am J Public Health 1997; 87:1207-1211.

The Essentials of Contraception

EFFICACY, SAFETY, AND
PERSONAL CONSIDERATIONS
James Trussell, PhD
Deborah Kowal, MA, PA

- Correct and consistent use of most contraceptive methods results in a low risk of pregnancy.
- Even a low annual risk of pregnancy implies a high cumulative risk of pregnancy during a lifetime of use. For example, an annual probability of pregnancy of 3% implies a 26% probability of pregnancy over 10 years.
- Emergency contraception provides a last chance to prevent pregnancy after unprotected intercourse.

- Contraceptives pose little risk to a user's health, although personal risk factors should influence personal choice.
- Half of all pregnancies are unintended: 3.2 million each year.
- Contraception saves medical care dollars by preventing unintended pregnancy. Ironically, women typically must pay for contraception while insurers, who pay for the cost of unintended pregnancy, reap the benefits of contraceptive use.

Choosing a method of contraception is an important decision. A method that is not effective for an individual can lead to the serious consequence of an unintended pregnancy. A method that is not safe for the user can create unfortunate medical consequences. A method that does not fit the individual's personal lifestyle is not likely to be used correctly or consistently. Who makes the choice? Individuals themselves should make the decision about the contraceptive method they use, taking into consideration the feelings and attitudes of their partners. The best method of contraception for an individual or couple is one that is safe and will actually be used correctly and consistently.

Through counseling, you can help your patient choose the most suitable contraceptive method. You also can influence the user's motivation and ability to use the method correctly.[19] Encourage clients to educate themselves about the various methods available. Simply stressing the "clinician's advice" makes women dependent upon a particular clinician's interpretation of current knowledge. Direct clients toward available literature. (See Chapter 11 on Selected Reproductive Health Resources.) Most people will use a variety of contraceptive methods throughout their lives and should be knowledgeable about various contraceptive methods. The patient's choice of a contraceptive method depends on several major factors: efficacy, safety, cost, noncontraceptive benefits, and personal considerations.

Information on levels and trends in contraceptive use in the United States is particularly good because it is based on the National Surveys of Family Growth (NSFG), periodic surveys conducted by the National Center for Health Statistics in which women age 15 to 44 are interviewed about topics related to childbearing, family planning, and maternal and child health. Among the 60.2 million women of reproductive age (age 15 to 44) in 1995, about 64% (38.6 million) were using some method of contraception, according to the 1995 NSFG. Among the 36% (21.6 million) who were not currently using a method, only about one-seventh were at risk of pregnancy. The remaining six-sevenths were not at risk because they had been sterilized for noncontraceptive reasons, were sterile, were trying to become pregnant, were pregnant, were interviewed within 2 months after the completion of a pregnancy, or were not having intercourse during the 3 months prior to the survey.[1]

Almost 93% of women at risk were using a contraceptive method. Seven percent of all women at risk of unintended pregnancy did not use any contraceptive method. Today, the most popular contraceptive methods are female sterilization (10.7 million), oral contraceptive pills (10.4 million), male condoms (7.9 million), and male sterilization (4.2 million).[1] See Table 9-1 for information on contraceptive method use by age of woman.[1,55]

Between 1988 and 1995, contraceptive method choices changed somewhat:

- Male condom use increased from 13.2% to 18.9% among all women age 15 to 44 at risk of pregnancy, generally because of the concern over acquired immune deficiency syndrome (AIDS) and sexually transmitted infections (STIs). Increases occurred in all age groups but were greatest among women age 20 to 24 (from 12.9% to 24.0%) and women age 25 to 29 (from 13.9% to 22.8%). Male condom use among women age 15 to 19 increased from 26.7% to 29.7%.
- Pill use among all women age 15 to 44 at risk declined slightly, from 27.7% to 24.9%. Pill use increased somewhat for women above age 30, but decreased among women below that age. Sub-

Table 9-1 Percentage and number of women at risk[1] and percentage at risk[1] currently using various methods from the 1995 National Survey of Family Growth

Age	Percent Using Among Women at Risk[1]						
	15–44	15–19	20–24	25–29	30–34	35–39	40–44
Female Sterilization	25.6	0.3	3.6	16.0	27.7	38.6	46.7
Pill	24.9	35.4	47.6	36.6	26.8	10.5	5.5
Male Condom	18.9	29.7	24.0	22.8	17.3	15.9	11.5
Male Sterilization	10.1	0.0	1.0	4.2	9.8	17.6	19.0
No Method	7.5	19.3	8.6	6.4	5.7	5.6	6.7
Withdrawal	2.9	3.3	3.0	3.5	2.7	3.0	1.8
Injectable	2.7	7.9	5.6	3.9	1.7	1.0	0.3
Periodic Abstinence	2.2	1.1	0.9	1.6	3.0	2.7	2.4
Natural Family Planning	0.3	0.0	0.1	0.3	0.4	0.5	0.3
Diaphragm	1.7	0.0	0.6	0.8	2.2	2.8	2.5
Implant	1.3	2.2	3.4	1.9	0.6	0.3	0.1
Spermicides	1.3	0.8	1.1	1.6	1.4	1.0	1.8
Intrauterine Device	0.7	0.0	0.3	0.7	0.8	0.9	1.2
Other[2]	0.1	0.0	0.1	0.0	0.3	0.1	0.5
Female Condom	0.0	0.0	0.1	0.0	0.0	0.0	0.0
Number of Women in Cohort, Percent and Number at Risk[1]							
Number (millions) of Women	60.2	9.0	9.0	9.7	11.1	11.2	10.2
Percent at Risk[1]	69.4	36.9	69.4	74.0	77.1	77.2	76.6
Number (millions) at Risk[1]	41.8	3.3	6.3	7.2	8.5	8.7	7.8

Source: Abma et al. (1997), Piccinino (1997).

Notes:
[1]At risk = those who EITHER are current contraceptive users OR are nonusers who have had sex in the past 3 months and are not trying to become pregnant, are not pregnant, or were not interviewed within 2 months after the completion of a pregnancy and are not sterile. Percentages may not add to 100 due to rounding.
[2]Other methods = cervical cap, sponge and other unspecified methods

stantial declines among women age 15 to 19 (from 47.1% to 35.4%) and 20 to 24 (from 59.8% to 47.6%) were compensated by use of two new methods, the implant and the injectable (used in 1995 by 10.1% and 9.0% of women age 15 to 19 and 20 to 24, respectively).

- Diaphragm use among all women age 15 to 44 at risk declined from 5.2% to only 1.7%, with the biggest decline observed among women age 30 to 34 (from 8.2% to 2.2%).

Actually, use of male condoms has increased more than these figures indicate. In the 1995 NSFG, women were asked to report all contraceptive methods used in the current month for any reason (for protection against either pregnancy or STDs). When more than one method was reported, only the most effective method is coded as the current method. Concomitant use of male condoms and sterilization, hormonal contraception, the intrauterine device (IUD), or diaphragm is coded in the NSFG as use of that other method, while concomitant use of male condoms and any contraceptive other than these methods is recoded as use of the male condom. When the data in Table 9-1 are recoded to capture all use of the male condom, the fraction using male condoms among all women at risk rises by 15%, from 18.9% to 21.6%. Increases are greatest among women age 20 to 24 (a 28% increase, from 24.0% to 30.7%) and women age 15 to 19 (a 25% increase, from 29.7% to 37.1%).[34]

The mix of methods shown in Table 9-1, including the 7.5% of women at risk who do not use any method, resulted in a staggering 3.04 million unintended pregnancies in 1994, the latest year for which data are available.[1,22,60] Nearly half (48.0%) of the 6.32 million pregnancies and nearly one-third (30.8% or 1.22 million) of the 3.95 million births in 1994 were unintended.[1,60] Every night in the United States, about 10 million couples at risk of unintended pregnancy have intercourse; among these, about 27,000 experience a condom break or slip, and over 700,000 are not protected against pregnancy at all.[1,39] (See Table 9-1 and Chapter 31.)

EFFICACY: "WILL IT WORK?"

"Is the condom really effective?"
"Which would be the most effective method for me?"
"Why did one magazine say diaphragms are 98% effective and another say they're 80% effective?"
"Can you still get pregnant if you take your pills every day on schedule?"

"Will it work?" is the question usually asked first and most frequently about any method of contraception. Because this question cannot be answered with certainty for any particular couple, most clinicians and counselors try to help patients understand something of the difficulty of quantifying efficacy.

It is useful to distinguish between measures of contraceptive effectiveness and measures of the risk of pregnancy during contraceptive use. If 20% of women using the diaphragm became accidentally pregnant in their first year of use, it does not follow that the diaphragm is 80% effective, because it is not true that 100% of these women would have become pregnant if they had not been using the diaphragm but had instead relied on chance. If 90% of these diaphragm users would have become pregnant had they relied on chance, the use of the diaphragm reduced the number of accidental pregnancies from 90% to 20%, a reduction of 78%. In this sense, the diaphragm could be said to be 78% effective at reducing pregnancy in the first year. But if only 60% of these women would have become pregnant if they did not use contraception, the diaphragm would be only 67% effective.* Because no study can ascertain the proportion of women who would have become pregnant had they not used the contraceptive method under investigation, it is simply not possible to measure effectiveness directly. Therefore, we focus attention entirely on pregnancy rates or probabilities of pregnancy during contraceptive use, which are directly measurable. However, we continue to use the term effectiveness in its loose everyday sense throughout this book. We also provide estimates of the proportion of women who would become pregnant if they did not use contraception, so the reader may calculate rough effectiveness rates if they are needed.

THE RISK OF PREGNANCY DURING TYPICAL AND PERFECT USE

Our current understanding of the literature on contraceptive efficacy is summarized in Table 9-2. More complete explanations of the derivations of the statistics in Table 9-2 are provided in Chapter 31. In addition, tables summarizing the efficacy literature for each method are contained in that chapter.

Typical use. In column 2 , we provide estimates of the probabilities of pregnancy during the first year of typical use of each method in the United States. For spermicides, periodic abstinence, the diaphragm, male condom, and pill, these estimates were derived from the experience of married women in the 1976 and 1982 National Surveys of Family Growth (NSFG) and of all women in the 1988 NSFG, so the information pertains to nationally representative samples of users.[24,50] We based the probabilities of pregnancy for the cervical cap and the sponge on results of two clinical trials in which women were randomly assigned to use the

---

*Strictly, effectiveness is the proportionate reduction in the probability per cycle of conception, c, when no contraception is used. If this per-cycle probability is constant across women and over time, then the proportion conceiving in 1 year with no contraceptive method use is $1-(1-c)^{13}$. Therefore, in the first example above $c = .162$ and in the second example $c = .068$. Using a contraceptive method with effectiveness e reduces the proportion becoming pregnant in 1 year to $1-\{1-c(1-e)\}^{13}$. Hence, in the first example, diaphragm effectiveness, strictly measured, is 90% and in the second example it is only 75%.

Table 9-2 Percentage of women experiencing an unintended pregnancy during the first year of typical use and the first year of perfect use of contraception and the percentage continuing use at the end of the first year: United States

Method (1)	% of Women Experiencing an Unintended Pregnancy within the First Year of Use		% of Women Continuing Use at One Year[3]
	Typical Use[1] (2)	Perfect Use[2] (3)	(4)
Chance[4]	85	85	
Spermicides[5]	26	6	40
Periodic Abstinence	25		63
Calendar		9	
Ovulation Method		3	
Symptothermal[6]		2	
Post-ovulation		1	
Cap[7]			
Parous Women	40	26	42
Nulliparous Women	20	9	56
Sponge			
Parous Women	40	20	42
Nulliparous Women	20	9	56
Diaphragm[7]	20	6	56
Withdrawal	19	4	
Condom[8]			
Female (Reality)	21	5	56
Male	14	3	61
Pill	5		71
Progestin only		0.5	
Combined		0.1	
IUD			
Progesterone T	2.0	1.5	81
Copper T 380A	0.8	0.6	78
LNg 20	0.1	0.1	81
Depo-Provera	0.3	0.3	70
Norplant and Norplant-2	0.05	0.05	88
Female Sterilization	0.5	0.5	100
Male Sterilization	0.15	0.10	100

Emergency Contraceptive Pills: Treatment initiated within 72 hours after unprotected intercourse reduces the risk of pregnancy by at least 75%.[9]
Lactational Amenorrhea Method: LAM is a highly effective, *temporary* method of contraception.[10]

(continued)

Table 9-2 Percentage of women experiencing an unintended pregnancy during the first year of typical use and the first year of perfect use of contraception and the percentage continuing use at the end of the first year: United States *(cont.)*

Source: Updated from Trussell and Kost (1987) and Trussell et al. (1990c). See Chapter 31.

[1]Among *typical* couples who initiate use of a method (not necessarily for the first time), the percentage who experience an accidental pregnancy during the first year if they do not stop use for any other reason.

[2]Among couples who initiate use of a method (not necessarily for the first time) and who use it *perfectly* (both consistently and correctly), the percentage who experience an accidental pregnancy during the first year if they do not stop use for any other reason.

[3]Among couples attempting to avoid pregnancy, the percentage who continue to use a method for 1 year.

[4]The percentages becoming pregnant in columns (2) and (3) are based on data from populations where contraception is not used and from women who cease using contraception in order to become pregnant. Among such populations, about 89% become pregnant within 1 year. This estimate was lowered slightly (to 85%) to represent the percentages who would become pregnant within 1 year among women now relying on reversible methods of contraception if they abandoned contraception altogether.

[5]Foams, creams, gels, vaginal suppositories, and vaginal film.

[6]Cervical mucus (ovulation) method supplemented by calendar in the pre-ovulatory and basal body temperature in the post-ovulatory phases.

[7]With spermicidal cream or jelly.

[8]Without spermicides.

[9]The treatment schedule is one dose within 72 hours after unprotected intercourse, and a second dose 12 hours after the first dose. The Food and Drug Administration has declared the following brands of oral contraceptives to be safe and effective for emergency contraception: Ovral (1 dose is 2 white pills), Alesse (1 dose is 5 pink pills), Nordette or Levlen (1 dose is 4 light-orange pills), Lo/Ovral (1 dose is 4 white pills), Triphasil or Tri-Levlen (1 dose is 4 yellow pills).

[10]However, to maintain effective protection against pregnancy, another method of contraception must be used as soon as menstruation resumes, the frequency or duration of breastfeeds is reduced, bottle feeds are introduced, or the baby reaches 6 months of age.

diaphragm or sponge or the diaphragm or cervical cap. Our estimates for methods such as the IUD, sterilization, Depo-Provera and Norplant were derived from large clinical investigations. The estimate for the female condom is based on the only clinical trial of this method. Finally, the estimates for withdrawal and chance were based on evidence from surveys and clinical investigations, respectively.

Pregnancy rates during typical use reflect how effective methods are for the average person who does not always use methods correctly or consistently. It is very important to understand typical use does not imply a contraceptive method was actually used. In the NSFG and in most clinical trials, a woman is "using" a contraceptive method if she considers herself to be using that method. So typical use of the condom could include actually using a condom only occasionally, and a woman could report she is "using" the pill even though her supplies ran out several months ago. In short, *use*—which is identical to *typical use*—is a very elastic concept that depends entirely on an individual woman's perception.

Perfect use. In column 3, we provide our best guess of the probabilities of *method* failure (pregnancy) during the first year of perfect use. A method is used perfectly when it is used consistently according to a specified set of rules. For many methods, perfect use requires use at every act of intercourse. Virtually all method failure rates reported in the literature have been calculated incorrectly and are too low. (See the discussion on Methodological Pitfalls.) Hence, we cannot justify our estimates rigorously except those for the ovulation method of periodic abstinence,[46] the cervical cap,[35,53] the diaphragm,[53] the sponge,[53] the male condom,[64] and the female condom,[15] those for methods with little scope for user error (implants, injectables, and sterilization), and those for the pill and IUD, which are based on extensive clinical trials with very low pregnancy rates. Even the estimates for the male condom, female condom, diaphragm, cervical cap, and sponge are based on only one or two studies. Our hope is that our understanding of efficacy during perfect use for these methods will be enhanced by additional studies, and that the total gap in our knowledge for methods such as spermicides, the male condom, withdrawal, and other variants of periodic abstinence will be closed by future research.

It is interesting to compare these estimates with pregnancy rates observed among women using isotretinoin, which is effective in treating severe acne but is also teratogenic. To minimize pregnancies among women undergoing treatment, the manufacturer and the U.S. Food and Drug Administration (FDA) implemented a pregnancy prevention program. Among 76,149 women who reported using contraception, 268 became pregnant, yielding a rate of 3.6 per 1,000 20-week courses of therapy;[32] this rate, if constant for a year, would be equivalent to an annual probability of pregnancy of 0.9%. Estimated annual probabilities of pregnancy were 0.8%, 2.1%, and 2.6% among women who reported using oral contraceptives, diaphragms, and condoms, respectively. Thus women using diaphragms achieved lower rates of pregnancy than we estimate would occur during perfect use, those using condoms experienced about the same pregnancy rate that would be expected during perfect use, while those using oral contraceptives had higher pregnancy rates than would be expected during perfect use. Pregnancy rates for women using any of these three methods, however, were substantially below rates generally observed during typical use; this finding would appear to indicate that understanding of the teratogenic risks of isotretinoin substantially enhanced correct and consistent use. It is also possible women in this study had lower than average fecundity because acne is a marker for excess androgen production resulting from anovulation,[41] that they lowered their coital frequency during treatment, or that they under-reported their number of pregnancies (and abortions).

Continuing use. Column 4 displays the first-year probabilities of continuing use. They are based on the same sources used to derive the estimates in the first column (typical use).

Alternative Estimates of Pregnancy During Typical Use

Alternative estimates of the probabilities of pregnancy during the first year of typical use are provided in Table 9-3. These are based on the 1976 and 1982 NSFGs,[50] the 1986 Australian Family Survey,[5] and the 1988 NSFG.[24] The estimates in the second column are standardized probabilities of pregnancy among married women based on the 1976 and 1982 NSFGs. They differ from the estimates in the other columns because they are based on the experience of married women only. They also are standardized to reflect the estimated probabilities of pregnancy that would be observed if users of each method had the same characteristics (the same age distribution, the same fraction seeking to prevent further childbearing instead of delaying the next wanted pregnancy, the same parity distribution, and the same fraction living in poverty), unlike the estimates in the third, fourth and fifth columns. The estimates in the third column are based on Australian women (62% of whom were married or cohabiting, ranging from only 45% of those using the pill to 92% of those using periodic abstinence or withdrawal) who were using a method for the first time. The estimates in the fourth column are based on all women age 15 to 44 in the 1988 NSFG regardless of marital or cohabitation status. Those in the fifth column are revised to reflect estimated under-reporting of induced abortion in the 1988 NSFG. The estimates in the sixth column are corrected for estimated under-reporting of abortion and standardized on a common distribution of age, poverty status and marital status.

The estimates from the 1976 and 1982 NSFGs are very similar to those from the Australian Family Survey and are slightly lower than the unstandardized estimates based on the 1988 NSFG corrected for under-reporting of abortion, even though the estimates pertain to different populations of users. We reason that the correction for under-reporting of abortion produces estimates (column 6) that are too high because women in abortion clinics (surveys of whom provided the information for the correction) over-report use of a contraceptive method at the time they became pregnant. Moreover, it seems likely that women in personal interviews for the NSFG also would tend to over-report use of a contraceptive method at the time of a conception leading to a live birth. Evidence for this suspicion is provided by a first-year probability of pregnancy of 6% for the IUD (a method with little scope for user error) among married women in the 1976 and 1982 NSFGs. This probability is much higher than rates observed in clinical trials of IUDs.[50] We would

Table 9-3 Percentage of women experiencing an unintended pregnancy in the first year of typical use of contraception: United States and Australia

Method (1)	United States 1976 and 1982 NSFGs. Married Women, Standardized (2)	Australia 1986 AFS. All Women, Not Standardized (3)	United States 1988 NSFG (uncorrected for abortion). All Women, Not Standardized (4)	United States 1988 NSFG (corrected for abortion). All Women, not Standardized (5)	United States 1988 NSFG (corrected for abortion). All Women, Standardized (6)
Pill	3	2	5	8	7
Male Condom	12	8	7	15	16
Diaphragm	18	21	10	16	22
Periodic Abstinence	20	18	21	26	31
Spermicides	21	22	13	25	30

Sources: 1976 and 1982 NSFGs, Trussell, et al. (1990c); 1986 AFS, Bracher and Santow (1992); 1988 NSFG, Jones and Forrest (1992).

naturally expect over-reporting of contraceptive method use in both the NSFG and in surveys conducted in abortion clinics: responsibility for the pregnancy is shifted from the woman (or couple) to the method. Thus, we suspect pregnancy rates based on the NSFG alone would tend to be too low because induced abortions (and contraceptive failures leading to induced abortions) are under-reported but would tend to be too high because contraceptive failures leading to live births are over-reported. These two sources of bias would tend to cancel, whereas adjustment for under-reporting of induced abortion would make the pregnancy rates too high. However, we would expect estimates based on married women only for the 1976 and 1982 NSFGs to be underestimates of the risk of pregnancy for all women, since unmarried women regularly having intercourse experience higher pregnancy rates during typical use of contraceptives than do married women.[24] We conclude the estimates in the second column of Table 9-3 are likely to be too low and those in the last column of Table 9-3 are likely to be too high; our final estimate (the second column in Table 9-2) is the average of these two.

SIMULTANEOUS USE OF METHODS

Using two methods at once dramatically lowers the risk of unintended pregnancy, provided they are used consistently. If one of the methods is a condom or vaginal barrier, protection from disease transmission is an added benefit. For example, the probabilities of pregnancy during the first year of perfect use of male condoms and spermicides are estimated to be 3% and 6%, respectively, in Table 9-2. It is reasonable to assume that during perfect use the contraceptive mechanisms of condoms and spermicides operate independently, since lack of independence during typical use would most likely be due to imperfect use (either use both methods or not use either). The annual probability of pregnancy during simultaneous perfect use of condoms and spermicides would be 0.1%, the same as that achieved by the combined pill (0.1%) and the Levonorgestrel (LNg) 20 IUD (0.1%) during perfect use. Even if the annual probabilities of pregnancy during perfect use for the condom and spermicides were twice as high—6% and 12%, respectively—the annual probability of pregnancy during simultaneous perfect use would be only 0.4%, comparable to that of the minipill (0.5%) and the Copper T 380A IUD (0.6%) during perfect use![25]

EFFICACY OVER TIME

We confine attention to the first-year probabilities of pregnancy solely because probabilities for longer durations are generally not available.

Pregnancy rates at these longer durations for most methods (but not Norplant) should be lower than pregnancy rates during the first year, primarily because those users prone to fail do so early, leaving a pool of more successful contraceptive users (or those who are relatively infertile) as time passes. Nevertheless, probabilities of pregnancy cumulate over time. Suppose 15%, 12%, and 8% of women using a method experience a contraceptive failure during years 1, 2, and 3, respectively. The probability of not becoming pregnant within 3 years is obtained by multiplying the probabilities of not becoming pregnant for each of the 3 years: 0.85 times 0.88 times 0.92, which equals 0.69. Thus, the percentage becoming pregnant within 3 years is 31% (=100% − 69%).

The lesson here is that the differences among probabilities of pregnancy for various methods will increase over time. For example, suppose each year the typical proportion becoming pregnant while taking the pill is 5% and while using the diaphragm is 20%. Within 5 years, 23% of pill users and 67% of diaphragm users would become pregnant.

CONTRACEPTIVE FAILURES IN A LIFETIME

Data from the 1982 NSFG indicate that from 1979 to 1982 there were 1.61 million contraceptive failures per year and that the typical woman would experience 0.81 contraceptive failures during her lifetime.[54] It is important this statistic be interpreted precisely. It is the average number of failures that a hypothetical woman would experience if during her life she faced at each age the risk of contraceptive failure actually observed in the 3 years from 1979 to 1981. These age-specific risks are governed by the proportions of women having intercourse, their frequency of intercourse, the mix of contraceptive methods, the consistency and correctness of contraceptive method use, the outcomes of pregnancies (births or induced abortions) and the underlying fecundity of the woman and her partner(s). Therefore, the estimate is very unlikely to pertain to any individual woman or even a cohort of women, because all the proximate determinants listed above are likely to change over time. Nevertheless, the estimate is a convenient summary statistic pertaining to a specific period of time.

Because the total fertility rate (TFR) between 1979 and 1981 averaged 1.82,[33] these results imply the typical woman will experience one contraceptive failure for every 2.25 live births during her lifetime, so contraceptive failures are not uncommon relative to live births. We suspect many readers will be surprised that the average lifetime number of contraceptive failures is so low, but several factors operate to make it smaller than one might expect.

- First, the average annual risk of contraceptive failure (which includes women at all durations of use) is much smaller than the first-year rates published in the literature and summarized in Table 9-2, because pregnancy rates decline with duration of use.[50,58,59,61]

- Second, substantial fractions of women are exposed to extremely small risks of contraceptive failure because they or their partners have been sterilized. In the preceding analysis, 39%, 54%, and 56% of the women age 30–34, 35–39, and 40–44, respectively, were protected by sterilization. If intervals during which women were protected by sterilization are removed when calculating the age-specific contraceptive failure rates, one obtains an estimate of 0.97 lifetime contraceptive failures for the typical woman who relies solely on reversible methods when she does use contraception.

- Third, contraceptive failures cannot be experienced by women who do not use contraception. The annual numbers of contraceptive failures experienced by teenagers are particularly low for this reason. If intervals during which contraception was not used (except during pregnancy following a contraceptive failure) are also removed from the denominators of the age-specific failure rates, one obtains an estimate of 1.96 lifetime failures for the typical woman who seeks to avoid pregnancy throughout her lifetime by relying solely on reversible methods.[54]

FACTORS THAT INFLUENCE EFFICACY

You and your patients can better understand why the answer to the simple question "Will it work?" is such a complicated issue if we recall that many factors influence efficacy. Factors that affect contraceptive failure rates and probabilities reported in the literature can be usefully divided into three categories: (1) the inherent efficacy of the method when used correctly and consistently (perfect use) and the technical attributes of the method that facilitate or interfere with proper use, (2) characteristics of the user, and (3) competence and honesty of the investigator in planning and executing the study and in analyzing and reporting the results.

Inherent Efficacy

For some methods, such as sterilization, implants, and the copper-T IUD, the inherent efficacy is so high and proper and consistent use is so nearly guaranteed that extremely low pregnancy rates are found in all studies, and the range of reported pregnancy rates is quite narrow. For other methods such as the pill and injectable, inherent efficacy is high, but there is still room for potential misuse (forgetting to take pills or failure to return on time for injections), so that the second factor can contribute to a wider range of reported probabilities of pregnancy. In general, the studies of sterilization, injectable, implant, pill, and IUD use have been very competently executed and analyzed. Studies of periodic abstinence, spermicides, and the barrier methods display a wide range of reported probabilities of pregnancy because the potential for misuse is high, the inherent efficacy is relatively low, and the competence of the investigators is mixed.

User Characteristics

Characteristics of the users can affect the pregnancy rate for any method under investigation, but the impact will be greatest when the pregnancy rates during typical use are highest, either because the method has less inherent efficacy or because it is hard to use consistently or correctly.

Imperfect use. The most important user characteristic is imperfect use of the method. Unfortunately, nearly all investigators who have attempted to calculate "method" and "user" failure rates have done so incorrectly. Investigators routinely separate the unintended pregnancies into two groups. By convention, pregnancies that occur during a month in which a method was used improperly are classified as user failures (even though, logically, a pregnancy might be due to failure of the method, if it was used correctly on some occasions), and all other pregnancies are classified as method failures. But investigators do not separate the exposure (the denominator in the calculation of failure rates) into these two groups.

For example, suppose there are two method failures and 8 user failures during 100 women-years of exposure to the risk of pregnancy. Then the common calculation is the user failure rate is 8% and the method failure rate is 2%; the sum of the two is the overall failure rate of 10%. By definition, however, method failures can occur only during perfect use and user failures cannot occur during perfect use. If there are 50 years of perfect and 50 years of imperfect use in the total of 100 years of exposure, the method failure rate would be 4% and the user failure rate would be 16%; the difference between the two rates (here 12%) provides a measure of how forgiving of imperfect use the method is. However, since investigators do not generally inquire about perfect use except when a pregnancy occurs, the proper calculations cannot be performed. The importance of perfect use is demonstrated in the few studies where the requisite information on quality of use was collected. For example, in a World Health Organization (WHO) study of the ovulation method of periodic abstinence, the proportion of women becoming pregnant among those who used the method perfectly during the first year was 3.1%, whereas the corresponding proportion failing during a year of imperfect use was 86.4%.[46] In a large clinical trial of the cervical cap conducted in Los Angeles, among the 5% of the sample who used the method perfectly, the fraction failing during the first year was 6.1%. Among the remaining 95% of the sample who at least on one occasion used the cap imperfectly, the first-year probability of pregnancy was nearly twice as high (11.9%).[35]

Frequency of intercourse.   Among those who use a method consistently and correctly (perfect users), the most important user characteristic that determines the risk of pregnancy is frequency of intercourse. For example, in a study in which users were randomly assigned to either the diaphragm or the sponge, diaphragm users who had intercourse four or more times a week became pregnant in the first year twice as frequently as those who had intercourse fewer than four times a week.[29] In that clinical trial, among women who used the diaphragm at every act of intercourse, only 3.4% of those who had intercourse fewer than three times a week became pregnant in the first year, compared with 9.7% of those who had intercourse three or more times per week.[53]

Age.   A woman's biological capacity to conceive and bear a child declines with age. This decline is likely to be pronounced among those who are routinely exposed to sexually transmitted infections such as chlamydia and gonorrhea. Among those not so exposed, the decline is likely to be moderate until a woman reaches her late thirties.[30] Although many investigators have found that contraceptive failure rates decline with age,[20,36,38,61] this effect almost surely overstates the pure effect of age because in many studies age primarily captures the effect of coital frequency, which declines both with age and with marital duration.[56] User characteristics such as race and income seem to be less important determinants of contraceptive failure.

Influence of the Investigator

The competence and honesty of the investigator also affect the published results. The errors committed by investigators range from simple arithmetical mistakes to outright fraud.[50] One well-documented instance of fraud involved the Dalkon shield. In a two-page article published in the *American Journal of Obstetrics and Gynecology*, for example, a first-year probability of pregnancy of 1.1% was presented and the claim made that "only the combined type of oral contraceptive offers slightly greater protection."[11] It was not revealed by the researcher that some women had been instructed to use spermicides as an adjunctive method to reduce the risk of pregnancy, nor that he was part-owner of the Dalkon Corporation. Furthermore, he never subsequently revealed (except to the A.H. Robins Company, which bought the shield from the Dalkon Corporation but did not reveal this information either) that as the original trial matured, the first-year probability of pregnancy more than doubled.[31]

The system of drug testing in the United States, which demands the company wishing to market a drug be responsible for conducting studies to assess its efficacy and safety, provides incentives for the unscrupulous to present less-than-honest results. Some actions that are not deliberately dishonest are, nevertheless, not discouraged by the incentives in the present system. For example, a woman who becomes pregnant may be discarded from a clinical trial if the researcher decides she did not fit the protocols after all. Or one can be less than vigilant in trying to contact patients lost to follow-up (LFU). The standard assumption made at the time of analysis is that women who are LFU experience unintended pregnancy at the same rate as those who are observed. This assumption is probably innocuous when the proportion LFU is small. But in many studies the proportion LFU may be 20% or higher, so what really happens to these women could drastically affect the estimate of the proportion becoming pregnant. Our strong suspicion is that women LFU are more likely to experience a contraceptive failure than are those remaining in the trial. For example, one study found the pregnancy rate for calendar rhythm rose from 9.4 to 14.4 per 100 women-years of exposure as a result of resolution of cases LFU.[43]

Methodological Pitfalls

Several methodological pitfalls can snare investigators. One of the most common is a misleading measure of contraceptive failure called the Pearl index, which is obtained by dividing the number of unintended pregnancies by the number of years of exposure to the risk of unintended pregnancy contributed by all women in the study. This measure can be misleading when one wishes to compare pregnancy rates obtained from studies with different average amounts of exposure. The likelihood of pregnancy declines over time because those most likely to become pregnant do so at earlier durations of contraceptive use and exit from observation. Those still using after long durations are unlikely to become pregnant, so an investigator could (wittingly or unwittingly) drive the reported pregnancy rate toward zero by running the trial "forever." Two investigators using the National Survey of Family Growth could obtain Pearl-index pregnancy rates of 7.5 and 4.4 per 100 women-years of exposure for the condom.[52] One (who got 4.4) allowed each woman to contribute a maximum of 5 years of exposure while the other (who got 7.5) allowed each woman to contribute only 1 year. Which investigator is incorrect? Neither. The two rates are simply not comparable. Life table measures of contraceptive failure are easy to interpret and control for the distorting effects of varying durations of use. (See Chapter 30 on Dynamics of Reproductive Behavior and Population Growth.) Another problem occurs when deciding which pregnancies to count. Most studies count only the pregnancies observed and reported by the women. If, on the other hand, a pregnancy test were administered every month, the number of pregnancies (and hence the pregnancy rate) would increase because early fetal losses not observed by the woman would be added to the number of observed pregnancies. Such routine pregnancy testing in the more recent contraceptive trials has resulted in higher pregnancy rates than would otherwise have been obtained and makes the results not comparable to those from other trials. Other, more technical, errors that have biased reported results are discussed elsewhere.[44,47,50]

The incentives to conduct research on contraceptive failure vary widely from method to method. Many studies of the pill and IUD exist because companies wishing to market them must conduct clinical trials to demonstrate their efficacy. In contrast, few studies of withdrawal exist because there is no financial reward for investigating this method. Moreover, researchers face differing incentives to report unfavorable results. The vasectomy literature is filled with short articles by clinicians who have performed 500 or 1,000 or 1,500 vasectomies. When they report pregnancies (curiously, pregnancy is seldom mentioned in discussions of vasectomy "failures," which focus on the continued presence of sperm in the ejaculate), their pregnancy rates are invariably low. Surgeons with high pregnancy rates simply do not write articles calling attention to their poor surgical skills. Likewise, drug companies do not commonly publicize their failures. Even if investigators prepared reports describing failures, journal editors would not be likely to publish them.

GOALS FOR TEACHING EFFICACY

Keep these thoughts in mind when counseling about contraceptive efficacy:

1. **What matters most is correct and consistent use.** For example, a 5% probability of pregnancy during the first year for typical use of the pill will not protect the careless user. The 20% probability of pregnancy during the first year of typical diaphragm use need not discourage a careful and disciplined woman who has infrequent intercourse from using a diaphragm.

2. **Make sure your staff provides consistent and correct information.** One study of the information provided by family planning staff indicated that providers tended to give the lowest reported probabilities of pregnancy for pills and IUDs, probabilities of pregnancy during typical use for diaphragms and spermicides, and higher-than-typical probabilities of pregnancy for condoms.[45] Thus, family planning providers may extensively bias their patient education in favor of methods they provide most frequently. In spite of their safety, condoms and withdrawal get an undeserved low efficacy score within many family planning clinics and offices. You can avoid unintentional bias by deciding carefully what pregnancy rates your clinic or staff members are going to use.

3. **Technology fails people just as people fail technology.** Patients are sometimes told that unintended pregnancies are their own fault because they did not use their method correctly or carefully. Contraceptive methods are imperfect and can fail even the most diligent user.

4. **Using two methods at once dramatically lowers the risk of unintended pregnancy,** provided they are used consistently. If one of the methods is a condom or vaginal barrier, protection from disease transmission is an added benefit.

5. **Emergency contraception provides a last chance to prevent pregnancy after unprotected intercourse.** Emergency contraceptive pills (ECPs) are an especially important second method for those relying on condoms, in cases of breakage or slippage, for those who do not actually use their ongoing method for whatever reason, and those who are forced to have unprotected intercourse.

6. **Methods that protect a person for a long time** (sterilization, implants, IUDs, and long-acting injections) **tend to be associated with lower pregnancy rates,** primarily because there is little scope for user error.

SAFETY: "WILL IT HURT ME?"

"I smoke. Won't the pill give me a heart attack?"
"Could the IUD puncture my womb?"
"Will I be able to get pregnant after stopping my method?"

In general, contraception poses few serious health risks to users. Moreover, the safety considerations of contraceptive methods are not as great as those of pregnancy-related complications. Unplanned and unwanted pregnancies place women at risk unnecessarily. Women in many developing countries will experience an even greater advantage in using contraceptive methods, especially in comparison to pregnancy-related mortality. Nonetheless, some contraceptive methods pose potential risk to the user.

- First, the method itself may have inherent dangers: it might be associated with death, hospitalization, surgery, medical side effects, infections, loss of reproductive capacity, or pain.
- Second, pregnancy itself is associated with risk: a woman must assess both the likelihood of contraceptive failure and the dangers a pregnancy would pose.
- Third, future fertility may be influenced by choice of a contraceptive method.

MAJOR HEALTH RISKS

When it comes to the most serious outcome of all—death—the absolute level of risk is extraordinarily low for most women (Table 9-4). Although the information in this table should not be used to dismiss the concerns of a woman who is worried about pills, abortion, or tampons, it may help her compare these risks with other risks she voluntarily faces in her life.

Other major health risks are not only uncommon, they are most likely to occur in women who have underlying medical conditions that may be influenced by hormonal contraception:

Cardiovascular disease. The pill has been associated with an increased risk of myocardial infarction and stroke. About 1.5 deaths per year in 100,000 nonsmoking users under the age of 45 have been attributable to use of the pill.[21] Risk increases with age because risk factors such as hypertension, thromboembolic disease, diabetes, and a sedentary lifestyle increase with age. Smoking definitely increases this risk, especially in women over age 35 who smoke more than 25 cigarettes a day.

Cancer. The pill appears to protect users against cancers of the endometrium and ovary.[37] The net effect of pill use on cancer is negligible.[37] The association between cancer of the breast and cervix and the use of the pill remains under scrutiny.

- Women face a slightly increased risk (about 20% higher) for having breast cancer diagnosed while they are using oral contraceptives and for 10 years after stopping use. Cancers diagnosed in these women are less advanced clinically than those diagnosed in women of the same age who have never used oral contraceptives.[10] The increased risk is apparent soon after exposure but does not increase with exposure and does not persist beyond 10 years

Table 9-4 Voluntary risks in perspective

Activity	Chance of Death in a Year
Risks per year for men and women of all ages who participate in:	
Motorcycling	1 in 1,000
Automobile driving	1 in 5,900
Power boating	1 in 5,900
Rock climbing	1 in 7,200
Playing football	1 in 25,000
Canoeing	1 in 100,000
Risks per year for women aged 15 to 44 years:	
Using tampons	1 in 350,000
Having sexual intercourse (PID)	1 in 50,000
Risks for women preventing pregnancy:	
Using oral contraceptives (per year)	
Nonsmoker	1 in 66,700
Age less than 35	1 in 200,000
Age 35–44	1 in 28,600
Heavy smoker (25 or more cigarettes per day)	1 in 1,700
Age less than 35	1 in 5,300
Age 35–44	1 in 700
Using IUDs (per year)	1 in 10,000,000
Using diaphragm, condom, or spermicides	None
Using fertility awareness methods	None
Undergoing sterilization:	
Laparoscopic tubal ligation	1 in 38,500
Hysterectomy	1 in 1,600
Vasectomy	1 in 1,000,000
Risk per pregnancy from continuing pregnancy	1 in 10,000
Risk from terminating pregnancy:	
Legal abortion	
Before 9 weeks	1 in 262,800
Between 9 and 12 weeks	1 in 100,100
Between 13 and 15 weeks	1 in 34,400
After 15 weeks	1 in 10,200

Sources: Berg, et al. (1996), Cates (1980), Dinman (1980), Escobedo, et al. (1989), Harlap, Kost and Forrest (1991), Lawson, et al. (1994), Lee (1981).

after exposure ceases. These patterns are not typical for a carcinogenic agent but could be consistent with promotion of already existing tumors or with earlier diagnosis of breast cancer in women who have used the pill.

- The incidence of cervical cancer is increased in women using oral contraceptives, particularly over the long-term.[42,62,63] Cervical cancer risk is strongly linked to infection with HPV.[4] It is possible pill use could affect cervical cancer directly, or indirectly by altering susceptibility to infection with HPV. Epidemiological studies indicate this excess risk persists after adjustment for potential confounding factors such as cigarette smoking, age at first intercourse, number of sexual partners, sexual behavior of male partners, and history of Papanicolaou smear screening.[6] Barrier methods used in conjunction with spermicides decrease the user's risk of cervical cancer.[9]

FUTURE FERTILITY

An important issue in helping a couple evaluate safety as they choose a contraceptive method may be their future childbearing aspirations. Several important considerations may help to protect the future fertility of patients:

- **Abstinence** from vaginal intercourse is the single most effective and risk-free means of protecting future fertility.
- **Pregnancy** and the outcomes of pregnancy carry risks to future fertility. About 20% of women undergo surgical (cesarean) delivery, which involves an increased risk of infection that could result in permanent tubal damage. Postpartum infection can also occur after vaginal delivery.
- **Oral contraceptives and other hormonal methods** do not provide protection against STIs, which can cause pelvic inflammatory disease (PID) and lead to infertility. When STI risk is a concern, avoiding intercourse, or using condoms correctly and consistently, is essential for preserving future fertility.
- **Mechanical and chemical barriers** reduce the risk of PID and of ectopic pregnancy, with the greatest risk reduction for those using a combination of both.[7]
- **The IUD** does not protect against STI. Women in recent IUD clinical trials who are presumed to have been at low risk of sexually transmitted infections have had no increased risk of pelvic infection except in the first few weeks following IUD insertion.[14]

- **Sterilization** must be considered permanent. It does not protect against STIs.

SIDE EFFECTS

Often the minor side effects of contraceptive methods, in addition to the more serious complications, influence whether an individual selects a certain method. "What physical changes will I undergo?" "Will I be annoyed by spotting, weight gain, cramping, or the sensation or messiness of using a given method?" Clinicians cannot dismiss the important role side effects play when an individual must repeatedly assess whether to continue using a method or whether to use it consistently.

Side effects can be hormonally, chemically, or mechanically induced. Headaches, weight gain, and depression can be side effects of hormonal methods. Menstrual changes such as spotting and decreased or increased bleeding can be caused by hormonal methods and IUDs. Physical sensations such as decreased penile sensitivity, pressure on pelvic walls, or uterine cramping are generally caused by mechanical methods. Other mechanically induced side effects include perforation of the uterus during IUD insertion and vaginal trauma from vaginal barrier methods. Use of a diaphragm and spermicide is strongly associated with an increased risk of urinary tract infection (UTI). Although the causal mechanism was long thought to be mechanical, it is now recognized as chemical, due to replacement of normal lactobacilli in the vagina by anaerobic organisms and vaginal irritation related to the detergent action of spermicides.[17,23] Other chemically induced side effects include allergic reactions to latex and to copper.

With the great majority of these side effects, patient education helps users accept and understand what is happening. The appearance of side effects that are not serious is not a medical contraindication to use of a method.

PRECAUTIONS

Some women are more likely than others to encounter problems with a specific method of contraception, so considering the precautions to the use of methods is important when a woman chooses her method. Most of the serious pill and IUD problems could be avoided by (1) not using the methods to which a woman has medical precautions and (2) teaching the user to recognize the early danger signals for serious complications.

The authors prefer to avoid the concept of contraindications to any given method. In the past, lists of contraindications have created barriers to provision and use of contraceptive methods. In place of contraindicating the use of a method, the authors suggest using a graded scale of precautions:

- Precautions — Refrain from providing the method to women with medical conditions that may increase their risk of serious complications.
- Exercise caution — Carefully follow the woman's health situation and monitor her for adverse side effects.
- Provide with care — Provide follow-up care and instruct the woman about early danger signals.

GOALS FOR TEACHING SAFETY

1. **Try to educate the patient about misconceptions**. People who are afraid do not respond well to rational persuasions. Many patients hold certain opinions about contraceptive methods—the pill is very dangerous even to healthy, nonsmoking young women or injectables lead to permanent sterility. If you see you are getting nowhere, stop. Help each client select a method that can be used correctly and consistently without fear.

2. **Make sure you and your staff know all about the major side effects** of contraceptive methods, such as the relation between pill use and blood clots or reproductive cancers. Give accurate information.

3. **Tell patients what they need to know** even if they do not ask. Patients do not always ask the questions they need answered.

4. **Compare risks of using contraception with pregnancy risks**. In general, the risks of pregnancy, abortion, and delivery are far greater than those for using a contraceptive method.

5. **Help patients make a contraceptive method choice that will protect them from both pregnancy and STIs**. Safety concerns often overlap with worries about infections. With the exception of abstinence, currently available methods that protect best against infection are not those that provide greatest protection against pregnancy. Conversely, the most highly effective methods of contraception provide *no* protection against infection. Therefore, highly effective protection against both risks requires use of two methods. Even abstinence has different rules for protection against pregnancy and protection against infection: oral and anal intercourse can result in STI transmission but not in pregnancy.

6. **Teach patients the danger signals** of the method they select. If a danger signal does appear, the informed user can quickly seek help.

NONCONTRACEPTIVE BENEFITS

Although the noncontraceptive benefits provided by certain methods are not generally the major determinant for selecting a contraceptive method, they certainly can help patients decide between two or more suitable methods (Table 9-5).

As the AIDS epidemic continues, methods that reduce the user's risk of acquiring HIV infection provide a noncontraceptive benefit that may weigh as heavily as the contraceptive benefit. Any sexually active person who may be at risk of acquiring infection with the HIV or other STIs should consider barrier methods, especially condoms.[16]

Fertility awareness methods provide key noncontraceptive benefits by educating women about their menstrual physiology. This knowledge can also help couples achieve a planned pregnancy.

The LNg 20 IUD has several noncontraceptive benefits, including markedly reduced menstrual blood loss and pain, very low ectopic pregnancy rate, and reduced risk of PID and endometritis.[28] It can be used to treat menorrhagia and to induce regression of endometrial hyperplasia or uterine fibroids. In addition, it may provide a new way of adding progestin in hormone replacement therapy.

Oral contraceptives offer several noncontraceptive benefits: protection against PID, cancers of the ovary and endometrium, recurrent ovarian cysts, and benign breast cysts and fibroadenomas.[21] As women who have suffered menstrual cramps and discomforts can attest, the pill eases their discomforts. The pill also provides relief from perimenopausal symptoms.

Make it a practice to tell your patients about the noncontraceptive benefits of the various methods. If patients have additional reasons for using the contraceptive method, their motivation to use the method correctly and consistently will probably be improved.

PERSONAL CONSIDERATIONS

A typical woman in the United States spends about 36 years—almost half of her lifespan of 79 years—at potential biological risk of pregnancy, during the time from menarche (at age 12.5) to natural menopause (at age 48.4).[18] What matters most to a woman when she considers a contraceptive method will ordinarily change over the course of her reproductive lifespan. Different reproductive stages are associated with distinct fertility goals and sexual behaviors (Table 9-6). From menarche to first birth, the primary fertility goal is to postpone pregnancy and birth. Between the first and last births, the primary goal is to space pregnancies leading to births. Between the last birth and menopause, the goal is to cease childbearing altogether. The biggest demands on a contraceptive method are generated

Table 9-5 Major methods of contraception and some related safety concerns, side effects, and noncontraceptive benefits

Method	Dangers	Side Effects	Noncontraceptive Benefits
Pill	Cardiovascular complications (stroke, heart attack, blood clots, high blood pressure), depression, hepatic adenomas, possible increased risk of breast and cervical cancers	Nausea, headaches, dizziness, spotting, weight gain, breast tenderness, chloasma	Decreases menstrual pain, PMS, and blood loss; protects against symptomatic PID, some cancers (ovarian, endometrial), some benign tumors (leiomyomata, benign breast masses), and ovarian cysts; reduces acne
IUD	PID following insertion, uterine perforation, anemia	Menstrual cramping, spotting, increased bleeding	None known except progestin-releasing IUDs, which decrease menstrual blood loss and pain
Male Condom	Anaphylactic reaction to latex	Decreased sensation, allergy to latex, loss of spontaneity	Protects against sexually transmitted infections, including HIV; delays premature ejaculation
Female Condom	None known	Aesthetically unappealing and awkward to use for some	Protects against sexually transmitted infections
Implant	Infection at implant site, complicated removals, depression	Tenderness at site, menstrual changes, hair loss, weight gain	Lactation not disturbed; may decrease menstrual cramps, pain, and blood loss
Injectable	Depression, allergic reactions, pathologic weight gain, possible bone loss	Menstrual changes, weight gain, headaches, adverse effects on lipids	Lactation not disturbed, reduces risk of seizures, may have protective effects against PID and ovarian and endometrial cancers
Sterilization	Infection; anesthetic complications; if pregnancy occurs after tubal sterilization, high risk that it will be ectopic	Pain at surgical site, psychological reactions, subsequent regret that the procedure was performed	Tubal sterilization reduces risk of ovarian cancer and may protect against PID
Abstinence	None known	Psychological reactions	Prevents infections, including HIV
Barriers: Diaphragm, Cap, Sponge	Vaginal and urinary tract infections, toxic shock syndrome	Pelvic pressure, vaginal irritation, vaginal discharges if left in too long, allergy	Provides modest protection against some sexually transmitted infections
Spermicides	Vaginal and urinary tract infections	Vaginal irritation, allergy	Provides modest protection against some sexually transmitted infections
Lactational Amenorrhea Method (LAM)	Increased risk of HIV transmission to infant if mother HIV+	Mastitis from staphylococcal infection	Provides excellent nutrition for infants under 6 months old

Table 9-6 The stages of reproductive life

	Adolescents/Young Adults		Later Reproductive Years	
	Menarche to First Intercourse	First Intercourse to First Birth	First Birth to Last Birth	Last Birth to Menopause
Fertility goals				
Births	postpone	postpone	space	stop
Ability to have children	preserve	preserve	preserve	irrelevant
Sexual behavior				
# of partners	none	multiple?	one?	one?
Coital frequency	zero	moderate to high	moderate	moderate to low
Coital predictability	low	moderate to high	high	high
Importance of Method Characteristics				
Pregnancy prevention		high	moderate	high
PID prevention		high	moderate	low
Not coitus-linked		high	low	moderate
Reversibility		high	high	low
Most common methods				
Most common		pill	pill	sterilization
Next most common		condom	condom	pill, condom

Source: Forrest (1993).

during the period between first intercourse and first birth, when the typical woman will have several sexual partners with periods of high coital frequency; the typical woman will attach great importance to preventing pregnancy and STIs and to a method's reversibility and ease of use. In the last stage of her reproductive lifespan, from the last birth to menopause, the most important factor is a method's efficacy at preventing pregnancy.

More than half the entire reproductive lifespan—18.4 years or 51% of the reproductive span of 35.9 years—is spent trying to avoid further childbearing, in the stage from the last birth to menopause (Figure 9-1). The typical woman accomplishes this goal via female or male sterilization. A further 13.5 years or 38% of the reproductive span, from menarche to the first birth, is characterized by no desire to become pregnant. Thus, of a total reproductive span of 35.9 years during which a woman is potentially biologically at risk of conception, only 4.0 years (11% of the total), from

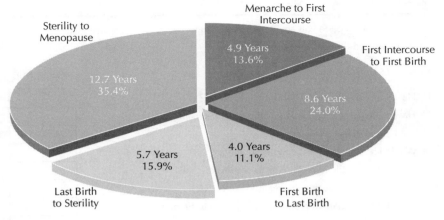

Source: Forrest (1993).

Figure 9-1 Time spent in the stages of reproductive life

the first to the last birth, is characterized by any desire to become pregnant. Even this figure is exaggerated since a great fraction of this stage is spent in the pregnant or lactating state or trying to postpone the next pregnancy.

The best method of contraception for patients is one that will be in harmony with their wishes, fears, preferences, and lifestyle. Table 9-7 lists questions designed to help patients determine whether or not a contraceptive method under consideration is a realistic choice. These questions may be used exactly as is or they may be adapted for local use without permission. "Don't know" answers point to a need for more thinking, more introspection, or more information. "Yes" answers may mean users might not like or be successful with the method. If they have more than a few "yes" responses, they may want to talk to their physician, counselor, partner, or friend. Talking it over can help them to decide whether to use this method, or how to use it so it will be effective for them. In general, the more "yes" answers they have, the less likely they are to use this method consistently and correctly.

Cost and cost-effectiveness of contraceptive methods. Tell a woman in advance what her ongoing expenses will be (Table 9-8). Currently, contraceptive method costs are generally not borne by third-party payers. With private insurers, contraceptive coverage varies dramatically. Virtually all cover surgical sterilization; some provide broad coverage for all methods, but most do not, leaving the individual to pay for contraception herself.[2] The public sector generally provides broader coverage

Table 9-7 Contraceptive method comfort and confidence scale

Method of contraception you are considering using: _____

Length of time you used this method in the past: _____

Answer YES or NO to the following questions:

	YES	NO
1. Have I had problems using this method before?		
2. Have I ever become pregnant while using this method?		
3. Am I afraid of using this method?		
4. Would I really rather not use this method?		
5. Will I have trouble remembering to use this method?		
6. Will I have trouble using this method correctly?		
7. Do I still have unanswered questions about this method?		
8. Does this method make menstrual periods longer or more painful?		
9. Does this method cost more than I can afford?		
10. Could this method cause me to have serious complications?		
11. Am I opposed to this method because of any religious or moral beliefs?		

Answer YES or NO to the following questions:

	YES	NO
12. Is my partner opposed to this method?		
13. Am I using this method without my partner's knowledge?		
14. Will using this method embarrass my partner?		
15. Will using this method embarrass me?		
16. Will I enjoy intercourse less because of this method?		
17. If this method interrupts lovemaking, will I avoid using it?		
18. Has a nurse or doctor ever told me NOT to use this method?		
19. Is there anything about my personality that could lead me to use this method incorrectly?		
20. Am I at any risk of being exposed to HIV (the AIDS virus) or other sexually transmitted infections if I use this method?		

Total number of YES answers: _____

Most individuals will have a few "yes" answers. "Yes" answers mean that potential problems may arise. If you have more than a few "yes" responses, you may want to talk with your physician, counselor, partner, or friend to help you decide whether to use this method or how to use it so that it will really be effective for you. In general, the more "yes" answers you have, the less likely you are to use this method consistently and correctly at every act of intercourse.

Table 9-8 Unit costs for contraceptive methods and associated services

	Unit Cost $	
Method	**Managed Care Setting**	**Public Provider Setting**
Tubal Ligation[a]	2466.80	1190.00
Vasectomy[a]	755.70	353.28
Oral Contraceptives		
Drug	21.00/cycle	17.70/cycle
Office Visit[a]	38.00	16.56
Implant		
Drug[a]	365.00	365.00
Insertion[a]	333.00	47.96
Removal	100.00	79.64
Injectable Contraceptive		
Drug	30.00/quarter	30.00/quarter
Office Visit	38.00/quarter	16.56/quarter
Progesterone-T IUD		
Device	82.00/year	82.00/year
Insertion	207.00/year	62.42/year
Removal	70.00/year	10.80/year
Copper-T IUD		
Device[a]	184.00	109.00
Insertion[a]	207.00	62.42
Removal	70.00	10.80
Diaphragm[b]		
Device	18.00/3 years	15.00/3 years
Office Visit (device fitting)	38.00	15.59
Spermicidal Jelly (12 acts of coitus)	12.00	8.75
Male Condom[b]	1.00	0.33
Female Condom[b]	3.66	1.25
Sponge[b]	1.50	0.83
Spermicides (12 acts)[b]	12.00	8.75

(continued)

Table 9-8 Unit costs for contraceptive methods and associated services *(cont.)*

Method	Unit Cost $	
	Managed Care Setting	**Public Provider Setting**
Cervical Cap[b]		
Device	31.00/3 years	19.00/3 years
Office Visit (device fitting)[a]	38.00	15.59
Spermicidal Jelly (12 acts)	12.00	8.75
Withdrawal	0.00	0.00
Periodic Abstinence	0.00	0.00
No Method	0.00	0.00

Source: Trussell et al. (1995), Smith (1993).

Notes:
[a]First year only.
[b]Method costs in Figures 9-2 and 9-3 were calculated based on 83 acts of intercourse per year among sexually active women aged 18-49, based on unpublished tabulations from the 1989, 1990, 1991 and 1993 General Social Surveys (Smith 1993).

than private payers although payment levels often are low, perhaps low enough to limit access.[40] If cost imposes a major hardship, offer an alternative contraceptive method or a means of obtaining the desired contraceptive method less expensively.

Remember the costs of contraceptive methods represent only part of the medical care dollars associated with use of contraception. To these must be added the net costs of treating side effects and the costs of unintended pregnancies resulting from a method or user failure. Unintended pregnancies result in births, induced abortions, spontaneous abortions, or ectopic pregnancies. The cost of a typical unintended pregnancy is extremely high: $3,795 in a managed care setting and $1,680 in a publicly funded program.[51] The total costs of using different methods are compared with the costs of using no method in a managed care setting over periods of 1 year in Figure 9-2 and 5 years in Figure 9-3. Four points emerge from examination of these figures.

- Use of any method of contraception is very cost-effective when compared with use of no method.
- Because unintended pregnancy is so expensive, those highly effective methods with high costs of acquisition actually save the most money; in particular, the long-term methods (sterilization, the implant, and the Copper T380A IUD) become especially cost-effective for longer durations of use.

Total Costs

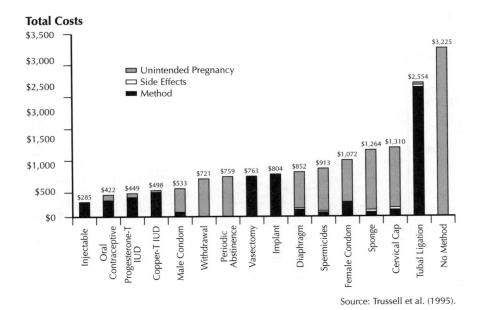

Source: Trussell et al. (1995).

Figure 9-2 One-year costs associated with contraceptive methods in the managed payment model

- Method costs (Table 9-8) are very misleading indications of the total costs.
- The net costs of treating side effects are a minuscule fraction of total costs. This conclusion holds even when STIs are included in the model.

The same conclusions emerge for publicly funded programs. Cost-savings for the less effective methods would increase substantially if they were used correctly and consistently at every act of intercourse. For an individual couple, methods that will be most cost-effective are those used correctly and consistently.

Emergency contraceptives are cost-effective whether they are provided when the emergency arises or in advance to be used as needed. A single treatment after unprotected intercourse saves $142 ($54) when emergency contraceptive pills and $119 ($29) when minipills are used in a managed care (public payer) setting. The copper-T380A IUD is not cost-effective as an emergency contraceptive alone but savings quickly exceed costs as use continues. Providing emergency contraceptive pills in advance to women using barrier contraceptives, spermicides, withdrawal, or periodic abstinence results in annual cost savings ranging from $263 to $498 in a managed care ($99 to $205 in a public payer) setting.[49] By

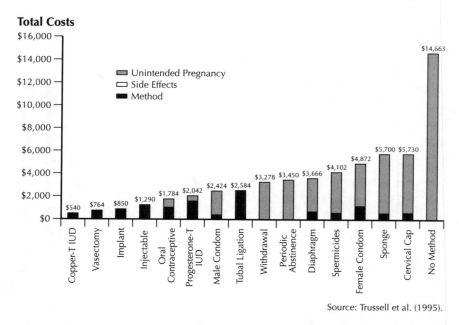

Total Costs

Legend:
- Unintended Pregnancy
- Side Effects
- Method

Values shown on bars:
Copper-T IUD: $540
Vasectomy: $764
Implant: $850
Injectable: $1,290
Oral Contraceptive: $1,784
Progesterone-T IUD: $2,042
Male Condom: $2,424
Tubal Ligation: $2,584
Withdrawal: $3,278
Periodic Abstinence: $3,450
Diaphragm: $3,666
Spermicides: $4,102
Female Condom: $4,872
Sponge: $5,700
Cervical Cap: $5,730
No Method: $14,663

Source: Trussell et al. (1995).

Figure 9-3 Five-year costs associated with contraceptive methods in the managed payment model

reducing unintended pregnancies, more extensive use of emergency contraception could save considerable medical and social costs.

Pattern of sexual activity. In choosing their contraceptive method, clients should consider their number of partners and their frequency of intercourse. The number of partners affects the risk of STIs. In more obvious cases, the individual will have more than one partner at any given time. Less obvious are the individuals who practice serial monogamy. That is, they have only one partner at a time; however, the relationships are not permanent and so at the end of one relationship, the individual will move on to a new partner. Having more than one partner in a life time is the norm, and it is not uncommon for unmarried men and women to have more than one partner per year. (See Chapter 2 on Sexuality and Reproductive Health.) The methods that would most protect individuals from STIs require commitment, understanding, and assertiveness on behalf of the client. The practitioner recommending the use of condoms (male or female) or other barrier protection must be prepared to take the time required to discuss risks, encourage behavioral change, and teach skills.

The frequency of intercourse also has bearing on a person's contraceptive method choice. For example, the woman who has infrequent intercourse may not wish to use a method that requires daily medication or continuous exposure to possible side effects posed by hormonal methods or IUDs. On the other hand, infrequent intercourse may also indicate that a client is at risk of intercourse at unpredictable times. These clients may need skills in "expecting the unexpected."

Pattern of childbearing. Couples who plan their families should choose their contraceptive method based on the number of and interval between desired children. For example, couples who plan on having a few children or having children early in their reproductive lifecycle may have more flexible requirements about the spacing before and between pregnancies and may be more willing to risk a mistimed, but not unwanted, pregnancy. Such flexibility may mean contraceptive method choices would not be limited to those with highest efficacy.

On the other hand, the couples who want only one child or want to delay childbearing until the woman is in her late 30s or early 40s may be less willing to choose any but the most highly effective methods. Among these couples, the reversible long-term methods may be more appealing than they would be for couples for whom a several-year span of protection is not an absolute necessity.

Access to medical care. Some people in our society have poor access to the health care system: they do not understand the system or cannot afford it or find that it shuns them. Others may find their access hampered by too long a wait at the clinic. Studies in other nations have shown that access has great bearing on contraceptive method compliance and choice.[57] Presumably, the degree of access can also influence women in the United States. Access can be eased for all clients by providing a full year's supply of contraceptives. While many clinicians do provide 13 cycles of pills, most do not offer sufficient quantities of condoms.

GOALS FOR TEACHING ABOUT PERSONAL CONSIDERATIONS

Key concepts for discussing contraceptive method choice and personal considerations include these:

1. **The patient decides which personal considerations matter**. Only the potential user can weigh the elements for personal choice: you will not be able to predict what matters. Privacy? Lubrication? Light periods? What big sister uses? Do not guess; ask.

2. **It is a long way from the exam room to the bedroom**. We offer methods as medicines in a clinical setting, and then our patients go home and use them in a sexual setting, be it a bedroom, motel room, car seat, or tent. Remember to help your patient think through the sexual aspects of contraception.

3. **Give patients permission to make a second (or third) contraceptive method choice**. They may not like the first method and will need to know it is acceptable to come back and try something else. Besides, it is always good to know how to use several methods.

4. **Encourage your patients to talk about contraceptive issues with their partners**. How can one person decide if a method of contraception will be compatible with a couple's personal and sexual styles? Help your clients practice discussing contraception with their partners if this is new territory for them.

5. **Personal considerations are likely to change over time**. Teenagers and 35-year-olds will use very different criteria as they evaluate their contraceptive method choices. Encourage patients to rethink their contraceptive method needs as life and sex and bodies change over time.

6. **Teach patients a wise and cautious approach to sexual activity**. All sexually active people need to know the risk factors for STIs and HIV infection. Moreover, they need to know how to avoid those risk factors.

SUGGESTED READING

Brown SS, Eisenberg L. *The best intentions: unintended pregnancy and the well-being of children and families*. Washington DC: National Academy Press, 1995.

Harrison PF, Rosenfield A. *Contraceptive research and development: looking to the future*. Washington DC: National Academy Press, 1996.

REFERENCES

1. Abma JC, Chandra A, Mosher WD, Peterson LS, Piccinino LJ. Fertility, family planning, and women's health: new data from the 1995 National Survey of Family Growth. Vital Health Stat 1997;Series 23, Number 19.

2. Alan Guttmacher Institute (AGI). Uneven and unequal: insurance coverage and reproductive health services. New York: The Alan Guttmacher Institute, 1994.

3. Berg CJ, Atrash HK, Koonin LM, Tucker M. Pregnancy-related mortality in the United States, 1987-1990. Obstet Gynecol 1996;88:161-167.

4. Bosch FX, Manos MM, Muñoz N, Sherman M, Jansen AM, Peto J, Schiffman MH, Moreno V, Kurman R, Shah KV, International Biological Study on Cervical Cancer (IBSCC) Study Group. Prevalence of human papillomavirus in cervical cancer: a worldwide perspective. J Natl Cancer Inst 1995;87:796-802.

5. Bracher M, Santow G. Premature discontinuation of contraception in Australia. Fam Plann Perspect 1992;24:58-65.

6. Brinton LA. Oral contraceptives and cervical neoplasia. Contraception 1991;43:581-595.

7. Cates W. Contraceptive choice, sexually transmitted diseases, HIV infection, and future fecundity. J Br Fertil Society 1996;1:18-22.
8. Cates W. Putting the risks in perspective. Contraceptive Technology Update 1980;1:111.
9. Coker AL, Hulka BS, McCann MF, Walton LA. Barrier methods of contraception and cervical intraepithelial neoplasia. Contraception 1992;45:1-10.
10. Collaborative Group on Hormonal Factors in Breast Cancer. Breast cancer and hormonal contraceptives: collaborative reanalysis of individual data on 53,297 women with breast cancer and 100,239 women without breast cancer from 54 epidemiological studies. Lancet 1996;347:1713-1727.
11. Davis HJ. The shield intrauterine device. A superior modern contraceptive. Am J Obstet Gynecol 1970;106:455-456.
12. Dinman BD. The reality and acceptance of risk. JAMA 1980;244:1226-1228.
13. Escobedo LG, Peterson HB, Grubb GS, Franks AL. Case-fatality rates for tubal sterilization in U.S. hospitals, 1979-1980. Am J Obstet Gynecol 1989;160: 147-150.
14. Farley TMM, Rosenberg MJ, Rowe PJ, Chen J-H, Meirik O. Intrauterine devices and pelvic inflammatory disease: an international perspective. Lancet 1992;339:785-788.
15. Farr G, Gabelnick H, Sturgen K, Dorflinger L. Contraceptive efficacy and acceptability of the female condom. Am J Public Health 1994;84:1960-1964.
16. Feldblum PJ, Morrison CS, Roddy RE, Cates W. The effectiveness of barrier methods of contraception in preventing the spread of HIV. AIDS 1995;9(Suppl A):S85-S93.
17. Fihn SD, Boyko EJ, Normand EH, Chen C-L, Grafton JR, Hunt M, Yarbro P, Scholes D, Stergachis A. Association between use of spermicide-coated condoms and Escherichia coli urinary tract infection in young women. Am J Epidemiol 1996;144:512-520.
18. Forrest JD. Timing of reproductive life stages. Obstet Gynecol 1993;82:105-110.
19. Gallen M, Lettenmaier C. Counseling makes a difference. Popul Rep 1987;15, Series J(35).
20. Grady WR, Hayward MD, Yagi J. Contraceptive failure in the United States: estimates from the 1982 National Survey of Family Growth. Fam Plann Perspect 1986;18:200-209.
21. Harlap S, Kost K, Forrest JD. Preventing pregnancy, protecting health: a new look at birth control choices in the United States. New York: The Alan Guttmacher Institute, 1991.
22. Henshaw SK. Unintended pregnancy in the United States. Fam Plann Perspect 1998;30:24-29, 46.
23. Hooton TM, Scholes D, Hughes JP, Winter C, Roberts PL, Stapleton AE, Stergachis A, Stamm WE. A prospective study of risk factors for symptomatic urinary tract infection in young women. N Engl J Med 1996;335:468-474.
24. Jones EF, Forrest JD. Contraceptive failure rates based on the 1988 NSFG. Fam Plann Perspect 1992;24:12-19.
25. Kestelman P, Trussell J. Efficacy of the simultaneous use of condoms and spermicides. Fam Plann Perspect 1991;23:226-227, 232.
26. Lawson HW, Frye A, Atrash HK, Smith JC, Schulman HB, Ramick M. Abortion mortality, United States, 1972 through 1987. Am J Obstet Gynecol 1994;171:1365-1372.

27. Lee BW. Risk assessment. JAMA 1981;246:1196-1197.
28. Luukkainen T, Toivonen J. Levonorgestrel-releasing IUD as a method of contraception with therapeutic properties. Contraception 1995;52:269-276.
29. McIntyre SL, Higgins JE. Parity and use-effectiveness with the contraceptive sponge. Am J Obstet Gynecol 1986;155:796-801.
30. Menken J, Trussell J, Larsen U. Age and infertility. Science 1986;233: 1389-1394.
31. Mintz M. At any cost: corporate greed, women, and the Dalkon shield. New York: Pantheon Books, 1985.
32. Mitchell AA, Van Bennekom CM, Louik C. A pregnancy-prevention program in women of childbearing age receiving isotretinoin. N Engl J Med 1995;333:101-106.
33. National Center for Health Statistics. Advance report of final natality statistics, 1989. Mon Vital Stat Rep 1991;40(8-Suppl).
34. Piccinino LJ. Personal communication to James Trussell, March 24, 1997.
35. Richwald GA, Greenland S, Gerber MM, Potik R, Kersey L, Comas MA. Effectiveness of the cavity-rim cervical cap: results of a large clinical study. Obstet Gynecol 1989;74:143-148.
36. Schirm AL, Trussell J, Menken J, Grady WR. Contraceptive failure in the United States: the impact of social, economic, and demographic factors. Fam Plann Perspect 1982;14:68-75.
37. Schlesselman JJ. Net effect of oral contraceptive use on the risk of cancer in women in the United States. Obstet Gynecol 1995;85:793-801.
38. Sivin I, Schmidt F. Effectiveness of IUDs: a review. Contraception 1987;36: 55-84.
39. Smith TW. Personal communication to James Trussell, December 13, 1993.
40. Sollom T, Gold RB, Saul R. Public funding for contraceptive, sterilization and abortion services, 1994. Fam Plann Perspect 1996;28:166-173.
41. Speroff L, Glass RH, Kase NG. Clinical gynecologic endocrinology and infertility (Fifth Edition). Baltimore MD: Williams & Wilkins, 1994.
42. Thomas DB, Ray RM, The World Health Organization Collaborative Study of Neoplasia and Steroid Contraceptives. Oral contraceptives and invasive adenocarcinomas and adenosquamous carcinomas of the uterine cervix. Am J Epidemiol 1996;144:281-289.
43. Tietze C, Poliakoff SR, Rock J. The clinical effectiveness of the rhythm method of contraception. Fertil Steril 1951;2:444-450.
44. Trussell J. Methodological pitfalls in the analysis of contraceptive failure. Stat Med 1991;10:201-220.
45. Trussell TJ, Faden R, Hatcher RA. Efficacy information in contraceptive counseling: those little white lies. Am J Public Health 1976;66:761-767.
46. Trussell J, Grummer-Strawn L. Contraceptive failure of the ovulation method of periodic abstinence. Fam Plann Perspect 1990a;22:65-75.
47. Trussell J, Hatcher RA, Cates W, Stewart FH, Kost K. A guide to interpreting contraceptive efficacy studies. Obstet Gynecol 1990b;76:558-567.
48. Trussell J, Hatcher RA, Cates W, Stewart FH, Kost K. Contraceptive failure in the United States: an update. Stud Fam Plann 1990c;21:51-54.
49. Trussell J, Koenig J, Ellertson C, Stewart F. Preventing unintended pregnancy: the cost-effectiveness of three methods of emergency contraception. Am J Public Health 1997;87:932-937.

50. Trussell J, Kost K. Contraceptive failure in the United States: a critical review of the literature. Stud Fam Plann 1987;18:237-283.
51. Trussell J, Leveque JA, Koenig JD, London R, Borden S, Henneberry J, LaGuardia KD, Stewart F, Wilson TG, Wysocki S, Strauss M. The economic value of contraception: a comparison of 15 methods. Am J Public Health 1995;85:494-503.
52. Trussell J, Menken J. Life table analysis of contraceptive failure. In: Hermalin AI, Entwisle B (eds). The role of surveys in the analysis of family planning programs. Liege, Belgium: Ordina Editions, 1982:537-571.
53. Trussell J, Strickler J, Vaughan B. Contraceptive efficacy of the diaphragm, the sponge and the cervical cap. Fam Plann Perspect 1993;25:100-105, 135.
54. Trussell J, Vaughan B. Aggregate and lifetime contraceptive failure in the United States. Fam Plann Perspect 1989;21:224-226.
55. Trussell J, Vaughan B. Selected results concerning sexual behavior and contraceptive use from the 1988 National Survey of Family Growth and the 1988 National Survey of Adolescent Males. Working Paper #91-12. Princeton NJ: Office of Population Research, Princeton University, 1991.
56. Trussell J, Westoff CF. Contraceptive practice and trends in coital frequency. Fam Plann Perspect 1980;12:246-249.
57. Tsui AO, Ochoa LH. Service proximity as a determinant of contraceptive behaviour: evidence from cross-national studies of survey data. In: Philips JF, Ross JA (eds). Family planning programmes and fertility. Oxford, England: Clarendon Press, 1992:222-256.
58. Vaughan B, Trussell J, Menken J, Jones EF. Contraceptive failure among married women in the United States, 1970-1973. Fam Plann Perspect 1977;9: 251-258.
59. Vaughan B, Trussell J, Menken J, Jones EF, Grady W. Contraceptive efficacy among married women aged 15-44 years, United States. Vital Health Stat 1980;Series 23, Number 5.
60. Ventura SJ, Martin JA, Matthews TJ, Clarke SC. Advance report of final natality statistics, 1994. Mon Vital Stat Rep 1996;44(11-Suppl).
61. Vessey M, Lawless M, Yeates D. Efficacy of different contraceptive methods. Lancet 1982;1:841-842.
62. WHO Collaborative Study of Neoplasia and Steroid Contraceptives. Invasive squamous-cell cervical carcinoma and combined oral contraceptives: results from a multinational study. Int J Cancer 1993;55:228-236.
63. Zondervan KT, Carpenter LM, Painter R, Vessey MP. Oral contraceptives and cervical cancer—further findings from the Oxford Family Planning Association contraceptive study. Br J Cancer 1996;73:1291-1297.

LATE REFERENCE

64. Nelson A, Bernstein GS, Frezieres R, Walsh T, Clark V, Coulson A. Study of the efficacy, acceptability and safety of a non-latex (polyurethane) male condom: revised final report (N01-HD-1-3109). Bethesda MD: National Institute of Child Health and Human Development, September 15, 1997.

Education and Counseling

Felicia Guest, MPH, CHES

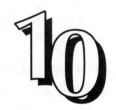

- Daily choices about personal risk taking exert a powerful influence on health. No care-giver task is more important than helping patients change their personal behavior to reduce health risks.
- People change behaviors more often as a result of new skills than of new knowledge. Teaching new skills to patients is most helpful when the care-giver matches the intervention to the patient's own readiness to change.
- Informed consent is an educational process, not a piece of paper. The consent form documents the educational process.
- Writing can be informative and simple at the same time. This chapter is deliberately written at grade level 13, while Chapter 9 is at grade 16, and Chapter 11 is at grade 14.*

FACTORS INFLUENCING EDUCATION AND COUNSELING

The success or failure of our communication efforts hinges in large part on our skill in *facilitating* patients' willingness and ability to let us know about their particular situations and needs. Then we can tailor an intervention that is compatible with the patient, the place and time, and the issue at hand. You need to know how to create a safe environment for discussing feelings and needs, coax insight out of a discussion, and clarify options and choices for the patient. Few people innately possess these

---

*The readability of these chapters was determined by using the Flesch-Kincaid formula provided on the Grammatik software.

skills; you may need training to master them. Patient characteristics—age, cultural background, literacy, emotional state, and readiness for behavior change—influence the encounter as well. Important characteristics of the situation can include the specific goals of both patient and care-giver, the time available for the encounter, and the need for a formal informed consent process.

AGE AND DEVELOPMENT

Patients may seek reproductive health care as children, adolescents, or adults. Cognitive and emotional capacities are strongly influenced by age. Developmentally, children move through early, middle, and late adolescence as they approach adulthood,[5] and educational strategies for one stage may be wrong for another. Young adolescents (age 11 to 13 or so) are still quite childlike, and older adolescents (age 16 or older) may have many adult characteristics. You may have only moments to ascertain whether a 14-year-old patient is more like a child or like an adult.

A substantial portion of patients making their first visit for reproductive care are in middle adolescence, about age 14 or 15. The stage can be distinctly characterized:

- Concrete thinking, oriented to the "here and now"
- Intense peer involvement around certain issues
- Idealized and romanticized first-love relationships

These young people often experiment with sexual activities, drugs, and alcohol. You can help by taking into account their special needs. For example, be respectful of concrete thinking by asking, "Exactly where would you keep your pills? What do you do every day that can remind you to take your pill?" Use the peer involvement issue. Ask, for example, "Do you have any friends who use pills? What do they say about them?" About romance you might say, "I know it's hard to imagine that Mike could have any infections that would hurt you, but it happens sometimes. I'd like to help you stay safe. Love doesn't protect anybody from infection!"

Stressful lives can retard cognitive and emotional growth,[5] so assess developmental status by what patients say and do more than by their chronological age.

The ability to plan ahead is a skill developed later in adolescence, usually about age 16 or older. All methods of contraception require at least some ability to plan ahead and are therefore incompatible with the developmental skills of early and middle adolescence. To be successful at reducing their risks of pregnancy and reproductive tract infection (RTI), these young people will need to practice new skills with you. For further insight into counseling young people, see "Compassionate Counseling for Adolescents" in this chapter.

PERSONAL AND CULTURAL VALUES

The values and ideas learned at home during childhood strongly influence each person. Cultures and families vary widely in many characteristics that influence reproductive lives. Learn the personal values of your patient:[13]

- What is the ideal family size?
- Who makes sexual decisions?
- What is the desirable marriage age?
- How is same-gender sexuality regarded and handled?
- How does the patient understand the causation of illness?
- Who are the highly respected healers? Medical doctors? Neighborhood lay healers? Lay midwives?
- What is safe to tell the care-giver?
- Is the general communication style direct or indirect? Formal or informal?

Balance an understanding of each patient's unique personality with an awareness of and respect for influential cultural values and characteristics. A study of interventions to teach young black women social skills to reduce sexual risk taking found that programs sensitive to gender and cultural values can enhance consistent condom use more effectively than other types of interventions.[2] For example, young women can attend weekly group sessions to discuss positive attributes of being a black woman and identify personal role models among black women.

Culturally competent communication skill begins with an awareness of how we are defined by our culture. For example, many clinics use an appointment system (based on Western European cultural values about the importance of punctuality) while serving a patient population that may not share that cultural value (such as a Latino[a] community where being hospitable to a drop-in visitor may be more important than getting to the clinic on time). In such settings, an appointment system can set up a no-win situation that frustrates everyone.

Remember that persons one or two generations removed from the immigration experience have already assimilated into the prevailing culture. In isolated communities with little exposure to other groups, strong cultural influences tend to persist. There is tremendous diversity within all cultures, so be careful not to stereotype individual patients.

COMPASSIONATE COUNSELING FOR ADOLESCENTS

SHARON SCHNARE, CNM, MSN, FNP

THE SILENT ADOLESCENT

Young people have the right to be silent and keep their feelings and views safe from adult intrusion. Often the most profound communication has no words. Occasionally you may feel frustrated that a silent adolescent seemed to get little from a clinical encounter, only to have the adolescent return, ready to share, at a later date. Set a fertile atmosphere for the relationship to grow.

Begin a clinical encounter by sharing general concerns of other adolescents. "Other young women and men have concerns and questions about having sex, masturbation, and contraception. Perhaps you can identify with these issues. I am here to talk to you about these or other issues you have questions about." If the adolescent remains quiet, consider choosing a topic of common concern: "Other young women have shared concerns about feeling pressured to have sex, and some are not sure how they feel about using contraception. One young woman, a little older than you, told me she was afraid her boyfriend would find another girlfriend if she didn't have sex with him. She told me she really loved him and didn't want to lose him, but she was also hurt that he didn't love her enough to respect her feelings. I asked her how she planned to solve this dilemma and this is what she told me . . ." (If your patients have not shared their solutions with you, then begin asking how they or their friends have solved sensitive situations.)

ANSWERING ADOLESCENT QUESTIONS

Be flexible with adolescent patients and respond to their "need to know right now." Adolescents need to know there is a person who will be honest and non-biased about sex. When adolescents are especially anxious about a situation, ask what concerns them most about the matter, or ask what they think would worry a friend about the topic. This technique can help elucidate a hidden agenda or an unspoken conflict.

Help the adolescent understand how information empowers us all. For example, "You now know a lot about contraception and especially about condoms. You can be a great teacher to your friends. What's the most important piece of information you can see yourself telling your friends about?"

SECRETS

Some adolescents may be struggling with sexual orientation. Never assume a sexual partner is of the opposite sex. Be aware of support and counseling available in your community for gay adolescents. Be vigilant in assessing for factors that suggest a possible history of molestation or abuse: first intercourse before age 14; a series of men (unrelated or related) living in the home; poor school performance; sexual acting out; running away from home; exchanging sex for money, food, or shelter; somatization and dissociation; substance abuse by the adolescent or family member; and cervical dysplasia in a woman younger than 25.

THE 14-YEAR-OLD WHO WANTS TO HAVE A BABY

Many adolescents fantasize about "a baby of my own." Adolescents need to share these longings and ambivalent feelings, and to hear from their care-giver that these feelings are normal and shared by women the world over. Once adolescents express their desire to have a baby, they can give up their denial and discuss their feelings without shame, guilt, or fear. A young woman is then free to take control, rather than to let pregnancy "just happen." Ambivalence can result in not using contraception or using it inconsistently.

Having a pregnancy is one of the most seductive ways for adolescents to feel grown up. A potent question to ask a adolescent is, "What will this baby *need* from you?" Sit quietly and wait for the question to ripen. Help the adolescent imagine the baby in a cradle across the room, and slowly begin: "The baby will need to be kept warm, to be fed and changed and vaccinated and to go to the doctor or clinic for checkups, to be kept safe and loved and never to be left alone." At this point, the adolescent may begin to see that it will not be her needs that are met by having a baby, because the baby has many, many needs beyond her own.

When an adolescent seems determined to become or remain pregnant, punitive or parental finger-wagging may simply reinforce her determination. Discuss the need to take preconceptual folic acid and vitamins and to make nutritional and behavioral changes (such as avoiding tobacco and alcohol and sexually transmitted infections). Ask the adolescent who will help her care for the baby and what her living situation will be like. Generally she will tell you she plans to live with her mother, who will also help her care for the baby. React to her plan positively. "That's great that you have talked with your mother about this, and that she is willing to help support you and your baby and also to help take care of your baby." The adolescent may look uncomfortable. "Well, I haven't talked with her yet." Respond with concern. "I see. I wonder how *fair* your mother will feel you are being, by not talking about your plans with her first? What if she promised a friend that *you* would care for *her* baby every day after school but didn't ask you first?" Adolescents can be wonderful moral warriors when it comes to injustices or unfairness, so use this quality to help her see it is unfair to expect her parent to support her and a baby without asking her first.

Remember that children generally meet the expectations society sets out for them, and these expectations sometimes seem to conflict:

- Yes, have our grandchildren . . . but not now.
- Yes, be popular and attractive to boys, especially older boys . . . but don't get sexually involved.
- Yes, society values women's bodies as sexual objects, especially young women's bodies . . . but your self-concept shouldn't be influenced by media images.

If we as health-care providers, family members, and adult models do not fill in the picture of what an authentic human being is, the unhealthy images will prevail.

LITERACY

Successful communication uses communication styles with which patients are comfortable and familiar. Perhaps the most common error is using print materials with patients who do not customarily read. A good screening question might be, "How many newspapers and magazines do you read in a typical week?"[15]

The 94 million illiterate and marginally literate adult Americans feel deep shame about their lack of reading skill and also have grave difficulties following medical instructions.[1,10] If in your judgment print materials are appropriate, match the readability of materials to the reading skill of the patient population. College students can usually read at almost any level. For other groups, aim for a seventh-grade reading level, the U.S. average. Use a tool such as the SMOG formula to determine the reading grade level of your materials.[7,8] The SMOG formula is a quick way to get an approximate idea of reading difficulty. A good place to start with a reading level assessment is your contraceptive consent forms, because they tend to be quite difficult to read.

SMOG FORMULA FOR READING LEVEL

When the text has at least 30 sentences:

1. Count three sets of 10 sentences each, one near the beginning, one in the middle, and one near the end.
2. Circle all words with three or more syllables, including repetitions of the same word. Total all circled words in the 30 sentences.
3. Find the nearest perfect square to your total. (Examples: total is 98, use 100; total is 51, use 49.) Take the square root. (Examples: 100 is 10; 49 is 7.)
4. Add 3 to your square root for the reading grade level. (Examples: 10 plus 3 = thirteenth grade; 7 plus 3 = tenth grade.)

When the text has fewer than 30 sentences:

1. Count all words in the text with three or more syllables. Next count the total number of sentences. Then divide to find the average number of long words per sentence. (Example: 40 circled words divided by 20 sentences = an average of 2 per sentence.)
2. Multiply your average number of long words per sentence by the number of sentences short of 30. (Example: 2 times 10 = 20.)
3. Add your answer to your total number of long words, find the square root, and then add 3. (Example: 20 plus 40 = 60. Nearest perfect square is 64. Square root is 8. 8 plus 3 = eleventh grade.)

The grade level tells you that two-thirds of the U.S. students in that grade could read the sample with 100% comprehension. The standard error of prediction is 1.5 grades in either direction. The most important strategies for lowering reading levels are to use short words and short sentences.[6]

EMOTIONAL STATE

Intense feelings of anger, anxiety, fear, disappointment, or even elation must be acknowledged and discussed before effective patient education can begin. "Yes, you are pregnant, and here are your options" is callous as well as ineffective. "Yes, you are pregnant. Can you tell me how this news feels to you?" gets off to a better start. In some situations, it may make sense to defer patient education until a later visit. People who learn their test for human immunodeficiency virus (HIV) is positive often say they remember nothing at all the counselor said after hearing the word "positive." When you and the patient think the likelihood of a return visit is low or unknown, take extra time to explore feelings.

Adolescents relieved at receiving negative pregnancy test results may be an especially important group of patients for prevention skills intervention. In one study, about 1 in 4 pregnant adolescents age 17 and younger had a previous clinic-based negative test result.[16]

CAPACITY FOR BEHAVIOR CHANGE

Not all patients are equally able to undertake the costly, perhaps even frightening, changes in personal daily life that promote health, such as abstaining from sex or using condoms when there is a risk of RTI, stopping smoking, or taking oral contraceptive pills diligently. Demonstration projects in HIV prevention have based educational interventions on stages of behavior change, in the theory that behavior change is incremental and that interventions must be tailored to the patient's (or target community's) particular position along a continuum of change.[9]

Perhaps the most thoroughly studied model was developed in psychotherapy and smoking cessation research,[11,12] where scientists describe sequential steps along a behavior-change continuum. Other interventions use models that include key elements of a number of accepted behavior-change theories. A model often used to train HIV counselors[3] explains the process of change using these key points:

- *Knowledge and awareness* come first. Behavior change begins in understanding the consequences of a behavior.
- Knowledge and awareness are not enough. *Significance to self,* or ownership of the new knowledge and awareness, is critical for progressing to action.

- *Self-efficacy* determines the ability to use new insights. Unless the patient sees herself or himself as *able* to change and *able* to be in control of a situation, the new insights are useless. Many people have low levels of self-efficacy and feel helpless to change. To undertake the change process, they will need your support as a care-giver, with praise for any steps they take toward better health behaviors, no matter how small.
- From the patient's perspective, the status quo has both pros and cons, just as healthier behavior does. Be careful not to short-change the pros of the status quo (risk-taking) or the cons of the healthier behavior, because they matter greatly to the patient who finds change difficult. For example, beginning condom use could carry these cons: loss of an important relationship, loss of self-esteem from being in a relationship, loss of economic support from a partner, and even risk of personal violence. Each patient undertakes a *cost-benefit analysis,* so take care to address all the costs and all the benefits.
- Change requires more than new knowledge. It requires new skills. This *capacity-building* must include help from you in communicating with a sexual partner and coping with both the patient's and the partner's fears and discomforts.
- Behavior change is rarely like flicking an on-and-off switch. Usually it takes a series of *provisional tries* at new behavior. Help by framing all attempts as successes, not failures, and by assisting with course corrections, boosting self-efficacy, and offering empathetic understanding.

In counseling, one or two questions ("What are you doing to protect yourself from accidental pregnancy?" "When would you like to become pregnant?") can help focus your efforts so that the limited time available for education can be used effectively and take into account the patient's readiness for new behaviors.

TIME CONSIDERATIONS

Because it is extremely rare to have all the time you and your patient need for talking, use *contracting* in the beginning of an encounter. Contracting makes clear from the outset what your priorities are for the time together, makes clear approximately how much time is available to talk, and encourages the patient to raise issues that are uppermost in her or his mind. For example, contracting with a first-time family planning patient might sound like this: "We have about 15 minutes to talk today, Linda. I will tell you about what we have to offer you here, and I'll ask you some questions about your health. What do *you* most want to talk about in our time together?"

When education and counseling issues are unfinished and more time is not immediately available, the following options can help:

- Schedule a return visit if possible for the patient.
- Schedule a telephone appointment for more discussion.
- Refer to a hotline for specific issues such as HIV or abuse.
- Offer reading material if the patient is able to read easily.
- Refer to another source of care, such as a prenatal clinic, mental health counselor, or substance abuse treatment center.

Table 10-1 distills some of the collected wisdom of reproductive health educators and counselors over the past three decades.

INFORMED CONSENT

Inform all patients about their complete range of options and allow them to choose freely. Once patients choose a course of action, give full disclosure about their choice. Only when these two steps have been completed can the patient provide an informed and documented consent to care. Help patients view informed choice and informed consent not as legal paperwork but as a serious process for ensuring voluntary, clearly understood medical care, beginning with the tone the care-giver sets as educator. Remember that you do not truly know what patients have learned until you hear them rephrase the information in their own words. This specialized aspect of patient education is the highest priority of all educational tasks in the health care setting.

Because contraceptive methods and medications are usually initiated at the request of a healthy person who has no traditional medical indications for treatment, informed choice and consent can sometimes be overlooked; however, informed choice and consent in family planning and reproductive health have three bases: ethical, pragmatic, and legal. Ethically, people have a right to thorough information about products or procedures that can affect health and a right to decide what is done to their bodies. Pragmatically, people are more likely to use their contraceptive method safely and effectively or undergo a medical procedure when they freely choose and thoroughly understand it. Legally, you must provide adequate information to help patients reach a reasonable and informed decision about contraceptive options, medications, procedures, and devices.

Legals standards for informed consent usually depend on the "reasonable person" standard. Did the patient receive all the information that a

Table 10-1 Collected wisdom on education and counseling

Education

- **The learner learns from what the learner does, not from what the teacher does.** Involve the patients in their own education, encouraging them to touch and handle medicines and supplies, repeat instructions in their own words, and practice anticipated conversations with partner or parent.

- **Limit take-home messages to about three.** Give your messages careful priority ranking and don't overload patients with data.

- **Honor the patient's agenda.** Allow time for patients to discuss their questions and concerns. There will almost certainly be questions you haven't thought of.

- **Evaluate patient learning.** You don't know what patients have learned until you hear what they say.

- **People learn best in an environment that feels safe and calm.** A person on the way to a medical exam rarely feels safe and calm. Allow time after the exam for more education, and invite call-backs later on.

- **Teens and adults may need different styles of education.** Learn about the cognitive and emotional developmental stages so you can frame your education to fit the patient.

Counseling

- **Listening is helpful. Almost always. All by itself.** Sometimes patients need to be heard and understood more than they need anything else.

- **With the exception of life-threatening emergencies, avoid making decisions for the patient.** You will almost certainly do harm, sooner or later, if you are authoritative. The best response to "What do you think I should do?" is, "What do *you* think? I'll help you sort out all your choices, and then we will look at the pros and cons for each choice."

- **Avoid thinking in "me" vs. "them" terms.** The successful counselor cherishes the common human ground shared with each patient.

- **Not all people are able to be "compliant."** When you and your patients are face to face, be honest, direct, and hold them accountable for their actions. Once they leave your office, *let it go.*

- **Denial and anger are common, normal responses to trouble.** Reflect and discuss these feelings when you encounter them in patients. Anger is usually a sane, healthy response to feelings of vulnerability and loss of control. Denial can be given up by the denier, but cannot be forcibly taken away by the counselor.

- **Be open to the broad variety of healthy, effective human coping styles.** Your way will almost never be the only way. People solve their own problems.

- **Assume nothing.** Discipline yourself to forestall labeling or stereotyping. Accept your patient where she or he is right now.

- **The patient knows what he or she wants from you.** Just ask! "Tell me how we can help you today," or "What do you most want to get out of this visit?"

Source: Collected from educators and counselors in reproductive health care, 1970–1997

reasonable person would need to make a sound decision and a truly informed choice and consent? Did the patient truly understand? It is your responsibility to ensure that patients sufficiently understand all reasonable alternatives and to determine whether the patient is competent to consent to the chosen medication, device, or procedure.

Federal regulations for informed consent to sterilization[14] provide helpful guidance to the contraceptive field in general for information that constitutes informed consent. According to these Department of Health and Human Services regulations, informed consent comprises seven basic elements. The word to remember is "BRAIDED":

Benefits of the method
Risks of the method (both major risks and all common minor ones), including consequences of method failure
Alternatives to the method (including abstinence and no method)
Inquiries about the method are the patient's right and responsibility
Decision to withdraw from using the method without penalty is the patient's right at any time
Explanation of the method is owed the patient, in a format that is understandable to the patient
Documentation that the care-giver has ensured understanding of each of the preceding six points, usually by use of a consent form

A voluntary decision—free from any coercion—is paramount. Although documentation is essential, a written consent form with a signature is not enough. It may also be helpful to document what print, audiovisual, or electronic aids you used to inform the patient.

COMPETENCE TO CONSENT

These are the basic criteria for competence to consent:

- Is the patient capable of understanding the proposed treatment, alternatives, and risks?
- Is the patient capable of making rational decisions?

In some situations, the patient's competence is difficult to evaluate. A very young teen, a person with a developmental disability, an intoxicated person, and a mentally ill person are examples of such patients. If you have any doubt regarding a patient's competence to consent, consult with other professionals to determine the appropriate course of action. Be sure to document your consultation in the patient's record.

EDUCATIONAL CONSIDERATIONS FOR CONSENT

Adults and adolescents best learn, and make considered decisions, under the following circumstances:

- In the absence of threat
- When information seems relevant
- When teaching takes cultural factors into account[4]
- When the learning process is interactive
- When having a chance to ask and receive answers to questions
- With time to digest, and room for insight

Provide audiotaped consent forms (in appropriate languages) for illiterate, marginally literate, and visually impaired patients, so they can learn by listening. Write consent forms at a manageable reading level, about grade seven or eight. Evaluate learning and comprehension by having patients *repeat* what they have learned.

CONSENT FORMS

A number of family planning programs view the consent form as an important piece of patient education literature and give each patient a copy to keep. This practice is entirely consistent with the philosophy of full disclosure, so consider using consent forms that include all the BRAIDED elements in simple language. Be sure to stress warning signs for serious complications on consent forms, especially for IUDs and hormonal methods.

REFERENCES

1. Baker DW, Parker RM, Williams MV, Pitkin K, Parikh NS, Coates W, Imara M. The health care experience of patients with low literacy. Arch Fam Med 1996;5:329-334.
2. DiClemente RJ, Wingood GM. A randomized controlled trial of an HIV sexual risk-reduction intervention for young African-American women. JAMA 1995;274:1271-1276.
3. Garrity JM, Jones SJ. HIV prevention counseling: A training program. Atlanta GA: Centers for Disease Control and Prevention, 1993.
4. Gostin LO. Informed consent, cultural sensitivity, and respect for persons. JAMA 1995;274:844-845.
5. Johnson R. Adolescent growth and development. In: Hofmann A, Greydanus D (eds). Adolescent medicine, 2nd ed. Norwalk CT: Appleton & Lange, 1989.
6. Manning D. Writing readable health messages. Pub Health Rep 1981;96: 464-465.

7. McLaughlin GH. SMOG grading—a new readability formula. J of Reading 1968;12:639-646.
8. Meade CD, Smith CF. Readability formulas: cautions and criteria. Patient Educ Couns 1991;17:153-158.
9. O'Reilly KR, Higgins DL. AIDS community demonstration projects for HIV prevention among hard-to-reach groups. Pub Health Rep 1991;106:714-720.
10. Parikh NS, Parker RM, Nurss JR, Baker DW, Williams MV. Shame and health literacy: the unspoken connection. Patient Educ Couns 1996;27:33-39.
11. Prochaska JO, DiClemente CC. Stages of change in the modification of problem behaviors. Prog in Behav Mod 1992;28:183-218.
12. Prochaska JO, Norcross JC, DiClemente CC. Changing for good. New York: William Morrow, 1994.
13. Randall-David E. Culturally competent HIV counseling and education. Rockville MD: National Hemophilia Program, 1994.
14. U.S. Food and Drug Administration. Sterilization of persons in federally assisted family planning projects. Federal Register 1978;43:52146-52175.
15. Wells JA, Sell RL. Learning AIDS: 1991 supplement: a special report on readability, literacy, and the HIV epidemic. New York: American Foundation for AIDS Research, 1991.
16. Zabin LS, Emerson MR, Ringers PA, Sedivy V. Adolescents with negative pregnancy test results: an accessible at-risk group. JAMA 1996;275:113-117.

Selected Reproductive Health Resources

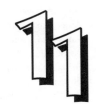

Robert A. Hatcher, MD, MPH
Deborah Kowal, MA, PA
James Trussell, PhD

- Providers and patients can select from a wide range of excellent resources on reproductive health issues.
- Many associations, organizations, government agencies, and pharmaceutical companies produce materials on contraception, sexually transmitted infections, sexuality, and pregnancy.

- If you tend to rely primarily on one medium (print, for example), try exploring the array of resources in other media, such as slide sets, audio or video tapes, CD-ROM, and the Internet.

Keeping current on reproductive health issues and finding answers to your and your patients' questions are more easily accomplished if you have on hand an array of resources and materials. This chapter presents some selected reproductive health resources developed by the authors of *Contraceptive Technology* and resources that colleagues have brought to our attention. The list is not complete, so if you have suggestions for future editions, please write to Contraceptive Technology Communications, P.O. Box 49643, Atlanta, GA 30359 (or send e-mail to ctcomm@mindspring.com).

Several organizations have a wealth of helpful and quality resources (Table 11-1). Materials from the Association of Reproductive Health Professionals, Bridging the Gap Foundation, Family Health International, and any branch of the federal government are not copyrighted and may be reproduced.

Table 11-1 Reproductive health organizations to call

Advocates for Youth	1-202-347-5700
American College Health Association	1-410-859-1500
American Medical Women's Association	1-703-838-0500
American Social Health Association	1-919-361-8400
American Society for Reproductive Medicine	1-205-978-5000
Association of Reproductive Health Professionals	1-202-466-3825
Bridging the Gap Foundation	1-404-373-0530
Education Training Research Associates (ETR)	1-800-321-4407
Family Health International (FHI)	1-919-544-7040
National Association of Nurse Practitioners in Reproductive Health	1-202-408-7025
Planned Parenthood Federation of America	1-212-261-4300
Program for Appropriate Technology in Health (PATH)	1-206-285-3500

PRINT MATERIALS

PROFESSIONAL EDUCATION

- *Guide to Clinical Preventive Services: Report of the United States Preventive Services Task Force.* How effective are the various periodic screening evaluations? This compendium details the quality of the research and the strength of the recommendations for performing Papanicolaou smears, conducting breast examinations, measuring blood pressure, counseling about sexually transmitted infections, and performing numerous other measures on patients of diverse age and risk groups. Available from Williams & Wilkins at book stores.

- *1998 Guidelines for Treatment of Sexually Transmitted Diseases.* The latest recommendations on preventing and treating sexually transmitted infections, by the Centers for Disease Control and Prevention (1-888-232-3228).

- *Clinical Gynecologic Endocrinology and Infertility,* 5th edition, by Speroff, Glass, and Kase. Available from Williams & Wilkins at book stores.

- *Federal Register* notice regarding emergency contraception. The publication describes the review by the Food and Drug Administration. Request document number 0265 at 1-800-342-2722.

- Annotated bibliographies of print materials. SIECUS offers a lengthy list of topics for which it has compiled annotated reference lists. Sexuality topics range from sexual abuse to sexual activities when you have disabilities, are in adolescence or middle and later ages; religion and spirituality and sexuality; and gay and lesbian issues. Available from the Publications Department at SIECUS (1-212-819-9770).

- *The World of Human Sexuality: Behaviors, Customs and Beliefs* by Gregarson. Sexuality around the world is viewed from an anthropological perspective. The book contains hundreds of photographs. Available from Ardent Media (see order form at end of book).
- *Lovemaps* by Money. This psychological perspective is written by one of the world's most prominent sex researchers. Available from Ardent Media (see order form at end of book).
- Fact sheets. Topics include male condom breakage and slippage, menstrual patterns after sterilization, postpartum IUD insertion, increasing effective pill use, role of progestin-only pills, use of spermicides and risk of cervical infection, and more. Call Family Health International for a complete listing (1-919-544-7040).
- "Emergency Contraception" provider resource packet. Prepared by the Program for Appropriate Technology in Health, the packet includes sample patient brochures, fact sheets, office poster, and a provider manual with prescribing information and sample protocols. Available from Planned Parenthood Federation of America (1-800-669-0156).
- *Sex and America's Teenagers*. Chock-full of graphs and tables, this slim book covers the breadth of adolescent sexual activity, pregnancy, and parenting. Available through the Alan Guttmacher Institute (AGI) (1-202-248-1111 ext. 2202).
- *The Best Intentions: Unintended Pregnancy and the Well-being of Children and Families*. This book details the causes, consequences, and costs of unintended pregnancy. The reference list is extensive. Available from the National Academy Press at book stores, by calling 1-800-624-6242, or by World Wide Web (http://www.nap.edu/).
- *Dubious Intentions: The Politics of Teenage Pregnancy* by Luker. One of the most articulate treatises on teenagers and pregnancy, the book takes an empathetic, myth-busting approach. Available from Harvard University Press at book stores.
- *Helping Women Keep Well* by Blum and Heinrichs. This book emphasizes the need to care for womens' physical as well as emotional health. Available from Ardent Media (see order form at end of book).
- *Readings on Men*. This volume brings together a compendium of articles on men's reproductive health and behavior from "Family Planning Perspectives," 1987 through 1995. Available from The Alan Guttmacher Institute (1-212-248-1111 ext. 2202).

- *Improving the Fit: Reproductive Health Services in Managed Care Settings*. This report synthesizes the latest research on reproductive health services covered by managed care plans, including the Medicaid managed care experience. Available from The Alan Guttmacher Institute (1-212-248-1111 ext. 2202).
- "Family Planning Perspectives." Each issue of this peer-reviewed monthly journal contains articles on reproductive health issues and their implications for policy, programs, and people's lives. Available from The Alan Guttmacher Institute (1-212-248-1111 ext. 2202).

PATIENT EDUCATION

- *The Planned Parenthood Women's Health Encyclopedia*. In this easily readable book, every woman can learn answers to her questions and also learn what questions to ask. Available from Planned Parenthood Federation of America (1-800-669-0156).
- *Safely Sexual* by the authors of *Contraceptive Technology*. This small handbook helps readers assess their own risks and benefits of using various contraceptive methods. Available from Ardent Media (see order form at end of book).
- Flip charts and leader's guides. Educate your patients with these exceptionally illustrated flip charts on "Birth Control," "Reproductive Anatomy and Physiology," "HIV/AIDS," and "Sexually Transmitted Diseases." Available from ETR Associates (1-800-321-4407).
- "Now What Do I Do?" and "Oh No! What Do I Do Now?" Designed to help parents communicate with pre-teens and pre-schoolers, respectively, these materials help answer the tough questions. Available from SIECUS (1-212-819-9770).
- "Emergency Contraceptive Kit." Conceived by Dr. Felicia Stewart, this kit provides instructions for how to use emergency contraceptives pills, background information on emergency contraceptives, and three condoms to avert the need for emergency contraception in the future. Available in large numbers through Bridging the Gap Foundation, Inc. (1-404-373-0530).
- *Emergency Contraception: The Nation's Best Kept Secret*. This book by Hatcher et al. provides practical information about emergency contraceptives—how they work, when to take them, and how to obtain them. Available through Bridging the Gap Foundation, Inc. (1-404-373-0530).
- *Alive and Well: A Path for Living in a Time of HIV* by Hendrickson. An HIV-positive psychologist offers practical guidelines for devel-

oping the emotional, social, and spiritual skills needed for living in a time of HIV. Available from Ardent Media (see order form at end of book).

- *Doctor, Am I a Virgin Again? Cases and Counsel for a Healthy Sexuality.* This book, written by Hatcher et al., presents anecdotes and instructions for teens and young adults. Available through Bridging the Gap Foundation, Inc. (1-404-373-0530).

- *The Quest for Excellence: From AIDS and Alcohol to Self-esteem and Healthy Sexuality.* This minibook by Hatcher et al. was written for teens. Available through Bridging the Gap Foundation, Inc. (1-404-373-0530).

- *Sexual Etiquette 101 ...and More.* Aimed at older teens and college students, this minibook was written by Hatcher et al. Available through Bridging the Gap Foundation, Inc. (1-404-373-0530).

M ULTIMEDIA RESOURCES

- Contraceptive Technology Expert slide sets. The Contraceptive Technology Update series covers topics such as injectables, lactational amenorrhea, postpartum contraception, and intrauterine devices. The sets include teaching modules with narrative, slides, audience handouts, references, and reprints of scientific articles. Available from Family Health International (1-919-544-7040).

- "Lactational Amenorrhea Method." This teaching/training packet includes a narrative, slides, audience handouts, and scientific articles. Available from Family Health International (1-919-544-7040).

- "Postpartum Contraception." Another teaching/training packet with narrative, slides, audience handouts, and scientific articles. Available from Family Health International (1-919-544-7040).

- "Listen Carefully." This audiotape by Hatcher describes how to take birth control pills, encourages condom use if needed, and describes proper condom use. Available in large numbers for your office through a local Parke Davis representative.

- "Planning for the Future: Norplant, a Contraceptive Option for Young Women." In this videotape, predominantly inner-city teenagers discuss Norplant. Available through Bridging the Gap Foundation, Inc. (1-404-373-0530).

- "Postponing Sexual Involvement: An Educational Series for Young Teens and One for Pre-teens." The series contains a leader's guide and a videotape for each age group. There is also a parent series for each age group. Available through Emory/Grady Teen Services Program (1-404-616-3513).

- "Choosing A Contraceptive." An interactive CD-ROM to help young people decide on a contraceptive. May be used to teach counselors and clinicians the essential information to provide clients who are deciding on a method. Available through Bridging The Gap Foundation, Inc. (1-404-373-0530).
- "Choices." A set of twenty-eight brief descriptions of contraceptive options may be used by high schools, colleges, medical and nursing schools, and family planning programs to provide brief summaries of each method. Each summary is not copyrighted, is reproducible without asking for permission, and may be translated. The emergency contraceptive pill sheet is available in 25 different languages (see also the emergency contraception website: http://opr.princeton.edu/ec/). Available through Bridging The Gap Foundation, Inc. (1-404-373-0530).

PHARMACEUTICAL HOUSE RESOURCES

Almost every contraceptive has a patient package insert. Some provide excellent information. Some are easier to read than others. All are free. Pharmaceutical houses are generally responsive to inquiries about educational materials for providers or patients (Table 11-2).

Table 11-2 Pharmaceutical company hotlines and "800" phone numbers

Alza Corporation	1-800-634-8977
Ansell Laboratories NJ (condoms)	1-800-524-1377
Apothecus (VCF)	1-800-227-2393
Berlex Laboratories (pills)	1-800-237-5391
Bristol-Meyers Squibb Drug Information (pills/ERT)	1-800-321-1335
Carter Wallace Laboratories (condoms)	1-800-833-9532
Glaxo Wellcome (AZT, antibiotics)	1-800-722-9292
Mayer Laboratories (condoms)	1-800-426-6366
Okamoto (condoms)	1-800-283-7546
Organon (pills/Time to Talk program for parents)	1-800-631-1253
Ortho-McNeil Pharmaceutical	1-800-524-5365
Paragard (Copper T 380-A)	1-800-322-4966
Parke Davis	1-800-223-0432
Pharmacia Upjohn	1-800-253-8600
Searle	1-800-323-4204
Smart Practice (non-allergenic condoms/gloves)	1-800-522-0800
3M Pharmaceuticals	1-800-328-0255
Wyeth Ayerst	1-800-777-6180

TELEPHONE HOTLINES AND SUPPORT

Among the new resources now available to women is a hotline to call should a couple have an unprotected act of intercourse. Several options are discussed and women are told phone numbers of the 5 nearest clinicians who will provide them an emergency contraceptive. The number is 1-888-NOT-2-LATE. Numerous organizations have set up hotlines and toll-free phone numbers for providers and patients.

Table 11-3 Hotlines and toll-free phone numbers

Disease/Condition	Organization	Phone Number
Abuse	Childhelp National Child Abuse Hotline	1-800-422-4453
	National Center for Kids in Crisis	1-800-334-4KID
	National Center for Missing & Exploited Children	1-800-843-5678
	National Committee to Prevent Child Abuse	1-312-663-3520
	National Resource Center on Domestic Violence	1-800-537-2238
Adoption	Adopt a Special Kid—America	1-202-388-3888
	Adoptive Families of America	1-612-535-4829
AIDS *(see also HIV/AIDS)*	CDC National HIV/AIDS Hotline	1-800-342-AIDS
	(Spanish)	1-800-344-7432
Alcoholism	Alcoholics Anonymous	1-212-870-3400
	Al-Anon & Al-Ateen Family Groups	1-800-356-9996
	American Council on Alcoholism	1-800-527-5344
	Children of Alcoholics Foundation	1-800-359-COAF
	Co-dependents Anonymous	1-212-685-3002
	National Organization on Fetal Alcohol Syndrome	1-800-66-NO-FAS
Anxiety *(see also Depression and Mental Illness)*	Anxiety Disorders Association of America	1-301-231-9350
	Agoraphobics in Motion (AIM)	1-248-547-0400
	Freedom from Fear	1-718-351-1717
	NIMH Panic Disorder Information Line	1-800-64-PANIC
Breast Cancer *(see also Cancer)*	Reach to Recovery (mastectomy patients)	1-800-ACS-2345
	Y-Me National Breast Cancer Organization	1-800-221-2141
	National Alliance of Breast Cancer Organizations	1-212-719-0154
Breastfeeding	La Leche League	1-800-LA-LECHE
Cancer *(see also specific cancers)*	American Cancer Society	1-800-ACS-2345
	National Cancer Institute's Cancer Information Service	1-800-4-CANCER
	Candlelighters Childhood Cancer Foundation	1-800-366-2223

(continued)

Table 11-3 Hotlines and toll-free phone numbers *(cont.)*

Disease/Condition	Organization	Phone Number
Contraception	Planned Parenthood	1-800-230-7526
Depression *(see also Mental Illness)*	National Depressive & Manic Depressive Association	1-312-642-0049
	National Foundation for Depressive Illness Recovery, Inc.	1-800-248-4344 1-312-337-5661
Drug Abuse	Narcotics Anonymous	1-212-929-6262
	Alcohol & Drug Helpline	1-800-821-4357
Eating Disorders	American Anorexia/Bulimia Association	1-212-575-6200
	National Association of Anorexia Nervosa and Associated Disorders	1-847-831-3438
Emergency Contraception	Emergency Contraception Hotline	1-800-584-9911 1-888-NOT-2-LATE
Endometriosis	Endometriosis Association	1-800-992-ENDO
Family/parenting	American Academy of Family Physicians	1-800-274-2237
	American Academy of Pediatrics	1-800-433-9016
	National Maternal & Child Health Clearinghouse	1-703-821-8955
Fitness	Aerobics and Fitness Association of America	1-800-225-2322
Headaches	National Headache Foundation	1-800-843-2256
Hepatitis	Hepatitis B Coalition	1-612-647-9009
Herpes	Herpes and HPV Hotline (ASHA)	1-800-230-6039
HIV/AIDS *(for health care professionals only)*	San Francisco General Hospital, clinical consultation	1-800-933-3413
	CDC National AIDS Clearinghouse	1-800-458-5231
Hospice	National Hospice Organization Helpline	1-800-658-8898
HPV	Herpes and HPV Hotline (ASHA)	1-800-230-6039
Hypertension	American Heart Association	1-800-AHA-USA-1
Infertility	National Resolve Helpline	1-617-623-0744
Interstitial Cystitis	Interstitial Cystitis Association of America	1-800-ICA-1626
Osteoporosis	National Osteoporosis Foundation	1-800-223-9994

(continued)

Table 11-3 Hotlines and toll-free phone numbers *(cont.)*

Disease/Condition	Organization	Phone Number
Ovarian Cancer (*see also* Cancer)	Roswell Park Cancer Institute	1-800-OVARIAN
Overweight	American Heart Association	1-800-AHA-USA-1
	Take Off Pounds Sensibly (TOPS)	1-800-932-8677
Pregnancy, crisis (*see also* Adoption)	Carenet	1-703-478-5661
	National Life Center Hotline	1-800-848-5683
Pregnancy, delivery and postpartum	Lamaze International	1-800-368-4404
	Bradley Method—Childbirth	1-800-422-4784
	Depression After Delivery—National	1-800-944-4773
	Postpartum Support, International	1-805-967-7636
Premenstrual Syndrome	PMS Access	1-800-222-4PMS
Sexually Transmitted Infections	CDC Sexually Transmitted Disease Hotline	1-800-227-8922
Smoking	American Cancer Society	1-800-ACS-2345
	American Lung Association	1-800-586-4872
Urinary Incontinence	National Association for Continence	1-800-BLADDER
Vulvodynia	National Vulvodynia Association	1-301-299-0775

INTERNET SITES

The Internet offers myriad resources for both professionals and patients. Newcomers to the Internet and World Wide Web should be aware that health and medical sites are not peer-reviewed. The sites listed in Table 11-4 have been checked by the authors and appear to be reliable sources; however, do not base clinical decisions on information found on the Internet.

Table 11-4 Online reproductive health resources

Webpages with Active Links to Many Other Websites
California Abortion and Reproductive Rights Action League:
http://www.caral.org/abortion.html
Center for Communication Programs: http://www.med.jhu.edu/ccp/webguid.htm
Department of Health and Human Services: http://www.healthfinder.gov
Family Health International: http://www.fhi.org/general/urlsrch.html#anchor37518
Princeton University: http://opr.princeton.edu/ec/contrac.html
Princeton University: http://opr.princeton.edu/resources/
Wwwomen: http://www.wwwomen.com

Selected Family Planning and Reproductive Health Websites
Abortion Clinics Online: http://www.gynpages.com/
The Abortion Report: http://www.apn.com/info/abortion/
Activists for Choice: http://www.choice.org/
Alan Guttmacher Institute (AGI): http://www.agi-usa.org/
American College of Obstetricians and Gynecologists (ACOG): http://www.acog.org
Ansell Public Sector: www.lifestyles.com
Association of Reproductive Health Professionals (ARHP): http://www.arhp.org/
At Risk: http://www.at-risk.com/
AltSex: http://www.altsex.org/health.html
AVSC International: http://www.avsc.org/avsc/
The Body Politic: http://www.enews.com:80/magazines/body/
Breast Cancer Information Clearinghouse: http://nysernet.org/bcic/
Campaign for Our Children: http://www.cfoc.org/
Canadian Women's Health Network: http://www.cwhn.ca/
Center for Reproductive Law and Policy (CRLP): http://www.echonyc.com/~jmkm/wotw/
Cinema Guild: http://www.cinemaguild.com/docs/human.htm
Condomania: http://www.condomania.com/
Contraceptive Research and Development (CONRAD) Program: http://www.conrad.org/
Emergency Contraception Website (Princeton University): http://opr.princeton.edu/ec/
Family Health International (FHI): http://www.fhi.org/
Family of the Americas: http://www.upbeat.com/family/om.html
Food and Drug Administration (FDA): http://www.fda.gov/cdrh/ode/ed_rp.html
Gaumard Scientific: http://www.gaumard.com/
Health Education Services: http://www.hes.org/
Healthwise at Columbia University: http://www.columbia.edu/cu/healthwise/
International Center for Research on Women: http://www.icrw.org/
International Planned Parenthood Federation (IPPF): http://www.oneworld.org/ippf/
International Women's Health Coalition: http://www.iwhc.org/index.html
INTRAH: http://www.med.unc.edu/intrah
JAMA Women's Health: http://www.ama-assn.org/special/womh/
JHPIEGO: http://www.jhpiego.jhu.edu/
Johns Hopkins University School of Public Health: http://www.jhuccp.org/
Management Sciences for Health: http://www.msh.org/

(continued)

Table 11-4 Online reproductive health resources *(cont.)*

Selected Family Planning and Reproductive Health Websites (Continued)

Medscape: http://www.medscape.com/

MedWeb: http://www.cc.emory.edu/WHSCL/medweb.html

NASCO: http://www.nascofa.com/

National Abortion and Reproductive Rights Action League (NARAL): http://www.naral.org/

National Abortion Federation (NAF): http://www.prochoice.org/naf/

National Library of Medicine: http://www.nlm.nih.gov

National Organization for Women (NOW): http://www.now.org/issues/abortion/

National Women's Health Organization: http://gynpages.com/nwho/

Natural Family Planning: http://www.usc.edu/hsc/info/newman/resources/nfp.html

Natural Family Planning: http://www.fertility uk.org/index.html

New York Times Women's Health: http://nytsyn.com/live/Women's_health/

North American Menopause Society: http://www.menopause.org/

Novela Health Education: http://weber.u.washington.edu/~novela/

OBGYN.net: http://www.obgyn.net/

Pan American Health Organization (PAHO): http://gopher.paho.org/

Pathfinder International: http://www.pathfind.org/

Planned Parenthood Federation of America (PPFA): http://www.plannedparenthood.org

Population and Reproductive Health Materials Working Group:
http://ww2.med.jhu.edu/ccp/

Population Council: http://www.popcouncil.org

Population Reference Bureau (PRB): http://www.igc.apc.org/prb/

Population Services International (PSI): http://www.psiwash.org/

Reproline: http://www.jhpiego.jhu.edu/ReproLine/repro.html

SaferSex: http://safersex.org/

Sexuality Information and Education Council of the United States (SIECUS):
http://www.siecus.org/

Sociometrics Corporation: http://www.socio.com/

SPOT Tampon Website: http://critpath.org/~tracy/spot.html

United Nations Children's Fund (UNICEF): http://www.unicef.org/

United Nations Population Fund (UNFPA): http://www.unfpa.org/

Wellness Web: http://www.wellweb.com/women/women.htm

Women's Health Action and Mobilization: http://www.echonyc.com/~wham/wham.html

Women's Health Interactive: http://www.womens-health.com/

World Health Organization (WHO): http://www.who.ch/

WRS Group: http://www.wrsgroup.com/

Selected HIV/STI Prevention Websites

AIDS Clinical Trials Information Service: http://www.actis.org/

AIDS Research and Information: http://www.CritPath.Org/aric/

AIDSCAP: http://www.fhi.org/aids/aidscap/aidscap.html

(continued)

Table 11-4 Online reproductive health resources *(cont.)*

Selected HIV/STI Prevention Websites (Continued)
  American Red Cross: http://www.redcross.org/hss/hivaids.html
  American Social Health Association: http://sunsite.unc.edu/ASHA/
  The Body: http://www.thebody.com/cgi-bin/body.cgi
  Canadian National AIDS Clearinghouse: http://www.cpha.ca/CPHA/ch/ch.html
  CDC National AIDS Clearinghouse: http://www.cdcnac.org/
  Centers for Disease Control and Prevention: http://www.cdc.gov/nchstp/dstd/dstdp.html
  Department of STD Control, Singapore: http://biomed.nus.sg/dsc/dsc.html
  Francois-Xavier Bagnoud Foundation: http://www.fxb.org
  Gay Men's Health Crisis: http://www.gmhc.org/
  Harvard University School of Public Health: http://www.hsph.harvard.edu/Register/fxb.html
  HIVNET: http://www.hivnet.org/english/e-hivnet.html
  International AIDS Society: http://www.ias.se/
  Institut Pasteur: http://www.pasteur.fr/Bio/rapports/Sida-uk.html
  JAMA: http://www.ama-assn.org/special/hiv/
  Mothers' Voices: http://www.mvoices.org/
  National Institute of Allergy and Infectious Diseases (NIAID): http://www.niaid.nih.gov/
  National Center for HIV, STD & TB Prevention: http://www.cdc.gov/nchstp/od/nchstp.html
  Population Services International (PSI): http://www.psiwash.org/
  PROCAARE: http://www.healthnet.org/programs/procaare.html
  Project Inform: http://www.projinf.org/
  Tulane University AIDS Database: http://www.Tulane.EDU/~aids_db/
  UNAIDS: http://www.unaids.org
  University of California at San Francisco: http://www.epibiostat.ucsf.edu/capsweb/

Population Centers
  Australian National University: http://coombs.anu.edu.au/CoombsHome.html
  Brown University: http://pstc3.pstc.brown.edu/
  Chulalongkorn University, Thailand: http://www.chula.ac.th/institute/ips/index.html
  City University, London: http://ssru.city.ac.uk/
  Cornell University: http://www.einaudi.cornell.edu/pdp/
  East West Center: http://www.ewc.hawaii.edu/pop/pop00000.htm
  Florida State University: http://mailer.fsu.edu/~popctr/
  Institut National d'Études Démographiques (INED), Paris: http://www.ined.fr/
  Johns Hopkins University: http://www.sph.jhu.edu/Departments/PopDyn/
  London School of Economics: http://www.lse.ac.uk/depts/spa/popstud.htm
  London School of Hygiene and Tropical Medicine:
    http://www.lshtm.ac.uk/eps/cps/cpsintro.htm
  Netherlands Interdiscplinary Demographic Institute, Netherlands: http://www.nidi.nl/
  Pennsylvania State University http://www.pop.psu.edu
  Princeton University: http://opr.princeton.edu
  RAND: http://www.rand.org/centers/population/
  Stockholm University: http://www.suda.su.se/

(continued)

Table 11-4 Online reproductive health resources *(cont.)*

Population Centers (Continued)

United Nations Population Information Network: http://www.undp.org/popin/infoserv.htm

Universite Catholique de Louvain: http://www.sped.ucl.ac.be/presdemo.htm

University of Helsinki: http://www.valt.helsinki.fi/sosio/pru/

University of Michigan: http://www.psc.lsa.umich.edu/pubs/

University of North Carolina: http://www.cpc.unc.edu/

University of Pennsylvania: http:/lexis.pop.upenn.edu/

University of Texas: http://www.prc.utexas.edu/

University of Washington: http://csde.washington.edu/csde.html

University of Wisconsin: http://www.ssc.wisc.edu/cde/

University of Western Ontario: http://yoda.sscl.uwo.ca/sociology/popstudies/

United States Census Bureau: http://www.census.gov/

Emergency Contraception

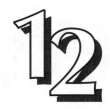

Paul F.A. Van Look, MD, PhD
Felicia Stewart, MD

- Emergency use of oral contraceptive pills containing ethinyl estradiol and norgestrel or levonorgestrel reduces the risk of pregnancy after unprotected intercourse by at least 74%.
- There are no medical contraindications to treatment with emergency contraceptive pills, except pregnancy. If a woman is already pregnant, treatment is ineffective.

- In the United States, emergency contraception could potentially prevent up to 1.7 million unintended pregnancies—about half of the estimated 3.5 million unintended pregnancies that occur annually.

Emergency contraception is defined as methods women can use after intercourse to prevent pregnancy.[2] The most commonly used option is a regimen of combined oral contraceptive pills (called ECPs, for emergency contraceptive pills) within 72 hours of unprotected intercourse (Table 12-1). Other options include use of progestin-only minipills within 48 to 72 hours or insertion of a copper-releasing intrauterine device (IUD) within 5 days. To describe these methods, terms such as postcoital contraception and morning-after pills are not satisfactory because they imply a need for immediate action, which could be misleading.

Given the chance, most women would prefer to prevent an unplanned pregnancy rather than decide what to do once one occurs. In some instances, unintended pregnancy is entirely unexpected, such as when a woman conceives while wearing an IUD or following sterilization. Often, however, unintended pregnancies occur after contraceptive failure that

Table 12-1 Oral contraceptives used for emergency contraception in the United States

Brand	Pills per Dose	Ethinyl Estradiol per Dose (mcg)	Levonorgestrel per Dose (mg)[a]
Nordette	**4** light-orange pills[b]	120	0.60
Levlen	**4** light-orange pills[b]	120	0.60
Lo/Ovral	**4** white pills[b]	120	0.60
Triphasil	**4** yellow pills[b]	120	0.50
Tri-Levlen	**4** yellow pills[b]	120	0.50
Ovral	**2** white pills[b]	100	0.50
Alesse	**5** pink pills[b]	100	0.50
Ovrette	**20** yellow pills[c]	0	0.75

Notes:
[a]The progestin in Ovral, Lo/Ovral, and Ovrette is norgestrel, which contains two isomers, only one of which (levonorgestrel) is bioactive; the amount of norgestrel in each dose is twice the amount of levonorgestrel.
[b]The treatment schedule is one dose within 72 hours after unprotected intercourse, and another dose 12 hours later.
[c]The treatment schedule in the only published prospective study of levonorgestrel was one 0.75 mg tablet (equivalent to 20 Ovrette pills) within 48 hours after unprotected intercourse, and another tablet 12 hours later. However, interim data from a large World Health Organization study indicate that the regimen is effective when initiated up to 72 hours after unprotected intercourse.

was recognized at the time it occurred. Typical examples of such situations include breakage or slippage of a barrier method, missing two or more combined oral contraceptive pills in a pill cycle, missing a single pill at the beginning or end of the no-hormone week so the pill-free interval is 8 or more days, or erring in practicing coitus interruptus or abstinence. In these instances, as well as in all situations in which sexual intercourse was unprotected, emergency contraception offers a second chance to avoid unintended pregnancy.

HISTORY

Today's hormonal methods of emergency contraception originated in the mid-1920s with the discovery that estrogenic ovarian extracts have an antifertility effect.[28] Human use of high-dose postcoital estrogen began in the 1960s as a treatment for rape victims.[15] The combined estrogen-progestin (Yuzpe) regimen was introduced in the early 1970s[35,36] and has replaced the high-dose estrogen approach. Postcoital insertion of a copper-releasing IUD for emergency contraception was first reported in 1976. Because no studies have been done for pills containing other progestins such as norethindrone, gestodene, or desogestrel in emergency contraception, such pills should not be used in routine practice.

Pills containing progestin alone have also been used for intermittent contraception in China,[13] and tablets containing 750 micrograms (mcg) levonorgestrel are marketed for this purpose in several countries under the trade name Postinor. Although this approach has proven to be unsuitable for ongoing postcoital use because of the high incidence of cycle disturbances,[17] single or infrequent use for emergency contraception is effective and well tolerated. Currently, no single levonorgestrel tablet of similar hormone content is available in the United States. To reach an equivalent dose would require taking 20 Ovrette tablets for each dose of 750 mcg levonorgestrel (Ovrette tablets contain 75 mcg norgestrel, equivalent to 37.5 mcg levonorgestrel).

In the future, antiprogestins may be another option for emergency contraception. This family of compounds, which includes mifepristone (RU 486), blocks the effects of progesterone by binding to its receptors; this effect prevents or stops ovulation and retards endometrial development, depending on whether the drug is administered before or after ovulation.[27] A single 600 milligram (mg) dose of mifepristone, initiated within 72 hours after unprotected intercourse, is highly effective in preventing pregnancy[7,30] and causes less nausea and vomiting and fewer side effects (except more menstrual cycle disruption) than does the Yuzpe regimen. A recently completed multinational trial indicates that a 10 mg dose of mifepristone may be equally effective.[26]

Older methods for emergency contraception, no longer recommended, include high-dose estrogen or danazol. Treatment with diethylstilbestrol (DES) 25 mg to 50 mg or ethinyl estradiol 5 to 10 mg given daily for 5 days provides efficacy similar to the Yuzpe method,[14,15,25] but with a high incidence of nausea. Studies of danazol, an androgenic steroid, were initially promising,[37] but this approach was abandoned when a subsequent study found an unacceptably low efficacy.[30]

FUTURE POTENTIAL FOR EMERGENCY CONTRACEPTIVE USE

Wider use of emergency contraception could prevent a substantial proportion of the millions of unplanned pregnancies that occur every year. Emergency contraception is also highly cost-effective. Comparing the cost of making emergency treatment available with health care costs for unintended pregnancies that would otherwise occur, ECP treatment provided to one woman results in a net saving of $54 to $124 based on care costs in a Medicaid or managed care setting respectively.[23] Educate women about this option during routine visits, provide information materials, provide a prescription or pills in advance for later use if needed, and make certain that office telephone and appointment procedures call for prompt response to any call for emergency contraceptive help.

In the United States, a dedicated product marketed specifically for emergency contraceptive use is not yet available, so treatment has involved use of tablets from oral contraceptive pill packets for a non-approved indication. Some practitioners have been reluctant to prescribe ECPs, and many are not familiar with this treatment option. Several important policy initiatives may help to change this situation.

The U.S. Food and Drug Administration (FDA) reviewed relevant research and published the following statement in the *Federal Register*:[6]

> Summary: The Food and Drug Administration (FDA) is announcing that the Commissioner of Food and Drugs (the Commissioner) has concluded that certain combined oral contraceptives containing ethinyl estradiol and norgestrel or levonorgestrel are safe and effective for use as postcoital emergency contraception. . . . The Commissioner bases this conclusion on FDA's review of the published literature concerning this use, FDA's knowledge of the safety of combined oral contraceptives as currently labeled, and on the unanimous conclusion that these regimens are safe and effective made by the agency's Advisory Committee for Reproductive Health Drugs at its June 28, 1996 meeting.

This action should reassure providers about using existing products for unlabeled, but now FDA-reviewed, indications. Additional reassurance can be drawn from the publication by the American College of Obstetricians and Gynecologists (ACOG) of a *Practice Pattern* detailing the use of emergency oral contraception,[1] and clinical guidelines that include emergency contraception options released by the International Planned Parenthood Federation[10] and by the World Health Organization for its Essential Drugs List.[34] In its clinical standards and guidelines, Planned Parenthood Federation of America now includes advance provision of ECPs for later use (adopted in 1996) or, for established clients, prescription given over the telephone (adopted in 1997). Family planning clinics in the federally funded Title X program received explicit authorization to provide emergency contraceptive treatment in April 1997.[12] These new policies should provide important encouragement for health care professionals to prescribe emergency contraception.

MECHANISM OF ACTION
EMERGENCY CONTRACEPTIVE PILLS AND MINIPILLS (ECPs)

When given before ovulation, the estrogen-progestin combination disrupts normal follicular development and maturation, resulting in anovulation or delayed ovulation with deficient luteal function. In contrast, when treatment is administered after ovulation has occurred and fertilization may have taken place, treatment has no effect on ovarian hormone secretion and only a limited effect on the morphologic characteristics of the endometrium.[19] These observations suggest that failure may be more likely if ovulation and fertilization have already taken place at the time of treatment and, thus, prevention of implantation may not be one of the primary modes of action.[26] The mechanism of action for ECPs is to prevent pregnancy, but not to interrupt or disrupt an already-established pregnancy. ECPs inhibit or delay ovulation to prevent fertilization, and they may possibly alter the endometrium to impair implantation.[19,31] It is also possible ECPs may alter the transport of sperm or ova.

COPPER-RELEASING IUDS

When used as a regular method of contraception, copper-releasing IUDs act primarily to prevent fertilization. In emergency contraception, the postcoital use of an IUD may involve the same mechanism in some cases, but it is more likely that the presence of an IUD or effects of copper ions may interfere with implantation. (See Chapter 21 on Intrauterine Devices.)

E FFECTIVENESS

Because emergency contraception is used only once or infrequently, traditional measures of contraceptive effectiveness such as the life-table pregnancy rate are not applicable. One way to measure effectiveness is the treatment failure rate: the number of pregnancies that occur in 100 treatment cycles. After ECP treatment, pregnancy rates are typically in the range of 0.5 to 2.5%.[5,22] A treatment failure rate of 1.0% does not mean, however, that the method was 99.0% effective. Actual efficacy is much lower because most of the women would not have become pregnant even without treatment. Even at the most fertile interval of the menstrual cycle (beginning 6 days before ovulation and ending the day after ovulation), the pregnancy risk is only 10% to 30%. It is close to 0% before and after that interval.[32] (See Chapter 27 on Impaired Fertility.)

Because treatment failure rate is strongly influenced by the specific day of the cycle that the women in the study had unprotected intercourse, failure rates of different studies cannot be meaningfully compared. A study in which all the women were treated after exposure to unprotected intercourse during the fertile phase of the cycle is bound to find a higher failure rate than a study in which women were treated irrespective of the cycle day when they had unprotected intercourse.

Comparing the number of pregnancies observed in a study with the number that would have been expected without treatment is therefore a more appropriate way of measuring efficacy. The expected number of pregnancies is computed by multiplying the number of women having unprotected intercourse at each day of the cycle by the probability of conception for that day. Using this approach, an analysis of the 10 published trials that included data on the cycle day of exposure yielded effectiveness rates for the Yuzpe regimen ranging from a low of 55% to a high of 94%. The weighted average of the effectiveness rates in all 10 studies was 74% (Table 12-2). In other words, this regimen prevented about three-fourths of the pregnancies that would have occurred had no treatment been given. Considering other methodological issues in these studies, however, the researchers concluded that the true effectiveness of ECP treatment is probably higher, at least 75% and perhaps higher than 80%.[22]

The effectiveness of progestin-only tablets containing 750 mcg levonorgestrel (one tablet followed 12 hours later by a second tablet) for emergency contraception has recently been tested against the Yuzpe regimen in a randomized trial; both treatment regimens were initiated within 48 hours after unprotected intercourse. The results showed the levonorgestrel regimen was as effective as the Yuzpe regimen but was associated with significantly less nausea and vomiting.[8] Interim data from a large multinational World Health Organization (WHO) trial with treatment time extended to 72 hours confirm the efficacy and low incidence of side effects of the levonorgestrel regimen and are expected to lead to the marketing of Postinor-2, a two-pill packet of 750 mcg levonorgestrel pills for emergency use.

Over 8,400 postcoital insertions of a copper-bearing IUD are known to have been carried out since its introduction in 1976. With only 8 failures, this approach probably has a pregnancy rate no higher than 0.1%, one-fifteenth that of the Yuzpe regimen.[20] The effectiveness of using the newer levonorgestrel-releasing IUD (LNg-20) for emergency contraception has not been studied.

A DVANTAGES AND INDICATIONS

Emergency contraceptives are the only methods a couple can use to prevent pregnancy after unprotected sexual intercourse or after a contraceptive "accident." Emergency contraception also is an essential part of treatment for victims of sexual assault who were not protected by an effective contraceptive method at the time. Emergency contraception is an appropriate option in the following circumstances:

- No contraceptive was used when intercourse took place.
- A male condom slipped, broke, or leaked.
- A woman's diaphragm or cervical cap was inserted incorrectly, dislodged during intercourse, was removed too early, or was found to be torn.

Table 12-2 Effectiveness rates of Yuzpe emergency contraceptive pill regimen

Reference	Number	Observed Pregnancies	Cycle Days of Unprotected Intercourse*	Expected Pregnancies	Effectiveness Rate	Comments
Yuzpe et al., 1977	152	1	−3 to +3	17.1	94.2	Expected pregnancies not reported by original investigators; estimate based on assumption that women are distributed uniformly across the reported range of days of intercourse.
Yuzpe et al., 1982	451	5	−8 to +5	31.8	84.3	Calculation of expected pregnancies include women lost to follow-up. Observed pregnancies exclude 4 women who had other unprotected intercourse.
Glasier et al., 1992	384	4	−8 to +5	23.0	82.6	Random assignment to Yuzpe or mifepristone.
Bagshaw et al., 1988	345	8	−3 to +3	38.8	79.4	Expected pregnancies not reported by original investigators; estimate based on assumption that women are distributed uniformly across the reported range of days of intercourse. Trial used both standard regimen and modified treatment (3 doses 12 hours apart).
Van Santen et al., 1985	461	5	−8 to +5	23.4	78.6	Combined data from open study and comparative study (Yuzpe versus high-dose estrogen); for Yuzpe regimen approximately half received norgestrel+EE and half received levonorgestrel+EE. One observed pregnancy omitted because subject took only one dose.
Percival-Smith et al., 1987	648	12	−8 to +5	40.2	70.1	Calculation of expected pregnancies includes women lost to follow-up.
Zuliani et al., 1990	407	9	−8 to +5	28.7	68.6	Random assignment to Yuzpe or danazol.
Ho et al., 1993	341	9	−8 to +5	22.0	59.1	Random assignment to Yuzpe or levonorgestrel-only regimen. Excludes 77 women who had subsequent unprotected intercourse.
Webb et al., 1992	191	5	−8 to +5	11.3	55.8	Calculation of expected pregnancies includes women lost to follow-up. Excludes 5 women who used ECPs twice in one cycle.
Tully, 1983	159	8	−3 to +3	17.9	55.3	
Total	3,539	66		254.2	74.0	

*Range of days on either side of ovulation

- A woman has missed one or more combined oral contraceptive pills at the beginning or end of a packet so the pill-free interval is prolonged beyond 7 days, or she has missed two or more pills during the pill cycle. Because combined pills act by suppressing ovulation, the risk of conception occurs some days after the missed pills when follicular development, freed from the inhibition by the oral contraceptive, is sufficient to allow ovulation. Ovulation is unlikely if only a few pills have been missed during a pill cycle. Nevertheless, treatment is reasonable if the woman is worried or wishes to avoid even a small risk of pregnancy.
- A woman has missed one or more progestin-only pills. In contrast to combined pills, ovulation is not consistently suppressed by progestin-only pills, and the risk of pregnancy after missing progestin-only pills is greater and more immediate than is the case with missed combined pills.
- A female condom was inserted or removed incorrectly leading to spillage of semen, or the penis was inserted mistakenly between the female condom and the vaginal wall resulting in intravaginal ejaculation.
- The couple erred in practicing coitus interruptus (ejaculation in vagina or on external genitalia).
- The couple erred in practicing periodic abstinence (sexual intercourse on a fertile day of the cycle).
- An IUD was partially or totally expelled.
- A woman was exposed to a possible teratogen such as a live vaccine or cytotoxic drug when she was not protected by effective contraception.

Because it can be used up to 5 days after intercourse, the IUD may be a useful option for women who present too late to take the Yuzpe regimen. It may also be a good choice for the woman who wishes to continue using an IUD as her long-term method of contraception.

D ISADVANTAGES AND CAUTIONS

SIDE EFFECTS—HORMONAL METHODS

Nausea and vomiting. Following treatment with ECPs, nausea occurs in 30% to 50% of women, and vomiting in 15% to 25%. Other reported complaints include fatigue, breast tenderness, headache, abdominal pain, and dizziness. Side effects subside within a day or two after treatment is completed. Routine use of anti-nausea or anti-emetic medication 1 hour before the first ECP dose may help reduce nausea and vomiting.[1] Nausea and vomiting are far less common among women using progestin-only pills for emergency contraception.

There is no research to indicate whether it is necessary to repeat the dose if the woman vomits within 1 to 3 hours after taking ECPs. Some practitioners take the view that a replacement dose should be given orally or, in the opinion of some, vaginally to prevent the tablets from being vomited a second time. Other providers, believing that nausea and vomiting are evidence of an estrogen-mediated effect on the central nervous system and thus of absorption of the drugs, conclude that a replacement dose is not necessary.

Ectopic pregnancy. No evidence suggests the Yuzpe regimen is associated with a higher relative risk of ectopic pregnancy. However, no studies have focused specifically on this issue and the possibility of an extrauterine implantation must be kept in mind whenever a treatment failure occurs.

Menstrual changes. ECPs change the amount, duration, and timing of the next menstrual period in about 10% to 15% of women treated. In most cases this effect is minor, and menstruation occurs a few days earlier or later than expected. If the delay in the onset of the menstrual period is greater than 7 days, consider the possibility of pregnancy. Menstrual cycle changes following progestin-only emergency treatment are similar to those seen after the Yuzpe regimen.[8]

SIDE EFFECTS—COPPER-RELEASING IUD

Side effects after postcoital insertion of an IUD are similar to those seen after routine insertion at other times and include abdominal discomfort and vaginal bleeding or spotting. (See Chapter 21 on Intrauterine Devices.)

CAUTIONS

There are no absolute medical contraindications to the use of ECPs, with the exception of pregnancy.[1,31,33] ECPs should not be used in pregnancy, not because they are thought to be harmful, but because they are ineffective. The advantages of ECP use generally outweigh the theoretical risks even for women who have one or more contraindications to the ongoing use of combined oral contraceptives, such as a history of heart disease, acute focal migraine, or severe liver disease. Use of progestin-only emergency treatment, however, may be preferable to use of ECPs for a woman who has a history of thromboembolic disease and wishes to be treated.

Eligibility criteria and contraindications for emergency insertion of an IUD are the same as for insertion at other times. (See Chapter 21 on Intrauterine Devices.) A particular concern is the risk of pelvic inflammatory disease, particularly in women requesting emergency contraception after intercourse with a new sexual partner and in victims of sexual assault, when the risk of sexually transmitted infection (STI) is high.

PROVIDING EMERGENCY CONTRACEPTION

About half of the women who request emergency contraception have not used contraception, 35% experienced a problem with a condom or other barrier method, and the remaining 10% experienced failed coitus interruptus, were raped, or missed oral contraceptive pills (Table 12-3). Although women who request emergency contraception come from all age groups and walks of life, the typical user is young (15 to 25 years of age), single, and nulliparous.

Although pregnancy can result from intercourse only during the fertile phase of the cycle, which begins 6 days before and ends the day after ovulation, any woman requesting emergency contraception after unprotected intercourse should be offered treatment unless there are sound medical grounds for not doing so. For example, a woman may present more than 72 hours (the time window for ECPs) after unprotected intercourse but have a contraindication to insertion of an IUD. In this case, offering ECPs may be considered: they may reduce the risk of pregnancy at least to some extent and are unlikely to be harmful. Some protocols for emergency contraception have rules that withhold treatment in situations involving more than one unprotected coital exposure or exposure on a low-risk day. Such limits may make sense in the context of research studies on efficacy but are not appropriate for routine clinical care. In reviewing the cycle day when exposure occurred, you may determine whether the risk of pregnancy is likely to be high or low, but what matters most is how the woman feels about her risk, no matter whether it is likely to be high or low.

Table 12-3 Reasons for requesting emergency contraception

| | | Reason | | |
| | | No Method Used | Barrier Method Failed | Other[a] |
Reference	Number	No Method Used	Barrier Method Failed	Other[a]
Tully, 1983	511	52%	34%	14%
Hoffman, 1983	737	46%	43%	11%
Bagshaw et al., 1988	1,200	57%	32%	11%
Kane et al., 1989	909	67%	25%	8%
Roberts et al., 1995	596	45%	48%	7%
Total	3,953	55%	35%	10%

[a]Missed pill(s), vomiting of pills, failed coitus interruptus, rape, etc.

Counseling

In counseling women who seek emergency contraceptive treatment, remember this is often a difficult and stressful situation. Be respectful of the woman and responsive to her needs. Reassure all women, regardless of age or marital status, that all information will be kept confidential. Be as supportive as possible of the woman's choices and refrain from making judgmental comments or indicating disapproval through body language or facial expressions. Supportive attitudes will help improve compliance and set the stage for effective follow-up counseling about regular contraceptive use and prevention of STI.[4]

After unprotected intercourse, some women may feel particularly anxious about becoming pregnant and missing the 72-hour window of opportunity for ECPs. They may feel embarrassed about failing to use regular contraception effectively. Rape victims will feel traumatized. Women may be very concerned about possible infection, especially in cases of rape. Counsel women and provide STI diagnostic services (or referrals) and information about preventive measures. Women must understand that emergency contraception offers no protection against STIs, including infection with the human immunodeficiency virus (HIV). Additional emergency treatment measures may be needed. (See Chapter 7 on HIV/AIDS and Reproductive Health and Chapter 8 on Reproductive Tract Infections.)

Based on the evidence available, women who would not plan to have an abortion in case of treatment failure can be reassured that pregnancies occurring despite treatment do not have an increased risk of adverse outcome.

Other Issues

Frequent use. Emphasize that ECPs are for emergency use only. They are not recommended for routine use because they are less effective than regular contraceptives. Note: Although not recommended, repeated ECP use is not known to pose health risks to users and is not a logical reason for denying women access to treatment.

Use after 72 hours. Although studies of ECP treatment have all specified treatment within 72 hours, it is unlikely that ECP effectiveness after this time drops immediately to zero. A woman seeking treatment shortly after 72 hours who cannot or does not want to have a copper-releasing IUD inserted may want to consider ECPs even though the timing is not optimal. Late treatment may reduce her risk for pregnancy and is unlikely to be harmful.[21]

Use after multiple acts of unprotected intercourse. If more than 72 hours have elapsed since the time of the first unprotected exposure,

ECPs may not be effective in preventing pregnancy that resulted from the first exposure. Providing ECPs, however, would not be expected to disrupt or harm subsequent pregnancy development, and would reduce the risk that pregnancy would result from later exposures that did occur within the preceding 72 hours.

Ongoing contraception refused. Women requesting emergency contraception should be offered information and services for regular contraception. Not all of them, however, will want contraceptive counseling. Thus, while counseling about regular contraceptives is recommended, it should not be a prerequisite for providing emergency treatment. If the reason for requesting emergency contraception is that the regular contraceptive method failed, discuss the reasons for failure and how it can be prevented in the future.

BEFORE PROVIDING EMERGENCY CONTRACEPTION TREATMENT

Exclude the possibility a woman may already be pregnant: assess the date of the last menstrual period and whether it was normal. Establish the time of the first episode of unprotected intercourse to ensure she is within the treatment time frame (72 hours for ECPs or emergency use of progestin-only minipills; 5 days for insertion of a copper-releasing IUD). Ask if the woman is currently using a regular method of contraception; this question can be a good starting point for a discussion of regular contraceptive use and how to use methods correctly.

Make certain the woman does not want to become pregnant and understands there is still a chance of pregnancy even after treatment. Describe common side effects. Advance counseling about possible side effects helps women know what to expect and may lead to greater tolerance. Provide anti-nausea medication or recommend an over-the-counter product to be taken 1 hour before starting ECP treatment (Table 12-4).

Make sure the woman understands that hormonal emergency contraception will not protect her from pregnancy if she engages in unprotected intercourse in the days or weeks following treatment. This is a common misperception among some women. If the woman wishes to use oral contraceptives as an ongoing method, she can begin taking one oral contraceptive tablet daily the day after emergency treatment is completed and continue with daily pills, as if the ECP treatment days had been the beginning of a new pill cycle. If the woman does not want to continue using oral contraceptives, but needs contraceptive protection, advise her to use a barrier method, such as condoms, for the remainder of her cycle. A different contraceptive method can be initiated at the beginning of her next cycle (Table 12-5).

Table 12-4 Anti-nausea treatment options

Drug	Dose	Timing of Administration
Non-prescription Drugs		
Meclizine hydrochloride (Dramamine II, Bonine)	One or two 25 mg tablets	1 hour before first ECP dose; repeat if needed in 24 hours
Diphenhydramine hydrochloride (Benedryl)	One or two 25 mg tablets	1 hour before first ECP dose; repeat as needed every 4–6 hours
Dimenhydinate (Dramamine)	One to two 50 mg tablets or 4-8 teaspoons liquid	30 minutes to 1 hour before first ECP dose; repeat as needed every 4–6 hours
Cyclizine hydrochloride (Marezine)	One 50 mg tablet	30 minutes before first ECP dose; repeat as needed every 4–6 hours
Prescription Drugs		
Meclizine hydrochloride (Antivert)	One or two 25 mg tablets	1 hour before first ECP dose; repeat if needed in 24 hours
Trimethobenzamide hydrochloride (Tigan)	One 250 mg tablet or 200 mg suppository	1 hour before first ECP dose; repeat as needed every 4–6 hours
Promethazine hydrochloride (Phenergan)	One 25 mg tablet or suppository	30 minutes to 1 hour before first ECP dose; repeat as needed every 8–12 hours

Source: Wells et al. (1997) with permission.

EMERGENCY CONTRACEPTION TREATMENT REGIMENS

Emergency contraceptive pills.   For maximum effectiveness, ECP treatment must start within 72 hours after unprotected intercourse (or within 72 hours of the first act if there have been several acts). Drugs and doses are shown in Table 12-1. To avoid making the woman take the second dose in the middle of the night, allow her to delay the first dose by a few hours, provided the 72-hour time limit is not exceeded.

Progestin-only pills.   The treatment schedule in the one published prospective study of a progestin-only regimen was one dose (0.75 mg levonorgestrel) provided within 48 hours after unprotected intercourse, and another dose 12 hours later. Interim data from a World Health Organization study indicate that the levonorgestrel regimen is also effective when initiated up to 72 hours after unprotected intercourse.

Intrauterine devices.   The IUD as an emergency contraceptive method can be inserted up to the time of implantation, about 5 days

Table 12-5 Initiating ongoing contraception after ECP use

Because ECPs can delay ovulation, a woman could be at risk of pregnancy in the first few days after treatment. Women should use a back-up method of contraception for the remainder of the treatment cycle then initiate a regular method of contraception with their next menstrual period.

Method	When to Initiate
Condom	Can be used immediately
Diaphragm	Can be used immediately
Spermicide	Can be used immediately
Oral Contraceptive (OC)	Initiate a new pack, either according to manufacturer's instructions after beginning the next menstrual cycle, or begin taking one OC tablet daily the day after ECP treatment is completed. Women using Lo/Ovral, Nordette, or Levlen for emergency contraception can continue taking one pill per day from the same pack.
Injectable	Initiate within 7 days of beginning the next menstrual period
Implants	Initiate within 7 days of beginning the next menstrual period
Intrauterine Device (IUD)	Initiate during the next menstrual period (If the patient intends to use an IUD for ongoing contraception, consider inserting a copper-releasing IUD for emergency contraception rather than using ECPs.)
Fertility Awareness	Initiate after onset of the next normal menstrual period and after the patient has been trained in using the method
Sterilization	Perform the operation any time after beginning the next menstrual period

Source: Wells et al. (1997) with permission.

after ovulation. Thus, if a woman had unprotected intercourse 3 days before the day ovulation is estimated to have occurred in that cycle, the IUD could, in principle, be inserted up to 8 days after the intercourse. Most family planning providers, however, limit insertion to the first 5 days after intercourse because it is difficult to reliably estimate the likely day of ovulation.

AFTER PROVIDING EMERGENCY CONTRACEPTIVE TREATMENT

If the woman has already adopted a method of contraception for regular use and wishes to continue using this method, no follow-up is needed unless she has a delay in her menstruation, suspects she may be pregnant, or has other reasons for concern. A follow-up appointment has several objectives:

- Record the menstrual data to verify the woman is not pregnant; if in doubt perform a pregnancy test.
- Discuss contraceptive options as appropriate and provide a contraceptive method.

If emergency contraception has failed and the woman is pregnant, advise her of the possible options. Refer her to other service providers as appropriate. If she decides to continue the pregnancy, reassure her there is no evidence of any teratogenic effect following the use of hormonal emergency contraception. *Be certain to rule out the possibility of ectopic pregnancy.* While emergency contraception methods are unlikely to increase the risk of ectopic pregnancy, women who become pregnant despite using emergency contraception may have a higher rate of ectopic pregnancy than do other pregnant women.

ESTABLISHING EMERGENCY CONTRACEPTIVE SERVICES

Additional information and materials that may be of help in establishing emergency contraception services are available from the following sources:

- Information about emergency contraception method options and access to the U.S. directory of providers via internet: http://opr.princeton.edu/ec/
- Toll-free telephone information about method options and referral to providers listed in the directory nearest the caller's telephone area code: call 1-888-NOT-2-LATE.
- Information about enrolling as a provider in the U.S. directory: call 1-888-NOT-2-LATE.
- Copy of the Food and Drug Administration *Federal Register* notice regarding emergency contraception: request document number 0265 at 1-800-342-2722.
- Summary of legal issues: order from the Center for Reproductive Law & Policy, 120 Wall Street, New York, NY 10005.
- Provider Resource Packet prepared by PATH (Program for Appropriate Technology in Health), including sample patient brochures, fact sheet, office poster, and a provider manual with prescribing information and sample protocols: order from Planned Parenthood

Federation of America, at 1-800-669-0156, or by mail at Marketing Department, PPFA, 810 Seventh Avenue, New York, NY 10019.

- Resource Packet for Health Care Providers and Programme Managers (in English and Spanish): Consortium for Emergency Contraception, 8930 Camp Road, Welcome, MD 20693 or any Consortium organization (Concept Foundation, International Planned Parenthood Federation, Pacific Institute for Women's Health, Pathfinder International, Population Council, PATH, or World Health Organization).

INSTRUCTIONS FOR USING EMERGENCY CONTRACEPTION

Instructions for women who have emergency insertion of an IUD are the same as for IUD insertion at other times (see Chapter 21 on Intrauterine Devices).

Women provided with ECPs or progestin-only emergency treatment should receive medication labeling that identifies the specific product prescribed and the number of tablets needed for each dose (see Table 12-1). The following instructions can be given to women to ensure correct use. For progestin-only emergency treatment, omit the anti-nausea medication instruction.

1. **Swallow the first dose no later than 72 hours after unprotected sex.** As long as the 72-hour time limit is not exceeded, you can delay the first dose by a few hours to avoid having to take your second dose in the middle of the night. **Do not take any extra pills.** More pills will not decrease the risk of pregnancy any further. More pills *may* increase the risk of nausea, possibly causing you to vomit.

2. Swallow the second dose 12 hours after taking the first dose.

3. **Take anti-nausea medication 1 hour before the first ECP dose.** About one-third to one-half of women who use ECPs have temporary nausea. It is usually mild and should stop in a day or so. If you vomit within 1 or 2 hours after taking a dose, call your clinician. You may need to repeat a dose.

4. **If your period does not start within 3 weeks, see your clinician for an exam and pregnancy test.** Your next period may start a few days earlier or later than usual. If you think you may be pregnant, see your clinician at once, whether or not you plan to continue the pregnancy. Emergency contraceptive pills may not prevent an ectopic pregnancy (in the tubes or abdomen), which is a medical emergency.

5. **Do not have unprotected intercourse in the days or weeks following treatment.** Hormonal emergency contraception will not protect you from pregnancy if you do so. Continue taking pills, one tablet daily, or use a barrier method, such as a condom, for the remainder of your cycle. After your menstrual period, continue using the condom or begin another method of contraception.

6. As soon as you possibly can, begin using a method of birth control you will be able to use on an ongoing basis. **Emergency contraceptive pills are not as effective as other forms of contraception.** They are meant for one-time, emergency protection. Discuss with your clinician which method may suit you best and when you can start it.

REFERENCES

1. American College of Obstetricians and Gynecologists. Emergency oral contraception. ACOG Practice Patterns. Washington DC: The American College of Obstetricians and Gynecologists, 1996.
2. Anonymous. Consensus statement on emergency contraception. Contraception 1995;52:211-213.
3. Bagshaw SN, Edwards D, Tucker AK. Ethinyl oestradiol and d-norgestrel is an effective emergency postcoital contraceptive: a report of its use in 1,200 patients in a family planning clinic. Aust NZ J Obstet Gynaecol 1988;28: 137-140.
4. Consortium for Emergency Contraception. Emergency contraceptive pills. A resource packet for health care providers and programme managers. Welcome MD: The Consortium for Emergency Contraception, 1996.
5. Fasoli M, Parazzini F, Cecchetti G, La Vecchia C. Post-coital contraception: an overview of published studies. Contraception 1989;39:459-468 and 39:699-700.
6. Food and Drug Administration. Prescription drug products; certain combined oral contraceptives for use as postcoital emergency contraception. Federal Register 1997;62:8610-8612.
7. Glasier A, Thong KJ, Dewar M, Mackie M, Baird DT. Mifepristone (RU 486) compared with high-dose estrogen and progestogen for emergency postcoital contraception. N Engl J Med 1992;324:1041-1044.
8. Ho PC, Kwan MSW. A prospective randomized comparison of levonorgestrel with the Yuzpe regimen in post-coital contraception. Hum Reprod 1993;8:389-392.
9. Hoffmann KOK. Postcoital contraception: experiences with ethinyloestradiol/ norgestrel and levonorgestrel only. In: Harrison RF, Bonnar J, Thompson W (eds). Fertility and Sterility. Lancaster UK: MTP Press Limited, 1983.
10. International Planned Parenthood Federation. Statement on emergency contraception. London: IPPF, 1994.
11. Kane LA, Sparrow MJ. Postcoital contraception: a family planning study. NZ Med J 1989;102:151-153.
12. Kring T (memorandum). OPA Program Instruction Series, OPA 97-2: Emergency Contraception. 23 April 1997.

13. Lei HP, Hu Z-Y. The mechanisms of action of vacation pills. In: Chang CF, Griffin D. Recent Advances in Fertility Regulation. Geneva: Atar SA, 1981.
14. Morris JM, van Wagenen G. Postcoital oral contraception. In: Hankinson RKB, Kleinman RL, Eckstein P, Romero H (eds). Proceedings of the Eighth International Conference of the International Planned Parenthood Federation, April 9-15, 1967; Santiago, Chile and London: International Planned Parenthood Federation, 1967.
15. Morris JM, van Wagenen G. Compounds interfering with ovum implantation and development. III. The role of estrogens. Am J Obstet Gynecol 1966;96:804-815.
16. Percival-Smith RKL, Abercrombie B. Postcoital contraception with dl-norgestrel/ethinyl estradiol combination: six years' experience in a study medical clinic. Contraception 1987;36:287-290.
17. Rinehart W. Postcoital contraception—an appraisal. Popul Rep 1976; Series J (No. 9).
18. Roberts RN, Moohan JM, McNeill S, Lyons MS. Audit of an emergency contraception service. Br J Fam Plann 1995;21:22-25.
19. Swahn M-L, Westlund P, Johannisson E, Bygdeman M. Effect of post-coital contraceptive methods on the endometrium and the menstrual cycle. Acta Obstet Gynecol Scand 1996;75:738-744.
20. Trussell J, Ellertson C. Efficacy of emergency contraception. Fertility Control Reviews 1995;4:8-11.
21. Trussell J, Ellertson C, Rodriguez G. The Yuzpe regimen of emergency contraception: how long after the morning after? Obstet Gynecol 1996;88:150-154.
22. Trussell J, Ellertson C, Stewart F. The effectiveness of the Yuzpe regimen of emergency contraception. Fam Plann Perspect 1996;28:58-64 and 87.
23. Trussell J, Koenig J, Ellertson C, Stewart F. Preventing unintended pregnancy: the cost-effectiveness of three methods of emergency contraception. Am J Publ Health 1997;87:932-937.
24. Tully B. Post-coital contraception—a study. Br J Fam Plann 1983;8:119-124.
25. Van Look PFA. Postcoital contraception: a cover-up story. In: Diczfalusy E, Bygdeman M (eds). Fertility Regulation Today and Tomorrow. New York: Serono Symposia Publications from Raven Press, 1987.
26. Van Look PFA. Emergency contraception: the Cinderella of family planning. In: Rodriguez O, Hedon B, Daya S (eds). Clinical Infertility and Contraception. International Federation of Fertility Societies. Carnforth UK: Parthenon Publishing, 1998.
27. Van Look PFA, von Hertzen H. Clinical uses of antiprogestogens. Hum Reprod Update 1995;1:19-34.
28. Van Look PFA, von Hertzen H. Emergency contraception. Br Med Bull 1993;49:158-170.
29. Van Santen MR, Haspels AA. Interception II: postcoital low-dose estrogens and norgestrel combination in 633 women. Contraception 1985;31:275-290.
30. Webb AMC, Russell J, Elstein M. Comparison of Yuzpe regimen, danazol and mifepristone (RU 486) in oral postcoital contraception. Br Med J 1992;305: 927-931.
31. Wells E, Crook B, Muller N. Emergency contraception: a resource manual for providers. Seattle: Program for Appropriate Technology in Health, 1997.

32. Wilcox AJ, Weinberg CR, Baird DD. Timing of sexual intercourse in relation to ovulation. Effects on the probability of conception, survival of the pregnancy, and sex of the baby. N Engl J Med 1995;333:1517-1521.

33. World Health Organization. Improving access to quality care in family planning. Medical eligibility criteria for contraceptive use. (Doc. WHO/FRH/FPP/96.9). Geneva: World Health Organization, 1996.

34. World Health Organization. The use of essential drugs. Seventh report of the WHO expert committee (including the revised model list of essential drugs). WHO technical report series no. 867. Geneva: World Health Organization, 1997.

35. Yuzpe AA, Lancee WJ. Ethinylestradiol and dl-norgestrel as a postcoital contraceptive. Fertil Steril 1977;28:932-936.

36. Yuzpe AA, Smith RP, Rademaker AW. A multicenter clinical investigation employing ethinyl estradiol combined with dl-norgestrel as a postcoital contraceptive agent. Fertil Steril 1982;37:508-513.

37. Zuliani G, Colombo UF, Molla R. Hormonal postcoital contraception with an ethinylestradiol-norgestrel combination and two danazol regimens. Eur J Obstet Gynecol Reprod Biol 1990;37:253-260.

Abstinence and the Range of Sexual Expression

Deborah Kowal, MA, PA

- Abstinence can be primary or secondary. Primary abstainers have not had a sexual experience with another person. Secondary abstainers are sexually experienced persons who have chosen to avoid some or all sexual activity with another person.
- Many abstainers choose to avoid intercourse but engage in other forms of sexual intimacy.
- Secondary abstinence, or celibacy, is the choice of many sexually experienced adolescents and adults. It is not an extremist position in the age of viral sexually transmitted infections.
- The care provider's role is to support the choice of abstinence and to teach negotiation and planning skills for using abstinence effectively and safely.

Some people define abstinence as refraining from all sexual behavior, including masturbation. Some people define abstinence as refraining from sexual behavior involving genital contact. Others define it as refraining from penetrative sexual practices. Still others would offer different definitions. For purposes of this discussion, abstinence is defined as refraining from vaginal or anal intercourse.

Asking clients what they define as abstinence is an important question with clinical implications. In a recent study of 2,206 male and female high-school students, many of those who reported never having had vaginal intercourse had engaged in other sexual practices. Overall, 47% reported that they were "virgins." Of these students, 30% had engaged in heterosexual masturbation of or by a partner, 9% had engaged in fellatio with ejaculation, and 10% had engaged in cunnilingus.[4]

Historically, sexual abstinence has probably been the single most important factor in curtailing human fertility.[2] Abstinence can be primary or secondary. Primary abstainers have never had sexual intercourse with another person. Secondary abstainers are sexually experienced persons who have chosen to avoid some or all sexual activity with another person. Secondary abstinence is the choice of many sexually experienced adolescents and adults.

Primary abstinence is not uncommon among young persons. Among never-married adolescent men age 15 to 19 years, 45% report never having had sexual intercourse.[5] Among adolescent women age 15 to 19 years, half report never having had voluntary sexual intercourse since menarche, according to the 1995 National Survey of Family Growth (NSFG).[1] After the teen years, the percentage of women who have not had sexual intercourse drops dramatically to 12% and below (Table 13-1).

About 17% of women age 15 to 44 years reported that they had not had sexual intercourse in the 3 months prior to the interview. Of these women, 11% had never had sexual intercourse and 6% had reported having had no sexual intercourse in those 3 months.[1] Whether these latter women deliberately chose to abstain, merely had a brief lapse in a relationship, or had other reasons for not having had sexual intercourse is not known.

At a number of times throughout their lives, however, people of all ages do deliberately choose to abstain. It is important that you regard these clients' abstinence as normal, common, and acceptable. Many persons

Table 13-1 Percentage of women age 15-44 who report having had no sexual intercourse in the 3 months prior to NSFG interview, 1995

	Age						
	15-44	15-19	20-24	25-29	30-34	35-39	40-44
No Intercourse in 3 Months Before Interview	17.1	56.9	18.9	9.9	7.6	7.6	8.2
Never had intercourse	10.9	49.8	12.1	4.2	2.7	1.4	1.4
Has had intercourse but not in 3 months before interview	6.2	7.1	6.8	5.7	4.9	6.2	6.8

Source: Abma et al. (1997).

Table 13-2 Teaching adolescents to say "no"

Technique	Example
Simple "no"	"No, thanks." or "No."
Emphatic "no"	"No! I don't want to do that!"
Repetitive "no"	"No." "No." "No."
Turn the tables	"You say that if I love you I would. But if you really love me, you wouldn't insist."
Give a reason	"I'm not ready." "We can't be too careful in this age of AIDS." "I've decided to wait until I've achieved my academic goals."
Leave the scene	Walk out of there.
Steer clear	If you suspect you will be pressured, do not go out with that person.
Call in the cavalry	Threaten to tell someone with authority (counselor, relative, police).
Safety in numbers	Double date; keep trusted friends nearby.

Source: Grossman et al. (1987).

freely and happily choose to be abstinent. They deserve respect, encouragement, and support. For others, abstinence is dysfunctional or involuntary. These individuals require help. Your role as care provider is to support the choice of abstinence and to teach negotiation and planning skills for using abstinence effectively and safely. Communication skills are also essential for clients, especially adolescents, to get across their intentions to partners (Table 13-2). Educate all abstemious persons about the other methods of contraception and safer sex available to them, including the following:

- Effective over-the-counter products
- Prescription methods
- Emergency contraception options
- Safer-sex practices

THE RANGE OF SEXUAL EXPRESSION

Although abstinence has become associated with saying "no," viewed from another perspective, abstinence can mean saying "yes" to a number of other sexual activities. All human beings need touching—for nurture, for solace, for communication, for simple affection. Most human beings enjoy erotic touching as well, a specialized language of sexual gratification and more intimate forms of affection.

For some people, erotic touching equals intercourse, nothing more or less. Most people, however, have a more expansive view of sexual expression, and other activities give them pleasure and meaning. Holding hands, kissing, massage, solo masturbation, mutual masturbation, dancing, oral-genital sex, fantasy, and erotic books and movies all fit along the sexual continuum, as do many other activities. Taste, smell, vision, and hearing may matter as much as touch for erotic pleasure.

INDICATIONS FOR ABSTINENCE OR OTHER FORMS OF SEXUAL EXPRESSION

When the only goal of abstinence is to avoid unwanted pregnancy, then all forms of sexual expression are available to a couple except for penis-in-vagina intercourse. When a goal of abstinence is to avoid sexually transmitted infections (STIs), then oral-genital sex, anal intercourse, and other practices that expose the partner to pre-ejaculatory fluid, semen, cervical-vaginal secretions, or blood must be reconsidered. Some couples avoid these practices altogether, and others use condoms, latex dams, or other barriers to inhibit body fluid transmission during these practices. The care provider's role is to offer factual, explicit guidance on safer-sex options. (See Chapter 7 on HIV/AIDS and Reproductive Health.)

Consider discussing abstinence even with adolescents who have experimented with intercourse and other sexual behaviors. Once young men and women have satisfied their initial curiosity about intercourse, and once they feel socially comfortable with their level of sexual sophistication, they may be willing to become abstinent, removing themselves at least for a while from the health risks of intercourse. You can help young people learn that the door between abstinence and sexual activity opens in both directions.

For times when vaginal or anal intercourse may be unwise from a medical standpoint for one or both partners, other forms of erotic touching may make more sense. Some situations in which insertive sex may be ill-advised and alternatives recommended include the following:

- Known or suspected STI (also avoid other sexual practices that transmit pre-ejaculatory fluid, semen, cervical-vaginal secretions, and blood)
- Post-operative pain or tenderness, such as from episiotomy, hemorrhoidectomy, vasectomy, and other procedures
- Pelvic, vaginal, or urinary tract infection
- Gastrointestinal illness or infection
- Dyspareunia or other pelvic pain
- Undiagnosed postcoital bleeding
- Late third trimester of pregnancy, postpartum, or postabortion
- Postmyocardial infarction

- Certain disabling physical conditions
- Known or suspected allergic sensitization to partner's semen

Therapy for a variety of sexual problems may include exploration of avenues of sexual gratification other than intercourse. Temporarily forbidding intercourse takes performance pressure off couples struggling with erection difficulty, orgasm difficulty, or rapid ejaculation. (See Chapter 2 on Sexuality and Reproductive Health.)

INSTRUCTIONS FOR USING ABSTINENCE

1. Decide what you want to do about sex at a time when you feel clearheaded, sober, and good about yourself. If you have a partner, decide together at a time when you feel close to each other but not sexual. For example, try talking while you take a walk and hold hands.
2. Decide in advance what sexual activities you will say "yes" to and discuss these with your partner.
3. Tell your partner, very clearly and in advance—not at the last minute—what activities you will not do.
4. Avoid high-pressure sexual situations, and stay sober.
5. If you say "no," say it so it is clear that you mean it.
6. Learn more about your body and how to keep it healthy.
7. Learn about contraception and safer sex, so you will be ready if you change your mind. Always keep condoms on hand.
8. Refrain from intercourse if you do not have a contraceptive method available. Learn about emergency contraception in case you have intercourse when you did not expect it. If your health care provider does not provide emergency contraception, call 1-888-NOT-2-LATE for a listing of emergency contraception providers in your area.

Emergency Contraceptive Pills: Treatment initiated within 72 hours of unprotected intercourse reduces the risk of pregnancy by at least 75%.

REFERENCES

1. Abma JC, Chandra A, Mosher WD, Peterson LS, Piccinino LJ. Fertility, family planning, and women's health: new data from the 1995 National Survey of Family Growth. Vital Health Stat 1997;Series 23, Number 19.
2. Grossman L, Kowal D. Kids, drugs, and sex. Preventing trouble. Brandon VT: Clinical Psychology Publishing Co., 1987.
3. Hajnal J. European marriage patterns in perspective. In: Glass DV, Eversley DEC (eds). Population in history: essays in historical demography. London: Aldine, 1986:101.

4. Schuster MA, Bell RM, Kanouse DE. The sexual practices of adolescent virgins: genital sexual activities of high school students who have never had vaginal intercourse. Am J Publ Health 1996:86:1570-1576.
5. Sonenstein FL, Pleck JH, Ku L, Lindberg LD, Turner CF. Changes in sexual behavior and contraception among adolescent males: 1988 and 1995. Unpublished manuscript. Washington DC: The Urban Institute, 1997.

Coitus Interruptus (Withdrawal)

Deborah Kowal, MA, PA

- Coitus interruptus does not eliminate the risk of sexually transmitted infections (STIs): the pre-ejaculate can contain HIV-infected cells, and lesions or ulcers on the genitals can transmit pathogens.

- Although popularly considered an ineffective method, coitus interruptus provides efficacy similar to that of barrier methods of contraception.

Coitus interruptus, or the withdrawal method, was a natural response to the discovery that ejaculation into the vagina caused pregnancy. The method was probably widely practiced throughout history, playing a predominant role in fertility declines occurring prior to the advent of the pill. Although the 1995 National Survey of Family Growth (NSFG) reports the prevalence of coitus interruptus is only 2.9%,[1] figures this low are probably a marked underestimate.[10] For example, single women may rely on the method more frequently than do married women who are the survey subjects. In addition, respondents may not regard coitus interruptus as a legitimate method and therefore fail to note its use.

MECHANISM OF ACTION

Coitus interruptus prevents fertilization by preventing the contact between spermatozoa and the ovum. The couple may have penile-vaginal intercourse until ejaculation is impending, at which time the male partner withdraws his penis from the vagina and away from the external genitalia of the female partner. The man must rely on his own sensations to determine when he is about to ejaculate. The pre-ejaculate, which is usually released just prior to full ejaculation, goes unnoticed by both the man and the woman during the course of intercourse and so is not a sign that ejaculation is about to occur.

EFFECTIVENESS

Although coitus interruptus has often been criticized as an ineffective method, it probably confers a level of contraceptive protection similar to that provided by barrier methods. Effectiveness depends largely on the man's ability to withdraw prior to ejaculation. How effective the method would be if used consistently and correctly is highly uncertain. Our best guess is that the probability of pregnancy among perfect users would be about 4% in the initial year of use (Table 14-1). Among typical users, the probability of pregnancy would be about 19% during the first year of use. Men who are less experienced with using the method or who have difficulty in foretelling when ejaculation will occur could have a greater risk of failure.

Table 14-1 First-year probability of pregnancy* for withdrawal, chance, condoms, and pills

Method	% of Women Experiencing an Unintended Pregnancy Within the First Year of Use		% of Women Continuing at 1 year
	Typical Use (%)	Perfect Use (%)	
Chance	85	85	
Condoms (male)	14	3	61
Pill	5		71
Combined		0.1	
Progestin Only		0.5	
Withdrawal	19	4	—

*See Table 9-2 for first-year probability of pregnancy for all methods.

Emergency Contraceptive Pills: Treatment initiated within 72 hours after unprotected intercourse reduces the risk of pregnancy by at least 75%. (See Chapter 12 for more information.)

ADVANTAGES AND INDICATIONS

As a method of contraception, withdrawal has several distinct advantages. It costs nothing, requires no devices, involves no chemicals, and is available in any situation. Practicing coitus interruptus causes no medical side effects. Couples who cannot or do not wish to use other contraceptive methods and who can accept the potential for unintended pregnancy may find withdrawal an acceptable alternative. It is a back-up contraceptive that is always available.

DISADVANTAGES AND CAUTIONS

The method is unforgiving of incorrect or inconsistent use, leading to a probability of pregnancy in typical users that is substantially higher than the rates for hormonal methods or intrauterine devices (IUDs). One reason for contraceptive failure may be a lack of self-control demanded by the method. With impending orgasm, men (and women) experience a mild to extreme clouding of consciousness during which coital movement becomes involuntary.[6] The man may feel the urge to achieve deeper penetration at the time of impending orgasm and may not withdraw in sufficient time to avoid depositing semen in his partner's vagina or on her external genitalia. In addition, some men have difficulty foretelling when they will ejaculate. For some couples, interruption of the excitement or plateau phase of the sexual response cycle may diminish pleasure.

Surface lesions, such as those from herpes genitalis or human papilloma virus, may be actively infective. In one prospective study, the condom failed to protect some users against gonorrhea because they were exposed to infectious secretions before the condom was used.[2]

SPECIAL ISSUES

Studies of stable couples in which the man was infected with human immunodeficiency virus (HIV) and the women was not demonstrate that coitus interruptus may reduce the risk of infection somewhat better than unprotected intercourse with ejaculation. Coitus interruptus cut the HIV conversion rate of women by half in one study,[7] and by a larger percentage in another study.[2] Because these studies examined only stable heterosexual couples, the findings may not hold true for women with several HIV-infected partners.

Coitus interruptus probably decreases HIV exposure by reducing the amount of semen that enters the woman's vagina. However, the seminal fluid that emerges from the penis prior to ejaculation may contain some HIV.[4,5,8] Although coitus interruptus may be less likely to transmit HIV than intercourse with ejaculation, women have become infected while their partners consistently practiced withdrawal. Coitus interruptus has not been studied as a way to reduce HIV transmission from woman to man.

Some concern exists that the pre-ejaculate fluid may carry sperm into the vagina. In itself, the pre-ejaculate, a lubricating secretion produced by the Littre or Cowper's glands, contains no sperm. A study examining the pre-ejaculate for the presence of spermatozoa found none in the samples of 16 men.[5] However, a previous ejaculation may have left some sperm hidden within the folds of the urethral lining. In examinations of the pre-ejaculate in a small study,[8] the pre-ejaculate was free of spermatozoa in all of 11 HIV-seronegative men and 4 of 12 seropositive men. Although the eight samples containing spermatozoa revealed only small clumps of a few hundred sperm, these could possibly pose a risk of fertilization. In all likelihood, the spermatozoa left from a previous ejaculation could be washed out with the force of a normal urination. However, this remains unstudied.

INSTRUCTIONS FOR USING COITUS INTERRUPTUS

1. Before intercourse, the man should urinate and wipe off the tip of his penis to remove any sperm remaining from a previous ejaculation.
2. When he feels he is about to ejaculate, the man should withdraw his penis from his partner's vagina, making sure that ejaculation occurs away from his partner's genitalia.
3. Withdrawal is not a good contraceptive method under the following conditions:

   - The man cannot predictably withdraw prior to ejaculation.
   - The man intends to have repeated orgasms, which may cause the pre-ejaculate to contain spermatozoa.

4. Withdrawal does not effectively protect against sexually transmitted infections (STIs), including infection with the human immunodeficiency virus (HIV). Abstinence or use of latex or plastic condoms provide far better protection.
5. Withdrawal is a considerably better method of contraception than no method at all.
6. As a couple, learn what options are available for postcoital protection should any ejaculate come in contact with the vagina. Try to have a supply of contraceptive foam or some type of spermicide available in case of unintentional ejaculation in or near the woman's vagina. Despite the seeming optimism of this suggestion, it is probably too late to stop some sperm from swimming up into the uterus.

If you think you may have been exposed to a risk of pregnancy, contact your clinician about emergency contraception. (You can also call the toll-free number 1-888-NOT-2-LATE [1-888-668-6528] for a listing of emergency contraception providers near you.)

REFERENCES

1. Abma JC, Chandra A, Mosher WD, Peterson LS, Piccinino LJ. Fertility, family planning, and women's health: new data from the 1995 National Survey of Family Growth. Vital Health Stat 1997;Series 23, Number 19.
2. Darrow WW. Condom use and use-effectiveness in high-risk populations. Sex Transm Dis 1989;16:157-160.
3. DiVincenzi I (for the European Study Group). A longitudinal study of human immunodeficiency virus transmission by heterosexual partners. N Engl J Med 1994;331:341-346.
4. Howe JE, Minkoff HL, Duerr AC. Contraceptives and HIV. AIDS 1994;8: 861-871.
5. Ilaria G, Jacobs JL, Polsky B, Koll B, Baron P, MacLow C, Armstrong D, Schlegel PN. Detection of HIV-1 DNA sequences in pre-ejaculatory fluid [Letter]. Lancet 1992;340:1469.
6. Kinsey AC, Pomeroy WB, Martin CE, Gebhard PH. Sexual behavior in the human female. Philadelphia PA: W.B. Saunders Co., 1953.
7. Musicco M, Nicolosi A, Saracco A, Lazzarin A (for the Italian Study Group on HIV Heterosexual Transmission). The role of contraceptive practices in HIV sexual transmission from man to woman. In: Nicolosi A (ed). HIV epidemiology: models and methods. New York: Raven Press, Ltd., 1994:121-135.
8. Pudney J, Oneta M, Mayer K, Seage G, Anderson D. Pre-ejaculatory fluid as potential vector for sexual transmission of HIV-1 [Letter]. Lancet 1992;340:1470.
9. Robertson W. An illustrated history of contraception. Park Ridge NJ: Parthenon Publishing Group, 1990.
10. Rogow D, Horowitz S. Withdrawal: a review of the literature and an agenda for research. Stud Fam Plann 1995;26:140-153.

Fertility Awareness Methods

Victoria H. Jennings, PhD
Virginia M. Lamprecht, RN, BSN, MSPH
Deborah Kowal, MA, PA

- Fertility awareness helps couples understand how to become pregnant and how to avoid pregnancy.
- Regardless of what method of family planning they use, every woman and man will find value in learning fertility awareness.

- Fertility awareness-based methods are effective when they are used correctly. However, they are not effective when used incorrectly because, with incorrect use, unprotected intercourse takes place when the woman is potentially fertile.

Fertility awareness-based methods of family planning depend on identifying days each menstrual cycle when intercourse is most likely to result in a pregnancy. Accurate identification of potentially fertile days is a skill that requires a woman to apply knowledge about fertility to herself:

- Recognizing men's and women's reproductive potential
- Observing and interpreting the signs and patterns of fertility that occur during the menstrual cycle
- Understanding how to use this information to avoid or to achieve a pregnancy

To avoid pregnancy, couples can either abstain, use a barrier method, or practice withdrawal during the fertile time. If couples use barriers or withdrawal during the fertile time, they are using fertility awareness-combined methods (FACM). If they abstain during the fertile time, they are using natural family planning (NFP). The term *natural* does not imply other methods are unnatural, only that the natural signs and symptoms associated with the menstrual cycle are observed, recorded, and interpreted to identify the fertile time.

MECHANISM OF ACTION

MFertility awareness-based methods of family planning use one or more indicators to identify the beginning and end of the fertile time during the menstrual cycle. To identify the start of the fertile time, women can observe cervical secretions, monitor the change in the position and feel of the cervix, or use a calendar calculation. To mark the end of the fertile time, women can use those same indicators as well as monitor the change in their basal body (resting) temperature (BBT).

The fertility signs during the woman's menstrual cycles are caused by changes in circulating hormone levels, primarily estrogen and progesterone. The female hormone estrogen, produced in increasing amounts by the growing follicle inside the ovary, changes cervical secretions. After menses, the cervical secretions are typically scant or absent. As the growing follicle releases more estrogen, cervical secretions appear. Initially, these secretions are sticky, thick, and cloudy. As estrogen levels peak at midcycle, the secretions become clear, stretchy, and slippery. The last day on which clear, stretchy, slippery secretions are observed is known as the peak day. These cervical secretions facilitate sperm transport through the cervix into the upper female genital tract where fertilization takes place. The presence of cervical secretions indicates the woman is fertile.

Near midcycle, the pituitary gland releases luteinizing hormone (LH). LH triggers ovulation and causes the follicle to transform into the corpus luteum. The corpus luteum begins to produce the female hormone progesterone while continuing to produce estrogen. Progesterone counteracts the effects of estrogen and causes cervical secretions in the cervix to dry up and form a mucus *plug* that prevents sperm from traveling through the cervix. By acting on the hypothalamus, progesterone also causes the BBT to rise around the time of ovulation.

Estrogen and progesterone also cause changes in the position and feel of the cervix itself. As ovulation approaches, the opening to the cervix becomes softer and wider, and the cervix pulls up higher in the vaginal vault. After ovulation, the cervix returns to a lower position, and its opening closes and feels more firm. Because fluctuating levels of hormones make fertility signs imprecise markers of the beginning and end of the fertile time, women must abstain or use a barrier method for several days longer than the actual fertile time.

Women can use calendar calculations to identify the fertile time. These calculations were developed in the 1930s to estimate the days the woman is fertile in the current cycle based upon her past cycle lengths. The calculations take into account the lifespan of the gametes and allow for variation in the timing of ovulation from one cycle to the next. If a woman uses a calendar calculation, the interval of time identified as potentially fertile is also longer than the actual time she is fertile. This is because most calendar calculations take into account the lifespan of the gametes and fluctuations in past cycle length. The more a woman's cycle length varies, the longer is the interval identified as potentially fertile.

Recent research shows that the actual fertile time lasts for only about 6 days each cycle. The length of the fertile time is related to the lifespan of the gametes: sperm can live up to 5 days inside the female genital tract, and the egg lives less than 1 day.[14]

EFFECTIVENESS

Successful use of fertility awareness-based methods depends upon (1) the accuracy of the method in identifying the woman's actual fertile days, (2) a couple's ability to correctly identify the fertile time, and (3) their ability to follow the rules of the method they are using. Training is essential for couples using fertility awareness-based methods.

Unintended pregnancies among women practicing fertility awareness-based methods are primarily related to user error. A sizable but unknown portion of the unintended pregnancies is attributable to improper teaching and poor use of the methods.[9,13] Experts at the World Health Organization (WHO) suspect that among users of NFP, sexual risk taking during fertile days—that is, having intercourse even when they know the woman is fertile—accounts for more unintended pregnancy than does inability to accurately identify the fertile time.[15] There are few data on the effectiveness of FACM, but similar principles may apply (i.e., most pregnancies probably occur because couples do not use a barrier method or withdrawal consistently or correctly during the fertile time). In a German study, for example, couples frequently had unprotected intercourse even though they had planned to abstain or use barrier methods during the fertile time.[5] Most had unprotected intercourse at the beginning of the woman's fertile time when they believed "nothing will happen this time."

Among typical users of fertility awareness-based methods, about 25% experience an unintended pregnancy during the first year of use (Table 15-1). Among perfect users, the first-year probabilities of pregnancy are substantially lower, ranging from 1% to 9%. (See Chapter 31 on Contraceptive Efficacy.) Some fertility awareness-based methods are inherently more effective than others.

Calendar method. Estimates of pregnancy rates for calendar calculations vary widely, partially because the estimates come from flawed studies.[8] One relatively recent comparative study reported a first-year pregnancy rate of only 5%.[4] The probability of pregnancy during the first

Table 15-1 First-year probability of pregnancy* for women using periodic abstinence, chance, and pills

Method	% of Women Experiencing an Unintended Pregnancy Within the First Year of Use		% of Women Continuing Use at One Year
	Typical Use	Perfect Use	
Chance	85	85	
Periodic Abstinence	25		63
Calendar		9	
Ovulation Method		3	
Sympto-Thermal		2	
Post-Ovulation		1	
Pill	5		71
Progestin Only		0.5	
Combined		0.1	

*See Table 9-2 for first-year probability pregnancy rates for all methods.

Emergency Contraceptive Pills: Treatment initiated within 72 hours after unprotected intercourse reduces the risk of pregnancy by at least 75%. (See Chapter 12 for more information.)

year of typical use of the calendar method is estimated to be about 13% when only well-designed studies are considered.[8] However, better studies need to be conducted to estimate the effectiveness of calendar-based methods.

BBT. Methods based on using BBT alone limit unprotected intercourse to the postovulatory infertile time. Among perfect users, the first-year probability of pregnancy is only about 2%. During typical use, the probability of pregnancy is about 20%.[7,12]

Cervical mucus. The first-year probability of pregnancy for methods based on using only cervical secretions to identify the beginning and end of the fertile time is about 3% among perfect users and 20% among typical users when who abstain reliably during the fertile time.[13,16]

Symptothermal. The first-year probability of pregnancy among couples who use two or more fertility indicators (usually cervical secretions and BBT, but others such as cervix position or a calendar calculation may also be used as a "double check" to identify the start and end of the fertile time) are about 2% to 3% among perfect users and as high as 13% to 20% among typical users.

COST

Obtaining charts and a thermometer for monitoring a woman's menstrual cycles entails minimal cost. Some programs offer training without any charge to the client, while others charge a nominal fee. The amount of time required to learn how to use fertility awareness-based methods depends on the woman. A woman who is younger and normally cycling generally has fertility signs that are easier to interpret than does a woman who has just discontinued taking oral contraceptives, is breastfeeding, or is approaching menopause. The cost would vary accordingly.

If a couple uses a barrier method during the fertile time, there are additional costs for obtaining and resupplying the barrier and, as appropriate, spermicides. A woman who plans to use a diaphragm or cervical cap during the fertile time will need to visit her health care provider for a fitting and for obtaining the device.

ADVANTAGES AND INDICATIONS

Fertility awareness is important for all men and women, regardless of which family planning method they use or whether they choose to use family planning at all. Fertility awareness increases the users' knowledge of their reproductive potential and enhances self-reliance. Some couples like the active involvement required of the male partner, who learns about his own and the woman's fertility and then abstains from intercourse or uses a condom (or possibly withdrawal) when the woman is fertile. Fertility awareness information can be used for a number of purposes:

1. **To conceive.** Couples have intercourse on days the woman is potentially fertile. These include the days she observes cervical secretions or notes that her cervix is relatively soft and open. The chances of achieving a pregnancy are greatest when the woman observes clear, stretchy, slippery secretions. Conception is most likely to occur within 1 to 2 days of peak mucus (secretions).[14]

2. **To detect pregnancy.** A postovulatory temperature rise (see the section on "Basal Body Temperature Charting") sustained for 18 or more days is an excellent early indicator that pregnancy is under way.

3. **To avoid pregnancy.** For maximum effectiveness, couples should abstain from intercourse or use a barrier method or withdrawal during the entire fertile time.

4. **To detect impaired fertility.** Charting fertility signs costs relatively little and can aid in diagnosing and treating fertility problems due to infrequent or absent ovulation. Women who do not ovulate

tend to have a meandering BBT pattern throughout the cycle, rather than the typical biphasic pattern (lower in the first part and higher in the second).

5. **To relieve premenstrual syndrome.** See Chapter 4 on The Menstrual Cycle.

6. **To detect a need for medical attention.** Changes in cervical secretions, abdominal pain, and other signs may indicate the need for medical attention. (See Chapter 8 on Reproductive Tract Infections.)

D ISADVANTAGES AND CAUTIONS

Fertility awareness-based methods produce no serious side effects. Foremost, however, they offer no protection against sexually transmitted infections (STIs), including infection with the human immunodeficiency virus (HIV). Also, lack of the male partner's cooperation will be a distinct obstacle for women who wish to practice abstinence or use a condom or withdrawal during the fertile time. Certain conditions may make fertility awareness methods more difficult to use and require more extensive counseling and follow-up:

- Recent discontinuation of hormonal contraceptive methods
- Recent menarche
- Approaching menopause
- Recent childbirth
- Current use of breastfeeding

Fertility awareness-based methods are not recommended for women with the following difficulties:

- Inability to interpret their fertility signs correctly
- Persistent reproductive tract infections that affect the signs of fertility

S PECIAL ISSUES

SAFETY

Because unintended pregnancies among couples who use fertility awareness usually result from having intercourse at the beginning or end of the fertile time, concerns have been raised about the risk of birth defects or poor pregnancy outcomes due to aged ovum or sperm. A prospective study showed no significant differences in rates of spontaneous abortion, low birthweight, or preterm birth among NFP-using women who had unintended pregnancies compared with women who had intended pregnancies.[1,6] However, women with a history of spontaneous abortion had a greater chance of having a spontaneous abortion when conception occurred very early or late in the fertile time (23% versus 10% to 15%). Reassure your clients that NFP does not pose a threat to the health of mothers and their offspring. However, to reduce their risk of pregnancy loss, counsel women with a history of spontaneous abortion to time intercourse as close as possible to ovulation if they are attempting to conceive.

SEX SELECTION

A study of about 1,000 births showed no association between timing of conception and the sex ratio at birth.[2] These results do not substantiate claims that couples can select the sex of their child by timing intercourse.

PROVIDING FERTILITY AWARENESS-BASED METHODS

To use fertility awareness-based methods, couples must adjust their sexual behavior according to their fertility intentions. Users of NFP will need to abstain from vaginal intercourse for about 10 to 14 days of the woman's menstrual cycle, depending on her cycle length and the method used. Users of FACM will need to use a barrier method or withdrawal on fertile days. Successful use of these methods therefore requires a couple be able to communicate effectively with each other about sexual matters.

The National Health Service in Great Britain estimates it takes 4 to 6 hours to teach a woman fertility awareness skills, including charting fertility signs and identifying the fertile time.[3] This estimate includes initial classes and follow-up until the woman can use the method without assistance.

Couples need an instructor's help to learn how to observe, chart, and interpret the woman's fertility signs and patterns. Follow users until they are able to identify the fertile time accurately and time intercourse according to their pregnancy intentions. They will need to seek additional counseling if they have difficulty identifying the woman's fertile time or if the woman's circumstances change, such as when the she is postpartum, breastfeeding, or approaching menopause.

Many couples who use NFP engage in noncoital sexual activities. In a series of more than 400 couples, 84% of the men and 80% of the women achieved orgasm with some regularity during periods of abstinence.[10,11]

Knowing alternative means are available to achieve sexual satisfaction may help some NFP-using couples abstain more successfully during the fertile time.

Tell couples about the various fertility indicators they can use to identify the fertile time. Some couples choose to use only one indicator to identify the fertile time—usually the length of the woman's previous cycles or the changes in her cervical secretions. Other couples prefer to use more than one indicator—usually a combination of the woman's previous cycle lengths, changes in cervical secretions, changes in her BBT, or changes in the position and feel of her cervix. In general, using more than one indicator helps a couple more accurately identify the woman's fertile time.

INSTRUCTIONS FOR USING FERTILITY AWARENESS-BASED METHODS

CALENDAR CALCULATIONS

Worldwide, the calendar calculation method is the oldest and most widely practiced of the fertility awareness-based methods.[17] Calculation of the fertile time using the rules developed by in the 1930s by Ogino and Knaus are based upon three assumptions: (1) Ovulation occurs on day 14 (plus or minus 2 days) before the onset of the next menses; (2) sperm remain viable for about 5 days; and (3) the ovum survives for about 1 day. Typically, a set number of days (usually a number between 18 and 21) are subtracted from the shortest cycle length in the past 6 to 12 cycles to identify the beginning of the fertile time, and a set number of days (usually a number between 9 and 11) are subtracted from the longest cycle to identify the beginning and end of the fertile time. Past cycle lengths give an estimate of the days the fertile time will occur.

Use the following calendar calculation to determine the fertile time:

1. Keep a record your past menstrual cycle lengths.
2. Find the longest and shortest of your past menstrual cycles. (A cycle begins on day 1 of menstrual bleeding and continues until the day before the next bleeding begins.
3. Look on the fertile days chart (see Table 15-2) and apply the "minus 18, minus 11" rule:*

---

*Some women may prefer to use another set of numbers, such as "minus 20, minus 10," or "minus 21, minus 9." The "minus 18, minus 11" rule is used here as an example.

- Use the shortest cycle to find the first fertile day; subtract 18 days from the length of your shortest cycle.
- Use the longest cycle to find the last fertile day; subtract 11 days from the length of your longest cycle.

For example, if your shortest cycle has been 27 days, the first fertile day will be day 9. If your longest cycle has been 30 days, the last fertile day will be day 19.

4. Next find the dates of the first and last fertile days for the current menstrual cycle. For example, if menses starts September 6 and the chart says the first fertile day will be day 9, then the first fertile day will be September 14. If the last fertile day will be day 19, then the last fertile day will be September 24.
5. **For conception**. Have intercourse during the fertile time.
6. **For contraception**. Abstain from sexual intercourse or use a barrier method (such as condoms, spermicides, or a diaphragm) during the fertile time.

Table 15-2 How to calculate your fertile period

If Your Shortest Cycle Has Been (# of Days)	Your First Fertile (Unsafe) Day is	If Your Longest Cycle Has Been (# of Days)	Your Last Fertile (Unsafe) Day is
21*	3rd	21*	10th Day
22	4th	22	11th
23	5th	23	12th
24	6th	24	13th
25	7th	25	14th
26	8th	26	15th
27	9th	27	16th
28	10th	28	17th
29	11th	29	18th
30	12th	30	19th
31	13th	31	20th
32	14th	32	21st
33	15th	33	22nd
34	16th	34	23rd
35	17th	35	24th

*Day 1 = First day of menstrual bleeding

Basal Body (Resting) Temperature (BBT)

The BBT is the body temperature of a healthy person on awakening. The BBT rises under the influence of progesterone. Most ovulatory cycles demonstrate a biphasic BBT pattern: lower in the first part of the cycle, rising to a higher level beginning around the time of ovulation, and remaining at the higher level for the rest of the cycle. By taking her temperature when she first wakes in the morning and recording her temperature on a chart each day of her menstrual cycle, a woman can retrospectively identify when she may have ovulated. However, because the BBT does not give adequate advance warning of ovulation, it cannot be used to identify the start of the fertile time. Therefore, it is of limited use for a woman who wants to achieve pregnancy.

Figure 15-1 illustrates the BBT variations during a model menstrual cycle of 28 days. In reality, the BBT may rise more suddenly or more gradually. The typical pattern of a lower temperature before ovulation, followed by a higher temperature immediately before, during, and after ovulation, can be disrupted by illness, stress, travel, or interrupted sleep.

Use the BBT to determine the postovulatory infertile time:

1. Take your BBT every morning at the same time before getting out of bed (after at least 3 hours of sleep). A special calibrated thermometer makes temperature reading easier. Take the BBT orally, rectally, or vaginally, but take it at the same site each day so changes in BBT can be detected accurately.

2. Record your BBT readings daily on a special NFP chart (Figure 15-1). Connect the dots for each day so a line connects dots from day 2 to day 3, and so on.

3. Your temperature will probably rise at least $0.4°$ F around the time of ovulation and remain elevated until the next menses begins.

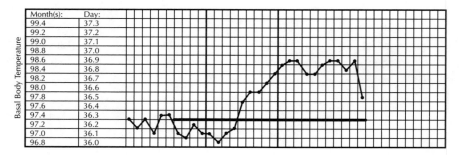

Figure 15-1 Basal body temperature variations during a model menstrual cycle

Your actual temperature and maximum temperature are not important, just the rise over the baseline (preovulatory) temperatures.

4. If you have 3 days of continuous temperature rise following 6 lower temperatures, you have ovulated and your postovulatory infertile time has begun. To see the baseline and rise clearly on the chart, draw a line just above (0.1 degree line) the lower (preovulatory) temperatures. When you record 3 continuous temperatures above this line and the last temperature is 0.4 degrees higher than this line, your postovulatory infertile time has begun.

5. If you cannot detect a sustained rise in BBT, you may not have ovulated in that cycle. A true postovulatory BBT rise usually persists 10 days or longer.

6. Some women notice a temperature drop about 12 to 24 hours before it begins to rise after ovulation, whereas others have no drop in temperature at all. A drop in your BBT probably means ovulation will occur the next day.

7. **For conception**. It is not possible to predict fertile days using BBT. By the time the rise is detected, you are probably in the infertile phase of your menstrual cycle and have missed the opportunity to become pregnant. A biphasic temperature pattern, however, can let you know you are probably normally ovulating.

8. **For contraception**. Because ovulation may occur as early as day 7 of the menstrual cycle, assume you may be fertile from just after menses (if your cycles are no less than 25 days in length) until your temperature has remained elevated for at least 3 consecutive days. The most effective way to use BBT charting when avoiding pregnancy is to avoid intercourse or use a barrier method of contraception all through the first part of your cycle, until the temperature rise indicates you have ovulated.

CERVICAL SECRETIONS

Cervical mucus changes signal the beginning and end of the fertile time, even among those who have irregular cycles. Observe your cervical secretions by "the look, the touch, and the feel":

- *Look* at the secretions on your panties, fingers, or toilet paper to determine its color and consistency.
- *Touch* the secretions to determine their stretch and slipperiness.
- *Feel* how wet the sensation is at your vulva when you are walking.

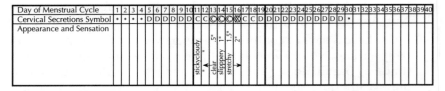

Figure 15-2 Cervical secretion variations during a model menstrual cycle

When they first appear, the secretions may be scant but sticky and thick with a cloudy or whitish color. Highly fertile secretions are abundant, clear, stretchy, wet, and slippery.

Ovulation most likely occurs within 1 day before, during, or 1 day after the last day of abundant, clear, stretchy, slippery cervical secretions. When you are observing your cervical secretions, do not douche, because it can wash out the secretions, making it very difficult to notice changes.

Use your cervical secretions to identify the beginning and end of the fertile time:

1. Observe your cervical secretions every day, beginning the day after your menstrual bleeding has stopped, and record them daily on a special chart (Figure 15-2). To help you avoid confusing cervical secretions with semen and normal sexual lubrication, some counselors advise complete sexual abstinence throughout the first cycle. Alternatively, you can use a condom.

2. Check secretions each time before and after you urinate by wiping (front to back) with tissue paper. Note and record the color and appearance (yellow, white, clear, or cloudy) and consistency (thick, sticky, or stretchy) of the secretions, and how they feel (dry, wet, or slippery). Record how much they stretch when pulled between your thumb and index finger. Also, note and chart the sensations of dryness, moistness, or wetness at your vulva. Always record the "most fertile" observations you see during the day.

3. Note the typical pattern in the cervical secretions:

   - *During menstruation*, blood masks any other sensations of wetness or secretions.
   - *After the menstruation*, the vagina may feel moist a few days, but not distinctly wet. There usually are no observable secretions. (Some women do not have any of these dry days, especially if they have very short cycles.)
   - *Next* may come secretions that are thick, cloudy, whitish or yellowish, and sticky. The vagina still does not feel distinctly

wet. This can last for several days. Consider these days as fertile.

- *As ovulation nears*, your secretions usually become more abundant, and you will have an increasingly wet sensation. Secretions become clear and slippery and can stretch 2 to 3 or more inches between the thumb and forefinger. The peak or last day of wetness and abundant, clear, slippery secretions is assumed to be about the time of ovulation.
- *After ovulation*, the secretions become thick, cloudy, and sticky or disappear until the time of the next menstrual period.

4. Douching, vaginal infection, semen, foam, diaphragm jelly, lubricants, medications, and even the normal lubrication of sexual arousal may interfere with the ability to notice a clear-cut secretion pattern.

5. **For conception**. Have intercourse when cervical secretions are present. The probability of conception is greatest when the secretions are abundant, clear, stretchy, and slippery.

6. **For contraception**. Check for secretions as soon as your menses are complete. (Some counselors recommend avoiding intercourse or using a barrier method during menses because it is difficult to detect secretions when they are mixed with menstrual blood.) You can have sexual intercourse on preovulatory days if no secretions are present. (Some counselors recommend abstaining the next day and night following intercourse to allow time for bodily fluids to drain out your body so you will not confuse semen and arousal fluids with cervical secretions. The following day, check your cervical secretions.) The fertile time begins when cervical secretions are first observed until 4 days past the peak day (the last day of clear, stretchy, slippery secretions).

7. Most women need help in the first few cycles to interpret their cervical secretion patterns and charts to determine the fertile time.

SYMPTOTHERMAL METHOD

Some couples prefer to observe more than one indicator of the woman's fertility. Most couples who use a combined or *symptothermal* approach use cervical secretions and BBT to identify the fertile time. Some women also check the position and feel of their cervix or use a calendar calculation as a "double-check" against cervical secretions to identify the start and end of the fertile time. Other minor indicators include noting ovulatory pain (mittelschmerz) or breast tenderness. Ovulatory pain refers to

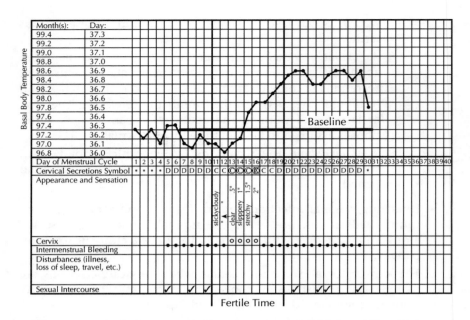

Figure 15-3 Symptothermal variations during a model menstrual cycle

lower abdominal pain or cramping some women feel around the time of ovulation. Couples using multiple indicators have a better chance of correctly identifying the start and end of the fertile time. See Figure 15-3 for an example of a chart completed by a woman using BBT, cervical secretions, cervical position and feel, and other minor indicators.

HOME TEST KITS FOR OVULATION PREDICTION AND DETECTION

Most research on ovulation prediction and detection devices has focused on helping women with fertility problems. Most ovulation prediction home tests kits measure LH, which can be detected the day before or the day of ovulation. Time intercourse to coincide with these days (or earlier in the fertile time if she is using a fertility awareness-based method).

A new test kit to help women avoid pregnancy is being developed by Unipath, Ltd. The test uses urinary metabolites and a computer chip to identify the beginning and end of the fertile time. Clinical trials are under way in Europe; U.S. trials are scheduled to begin.

REFERENCES

1. Bitto A. The effect of planning on pregnancy outcome: a prospective multi-center study of natural family planning users. DRPH thesis. Baltimore MD: The Johns Hopkins University School of Hygiene and Public Health, 1994.
2. Bitto A, Gray RH, Simpson JL, Queenan JT, Kambic RT, Perez A, Mena P, Barbato M, Jennings V. Effects of cycle length, timing of conception and planning status on sex ratio in natural family planning users. Washington DC: Georgetown University, 1996. Cooperative agreement no. DPE-3040-00-5064-00. Sponsored by the United States Agency for International Development.
3. Clubb EM, Pyper CM, Knight J. A pilot study on teaching natural family planning in general practice. Natural family planning: current knowledge and new strategies for the 1990s, Part II 1992: 130-132.
4. Dicker D, Wachsman T, Feldbergt D. The vaginal contraceptive diaphragm and the condom: a reevaluation and comparison of two barrier methods with the rhythm method. Contraception 1989;40:497-503.
5. Frank-Herrmann P, Freundl G, Baur S, Bremme M, Doring GK, Godehardt EAJ, Sottong U. Effectiveness and acceptability of the symptothermal method of natural family planning in Germany. Am J Obstet Gynecol 1991;165: 2052-2054.
6. Gray RH, Simpson JL, Kambit RT, Queenan JT, Mena P, Perez A, Barbato M. Timing of conception and the risk of spontaneous abortion among pregnancies occurring during use of natural family planning. Am J Obstet Gynecol 1995;172:1567-1572.
7. Hartzen P. Effectiveness of the temperature rhythm system of contraception. Fertil Steril 1967;18:694-706.
8. Kambic RT, Lamprecht V. Calendar rhythm efficacy: a review. Adv Contracept 1996;12:123-128.
9. Labbok MH, Klaus H, Barker D. Factors related to ovulation method efficacy in three programs: Bangladesh, Kenya, and Korea. Contraception 1988;37:577-589.
10. Marshall J, Rowe B. The effect of personal factors on the use of basal body temperature method of regulating births. Fertil Steril 1972;23:417-421.
11. Marshall J, Rowe B. Psychological aspects of the basal body temperature method of regulating births. Fertil Steril 1970;21:14-19.
12. Marshall J. A field trial of the basal body temperature method of regulating births. Lancet 1968;316:8-10.
13. Trussell J, Grummer-Strawn L. Contraceptive failure of the ovulation method of periodic abstinence. Fam Plann Perspect 1990;22:65-75.
14. Wilcox AJ, Weinberg CR, Baird DD. Timing of sexual intercourse in relation to ovulation. N Engl J Med 1995;333:1517-1521.
15. World Health Organization. A prospective multicentre trial of the ovulation method of natural family planning. V. Psychosexual aspects. Fertil Steril 1987;47:765-772.
16. World Health Organization. A prospective multicentre trial of the ovulation method of natural family planning. II. The effectiveness phase. Fertil Steril 1981;36:591-598.
17. World Health Organization. Fertility awareness methods: report on a WHO workshop, August 26-29, 1986, in Jablonna, Poland.

Male Condoms

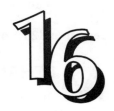

D. Lee Warner, MPH
Robert A. Hatcher, MD, MPH

- When used consistently and correctly, latex or plastic male and female condoms with or without spermicide can prevent pregnancy and many sexually transmitted infections (STIs) including infection with the human immunodeficiency virus (HIV).
- Condoms are inexpensive, available without a prescription, and easy to use.

- By preventing STIs and their long-term sequelae, condoms help protect future fertility.
- Clients at risk for an STI should be encouraged to wear condoms even if they already rely on oral contraceptives, Norplant, Depo Provera, intrauterine devices (IUDs), fertility awareness, or sterilization (including hysterectomy) for contraception.

The condom remains the most widely available and popular male contraceptive method in the United States. According to the 1995 National Survey of Family Growth (NSFG), more than 9 million reproductive-age women in the United States reported using condoms for contraception or protection from sexually transmissible infections (STIs).[1] During the last decade, condom use has become an important part of public health efforts to prevent new cases of infection with human immunodeficiency virus (HIV) as well as other other STIs. In the year following the 1986 U.S. Surgeon General's report, which stated that latex condoms should be used to prevent AIDS, condom sales, the best indicator of condom use, rose by 20%.[60] By the early 1990s, consumers purchased more than 450 million condoms per year.[21] Between 1988 and 1995, the percentage of reproductive-age women who reported using male condoms for contraception rose from 13% to 19%, with marked increases reported by women age 20 to 29. Among adolescent women age 15 to 19, condom use rose slightly from 27% to 30%.

The public's awareness and perception of the condom have also improved. Most Americans correctly believe latex condoms can be effective at preventing sexually transmitted HIV infection.[76] Moreover, 75% of men agree that using a condom "shows you are a caring person," while 32% agree that using a condom "makes sex last longer." Nevertheless, about 25% of men are still embarrassed to buy condoms.[39]

MECHANISM OF ACTION

The male condom, a thin sheath placed over the glans and shaft of the penis, acts as a physical barrier. The condom prevents pregnancy by blocking the passage of semen and is effective only when used from "start to finish" during every act of intercourse. Among barrier contraceptive methods, the condom provides the most effective protection of the genital tract and is thus the most effective method for preventing STIs.[84]

A sheath worn over the penis can be traced as far back as 1350 B.C., when Egyptian men wore decorative covers for their penises. In 1564 A.D., Fallopius first described linen sheaths used to protect against syphilis.[90] Protective sheaths made from dried animal intestines followed in the 18th century, when they were first given the name "condom," presumably after inventor Colonel Cundum.[90] With the advent of vulcanized rubber in 1843 came the mass production of synthetic condoms.[61] In the 1990s, manufacturers began to use plastics (e.g., polyurethane).

CONDOM OPTIONS

Until recently, most commercially available condoms were manufactured from latex ("rubber" condoms), while about 5%[61] were made from the intestinal caecum of lambs ("natural skin," "natural membrane," or "lambskin" condoms).[20] Natural membrane condoms may not offer the same level of protection against STIs as latex condoms, however. Unlike latex condoms, natural membrane condoms contain small pores that may permit passage of viruses, including hepatitis B virus, herpes simplex virus, and HIV,[12] and are recommended for contraceptive use only.

New condoms manufactured from polyurethane are thinner and stronger than those manufactured from latex, provide a less constricting fit, are more resistant to deterioration, and may enhance sensitivity. Unlike latex condoms, condoms made of polyurethane are compatible with oil-based lubricants.[70] Plastic condoms have not been well studied for protection against STIs but are believed to provide protection similar to that of latex condoms. Current studies of their effectiveness are under way. As of mid-1997, two polyurethane condoms have been approved by the U.S. Food and Drug Administration (FDA) for latex-sensitive persons and are commercially available in the United States: the Avanti condom (Durex

Table 16-1 Characteristics of latex, natural membrane, and plastic condoms

Type	Latex	Natural membrane	Plastic
Brand Names	Numerous	Fourex, Naturalamb	Avanti, Reality
Material	Natural rubber	Lamb caecum	Polyurethane*
Lubricant Use	Water-based only	Any	Any
Cost	Low	Moderate	Moderate/high
Prevention of Pregnancy	Yes	Yes	Yes
Prevention of STIs and HIV	Yes	No	Likely

Source: Modified from Contraceptive Technology Update (March, 1995).

* Non-polyurethane plastic condoms may become available soon.

Consumer Products) and the Reality female condom (The Female Health Company). (A detailed discussion of the female condom can be found in Chapter 18 on Vaginal Barriers.) Two new polyurethane condoms with a loose fit are also being developed. Acceptability studies have been encouraging for both condoms.[27] Plastic condoms manufactured from materials other than polyurethane will soon be marketed. The Tactylon condom (Sensicon Corporation), manufactured from a plastic material used in non-allergenic examination gloves,[88] recently received clearance from the FDA and may be available in 1998.[41] See Table 16-1 for a comparison of condom types.

Spermicidal condoms

Some condoms are lubricated with a small amount of nonoxynol-9, ranging in concentration from 1% to 12%.[20] Although spermicidally lubricated condoms have been available in the United States since 1983, there is no evidence that these condoms are more effective than condoms without spermicide.[13] Use of a separate vaginal spermicide is recommended as a back-up method superior to spermicide applied to the surface of the condom or use of a spermicidal condom. Vaginally applied spermicide guarantees its presence in the vaginal area should the condom break or fall off. Although sperm are quickly inactivated when injected into a spermicidally lubricated condom in vitro,[6] the dose of active ingredient delivered by a spermicidal condom is much less than that provided by a separate spermicide such as vaginal cream, foam, or suppository.

Moreover, the spermicide in latex condoms may cause potentially allergenic proteins to leach out of the latex.[85] High-frequency use of spermicides may cause genital ulceration and irritation, thereby facilitating transmission of STIs,[53] although the exact frequency and dose resulting in genital ulceration is not known. One study found that use of spermicide-coated condoms significantly increased the risk of urinary tract infections among young women.[29] (See Chapter 17 on Vaginal Spermicides.)

EFFECTIVENESS (AGAINST PREGNANCY)

Method failure of the male condom resulting in unintended pregnancy is uncommon, estimated to occur in about 3% of couples using condoms consistently and correctly during the first year of use (Table 16-2). A summary of studies of contraceptive failure for the male condom, as well as a detailed discussion of the estimates used to derive these rates, can be found in Chapter 31.

The 3% probability of pregnancy during a year of perfect use of the male condom does not mean that 3 of every 100 condoms used will result in unintended pregnancy. What this means is that only 3 of 100 couples who use condoms perfectly for 1 year will experience an unintended pregnancy. If each couple had intercourse at the average coital frequency for U.S. women of 83 acts per year,[87] then the 100 couples would have had intercourse a combined total of 8,300 times over the course of a year. Three pregnancies resulting from 8,300 acts of condom

Table 16-2 First year probability of pregnancy* for couples using condoms, withdrawal, diaphragm, and pill

Method	% of Women Experiencing an Unintended Pregnancy Within the First Year of Use		% of Women Continuing Use at One Year
	Typical Use	Perfect Use	
Withdrawal	19	4	
Diaphragm	20	6	56
Condom			
Male	14	3	61
Female (Reality)	21	5	56
Pill	5		71
Progestin Only		0.5	
Combined		0.1	

*See Table 9-2 for first-year probability pregnancy of all methods.

Emergency Contraceptive Pills: Treatment initiated within 72 hours after unprotected intercourse reduces the risk of pregnancy by at least 75%. (See Chapter 12 for more information.)

use (or about one pregnancy per 2,800 acts of intercourse) is a remarkably low pregnancy rate (0.04%) when calculated on a per-condom basis.

However, couples vary widely in their ability to use condoms consistently and correctly. Among those using condoms for contraception, about 14% will experience an unintended pregnancy during the first year of typical use. The marked difference between the condom's probability of pregnancy during typical use and during perfect use generally reflects errors in use, most notably the failure of couples to use condoms during every act of sexual intercourse. Several user behaviors, described later, likely contribute to the risk of unintended pregnancy and the transmission of infection despite condom use. Detailed instructions for proper condom use are provided at the end of this chapter.

CONDOM BREAKAGE

Although users often fear the condom will break or fall off during use,[20,39,51,54,89,92] studies indicate these events rarely occur during proper use. A recent prospective study of female sex workers in Nevada brothels, where condom use is required by law, demonstrated high condom proficiency. Of 353 condoms used by the sex workers during the study, none broke and none fell off during intercourse, and only 2 (0.6%) slipped off during withdrawal.[2] In prospective studies, reported breakage rates during vaginal intercourse range from 0% to 6.7%, although most studies report that condoms break less than 2% of the time during intercourse or withdrawal (Table 16-3). Not all condom breaks are equally risky. As many as 24% to 65% occur before intercourse [81,83,88,89] and pose no biological risk of pregnancy or infection if a new condom is used for intercourse.[82] Thus, *advise users to have several condoms available in case a condom is torn or put on incorrectly, intercourse is postponed until later, or repeated intercourse is desired.*

Little research has been conducted on condom breakage during anal intercourse. Breakage rates during anal sex among gay men in four prospective studies range from 0.5% to 12%, with rates less than 2% in three of the studies.[7,37,67,97] Rates from retrospective studies range more widely, from 1% to 8%.[18,20,36,68,86] Although condoms designed for anal intercourse are now marketed in Europe, these have not been well studied and are not available in the United States.[78]

CONDOM SLIPPAGE

Condoms fall off the penis in 0.6% to 5.4% of acts of vaginal intercourse and may slip down the penis without falling off in 3.4% to 13.1% of acts of vaginal intercourse—suggesting that slippage may be more common than breakage (Table 16-3). In three prospective studies of condom use

Table 16-3 Prospective studies of condom breakage and slippage

| Population | No. | Study Period (Total Condoms) | Type of Sex | Breakage Rate (%) | | | Slippage Rate (%) | | |
				Clinical	Nonclinical	Total	Complete	Partial	Undefined
Brothel prostitutes[2] (Nevada)	41	3 days (353)	Vaginal	0.0	0.0	0.0	0.6	3.4–4.3	…
Monogamous couples[103] (US)[cm]	92	… (4,632)	Vaginal	0.3[h]	0.1	0.4[h]	0.6	…	…
Female and male prostitutes[67] (Sidney)	4 30	4 mo (605) 4 mo (664)	Vaginal Anal	0.5 0.5	…	…	…	…	…
Clinical research participants[54] (US)	49	… (147)	Vaginal	0.7[h]	…	…	5.4	2.0	…
Gay male recruits[37] (London)[k]	86	… (772)	Anal	1.8% combined slippage and breakage rate				9.5–16.6	…
Family planning recruits[88] (Atlanta) [b,c]	49	21 days (478)	Vaginal	1.3[h]	2.4	3.7[h]	0.6	9.5–16.6	…
Family planning recruits[89] (Atlanta)[c,d]	68	16 days (405)	Vaginal	1.7[h]	0.7	2.4[h]	…	…	13.1
Gay men[7] (San Francisco)	1,773	18 mo (84,202)	Anal	1.8% combined slippage and breakage rate					
Male STI clinic attendees[68] (Sidney)	36	3 mo (529)	Vaginal and anal	1.9	0.9	2.8	…	…	3.4

(continued)

Table 16-3 Prospective studies of condom breakage and slippage *(cont.)*

Population	No.	Study Period (Total Condoms)	Type of Sex	Breakage Rate (%)			Slippage Rate (%)		
				Clinical	Nonclinical	Total	Complete	Partial	Undefined
Monogamous couples[101] (Southern California)[c]	759	...(3,717)	Vaginal	2.2[h]	0.8	3.0[h]	2.9	...	...
Monogamous couples (N. Carolina)[c,e]	268	...(1,072)	Vaginal	2.4[f]	0.8	3.3[f]	5.4	...	...
Monogamous couples (N. Carolina)[f]	262	4 mo (4,589)	Vaginal	...	...	3.5–18.6	...	...	...
Monogamous couples (N. Carolina)[c]	177	4 mo (1,947)	Vaginal	3.7[i]	1.6	5.3[i]	...	...	3.5
Monogamous couples[102] (Southern California)[c]	348	...(2,059)	Vaginal	4.2[h]	0.2	4.3[h]	2.2	...	...
Couples recruited by mail (N. Carolina)	188	...(752)	Vaginal	...	...	4.1	...	...	...
Female prostitutes and male and female hospital staff (Denmark)	40	...(385)	Vaginal	...	...	5.0	...	...	...
Male and female family planning clinic clients (New Zealand)[c-g]	540	1 mo (3,685)	Vaginal	...	...	5.3	...	...	5.1

(continued)

Table 16-3 Prospective studies of condom breakage and slippage *(cont.)*

Population	No.	Study Period (Total Condoms)	Type of Sex	Breakage Rate (%)			Slippage Rate (%)		
				Clinical	Nonclinical	Total	Complete	Partial	Undefined
Local recruits (N. Carolina)	45	6 wk (358)	Vaginal	...	...	6.7	...	...	...
Gay men[97] (Netherlands)[l]	17	...(200)	Anal	...	...	12.0	...	...	15.0

Source: Modified from Albert et al. (1995) with permission.

Note: Clinical breakage refers to breakage occurring during either intercourse or withdrawal; nonclinical breakage refers to breakage occurring before intercourse.
[b]Rates of condoms slipping down without falling off were 9.5% during intercourse and 16.6% during withdrawal.
[c]In these studies, events of breakage and slippage were unambiguously not double counted; in other studies, some condoms that broke may have also slipped.
[d]Slippage rate recalculated from original article and reflects condoms that fell off or slipped down during intercourse or withdrawal.
[e]Among new condoms used with either no additional lubricant or water-based lubricant. Rates recalculated from original article.
[f]Breakage rates ranged from 3.5% for a new lot to 18.6% for an 81-month-old lot.
[g]In addition, 6 condoms broke and 4 condoms slipped in a total of 19 episodes of anal intercourse when condoms were used.
[h]Excludes breakage when removing the condom from the penis after withdrawal.
[i]Includes breakage when removing the condom from the penis after withdrawal.
[j]In addition, no condoms broke or fell off in 19 episodes of fellatio when condoms were used.
[k]Participants used anal-qualified condoms 30% thicker than standard condoms.
[l]Seven different combinations of condoms and lubricants assessed. Stiffest condoms did not break or slip off.
[m]In addition, no condoms broke when condoms were used for anal intercourse.

for anal intercourse, rates of slippage ranged from 2% to 15%.[6,37,97] Retrospective studies suggest slippage occurs in about 5% of condom uses during anal intercourse.[36,68] Unfortunately, many studies do not distinguish between partial and complete slippage, which pose different risks for pregnancy and STIs. The degree to which partial or complete slippage during vaginal or anal intercourse increase the risk of pregnancy or STIs due to semen leakage or exposure to genital lesions is unknown and warrants further study.

CONDOM TESTING

Since 1976, condoms have been regulated as medical devices by the U.S. Food and Drug Administration (FDA). Manufacturers test each lot of condoms according to voluntary performance standards established by the American Society for Testing and Materials (ASTM) and recommended by the FDA.[5] As new technologies and testing procedures develop, these standards undergo periodic review.[64]

Every condom manufactured in the United States is tested electronically for holes and weak spots before it is released for sale.[15,21] Samples of condoms from each batch that pass electronic testing then undergo a series of standardized laboratory tests for leaks and breakage. If the sample condoms fail these tests, the entire batch is destroyed and not permitted for sale.[15] Imported condoms are required to pass the same tests as domestic condoms and should be equally safe. In the water leakage test, randomly selected condoms are filled with 300 ml of water and checked for holes. Moisture detected on the outside of the condom is considered a failed test. Batches with more than 4 failed tests per 1,000 sampled condoms are not permitted for sale in the United States. In the air-burst test adopted by ASTM in 1994, samples of condoms are inflated until they burst; the volume at burst point is documented. The tensile test was dropped in 1996 because of its poor ability to predict deterioration or breakage during actual use.

COST

The condom is among the most inexpensive and cost-effective contraceptives, especially considering the added protection against STIs and HIV. U.S. consumers pay about 50 cents per condom,[56] and few men complain that condoms cost too much.[39] In a recent *Consumer Reports* survey, high-quality latex condoms ranged in price from $0.31 to $1.08 per unit.[21] There is no evidence suggesting that less expensive condoms are of lower quality. Based on the average coital frequency for U.S. women,[87] the cost to a couple using condoms with every act of intercourse amounts to about

$40 annually. Non-profit facilities may purchase condoms in bulk at reduced cost to encourage distribution to family planning clients (often for 5 cents to 10 cents per condom). Both natural skin condoms and plastic condoms are more expensive than latex condoms. Natural membrane condoms are expensive to manufacture because each lamb caecum produces only one condom.[61] The average retail cost for the only polyurethane male condom available is about $1.75.[21]

A DVANTAGES AND INDICATIONS

Condom use offers several noncontraceptive benefits. Emphasize that the condom can be fun for both partners when it is made a part of sexual intercourse.

1. **Protection against STIs**. When used consistently and correctly, condoms effectively reduce the risk of STIs including HIV.

2. **Prevention of infertility**. By preventing STIs and their long-term sequelae, condoms protect fertility. (See Chapter 27 on Impaired Fertility.)

3. **Accessibility**. Usage does not require medical examination, prescription, or fitting. Condoms can be obtained from many sources, including drug stores, grocery stores, family planning clinics, vending machines, gas stations, bars, and mail-order services.

4. **Low cost.** Condoms are available at low cost in both the private and public sectors. Users can often obtain condoms for free from some publicly funded programs.

5. **Male participation**. Condom use allows men to participate actively in contraception and infection protection.

6. **Erection enhancement**. Condoms can help men maintain their erections longer and prevent premature ejaculation.

7. **Hygiene**. Postcoital leakage of semen from the vagina or anus, a bothersome aftermath for some persons, is avoided by using condoms.

8. **Prevention of sperm allergy**. Women are occasionally allergic to the sperm or semen of their partner to the extent that they have urticarial and anaphylactic reactions. In some infertile couples, the woman's body produces antibodies to her partner's sperm; use of condoms for 3 to 6 months may prevent the release of sperm antigens into the vagina.

9. **Proof of protection**. Condoms provide immediate, visible proof of effectiveness when ejaculate is contained within the condom.

10. **Personal concerns**. Men or women who do not wish to have the penis in direct contact with the mouth, vagina, or anus may find that condom use makes intercourse more pleasurable.

11. **Portability**. Condoms can be easily and discretely carried by men or women.

12. **Minimal side effects**. Because condoms are non-hormonal, they cause few medical problems among users. The most frequent side effect is most likely latex sensitivity; men or women with this condition can be directed to use plastic condoms.

PROTECTION AGAINST STIs AND HIV

When used consistently and correctly, latex or plastic condoms with or without spermicide provide highly effective protection against bacterial and viral STIs. When placed on the penis before any genital contact, the condom prevents contact with semen; genital lesions on the shaft of the penis; and penile, vaginal, or anal discharges. In vitro laboratory studies show latex condoms provide a highly effective mechanical barrier to bacterial and viral STIs[12] including HIV.[9,12,57] In vivo, condoms have proven to be highly effective against a wide variety of STIs such as gonorrhea, ureaplasma infection, herpes simplex virus, and HIV infection.[11,12,13,28,93,96] Of 10 cohort studies to date evaluating condom use and HIV infection among heterosexual couples, all showed a protective effect for the consistent use of condoms (Figure 16-1).[10]

In one European study,[25] no uninfected partners in the 124 serodiscordant couples who used condoms consistently became infected. Conversely, among 121 couples who reported using condoms inconsistently, 12 (10%) of uninfected partners seroconverted. In a second European study,[74] among 171 serodiscordant couples who used condoms with every act of intercourse, 3 (2%) uninfected partners became infected with HIV. In contrast, 16 uninfected partners (12%) of 134 discordant couples who used condoms inconsistently or not at all became infected. A third study in Haiti[24] found that only 1 (2%) of 42 couples using condoms consistently became infected in contrast to 19 (14%) of 135 couples who used condoms inconsistently. A troubling finding in each study was the high percentage of serodiscordant couples who used condoms inconsistently despite a known risk of exposure to HIV.

D ISADVANTAGES AND CAUTIONS

Male condom use does have disadvantages that may cause men and women to use them inconsistently or not at all. Many of the barriers to condom use can likely be overcome with practice and experience. Encour-

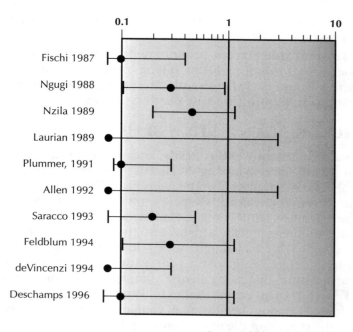

**Relative Risk (log scale) and
95% Confidence Interval**

Source: Feldblum et al., (1995).

Figure 16-1 Condom use and HIV infection in heterosexuals, 10 studies

age men or women to try different brands of condoms and lubricants until they find one most suitable for them.

1. **Sensitivity**. Many men and their partners complain that condoms reduce sensitivity. Men can try different types of condoms and add water-based lubricant to the outside of the condom (or even a few drops to the inside of the condom) to increase sensation.

2. **Spontaneity**. Some men and their partners dislike interrupting foreplay to put on the condom. One solution may be for the partner to put the condom on the penis as part of foreplay.

3. **Problems with erection**. Some men cannot consistently maintain an erection during condom use, so condom use becomes impossible. To help overcome this obstacle, couples may integrate condom use into foreplay. Female condom use may be appropriate in some cases.

4. **Embarrassment**. Some men and women may be embarrassed to obtain condoms from a drug-store shelf or a health clinic. Others

may be embarrassed to suggest or initiate using condoms because they perceive condom use implies a lack of trust or intimacy. Counsel clients about their embarrassment and teach clients about condoms and how to negotiate their use. Include clients' partners in these discussions when possible.

5. **Coital dependent.** Some men and their partners may find it inconvenient to use a condom with every act of intercourse.

6. **Lack of cooperation**. In some instances, men will not accept responsibility for contraception or prevention of infection, thus making condom use impossible. Encourage clients whose partners are resistant to condom use to communicate their concerns to their partners and teach them the skills necessary to negotiate condom use.

7. **Latex allergy**. Some men and women, especially health care workers repeatedly exposed to latex, may be allergic or sensitive to latex and thus unable to use latex condoms. Plastic condoms are excellent alternatives. (See the section on Managing Problems and Follow-Up.)

PROVIDING CONDOMS

COUNSELING

While men perceive several advantages to condom use (e.g., peace of mind, ease of use, and prolonging of sex,[20,39]), men also express concern that condoms reduce sensation, decrease spontaneity, interfere with erection, make intercourse unnatural, and imply a lack of trust between partners.[21,33,39,92,95,98] In the National Survey of Men, for example, 75% of respondents agreed that condoms decreased sensation.[39] Such concerns likely affect men's decisions to use condoms consistently during intercourse. (See the sections on Advantages and Indications and Disadvantages and Cautions.) All clients should understand when to use condoms, how to use them most effectively, how to discuss condom use with their partner(s), and how to make condom use an exciting part of intercourse:

STI protection. Recommend condoms to at-risk clients using contraceptive methods that offer little or no protection against STIs or HIV. At-risk clients using another method (oral contraceptives, Norplant, Depo-Provera, IUDs, fertility awareness, or sterilization) or who have had hysterectomies should be strongly and frequently encouraged to use condoms. Although women using these methods are believed to be less likely to use condoms for prevention of infection,[3] a recent study found increases in consistent condom use among STI clinic clients following an intervention to promote condoms, regardless of their contraceptive method at enrollment.[17]

Emphasize the need for condom use during *all* sexual activities that can transmit STIs and HIV. Recommend that clients use a new condom for each act of anal, vaginal, or oral intercourse when any risk of infection exists.[14] (See the section on Effectiveness Against STIs and HIV).

Dual method use. Use caution when recommending dual method use to clients. Although using a condom plus another contraceptive method dramatically reduces the risks of pregnancy and STI, simultaneous use of multiple methods can be overly complicated for some couples, who may instead opt to use no method of contraception at all. Follow the client's lead and perhaps suggest a brief trial period of dual method use. If this proves difficult for the client, consider recommending consistent and correct use of condoms *alone* to provide adequate protection against both pregnancy and infection. Emergency contraception can be a back-up method against pregnancy in case a condom breaks, falls off, or is not used.

Tailored counseling. Adapt counseling messages on condom use to each clients' needs. Clients may have formed their own attitudes about condom use and may have had varying experiences with condoms. Tailor the counseling session to each client's risk factors, abilities, needs, and readiness to change. Many clinicians use behavioral change models[65] to assess the ability of their clients to use condoms consistently and to guide the content of the counseling session, a process which makes effective use of time.[22] (See Chapter 10 on Education and Counseling.)

Personal benefits. Make sure clients understand how condom use benefits them *personally*. Explain that condoms protect future fertility by preventing long-term sequelae of STIs. (See Chapter 8 on Reproductive Tract Infections.) Strongly encourage pregnant women at high risk for STIs to use latex or plastic condoms to protect their fetus, their partner(s), and themselves against STIs.

Partner negotiation. Teach clients how to negotiate condom use with partners. Many clients may have contemplated using condoms but may be uncomfortable suggesting condom use to their partners, especially when beginning a new relationship, when involved in an existing relationship, or when trying to sustain condom use in an ongoing relationship. Teach clients how to negotiate condom use with their partner(s) and help clients develop replies they can use when a partner objects to condoms [8,40,73] (Table 16-4). Assess the likelihood of a partner's negative reaction to the suggestion of condom use; some clients fear that they will be abused or abandoned if they insist on using condoms. Counsel or refer as appropriate if you detect battering or other forms of abuse.

Effective use. Make sure clients understand how to use condoms effectively. Emphasize that condoms are most effective when used correctly during every act of intercourse. Assessing condom use among

Table 16-4 Dialogues for negotiating condom use with sex partners

Objection	Response
Sensation	
"I won't feel as much if I have a condom on."	"You won't feel anything if you don't have a condom on."[40]
"It doesn't feel good."	"I think it's really sexy when a guy uses a condom. It shows he cares. What if I put it on for you?"[73]
	"I'd feel better"[8]
Availability	
"I don't have one."	"I do, and it's ribbed inside for your pleasure."[73]
Disease prevention	
"If you trusted me, you wouldn't ask me to use one."	"I trust that you're telling me the truth, the best you can. But with some STIs, you can't tell if you have them just by looking. Let's be safe and use condoms."[73]
"You won't catch anything from me."	"If you love me, respect my health."[8]
	"Condoms protect. Love doesn't."[8]
Spontaneity	
"It will interrupt sex."	"Let me put it on you. You'll love it."[40]
	"I'll wait."[8]
"It spoils the mood."	"It puts me in the mood."
	"Not if I help."
	"We could always go to a movie."[8]

Adapted from California Office of AIDS, Grieco (1987), and Sapsis (1996).

clients is a two-tiered process. First ask clients how often they are using condoms (e.g., always, most of the time, sometimes, never). Then ask clients to explain (and perhaps demonstrate on an appropriate model of a penis) how they use condoms to recognize potential misuse. (See the section on Minimizing User Errors and on Instructions for Condom Use.) Encourage clients to use condoms consistently and correctly with every act of anal, vaginal, and oral intercourse.

Suitability. Encourage clients who experience problems using condoms to try different brands, until they find one most suitable for them. Ask clients what does not work about using condoms and offer to help them select a condom most suitable to their needs (Table 16-5). Remember that all condoms are not the same, and clients will undoubtedly find some condoms more acceptable than others. Some clinics now provide a variety of condoms to clients, including male and female condoms. Although cost is often the primary factor when deciding which condom to distribute in the clinic, many condom brands are similarly priced when purchased in bulk.

Practice.   Encourage clients to practice using condoms. Many problems occurring during condom use can be attributed to inexperience [81] and can be overcome with practice. Users who have had negative experiences with condoms may be at risk of discontinuing condom use altogether;[62] encourage them to continue practicing with condoms. When providing instruction on how to use condoms, have the client unroll a condom onto a model of a penis or similarly shaped object, both with eyes open and then again in the dark. Men can also practice using condoms during masturbation, either while alone or with a partner. Condom use during masturbation may provide men with visible proof that they can successfully ejaculate while wearing a condom. With practice, condoms can become an exciting part of intercourse for both partners, particularly when integrated into sexual activity.

CONDOM PREFERENCES

According to a survey of condom manufacturers, more than 100 brands of condoms are available in the United States.[43] Condoms are available in a wide variety of shapes, sizes, colors, and thicknesses, as well as with or without lubricants or spermicides, and with or without reservoir-tip or nipple-ends (Table 16-5). Condoms can be straight-sided or tapered toward the closed end, textured (e.g., ribbed) or smooth, solid-colored or nearly transparent, and odorless or scented or flavored. Most condoms are about 7 inches (170 mm) long, 2 inches (50 mm) wide, and .003 inches (.07 mm) thick. More comprehensive listings of the names and characteristics of available condoms can be found in the 16th revised edition of *Contraceptive Technology*[43] and in a recent article from *Consumer Reports*.[21]

Recent attention has focused on the characteristics that men, women, and their partners seek when choosing a condom. In a *Consumer Reports* survey of self-selected readers, lubrication and the reservoir tip were named as the two most important condom features. Some men also preferred natural membrane condoms because they reported more sensitivity with these condoms.[20] In the more representative National Survey of Men, those surveyed preferred condoms that stayed on during sex, were easy to put on, and contained the right amount of lubrication. Few men considered color, ribbing, or cost when purchasing condoms (Table 16-6).[39]

Table 16-5 Resource guide for condoms available in the United States

Manufacturer Name	Institutional Sales Phone Number	Condom Types					Features Available	Examples of Brands
		Latex	Natural Skin	Plastic Male	Plastic Female			
Ansell Public Sector	1-800-327-8659 *www.lifestyles.com*	x					a, b, c, d, e, g, i, j	Kiss of Mint, Lifestyles, Prime, Rough-Rider
Carter-Wallace, Inc.	1-800-828-9032 *www.trojancondoms.com*	x	x				a, b, c, f, h	Trojan, Trojan-Enz, Trojan Magnum, Class Act, *Naturalamb*
Durex Consumer Products	1-888-266-3660 *www.durex.com*	x	x	x			a, b, c, d, e, h	<u>Avanti</u>, Circle Coin, *Fourex* Ramses, Saxon, Sheik
Female Health Company	1-800-274-6601				x		a, e	<u>Reality female condom</u>
Mayer Laboratories	1-800-426-6366 *www.MayerLabs.com*	x					a, b, c, e, f, h	Kimono, MAXX, P.S., Sensation
Okamoto U.S.A., Inc.	1-800-283-7546	x					a, b, c, e, h	Beyond Seven, Crown
Sagami Inc.	1-800-551-1888	x					a, b, e	Excalibur, Sagami Type E, Vis-A-Vis

Source: U.S. condom manufacturers (1997).

Natural skin condoms are italicized; plastic condoms are underlined.

Feature codes:

a Lubricated	c Spermicidal lubricant	e Thin (≤ .05 mm.)	g Narrow (≤ 2.0 in.)	i Short (≤ 6.5 in.)
b Reservoir end	d Thick (≥ .10 mm.)	f Wide (≥ 2.2 in.)	h Long (≥ 7.5 in.)	j Scented

Table 16-6 Characteristics men seek when selecting a condom, 1991 National Survey of Men

Characteristic	% of Men Agreeing
Stays on	58
Easy to put on	57
Right amount of lubrication	54
Easy to obtain	47
Reservoir tip	43
Thin, greater sensation	42
Spermicidal	33
No unpleasant odor	32
Partner likes it	27
Low cost	18
Ribbing	13
Color	7

Source: Grady et al. (1993).

MINIMIZING USER ERROR

Misuse of the condom, rather than poor condom quality, accounts for the majority of breakage and slippage. Most users rarely experience breakage or slippage. Condom effectiveness depends heavily on the skill level and experience of the user.[2,13,38,81,83,92] In the study of Nevada sex workers,[2] techniques for avoiding breakage and slippage included putting the condom on correctly for the client, using adequate amounts of water-soluble lubricant, using appropriately sized condoms, monitoring the condom throughout intercourse, and using multiple condoms simultaneously. The absence of HIV[94] and STIs in the Nevada brothel population[2] further suggests these women are using condoms consistently and correctly during intercourse.

Common errors with condoms facilitate exposure to STIs and pregnancy:

- **Failure to use the condom with every act of intercourse**. Rather than breakage or slippage, non-use accounts for most pregnancies attributed to condom use.
- **Failure to use condoms throughout intercourse**. Some men put condoms on after starting intercourse or may remove

condoms before ejaculating, practices that expose men and their partners to risks of pregnancy or STIs.[30,92] In one study, men acquired gonorrhea despite condom use because they failed to put the condom on before starting intercourse.[23] *Clients should be encouraged to use condoms every time from "start to finish."*

- **Improper lubricant use with latex condoms**. Unlike water-based lubricants (e.g., K-Y Jelly), oil-based lubricants (e.g., petroleum jelly, baby oil, and hand lotions) reduce latex condom integrity[91] and facilitate breakage[83] (Table 16-7). Some clients use oil-based products as condom lubricants, mistaking them for water-based lubricants because they readily wash off with water.[83,89] Because vaginal medications (e.g., for yeast infections) often contain oil-based ingredients that can damage latex condoms, clients who are using or prescribed these medications should be advised to remain abstinent, use plastic condoms, or use other contraceptives until the medication is fully completed and the infection is cured. *Note: oil-based products may be safely used as lubricants with polyurethane condoms.*

- **Incorrect placement of the condom on the penis.** Condoms may tear if clients are not careful when removing the condom from the package, test condoms for holes by filling them

Table 16-7 Examples of products which can and cannot be used as lubricants with latex condoms[1]

Safe	Unsafe
Egg whites	Baby oil
Glycerine	Cold creams
Spermicide (Nonoxynol-9)	Edible oils (olive, peanut, corn, sunflower)
Saliva	
Water	Hand and body lotions
	Massage oil
Examples of products:	Petroleum jelly
• Aloe-9 • K-Y Jelly	Rubbing alcohol
• Aqua Lube • Prepair	
• Astroglide • Probe	Suntan oil and lotions
• ForPlay Lubricants • Ramses Personal Spermicidal	Vegetable or mineral oil
• Gynol II • Touch Personal Lubricant	Vaginal yeast infection medications in cream or suppository form
• H-R Lubricating Jelly • Wet	

[1]All lubricants, including oil-based products, may be used with polyurethane condoms.

with air or water, or unroll condoms before putting them on.[26,89,92] Some men accidentally place the condom upside-down on the penis and then flip the condom over and use it for intercourse,[30,92] a practice that may expose their partner to pre-ejaculatory fluid or infectious penile secretions. Although pregnancy is unlikely to result from exposure to pre-ejaculate, HIV has been detected in the pre-ejaculatory fluid of infected men.[45,66] Whether the amount of HIV in pre-ejaculate is sufficient to cause infection has not been established. On the horizon is an applicator for putting the condom on the penis in a single-handed motion.[77]

- **Poor withdrawal technique.** Although slippage during withdrawal, normally considered user error, may be prevented if the condom's rim is held against the base of the erect penis soon after ejaculation, one study found only 71% of men held the rim during withdrawal and only 50% withdrew immediately after ejaculation.[92]

CONDOM USE DURING ANAL AND ORAL INTERCOURSE

Latex and plastic condoms can also be used during anogenital and orogenital intercourse to prevent STIs. The risk of HIV transmission during anal intercourse can be reduced with the use of latex or plastic condoms, although the FDA has not approved condom use for this purpose. The use of a thicker condom or two condoms simultaneously, or the application of an adequate amount of water-based lubricant, may minimize the risk of breakage during anal intercourse or rigorous vaginal intercourse. Oral HIV transmission appears possible.[48,55,71,75,79] Mouth-to-penis contact (fellatio) and mouth-to-vulva contact (cunnilingus) can also transmit other bacterial and viral pathogens. Unlubricated, scented, or flavored latex or plastic condoms are recommended for use during fellatio. Household plastic wrap can be used during cunnilingus and anilingus, although it has not been manufactured, intended, or approved by the FDA for medical applications. Household plastic wrap offers many advantages for persons having oral intercourse in that it is safe, cheap, widely available, conducts heat, and is large enough to cover large areas. Although research on barrier properties of household plastic wrap against viral transmission is extremely limited, one study found it effectively blocked the passage of herpes simplex virus,[34] which is comparable in size to HIV. Dental dams and condoms adapted to form a barrier sheet have also been proposed as barriers for cunnilingus; however, their limited size may allow potentially infectious fluids to roll onto adjacent tissues, and these products also have not been evaluated or approved for this use.

Innovative Programs

During the 1990s, many creative social marketing and public awareness efforts have been implemented in the United States and abroad to promote condom use. One feature common to successful condom distribution programs is the provision of large numbers of condoms to each client at low or no cost. Providing a few condoms is only a short-term solution for clients who find the health care system inaccessible or who find it embarrassing to return repeatedly for condoms.

- To attract younger audiences, several U.S. condom manufacturers now advertise their products on the World Wide Web. These sites permit visitors to purchase condoms discretely on the Internet, and often contain interesting and useful information regarding the history of the condom, instructions for proper use, question-and-answer forums, and condom promotions (Table 16-5).

- Many retailers specializing in condoms and other "safer sex" products have opened in large cities throughout the United States and can also be accessed for mail-order purchases. Condomania, for example, has developed an interactive Web site to help users select a condom that best satisfies their needs (*http://www.condomania.com*). (See Chapter 11 on Selected Reproductive Health Resources.)

- In Louisiana, the State Department of Health has developed "Operation Protect," a social marketing program designed to make condoms more accessible in neighborhoods with high rates of STIs. Through the participation of more than 1,200 businesses, "Operation Protect" has distributed more than 20 million condoms free or at low cost during its first 2 years.[19]

- In Oregon, "Project Action"—an HIV prevention program for young adults—has developed a social marketing program to encourage condom use through a television campaign and strategic placement of condom vending machines.[63]

- The Thai Ministry of Health implemented a national "100% condom campaign" to encourage widespread condom use during commercial sex.[72] As a result, condom use increased from 25% to more than 90% during the program, and the rate of curable STI decreased.[10]

Promotion among Adolescents

Despite their increasing popularity, condom promotion programs may be difficult to implement in some settings. Among the most controversial questions are whether adolescents, who may be too embarrassed to purchase or otherwise obtain condoms, should be able to obtain condoms and contraceptive counseling through schools.[58] Although schools are the primary source of information on STIs and HIV for most adolescents,[46] only 2% of public high schools make condoms available to students[50] despite public support for such programs. No evidence clearly suggests that condom availability programs in high schools hasten the onset or frequency of sexual intercourse among students.[46,49]

A need clearly exists for increased condom promotion among adolescents, given that many youth engage in behaviors that place them at increased risk of STIs, including HIV. Three million new cases of STIs are diagnosed among adolescents each year.[46] Additionally, national surveys have found that 53% of high school students report having had sexual intercourse and 19% report having had four or more lifetime sex partners, yet only 53% report using a condom at last intercourse.[47] Access, availability, confidentiality, and cost may all be important determinants of condom use among adolescents.[46] Whether a condom is used at first sexual intercourse may also predict subsequent condom use patterns among adolescents.[59]

M ANAGING PROBLEMS AND FOLLOW-UP

Persons sensitive or allergic to natural rubber latex may experience irritation, allergic contact dermatitis, or systemic anaphylactic symptoms when exposed to latex-containing products.[4,100] While only 1% of the U.S. population are believed to be allergic to latex,[80] the prevalence of latex sensitivity is much higher among health care workers (up to 17%[99]) who have repeated exposure to latex- containing medical devices (e.g., surgical and examination gloves, catheters, intubation tubes, anesthesia masks, and dental dams).[32,100] Proteins in the latex appear to be the primary source of allergic reactions.[32]

The FDA has recommended that all patients be questioned for potential latex allergy. Ask whether the client experiences itching, rash, or wheezing after wearing latex gloves or inflating a balloon.[32] If you suspect a client has generalized latex sensitivity, consider using medical devices made of alternative materials such as plastic [32] and refer the client for allergy skin testing.[99] From a family planning and STI prevention standpoint, the implications of latex allergy also extend to the use of condoms.[31] While latex condom use is contraindicated for clients with general latex sensitivity, both plastic or natural membrane condoms can be recommended for prevention of pregnancy, but only plastic condoms for prevention of STIs, including HIV.

Allergic reactions that occur only after exposure to latex condoms and not after exposure to other latex-containing products may be attributable to brand-specific condom attributes such as spermicides, lubricants, perfumes, local anesthetics, or other chemical agents added during the manufacturing process.[42] Advise clients to try different brands of latex and plastic condoms. In any case, clients should immediately contact their health care provider for follow-up if they or their partner(s) experience a severe allergic reaction while using latex condoms or spermicides.

INSTRUCTIONS FOR USING CONDOMS

Use latex or plastic condoms when you have any concern about reproductive tract infections, including infection with the human immunodeficiency virus (HIV). When used consistently and correctly, condoms also provide good protection against unintended pregnancy.

BEFORE INTERCOURSE

1. Have on hand an adequate supply of latex or plastic condoms and water-based lubricant if you might use one for intercourse, even if you plan to use another contraceptive. Have extra condoms available in case the first is damaged or torn before use or put on incorrectly or if you have repeated intercourse.
2. Discuss condom use *before* you have intercourse.

AT TIME OF INTERCOURSE

1. Open the condom package carefully to avoid damaging it with fingernails, teeth, or other sharp objects.
2. Put on the condom before the penis comes in contact with the partner's mouth, anus, or vagina. If the penis is uncircumcised, pull the foreskin back before putting on the condom. Keep the condom on the penis until after intercourse or ejaculation.
3. Unroll the condom a short distance to make sure the condom is being unrolled in the right direction. The rolled ring should be on the outside. Then hold the tip of the condom and unroll it down to the base of the erect penis. If the condom does not unroll easily, it is on upside-down and may expose the partner to infectious organisms contained in the pre-ejaculate. Discard and begin with a new condom.
4. Adequate lubrication is important. For latex condoms, use only water-based lubricants like water; lubricating jellies (e.g., K-Y Jelly);

or spermicidal creams, jellies, foam, or suppositories. Avoid oil-based lubricants like cold cream, mineral oil, cooking oil, petroleum jelly, body lotions, massage oil, or baby oil that can damage latex condoms (Table 16-7). For plastic condoms, any type of lubricant can be used.

5. If the condom breaks or falls off during intercourse but before ejaculation, stop and put on a new condom. A new condom can also be used when you have prolonged intercourse or different types of intercourse within a single session (e.g., vaginal and anal).

AFTER INTERCOURSE

1. Soon after ejaculation, withdraw the penis while it is still erect. Hold the condom firmly against the base of the penis to prevent slippage and leakage of semen.

2. Check the condom for visible damage such as holes, then wrap it in tissue and discard. Do not flush condoms down the toilet.

3. If the condom breaks, falls off, leaks, or is not used—

   a. Discuss the possibility of pregnancy or infection with your partner and contact your health care provider as soon as you can. *Do not douche.* Emergency contraception may be used to prevent pregnancy if started within 72 hours of having unprotected intercourse. Call 1-888-NOT-2-LATE to learn more about emergency contraceptives and to obtain phone numbers of providers of emergency contraception nearest to you, or obtain this information from the World Wide Web at http://opr.princeton.edu/ec. (See Chapter 12 on Emergency Contraception.)

   b. Gently wash the penis, vulva, anus, and adjacent areas with soap and water immediately after intercourse to help reduce the risk of acquiring an STI.[44] Then insert an applicator full of spermicide into the vagina as soon as possible.

REPEATED INTERCOURSE

1. Use a new condom from "start to finish" with each act of anal, vaginal, or oral intercourse. Do not reuse condoms.

TAKING CARE OF SUPPLIES

1. Store condoms in a cool and dry place out of direct sunlight (heat may weaken latex). Latex condoms can probably be stored in a wallet for up to 1 month when kept away from heat and sunlight.[35]

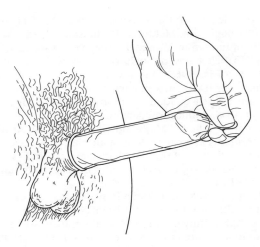

Figure 16-2 Unroll the condom over the penis

2. Check the expiration or manufacture date on the box or individual package of condoms. Expiration dates are marked as "Exp"; otherwise, the date is the manufacture date (MFG). Latex condoms should not be used beyond their expiration date or more than 5 years after the manufacturing date. Latex condoms with spermicide should probably be used within 2 years of the manufacture date. Condoms in damaged packages or that show obvious signs of deterioration (e.g., brittleness, stickiness, or discoloration) should not be used regardless of their expiration date.

REFERENCES

1. Abma JC, Chandra A, Mosher WD, Peterson LS, Piccinino LJ. Fertility, family planning, and women's health: new data from the 1995 National Survey of Family Growth. Vital Health Stat 1997;Series 23, Number 9.
2. Albert AE, Warner DL, Hatcher RA, Trussell J, Bennett C. Condom use among female commercial sex workers in Nevada's legal brothels. Am J Publ Health 1995;85:1514-1520.
3. Anderson JE, Brackbill R, Mosher WD. Condom use for disease prevention among unmarried U.S. women. Fam Plann Perspect 1996;28:25-28,39.
4. Anglia and Oxford Regional Health Authority. Latex allergy: implications for patients and health care workers. Bandolier 1994;7:1-3.
5. ASTM (American Society for Testing Materials). Annual book of ASTM standards: Easton MD: ASTM: section 9, rubber. Volume 09.02 Rubber products; standard specifications for rubber contraceptives (male condoms). Philadelphia: American Society for Testing Materials 1996.

6. Brown MD. Spermicidal condoms. Kansas Med 1988;89:114-115.
7. Buchbinder SP, Douglas JM, McKirnan DJ, Judson FN, Katz MH, MacQueen KM. Feasibility of human immunodeficiency virus vaccine trials in homosexual men in the United States: risk behavior, seroincidence, and willingness to participate. J Infect Dis 1996;174:954-61.
8. California Office of AIDS. Condom comebacks: what to say when your partner doesn't want to use a condom. California AIDS Clearinghouse and California Office of AIDS, publication date unknown.
9. Carey RF, Herman WA, Retta SM, Rinaldi JE, Herman BA, Athey TW. Effectiveness of latex condoms as a barrier to human immunodeficiency virus-sized particles under conditions of simulated use. Sex Transm Dis 1992;19:230-234.
10. Cates W. How much do condoms protect against sexually transmitted diseases? IPPF Bulletin 1997;31:2-3.
11. Cates W Jr., Holmes KK. Re: condom efficacy against gonorrhea and nongonococcal urethritis. Am J Epidemiol 1996;143:843-844.
12. Cates W, Stone KM. Family planning, sexually transmissible infections and contraceptive choice: a literature update – Part I. Fam Plann Perspect 1992;24:75-84.
13. Centers for Disease Control and Prevention. Update: barrier protection against HIV infection and other sexually transmitted diseases. MMWR 1993;42:589-591, 597.
14. Centers for Disease Control and Prevention. Facts about condoms and their use in preventing HIV infection and other STDs. Atlanta GA: CDC, 1995.
15. Centers for Disease Control and Prevention. CDC national AIDS hotline training bulletin (#138). Atlanta: CDC, 1995.
16. Centers for Disease Control and Prevention. Update: questions and answers about male latex condoms to prevent sexual transmission of HIV. Atlanta: CDC, 1997.
17. Centers for Disease Control and Prevention. Contraceptive practices before and after an intervention promoting condom use to prevent HIV infection and other sexually transmitted diseases among women—selected U.S. sites, 1993-1995. MMWR 1997;46:373-377.
18. Chan-Chee C, de Vincenzi I, Sole-Pla MA, Ancelle-Park R, Brunet JB. Use and misuse of condoms. Genitourin Med 1991;67:173-175.
19. Cohen DA. How to implement a community-based condom accessibility program (Session A1). Proceedings of the National STD Prevention Conference, December 9-12, 1996. Tampa FL.
20. Consumers Union. Can you rely on condoms? Consum Rep 1989;March: 135-142.
21. Consumer's Union. How reliable are condoms? Consumer Reports 1995; May:320-325.
22. Contraceptive Technology Update. Can't get patients to use condoms? Try mix of staging and counseling. Contraceptive Technology Update 1997; 18:1-12.
23. Darrow W. Condom use and use-effectiveness in high-risk populations. Sex Transm Dis 1989;16:157-160.
24. Deschamps MM, Pape JW, Hafner A, Johnson WD Jr. Heterosexual transmission of HIV in Haiti. Ann Intern Med 1996;125:324-330.

25. De Vincenzi I. A longitudinal study of human immunodeficiency virus transmission by heterosexual partners. European Study Group on Heterosexual Transmission of HIV. N Engl J Med 1994;331:341-346.

26. Family Health International. How human use affects condom breakage. Network 1991;12:10-14.

27. Feldblum P, Joanis C. Modern barrier methods: effective contraception and disease prevention. Research Triangle Park NC: Family Health International, 1994.

28. Feldblum PJ, Morrison CS, Roddy RE, Cates W Jr. The effectiveness of barrier methods of contraception in preventing the spread of HIV. AIDS 1995;9(suppl A):585-593.

29. Fihn SD, Boyko EJ, Normand EH, Chi-Ling C, Grafton JR, Hunt M, Yarbro P, Scholes D, Stergachis A. Association between use of spermicide-coated condoms and Escherichia coli urinary tract infection in young women. Am J Epidemiol 1996;144:512-520.

30. Fishbein M, Aral S, Collins J, Peterman T. Issues concerning the use of behavioral and biological outcome measures in STD/HIV prevention (Session A6). Procedings in the National STD Prevention Conference, December 9-12, 1996. Tampa FL.

31. Fisher AA. Condom dermatitis in either partner. Cutis 1987;39:284-285.

32. Food and Drug Administration. Allergic reactions to latex-containing medical devices [press release]. Rockville MD; Food and Drug Administration, March 29, 1991.

33. Forrest JD, Singh S. The sexual and reproductive behavior of American women, 1982-1988. Fam Plann Perspect 1990;22:206-214.

34. Garland SM, Newnan DM, de Crespigny LC. Plastic wrap for ultrasound transducers. J Ultrasound Med 1989;8:661-663.

35. Glasser G, Hatcher RA. The effect on condom integrity of carrying a condom in a wallet for three months [abstract]. Proceedings of the American College of Obstetricians and Gynecologists District IV Conference, November 1992. San Juan PR.

36. Golombok S, Sketchley J, Rust J. Condom failure among homosexual men. J AIDS 1989;151:318-322.

37. Golombok S, Sheldon J. Evaluation of a thicker condom for use as a prophylactic against HIV transmission. AIDS Educ Prev 1994;6:454-458.

38. Grady WR, Klepinger DH, Billy JOG, Tanfer K. Condom characteristics: the perceptions and preferences of men in the United States. Fam Plann Perspect 1993;25:67-73.

39. Grady WR, Tanfer K. Condom breakage and slippage among men in the United States. Fam Plann Perspect 1994;26:107-112.

40. Grieco A. Cutting the risks for STDs. Med Aspects Hum Sex 1987;21:70-84.

41. Hamann CP. Personal communication to David Lee Warner, April 1997.

42. Hamann CP, Kick SA. Update: immediate and delayed hypersensitivity to natural rubber latex. Cutis 1993;52:307-311.

43. Hatcher RA, Trussell J, Stewart F, Stewart G, Kowal D, Cates W, Guest F. Contraceptive technology. Rev. 16th ed. New York: Irvington Publishers, 1994.

44. Hooper RR, Reynolds GH, Jones OG, Zaidi A, Wiesner PJ, Latimer KP, Lester A, Campbell AF, Harrison WO, Karney WW. Holmes KK. Cohort study of

venereal disease. I: the risk of gonorrhea transmission from infected women to men. Am J Epidemiol 1978;108:136-144.

45. Ilaria G, Jacobs JL, Polsky B, Koll B, Baron P, Maclow C, Armstrong D. Detection of HIV-1 DNA sequences in pre-ejaculatory fluid. Lancet 1992;340(8833):1469.

46. Institute of Medicine. The hidden epidemic: confronting sexually transmissible infections. In: Eng TR, Butler WT (eds). Washington DC: National Academy Press, 1997.

47. Kann L, Warren CW, Harris WA, Collins JL, Williams BI, Ross JG, Kolbe LJ. Youth risk behavior surveillance—United States 1995. MMWR 1996;45(SS-4).

48. Keet IPM, Van Lent NA, Sandfort TGM, Coutinho RA, Van Griensven GJP. Orogenital sex and the transmission of HIV among homosexual men. AIDS 1992;6:223-226.

49. Kirby D, Short L, Collins J, Rugg D, Kolbe L, Howard M, Miller B, Sonenstein F, Zabin LS. School-based programs to reduce sexual risk behaviors: a review of effectiveness. Public Health Reports 1994;109:339-60.

50. Kirby DB, Brown NL. Condom availability programs in U.S. schools. Fam Plann Perspect 1996;28:196-202.

51. Kirkman RJE, Morris J, Webb AMC. User experience: Mates v. Nuforms. Br J Fam Plann 1990;15:107-111.

52. Koop CE. Surgeon General's report on acquired immune deficiency syndrome. Washington DC: US Department of Health and Human Services, 1986.

53. Kreiss J, Ngugi E, Holmes K, Ndinya-Achola J, Waiyaki P, Roberts PL, Ruminjo I, Sajabi R, Kimata J, Fleming TR, Anzala A, Holton D, Plummer F. Efficacy of nonoxynol-9 contraceptive sponge use in preventing heterosexual acquisition of HIV in Nairobi prostitutes. JAMA 1992;268:477-482.

54. Leeper MA, Conrardy M. Preliminary evaluation of REALITY, a condom for women to wear. Adv Contracept 1989;5:229-235.

55. Lifson AR, O'Malley PM, Hessol NA, Buchbinder SP, Cannon L, Rutherford GW. HIV seroconversion in two homosexual men after receptive oral intercourse with ejaculation: implications for counseling concerning safe sexual practices. Am J Publ Health 1990;80:1509-1511.

56. Liskin L, Wharton C, Blackburn R, Kestelman P. Condoms: now more than ever. Pop Rep 1990;8(Series H).

57. Lytle CD, Routson LB, Seaborn GB, Dixon LG, Bushar HF, Cyr WH. An in vitro evaluation of condoms as barriers to a small virus. Sex Transm Dis 1997;24:161-164.

58. Mahler K. Condom availability in the schools: lessons from the courtroom. Fam Plann Perspect 1996;28:75-77.

59. Miller, KS. Personal communication to David Lee Warner, April, 1997.

60. Moran JS, Janes HR, Peterman TA, Stone KM. Increase in condom sales following AIDS education and publicity, United States. Am J Public Health 1990;80:607-608.

61. Murphy JS. The condom industry in the United States, 1990. Jefferson NC: McFarland & Company, Inc., Publishers, 1990.

62. Norris AE, Ford K. Associations between condom experiences and beliefs, intentions, and use in a sample of urban, low-income, African-American and Hispanic youth. AIDS Education Prevention 1994;6:27-39.

63. Population Services International. Personal communication to David Lee Warner, 1993.

64. Price HC. A contraceptive and prophylactic barrier: current concepts for the male condom. In: Mauck CK, Cordero M, Gabelnick HL, Spieler JM, Rivera R (eds). Barrier contraceptives: current status and future prospects. New York: Wiley-Liss, Inc., 1994.

65. Prochaska JO, Norcross JC, DiClemente CC. Changing for good. New York: Avon Books, 1994.

66. Pudney J, Oneta M, Mayer K, Searge G (III), Anderson D. Pre-ejaculatory fluid as potential vector for sexual transmission of HIV-1. Lancet 1992;340:1470.

67. Richters J, Donovan B, Gerofi J, Watson L. Low condom breakage rate in commercial sex [letter]. Lancet 1988;2:1487-1488. Correction by John Gerofi in personal communication to Philip Kestelman, July 1989.

68. Richters J, Donovan B, Gerofi J. How often do condoms break or slip off in use? Int J Sex Transm Dis 1993;4:90-94.

69. Roddy RE, Zekeng L, Ryan KK, Tamoufi U, Weir SS, Din E. Effectiveness of nonoxynol-9 film in preventing transmission of human immunodeficiency virus. Proceedings of the NIAID Ad Hoc Conference on N-9 Film, April 9, 1997. Bethesda MD.

70. Rosenberg MJ, Waugh MS, Solomon HM, Lyszkowski ADL. The male polyurethane condom: a review of current knowledge. Contraception 1996;53:141-146.

71. Rozenbaum W, Gharakhanian S, Cardon B, Duval E, Coulaud JP. HIV transmission by oral sex. Lancet 1988;1:1395.

72. Rugpao S, Beyrer C, Touanabutras S, Natpratan C, Nelson KE, Celentano DD, Khamboonruang C. Multiple condom use and decreased condom breakage and slippage in Thailand. J Acq Imm Def Syndr Hum Retro 1997;14:169-173.

73. Sapsis K. Putting theory into practice: tools for change. January, 1996.

74. Saracco A, Musicco M, Nicolosi A, Angarano G, Arici C, Gavazzeni G, Costigliola P, Gafa S, Gervasoni C, Luzzati R. Man-to-woman sexual transmission of HIV: longitudinal study of 343 steady partners of infected men. J Acq Imm Def Synd 1993;6:497-501.

75. Schacker T, Collier AC, Hughes J, Shea T, Corey L. Clinical and epidemiologic features of primary HIV infection. Ann Intern Med 1996;125:257-264.

76. Schoenborn CA, Marsh SL, Hardy AM. AIDS knowledge and attitudes for 1992: data from the National Health Interview Survey. Advance Data 1994;243:13.

77. Siegel H. Personal communication to David Lee Warner, April, 1997.

78. Silverman BG, Gross TP. Use and effectiveness of condoms during anal intercourse. Sex Transm Dis 1997;24:11-17.

79. Spitzer PG, Weiner NJ. Transmission of HIV infection from a woman to a man by oral sex. N Engl J Med 1989;320:251.

80. Sprouls LS. When latex gloves aren't a perfect fit: reactions, sensitivity plague 12 percent of HCWs. Dental Teamwork 1992;November-December:28-31.

81. Steiner M, Piedrahita C, Glover L, Joanis C. Can condom users likely to experience condom failure be identified? Fam Plann Perspect 1993;25:220-223,226.

82. Steiner M, Trussell J, Glover L, Joanis C, Spruyt A, Dorflinger L. Standardized protocols for condom breakage and slippage trials: a proposal. Am J Publ Health 1994;84:1897-1900.

83. Steiner M, Piedrahita C, Glover L, Joanis C, Spruyt A, Foldesy R. The impact of lubricants on latex condoms during vaginal intercourse. Int J STD AIDS 1994;5:29-36.
84. Stone, KM. HIV, other STDs, and barriers. In: Mauck CK, Cordero M, Gabelnick HL, Spieler JM, Rivera R (eds). Barrier contraceptives: current status and future prospects. New York: Wiley-Liss, Inc., 1994.
85. Stratton P, Hamann C, Beezhold D. Nonoxynol-9 lubricated latex condoms may increase release of natural rubber latex protein [abstract Th.C.433]. XI International Conference on AIDS, Vancouver, July 1996.
86. Tindall B, Swanson C, Donovan B, Cooper DA. Sexual practices and condom usage in a cohort of homosexual men in relation to human immunodeficiency virus status. Med J Aust 1989;151:318-322.
87. Trussell J, Leveque JA, Koenig JD, London R, Borden S, Henneberry J, LaGuardia KD, Stewart F, Wilson TG, Wysocki S, Strauss M. The economic value of contraception: a comparison of 15 methods. Am J Publ Health 1995;85:494-503.
88. Trussell J, Warner DL, Hatcher RA. Condom performance during vaginal intercourse: comparison of Trojan-Enz and Tactylon condoms. Contraception 1992;45:11-19.
89. Trussell J, Warner DL, Hatcher RA. Condom slippage and breakage rates. Fam Plann Perspect 1992;24:20-23.
90. Valdiserri RO. Cum hastis sic clypeatis: the turbulent history of the condom. Bull NY Acad Med 1988;64:237-245.
91. Voeller B, Coulson A, Bernstein GS, Nakamura R. Mineral oil lubricants cause rapid deterioration of latex condoms. Contraception 1989;39:95-101.
92. Warner DL, Hatcher RA, Boles J, Goldsmith J. Practices and patterns of condom usage for prevention of infection and pregnancy among male university students (Session PS-12). Proceeding of the Eleventh Annual National Preventive Medicine Meeting. March 1994.
93. Warner DL, Hatcher RA. A meta-analysis of condom effectiveness in reducing sexually transmitted HIV. Soc Sci Med 1994;38:1169-1170.
94. Weber JT, Reich R, Todd R, Horsley R. Absence of HIV seroconversion among sex workers at legal brothels, Nevada, 1990-1995 (Session 1203). Proceedings of the 124th Annual Meeting of the American Public Health Association, November 17-21, 1996. New York.
95. Weinstock HS, Lindan C, Bolan G, Kegeles SM, Hearst N. Factors associated with condom use in a high-risk heterosexual population. Sex Transm Dis 1993;20:14-20.
96. Weller S. A meta-analysis of condom effectiveness in reducing sexually transmitted HIV. Soc Sci Med 1993;36:1635-44.
97. Wigersma L, Oud R. Safety and acceptability of condoms for use by homosexual men as a prophylactic against transmission of HIV during anogenital sexual intercourse. BMJ 1987;295:94.
98. Williamson NE, Joanis C. Acceptability of barrier methods for prevention of unwanted pregnancy and infection. In: Mauck CK, Cordero M, Gabelnick HL, Spieler JM, Rivera R (eds). Barrier contraceptives: current status and future prospects. New York: Wiley-Liss, Inc., 1994.
99. Yassin MS, Lierl MB, Fischer TJ, O'Brien KO, Cross J, Steinmetz C. Latex allergy in hospital employees. Ann Allergy 1994;72:245-249.

100. Zaza S, Reeder JM, Charles LE, Jarvis WR. Latex sensitivity among perioperative nurses. AORN 1994;60:806-812.

LATE REFERENCES

101. Nelson A, Bernstein GS, Frezieres R, Walsh T, Clark V, Coulson A. Study of the efficacy, acceptability and safety of a non-latex (polyurethane) male condom: revised final report (N01-HD-1-3109). Bethesda MD: National Institute of Child Health and Human Development, September 15, 1997.
102. Nelson A, Frezieres R, Walsh T, Clark V, Coulson A. Controlled randomized evaluation of a commercially available polyurethane and latex condom (Avanti™ versus Ramses Sensitol™): final report (N01-HD-1-3109). Bethesda MD: National Institute of Child Health and Human Development, November 6, 1996.
103. Rosenberg MJ, Waugh MS. Latex condom breakage and slippage in a controlled clinical trial. Contraception 1997;56:17-21.

Vaginal Spermicides

Willard Cates Jr., MD, MPH
Elizabeth G. Raymond, MD, MPH

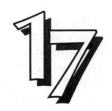

- Spermicides are simple, free of systemic side effects, and available without prescription. They can be used intermittently with little advance planning.
- Spermicides are an integral component of vaginal barrier methods (diaphragm, sponge, cap, and shield).
- Using spermicide may provide modest protection (up to 25%) against transmission of some STIs including gonorrhea and chlamydia. No evidence to date, however, shows that spermicide protects against HIV.
- Any woman who is at risk for an STI is also at risk for HIV. Abstinence is her safest choice, although use of condoms greatly reduces HIV risk and should be encouraged.

Spermicide products can be purchased without prescription in pharmacies and supermarkets. They can be used alone, with a vaginal barrier method, or as an adjunct to any of the other contraceptive methods for added protection against both pregnancy and some sexually transmitted infections (STIs).

MECHANISM OF ACTION

Spermicidal preparations consist of two components:

- Formulation (gel, foam, cream, film, suppository, or tablet), also called a carrier or base
- Chemical that kills the sperm in different doses and concentrations

For some products, the formulation helps disperse the spermicide. In the case of viscous gel and foam, the formulation itself may provide both lubrication and an additional barrier effect. Nonoxynol-9 (N-9), the active chemical agent in spermicide products available in the United States (Table 17-1), is a surfactant that destroys the sperm cell membrane. Other surfactant products, including octoxynol and benzalkonium chloride, are widely used in other parts of the world. Because of the recent emphasis on providing microbicides that are female-controlled, more than 20 chemical barrier methods are in various stages of development and evaluation.[8]

Table 17-1 U.S. marketed spermicides containing nonoxynol-9

Product Name and Manufacturer	Dose N-9	Delivery Device	Duration of Action
Soluble Films			
VCF Apothecus Pharmaceutical Corp.	70 mg	n/a	15 minutes after insertion up to 1 hour
Suppositories			
Encare Thompson Medical Company, Inc.	100 mg	n/a	10 minutes after insertion up to 1 hour
Semicid Insert Whitehall/Robins, American Home Products	100 mg	n/a	15 minutes after insertion up to 1 hour
Conceptrol Vaginal Insert Advanced Care Products, Division of J&J	100 mg	n/a	
Sweet and Fresh AID-PACK, Div. of NutraMax Prod.	100 mg	n/a	15 minutes after insertion up to 1 hour
Koromex Contraceptive Insert Quality Health Products, Inc.	125 mg	n/a	10-15 minutes after insertion up to 1 hour
Conceptrol Contraceptive Insert Advanced Care Products, Division of J&J	150 mg	n/a	Discontinued

(continued)

Table 17-1 U.S. marketed spermicides containing nonoxynol-9 *(cont.)*

Product Name and Manufacturer	Dose N-9	Delivery Device	Duration of Action
Gels			
Advantage-S Columbia Research Laboratories	52.5 mg	Pre-filled applicator	Immediately after insertion
Conceptrol Advanced Care Products, Division of J&J	100 mg	Pre-filled applicator	Immediately after insertion up to 1 hour
Gynol II Original Formula Advanced Care Products, Division of J&J	100 mg	Applicator	*To be used with diaphragm only, not alone*
KY Plus Advanced Care Products, Division of J&J	110 mg	Applicator	Immediately after insertion up to 1 hour
Shur Seal Gel Milex Products, Inc.	120 mg	Applicator	*To be used with diaphragm only, not alone*
Gynol II Extra Strength Advanced Care Products, Division of J&J	150 mg	Applicator (Prefillable)	*Alone or with condom:* immediately after insertion up to 1 hour
Koromex Jelly Quality Health Products, Inc.	150 mg	Applicator	Immediately after insertion up to 1 hour
Aerosol Foams			
Emko/Prefil/Because Schering Corp.	60 or 100 mg	Applicator	Immediately after insertion up to 1 hour
Delfen Advanced Care Products, Division of J&J	85 mg	Applicator	Immediately after insertion up to 1 hour
Koromex Quality Health Products, Inc.	125 mg	Applicator	Immediately after insertion up to 1 hour

Gels and creams. Gels, creams, and foam are commonly marketed for use with a diaphragm, but they can also be used alone. One application delivers 50 mg to 150 mg of spermicide, depending on the product: the spermicide concentration ranges from 8% to 12% in foam and from 2% to 5% in gels and creams.

Suppositories. Spermicide suppositories can be used alone or with a condom. Suppositories have a spermicide concentration of 2.3% to 5.6% and provide 50 mg to 125 mg of spermicide. Adequate time between insertion and intercourse (10 to 15 minutes depending on the product) is essential for the spermicide to dissolve and disperse. Incomplete dissolution of the suppository may reduce its contraceptive efficacy and may cause an uncomfortable gritty sensation or friction for the woman or the man.

Film. Vaginal contraceptive film (VCF) can be used alone or with a diaphragm. Each 2" × 2" paper-thin sheet of film has a spermicide concentration of 28% and contains 72 mg of N-9. The sheet must be inserted on or near the cervix (or inside the diaphragm) at least 15 minutes before intercourse to allow time for the sheet to melt and disperse. Placing film on the tip of the penis for insertion is not recommended; the film will not have adequate time to dissolve, and it may not be properly placed so as to cover the cervical os.

Spermicidal condoms. Latex condoms coated with N-9 have been available in the United States since 1983. (See Chapter 16 on Male Condoms.)

EFFECTIVENESS

Pregnancy rates among typical users cover a wide range, from less than 5% to more than 50% in the first year of use. Most published clinical trials of spermicide used alone do not meet modern standards for study design and analysis; thus, we must be cautious when comparing the efficacy of spermicides with the efficacy of either other contraceptive methods or other spermicide preparations.

The effectiveness of spermicides, like any barrier method, depends on consistent and correct use. For spermicide to be effective, it must be placed correctly in the vagina no longer than 1 hour before intercourse. The spermicide applicator, tablet, suppository, or film needs to make contact with the cervix, which for most women is deep in the vagina. Suppositories, foaming tablets, and films require adequate time for dissolution and dispersion. A method's characteristics (timing, degree of lubricating effect, or required delay for suppository to melt) may influence a couple's ability to use the spermicide effectively.[9] A couple is most likely to succeed with a method that is compatible with their sexual routines.

Using a physical and a chemical barrier method together increases contraceptive efficacy. For example, diaphragm users have less risk of pregnancy when they also use a spermicide. (See Chapter 9 on Essentials of Contraception.) Likewise, using emergency contraception to back up spermicides in situations of incorrect or non-use will increase effectiveness.

Douching is not a reliable contraceptive, even when a spermicide is in the douching solution, because sperm enter the cervical canal soon after ejaculation. Moreover, women who routinely douche for hygiene have an increased risk of both pelvic inflammatory disease (PID) and ectopic pregnancy. (See Chapter 8 on Reproductive Tract Infections.) A woman who has used a vaginal spermicide for contraception should not douche until at least 6 hours after sexual intercourse to avoid washing away the spermicide prematurely.

COST

Retail prices for spermicidal supplies range from less than $0.35 (for discount suppositories or gel) to $1.30 (for single-use gel packets). Users must make a small initial investment to purchase a container of foam ($12.00), a package of film ($9.25 for 12 sheets), a package of suppositories ($4.00 for 12 suppositories), or a tube of gel or cream ($12.00). The more frequently a woman uses spermicide for intercourse, the greater her cost.

ADVANTAGES AND INDICATIONS

Spermicides are a useful short-term contraceptive option and may be a reasonable long-term choice for couples who use them consistently.

1. Spermicide (used with a barrier method) and backed up by abortion in case of failure is one of the safest contraceptive options.
2. Spermicide use may lower the chance of becoming infected with a bacterial STI by an estimated 25%.
3. Spermicides can be purchased over-the-counter and do not require the user to seek medical consultation.
4. A male partner need not be involved in the decision to use or in the use of spermicide.
5. Spermicides can be kept available for immediate protection, for those who have intercourse infrequently or after long intervals.
6. Spermicides are a simple back-up option for a woman who is waiting to start oral contraceptives or have an intrauterine device (IUD) inserted, who forgets two or more pills or runs out of pills, or who suspects her IUD has been expelled.

7. Spermicides can be used to augment the effectiveness of fertility awareness methods.

8. Spermicides can be used to provide lubrication during intercourse, including intercourse involving a condom.

PROTECTION AGAINST STIS AND HIV

How well spermicides work as microbicides is a central issue in the reproductive health field.[1,8,21] In the laboratory, N-9 is lethal to organisms that cause gonorrhea, genital herpes, trichomoniasis, syphilis, and acquired immune deficiency syndrome (AIDS).[8] Microbicide activity in the test tube, however, does not mean spermicides can provide reliable protection in actual human use.

Findings from human studies on the efficacy and the safety of N-9 have been inconsistent.[2,12] These studies have used different study designs, different spermicide formulations and concentrations, and different populations, making it complicated to draw clinically meaningful conclusions. For example, most investigations of spermicides and their effect on STIs have been observational—namely cross-sectional, case-control, or cohort studies. Cross-sectional and case-control studies are retrospective, so it is difficult to determine when users acquired an STI in relation to spermicide use. Cohort studies are also limited because sexual behaviors that increase or decrease STI risk may influence contraceptive choice.[6] Therefore, any study of the association between contraceptive use and the risk of STI transmission should carefully control for all potential confounders. Behavioral risk factors may be more important than biologic influences such as contraceptive use in affecting the overall risk of STI. Because flaws in study design can be larger than the effect from the spermicide itself, it is not surprising our current studies do not agree.

The optimal study designs are randomized controlled trials (RCT), also referred to as level I scientific evidence. (See Chapter 1 on Expanding Perspectives on Reproductive Health.) Because both randomization and masking help eliminate behavioral and other differences among the study populations being compared, bias and confounding are greatly reduced. Through 1997, the four highest-quality RCTs (Figure 17-1) have studied three different products—a gel,[18] the film,[20,23] and the sponge.[17] In the aggregate, these studies have shown that N-9 spermicide used alone reduces the risks of bacterial infection only modestly. The users' relative risk of acquiring gonorrhea, chlamydia, trichomoniasis, or bacterial vaginosis was about 0.75 (a 25% reduction in risk). However, even this modest risk reduction may be questionable because the range for statistical variation could not rule out chance.

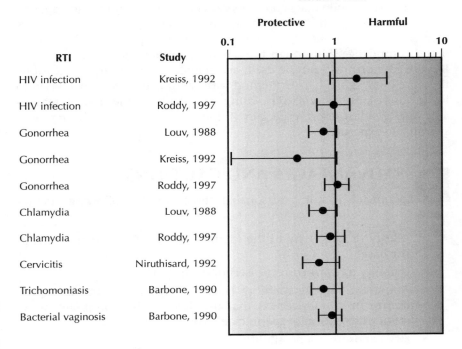

*Indicates 95% confidence interval

Figure 17-1 Relation of nonoxynol-9 spermicide use to risk of reproductive tract infection (RTI)

In addition, no evidence indicates that N-9 provides any protection against HIV. The most recent investigation of N-9 in Cameroon found that vaginal contraceptive film containing 72 mg of N-9 provided no additional protection against HIV and other STIs when provided as part of an overall HIV/STI prevention program.[23] This comprehensive program included behavioral change counseling, promotion and distribution of male latex condoms, and monthly screening and treatment of STI. Until the association between spermicide use and HIV risk is better understood, do not recommend the use of spermicide alone to prevent HIV. Furthermore, frequent use of spermicides can cause vulvovaginal epithelial disruption, which theoretically could increase susceptibility to HIV. Therefore, advise caution about frequent use of spermicide when HIV exposure is a concern. (See Chapter 7 on HIV/AIDS and Reproductive Health.)

We have a critical need for female-controlled methods to prevent STIs, including HIV. While male condoms provide excellent protection against STIs, their use is low among many couples at high risk.[14,27] Methods women can use autonomously may improve their protection because of better compliance,[24] although the science on this topic is still unclear.[3,4] If male condoms will not be used, and female condoms are not feasible, then use of a vaginal barrier method with spermicide has been advised to lower the risk of bacterial STIs. Using spermicides alone may be reasonable only as a last resort, especially if doing so does not involve repeated spermicide exposure.

D ISADVANTAGES AND CAUTIONS

Spermicide is not a reasonable choice in the following circumstances:

- Allergy or sensitivity to the spermicidal agent or to ingredients in the base
- Inability to learn correct insertion technique
- Abnormal vaginal anatomy (such as vaginal septum, prolapsed uterus, or double cervix) that interferes with appropriate placement or retention of spermicide
- HIV exposure is a possibility

Irritation.   Temporary skin irritation involving the vulva, vagina, or penis caused by either local toxicity or allergy is the most common problem associated with spermicide use. Vaginal epithelial disruption has been associated with frequent use (once-a-day or more).[13,22] However, symptoms of irritation do not necessarily indicate epithelial disruption. When an allergy is suspected, suggest the client try another contraceptive method. If epithelial disruption is found, advise the client to use spermicides less frequently or to discontinue their use.

Common dislikes.   Some couples find the taste of spermicide unpleasant when they engage in oral-genital sex. Some women find the effervescence of foaming vaginal suppositories is unpleasant or vaginal suppository products do not melt or disperse as intended.

Yeast vaginitis.   Women who use sponges have an increased incidence of symptomatic candidiasis.[25] Use of a diaphragm with spermicide can also increase vaginal colonization with Candida species.[15]

Bacterial vaginosis.   Spermicide use can encourage selective colonization of the vagina with anaerobic bacteria and uropathogens relatively resistant to N-9.[16] This mechanism may also explain the increased incidence of urinary tract infection reported among women who use the diaphragm, since wearing this device entails spermicide exposure for most women.

Systemic effects. No serious adverse reactions to the spermicide products now marketed in the United States have been reported. In 1980, an advisory panel for the U.S. Food and Drug Administration (FDA), reviewing published information and information from manufacturers, approved them as safe and effective. However, toxicology studies to determine the degree of vaginal absorption and to detect possible systemic effects are limited. Intravaginal exposure to large doses of N-9 has been associated with abnormalities such as liver toxicity.[5,19]

Spermicide use and pregnancy. Several studies have reported possible adverse associations between spermicide exposure and birth defects; however, serious methodologic problems weakened the investigations and questioned the conclusions.[28] Subsequent research has *not* confirmed an association between adverse fetal effects and spermicide use.[7,26] Thus, no apparent causal association exists between spermicide use and fetal defects.

PROVIDING SPERMICIDES

Spermicides are currently available over-the-counter. When providing spermicides in a clinical setting, reinforce instructions for proper use and remind users about common errors that can lead to unintended pregnancy. (See the section on Instructions for Using Spermicides). Counsel users about emergency contraception as a back-up. Warn women who have abnormalities of vaginal anatomy (such as a septate vagina or a severe uterine prolapse), which may interfere with proper spermicide placement, that spermicide use may not be effective for them.

Spermicide acceptability affects correct and consistent use, which in turn determines contraceptive effectiveness.[12] Women have found the N-9 film and gel formulations preferable to suppositories.[27] Men have found spermicides to be at least as acceptable as women have.[12] Given men's influence in sexual decision making, encouraging them to suggest spermicide use or at least to cooperate with their partner's desire to use spermicides could be a helpful approach for increasing spermicide prevalence.

MANAGING PROBLEMS AND FOLLOW-UP

Spermicide use does not require any special follow-up. Women who experience irritation may seek care. If symptoms persist more than a day or two after the patient discontinues using spermicides, evaluate the underlying factors, such as STI exposure, yeast vaginitis, or bacterial vaginosis. If irritation occurs immediately after insertion of spermicide, sensitivity rather than true allergy is the likely diagnosis. Changing to an alternative product with a different formulation or changing to a less concentrated product may help (Table 17-1).

INSTRUCTIONS FOR USING SPERMICIDES

1. Use spermicide every time you have intercourse. Be sure spermicide is in place before your partner's penis enters your vagina.
2. If you have subsequent problems with vaginal or penile irritation, you may want to try a different spermicide product. You could switch to condoms or see your clinician for another method of birth control.
3. You can use condoms along with spermicide if you wish. By using this combination, contraceptive protection should more effective and your risk of sexually transmitted infection is greatly reduced.

COMMON ERRORS IN SPERMICIDE USE

Common errors can lead to unintended pregnancy:

- Failing to use spermicide or an alternative method such as condoms each and every time intercourse occurs, even when menstrual bleeding is present
- Failing to place spermicide high enough in the vaginal vault to be effective
- Failing to wait long enough after insertion for suppositories or film to dissolve and disperse
- Failing to use another application of spermicide if more than 1 hour has elapsed between insertion and intercourse
- Using too little spermicide or foam, or failing to shake the foam can vigorously enough
- Failing to use another applicator with every repeated act of intercourse
- Failing to recognize that the foam bottle or spermicide tube is empty
- Failing to have spermicide available

Before Intercourse

1. Check to be sure you have all the supplies you need. If you are using foam, cream, or gel, you may also need a plastic applicator. If you use foam, keep an extra container on hand. You may not be able to tell when your current container is running low.

2. Plan ahead about when to insert your method. Try to find a routine that is comfortable for you and your partner. If you are using suppositories, or film, a waiting period between insertion and intercourse is essential to allow the product to melt or spread inside your vagina. The package instructions explain the exact time required. One dose of most spermicide formulations remains effective for 1 hour. If a longer time has passed, or if you have intercourse again, you must use a new dose of spermicide.

For Insertion

1. Wash your hands carefully with soap and water.

2. *Foam.* Shake the foam container vigorously at least 20 times then use the nozzle to fill the plastic applicator.

   Gel, Cream, or Foam. Fill the applicator by squeezing the spermicide tube. Next insert the applicator into your vagina as far as it will comfortably go; then, holding the applicator still, push the plunger to release the gel, cream, or foam. The spermicide should be deep in your vagina, close to your cervix.

   Suppository. Remove the wrapping and slide the suppository into your vagina. Push it along the back wall of your vagina as far as you can so it rests on or near your cervix.

   Film. Be sure your fingers are completely dry. Place one sheet of film on your finger tip and slide it along the back wall of your vagina as far as you can so the film rests on or near your cervix.

3. **Repeated intercourse**. Apply a new application of spermicide each time you have intercourse. Alternatively, you can switch to condoms for repeated intercourse if you wish.

4. **After intercourse**. Leave spermicide in place for at least 6 hours after intercourse; do not douche or rinse your vagina. Douching is not recommended, but if you choose to douche you must wait at least 6 hours.

Caring for Spermicide Supplies

1. Store your spermicide in a convenient location that is clean, cool, and dark.
2. After each use wash your reusable applicator with plain soap and warm water. Do not use talcum powder on your applicator.

References

1. Alexander NJ. Barriers to sexually transmitted diseases. Sci Med 1996;2(Mar/Apr):32-41.
2. Cates W Jr, Stone KM. Family planning, sexually transmitted diseases, and contraceptive choice: a literature update. Part I. Fam Plann Perspect 1992;24:75-84.
3. Cates W Jr, Stewart FH, Trussell J. The quest for women's prophylactic methods: hopes vs. science. Am J Public Health 1992;82:1479-1482.
4. Centers for Disease Control and Prevention. What do we know about nonoxynol-9 for HIV and STD prevention? CDC Update. Atlanta GA: CDC, April 1997.
5. Chvapil M, Droegemueller W, Earnest DL. Liver function tests in women using intravaginal spermicide nonoxynol-9 [letter]. Fertil Steril 1982;37:281-282.
6. Costello Daly C, Helling-Giese GE, Mati JK, Hunter DJ. Contraceptive methods and the transmission of HIV: implications for family planning. Genitourin Med 1994;70:110-117.
7. Einarson TR, Koren G, Mattice D, Schechter-Tsafriri O. Maternal spermicide use and adverse reproductive outcome: a meta-analysis. Am J Obstet Gynecol 1990;162:655-660.
8. Elias CJ, Coggin C. Female-controlled methods to prevent sexual transmission of HIV. AIDS 1996;10(suppl 3):S43-S51.
9. Family Health International. Barrier methods. Network 1996;16:1-23.
10. Feldblum P, Joanis C. Modern barrier methods: effective contraception and disease prevention. Research Triangle Park NC: Family Health International, 1994.
11. Feldblum PJ, Morrison CS, Roddy RE, Cates W Jr. The effectiveness of barrier methods of contraception in preventing the spread of HIV. AIDS 1995;9(suppl A):S85-S93.
12. Feldblum PJ, Weir SS. The protective effect of nonoxynol-9 against HIV infection [letter]. Am J Public Health 1994;84:1032-1034.
13. Goeman J, Ndoye I, Sakho LM, et al. Frequent use of menfegol spermicidal vaginal foaming tablets associated with a high incidence of genital lesions. J Infect Dis 1995;171:1611-1614.
14. Hira SK, Spruyt AB, Feldblum PJ, et al. Spermicide acceptability among patients at a sexually transmitted disease clinic in Zambia. Am J Public Health 1995;85: 1098-1103.
15. Hooton TM, Fennell CL, Clark AM, Stamm WE. Nonoxynol-9: differential antibacterial activity and enhancement of bacterial adherence to vaginal epithelial cells. J Infect Dis 1991;164:1216-1219.

16. Hooton TM, Scholes D, Hughes JP, et al. A prospective study of risk factors for symptomatic urinary tract infection in young women. N Engl J Med 1996;335:468-474.
17. Kreiss J, Ngugi E, Holmes K, Ndinya-Achola J, Waiyaki P, Roberts PL, Ruminjo I, Sajabi R, Kimata J, Fleming TR, Anzala A, Holton D, Plummer F. Efficacy of nonoxynol-9 contraceptive sponge use in preventing heterosexual acquisition of HIV in Nairobi prostitutes. JAMA 1992;268:477-482.
18. Louv WC, Austin H, Alexander WJ, Stagno S, Cheeks J. A clinical trial of nonoxynol-9 for preventing gonococcal and chlamydial infections. J Infect Dis 1988;158:518-523.
19. Malyk B. Preliminary results: serum chemistry values before and after the intravaginal administration of 5% nonoxynol-9 cream. Fertil Steril 1981;36:647-652.
20. Niruthisard S, Roddy RE, Chutivongse S. Use of nonoxynol-9 and reduction in rate of gonococcal and chlamydial cervical infections. Lancet 1992;339:1371-1375.
21. Pauwels R, DeClercq E. Development of vaginal microbicides for the prevention of heterosexual transmission of HIV. J AIDS Hum Retrov 1996;11: 211-221.
22. Roddy RE, Cordero M, Cordero C, Fortney JA. A dosing study of nonoxynol-9 and genital irritation. Int J STD AIDS 1993;4:165-170.
23. Roddy RE, Zekeng L, Ryan KA, Tamoufe U, Weir SS, Din E, Wong E, Dominik R, Taylor D, Wheeless A. A randomized controlled trial of the effect of nonoxynol-9 film on male-to-female transmission of HIV-1. Presented at National Institute of Allergy and Infectious Disease Ad Hoc Meeting, Bethesda MD, April 9, 1997.
24. Rosenberg MJ, Gollub EL. Commentary: methods women can use that may prevent sexually transmitted disease, including HIV. Am J Public Health 1992;82:1473-1478.
25. Rosenberg MJ, Rojanapithayakorn W, Feldblum PJ, Higgins JE. Effect of the contraceptive sponge on chlamydial infection, gonorrhea, and candidiasis: a comparative clinical trial. JAMA 1987;257:2308-2312.
26. Simpson JL, Phillips OP. Spermicides, hormonal contraception and congenital malformations. Adv Contracept 1990;6:141-167.
27. Steiner M, Spruyt A, Joanis C, et al. Acceptability of spermicidal film and foaming tablets among women in three countries. Int Fam Plann Perspect 1995;21:104-107.
28. Strobino B, Kline J, Warburton D. Spermicide use and pregnancy outcome. Am J Public Health 1988;78:260-263.

Vaginal Barriers

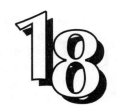

THE DIAPHRAGM, CONTRACEPTIVE SPONGE, CERVICAL CAP, AND FEMALE CONDOM

Felicia Stewart, MD

- Vaginal barriers are simple to use and non-invasive. They can be used intermittently with little advance planning.
- Reduced risks for some sexually transmitted infections (STIs) have been reported for diaphragm and sponge users, and using spermicide may reduce the transmission of some STIs including gonorrhea and chlamydia, albeit at modest levels (as much as 20%). Protection against human immunodeficiency virus (HIV) has not been documented for spermicide or vaginal barriers used with spermicide.
- Except for the female condom, using barrier methods does not require the direct involvement of the male partner and does not interrupt lovemaking.
- Consistent and correct use is essential for vaginal barrier effectiveness; most pregnancies occur because the method is not used.

When Margaret Sanger and Emma Goldman visited Europe in the early 1900s, they found a wide variety of cap and diaphragm models being used. The diaphragm soon became "the" modern contraceptive method in the United States. In 1925, Sanger's husband established Holland Rantos, the first U.S. diaphragm manufacturer.[9] Except for improvements in spermicides used with it, diaphragm technology changed little during its first 60 years in the United States. The most recent development was the 1983 introduction of a new model, the wide-seal style, with a soft latex flange attached to the inner side of the rim.

Earlier in this century, cervical caps were made of silver, copper, or impermeable plastic. Inserted and removed by the woman's physician, they were left in place for as long as 3 to 4 weeks. These have been replaced by latex caps now manufactured in England. In 1988 the Food and Drug Administration (FDA) approved one such product, the Prentif Cavity Rim Cervical Cap, for general use in the United States.

In 1983, the FDA approved a vaginal contraceptive sponge for use in the United States. The Today Sponge, containing nonoxynol-9 spermicide, was marketed in the U.S. until 1995 when its distribution was stopped because the manufacturer decided not to invest in needed modernization of production equipment. Vaginal contraceptive sponges containing nonoxynol-9 continue to be marketed in other countries, as are similar products containing other spermicides, such as benzalkonium chloride.

The first female condom, called Reality, was approved by the FDA in 1993 for over-the-counter sale in the United States. For ethical reasons, researchers did not include women at risk for sexually transmitted infection (STI) in the efficacy research that was required for FDA approval. Thus, available research provides only indirect evidence of its likely efficacy in reducing STI risk. Design of the female condom, and its physical properties, however, are appropriate to the task.

M ECHANISM OF ACTION

The female condom provides a physical barrier that lines the vagina entirely and partially shields the perineum. Diaphragms, caps, and sponges combine two contraceptive mechanisms: a physical barrier to shield the cervix and a chemical to kill sperm. These devices also may help to hold spermicide in place against the cervix, and in the case of the sponge, absorb and trap sperm.

VAGINAL BARRIER OPTIONS

Female condom. The Reality Female Condom is a soft, loose-fitting polyurethane sheath, 7.8 cm in diameter and 17 cm long. It contains two flexible polyurethane rings. One ring lies inside, at the closed end of the sheath, and serves as an insertion mechanism and internal anchor. The other ring forms the external, open edge of the device and remains outside the vagina after insertion (Figure 18-1). The external portion of the device provides some protection to the labia and the base of the penis during intercourse. The sheath is coated on the inside with a silicone-based lubricant; additional lubricant for the outside is provided with the device. The lubricant does not contain spermicide. Reality, approved for over-the-counter sale without prescription, is intended for one-time use. It can be inserted up to 8 hours before intercourse. Female and male condoms should not be used together; they can adhere to each other, causing slippage or displacement of one or both devices.

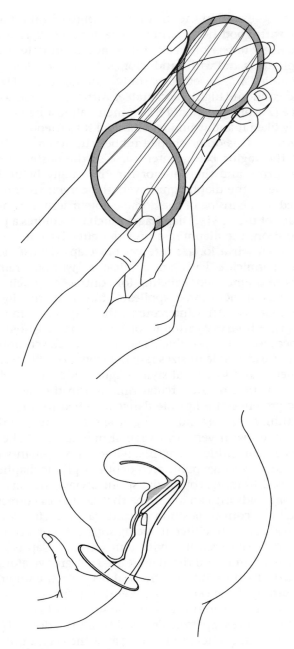

Figure 18-1 Reality Female Condom

The polyurethane used in the sheath is a thin (0.05 mm) but impermeable material with good heat-transfer characteristics. It is stronger than latex and less likely to tear or break. It does not deteriorate with exposure to oil-based products and withstands storage better than latex does.

Couples enrolled in the efficacy study conducted for FDA approval found female condoms highly acceptable. Although some users did not like the device (7% of women and 8% of men), almost half of the couples indicated they liked it and would recommend it to friends.[17]

Diaphragm.   This dome-shaped rubber cup has a flexible rim; it is inserted into the vagina before intercourse so the posterior rim rests in the posterior fornix and the anterior rim fits snugly behind the pubic bone. The dome of the diaphragm covers the cervix; spermicidal cream or jelly applied to the inside of the dome before insertion is held in place near the surface of the cervix. Diaphragm purchase requires a prescription.

Once in position, the diaphragm provides effective contraceptive protection for 6 hours. If a longer interval has elapsed, insertion of additional, fresh spermicide with an applicator (without removing the diaphragm) is recommended. Labeling for contraceptive jelly and cream also recommends an additional applicator-full of spermicide whenever intercourse is repeated. After intercourse, the diaphragm must be left in place for at least 6 hours. Wearing it for longer than 24 hours is not recommended because of the possible risk of toxic shock syndrome (TSS).

Diaphragms are available in sizes ranging from 50 millimeters (mm) to 95 mm (diameter) and in several styles (Figure 18-2). The styles differ in the inner construction of the circular rim, and in the case of the wide-seal style, the presence of a flexible flange attached to the inner edge of the rim. The thin, *flat spring* rim has a gentle spring strength that is comfortable for women with very firm vaginal muscle tone. The sturdy *coil spring* rim has a firm spring strength suitable for a woman with average muscle tone and an average pubic arch depth. A plastic diaphragm introducer can be used to insert coil or flat spring styles. The very sturdy and firm *arcing spring* folds into an arc shape that facilitates correct insertion; it can maintain a correct position despite lax muscle. Wide-seal diaphragms are available with either an arcing spring rim or a coil spring rim.

Cervical cap.   The Prentif Cavity Rim Cervical Cap is a soft, deep rubber cup with a firm round rim (Figure 18-3). A groove along the inner circumference of the rim improves the seal between the inner rim of the cap and the surface of the cervix. The Prentif cap fits with its rim snugly around the base of the cervix, close to the junction between the cervix and the vaginal fornices. Spermicide, used to fill the dome 1/3 full prior to insertion of the cap, is held in place against the cervix until the cap is removed.

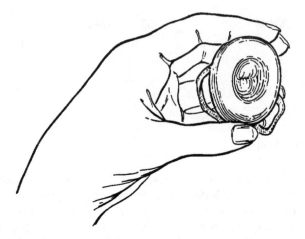

Figure 18-2 Contraceptive sponge

The cap provides continuous contraceptive protection for 48 hours, no matter how many times intercourse occurs. Additional spermicide is not necessary for repeated intercourse. Because of the possible risk of TSS, wear for longer than 48 hours is not recommended. Some women experience odor problems with more prolonged use.

Contraceptive sponge. The Today Sponge is a small, pillow-shaped polyurethane sponge containing 1 gram of nonoxynol-9 spermicide. The

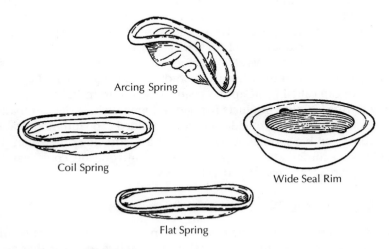

Arcing Spring

Coil Spring

Wide Seal Rim

Flat Spring

Figure 18-3 Types of diaphragms

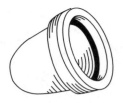

Prentif Cavity Rim Cervical Cap

Figure 18-4 Cervical cap

concave dimple on one side was designed to fit over the cervix and decrease the chance of dislodgement during intercourse (Figure 18-4). The other side of the sponge incorporates a woven polyester loop to facilitate removal. The sponge is a one-size, over-the-counter product. It is moistened with tap water prior to use and inserted deep into the vagina.

The sponge protects for up to 24 hours, no matter how many times intercourse occurs. After intercourse, the sponge must be left in place for at least 6 hours before it is removed and discarded. Wearing the sponge for longer than 24 to 30 hours is not recommended because of the possible risk of TSS.

Future barrier devices. Several new vaginal barrier devices are on the horizon. Lea's Shield, an oval, silicone rubber device (Figure 18-5) is used with spermicide with rules similar to those for the diaphragm, but it has only one size so fitting is not required. Participants in an efficacy study found the Lea's Shield comfortable and acceptable, and the failure rate of 8.7 pregnancies per 100 women over the 6-month study was similar to rates observed in previous efficacy studies for the cervical cap, diaphragm and sponge when standardized for parity in the study populations.[37] An FDA committee recommended further research be reported before approval, but found results from the study promising. A hat-shaped silicone rubber cap called FemCap has been successful in initial contraceptive efficacy testing.[52] Other products being developed include devices made of polymers that release spermicide, a custom-molded cap, and modifications of the contraceptive sponge. A sponge with a spermicide other than non-oxynol-9, or a combination of spermicide and microbicide, could have significant advantages, especially in STI protection.

E FFECTIVENESS

Parity affects vaginal barrier efficacy significantly. For parous women, the sponge and the cap are substantially less effective than the diaphragm or female condom (Table 18-1).[62] For nulliparous women, the female condom, diaphragm, cervical cap, and sponge all provide similar contraceptive efficacy during typical use; with perfect use, the female condom and diaphragm are somewhat more effective than the cap or sponge.

Efficacy and diligence. To make an informed choice, a woman needs to understand what correct use of the method requires, and what success she can expect if she is able to use it consistently and correctly. About half of the women who become pregnant while using vaginal barrier methods report contraceptive failure has occurred in a context of imperfect use. The other half experience method failure despite correct use. From 5% to 9% of nulliparous users and from 5% to 26% of parous users of these methods will become pregnant during the first year of perfect use.[3,13,61] So it is misleading to teach patients that all conscientious barrier users can achieve high efficacy. The difference between low failure rates reported in some studies and high rates reported in others is not accounted for entirely by patient diligence. The wide range reflects the profound effect of differences between study populations in fertility characteristics as well as in patient compliance. Differences in study design and analysis methods also are important factors.

Table 18-1 First-year probability of pregnancy* for women using vaginal barrier methods

Method	% of Women Experiencing an Unintended Pregnancy Within the First Year of Use		% of Women Continuing Use at One Year
	Typical Use	Perfect Use	
Cap			
Parous Women	40	26	42
Nulliparous Women	20	9	56
Sponge			
Parous Women	40	20	42
Nulliparous Women	20	9	56
Female Condom	21	5	56
Diaphragm	20	6	56

*See Table 9-2 for first-year probability of pregnancy of all methods.

Emergency Contraceptive Pills: Treatment initiated within 72 hours after unprotected intercourse reduces the risk of pregnancy by at least 75%. (See Chapter 12 for more information.)

Efficacy and fertility characteristics. A woman who uses a diaphragm with typical diligence but has characteristics associated with high fertility, such as age less than 25 years and frequent intercourse (three times weekly or more), is more likely to experience contraceptive failure than is the average woman. In effect, the failure rate for her is greater than the 20% overall "typical-user" rate for the diaphragm. On the other hand, citing an 20% failure rate significantly overestimates the pregnancy risk for a 30-year-old diaphragm user who has intercourse less often. Available research data are limited, but they do show the effect of such factors is substantial. For example, in the diaphragm/cap comparison study, women who used the diaphragm consistently, and had intercourse three times weekly or more, were almost three times as likely to experience failure compared with women who had intercourse less than three times weekly (Table 18-2).

Efficacy and research design. Because the 1976 study by Lane, et al., is so often cited as evidence that conscientious diaphragm users can achieve highly effective contraceptive protection, it deserves special comment.[33] Lane reported an overall failure rate of 2.1% for 2,168 women using the diaphragm for 1 year. At the time this estimate was calculated, however, the accepted procedures for data analysis were different from those used in more recent studies. Subjects who were no more than 2 months late for a follow-up visit were assumed to be continuing, successful users. Consequently, up to 14 months of successful diaphragm use were counted for women who had been enrolled in the study and were no more than 2 months late for their follow-up visit (a 1-year visit) when the study ended. Data analysis procedures used in more recent studies would have credited months of successful use only for patients who actually did return for follow-up. Using current analysis methods, Lane would have reported a substantially higher failure rate.

Spermicide: essential or not essential? Several researchers and no doubt many vaginal barrier users have wondered whether using spermicide with a diaphragm or cap is really necessary. An enthusiastic 1980

Table 18-2 Intercourse frequency and diaphragm failure

	Contraceptive Failure Within One Year (%)
Consistent diaphragm user Intercourse less than 3 times weekly	3.4%
Consistent diaphragm user Intercourse 3 times weekly or more	9.7%

Source: Trussell, et al., (1993).

article described spermicide-free diaphragm use and has been the subject of considerable speculation.[7,58] Recently reported research, however, indicates that spermicide may be important in achieving satisfactory contraceptive efficacy with these devices. Results of a pilot study that replicated the 1980 study design found women using the diaphragm without spermicide had a failure rate of 24 pregnancies per 100 women within 12 months.[54] Similarly, women using the new diaphragm-like Lea's Shield device without spermicide experienced almost twice as many pregnancies as those who used spermicide (9.3 pregnancies over the 6-month study interval compared with 5.6 pregnancies).[37]

COST

The cost for obtaining a diaphragm or cap ranges from $50 to $150, depending on the fee for the necessary medical visit and device fitting. Purchase of a cap or diaphragm alone is about $30 to $40; replacement is recommended every 2 years for the diaphragm, and annually for the cap. The only ongoing cost for these methods is for spermicide; the amount of spermicide needed depends on intercourse frequency. Cream or jelly cost is minimal, about $0.25 per application. Reality Female Condoms cost $2.50 each. Sponges, not currently marketed in the U.S., cost $1.25 to $1.50 each when last sold here. A similar sponge product, called Protectaid, is available in Canada. Protectaid sponges contain benzalkonium chloride, sodium cholate, and nonoxynol-9. Protectaid sponges for personal use (small quantities) can be ordered legally from Canada through the supplier's website: http://www.birthcontrol.com.

ADVANTAGES AND INDICATIONS

Vaginal barrier methods have many advantages that make them reasonable for both short-term and long-term contraception. Apart from the issue of sexually transmitted infection protection, the overall medical safety of these methods, backed up by abortion in case of failure, is comparable to consistent use of male condoms. They do not cause systemic side effects and do not alter a woman's hormone patterns.

For many women, relying on a partner to use condoms is not a realistic option. Except for the female condom, vaginal barrier methods do not require partner involvement in the decision to use them or in their implementation.

For women who need contraception only intermittently, a vaginal barrier can be available for immediate protection whenever needed, no matter how long the interval between uses. No doubt many pregnancies have been prevented because a woman had available a vaginal barrier device obtained long before.

Sexually transmitted infection (STI) protection. The female condom lines the vagina completely, preventing contact between the penis and vagina. The condom traps semen and is then discarded. Polyurethane is strong and impermeable to organisms as small as the HIV virus.[12] In a study of postcoital leakage designed to detect pinholes and tears after actual condom use, 3.5% of male latex condoms showed leakage when tested after use compared with 0.6% of Reality condoms.[34] Unless the female condom slips out of place or is torn, it should provide protection against STI exposure that is as least as good as that provided by latex male condoms. Research documentation, however, is limited. A small study confirmed that consistent, correct use of female condoms is effective in preventing trichomonas reinfection.[55]

With the exception of the female condom, all vaginal barrier methods involve use of spermicide. Laboratory research shows nonoxynol-9 is lethal to the organisms that cause gonorrhea, genital herpes, trichomoniasis, syphilis, and acquired immunodeficiency syndrome (AIDS). (See Chapter 7 on HIV/AIDS and Reproductive Health.) Unfortunately nonoxynol-9's lethal effect in the test tube has not translated directly to effective protection in human studies. Factors such as even dispersion of spermicide in the vagina, or thorough mixing of semen and vaginal fluids with the spermicide, may influence infection protection. Spermicide use also may alter vaginal flora or acidity, which could affect susceptibility to infection.[1]

Potentially, protection against spread of STIs could be the most important noncontraceptive benefit of vaginal barrier use. Unfortunately, uncertainty about the effect of spermicide on HIV risk clouds this issue for barriers used with spermicide (see the section on Special Issues).

Gonorrhea, chlamydia, trichomoniasis, and sequelae. The degree of risk reduction for gonorrhea, chlamydia, and trichomoniasis reported for women who use a diaphragm or sponge with spermicide differs across various studies (Table 18-3). Although some researchers have reported very effective protection, most have concluded the risk reduction is modest.[11,47] One of the few randomized studies able to distinguish between the effect of spermicide versus the effect of self-selection bias—an important issue in studies of women who have voluntarily chosen to use a method—found spermicide users had a 20% reduction in risk.[36] A reduced risk for STI consequences such as pelvic inflammatory disease (PID) and tubal infertility has also been documented for diaphragm users.[10,30] In both the PID study and in the tubal infertility study, women

Table 18-3 STI protection with use of vaginal barrier methods

Reference[a]	STI Studied	Relative Risk 95% Confidence Interval	
Soper (1992) US Gyn Clinics Female Condom	Trichomoniasis (Reinfection)	0.00***	
Rosenberg (1992) Colorado STD Clinic* Diaphragm	Gonorrhea Trichomoniasis Chlamydia Bacterial Vaginosis	0.35 0.29 0.28 0.99	(0.16–0.75) (0.15–0.58) (0.05–1.54) (0.63–1.55)
Kjaer (1990) Greenland and Denmark** Condom or Diaphragm	Cervical HPV Herpes 2 Seropositivity	1.00 0.90	(0.70–1.40) (0.60–1.30)
Magder (1988) Colorado STD Clinic Diaphragm	Gonorrhea Chlamydia	Protective (p less than 0.001) 0.00	(0.00–0.20)
Cramer (1987) US Infertility Centers* Diaphragm	Tubal Infertility	0.50	(0.30–0.70)
Rosenberg (1987) Thailand Prostitutes*** Sponge	Gonorrhea Chlamydia	0.67 0.31	(0.42–1.07) (0.16–0.60)
Quinn (1985) Tennessee STD Clinic*** Diaphragm or Condom	Gonorrhea	0.11	(0.08–0.17)
Austin (1982) Alabama STD Clinic* Diaphragm	Gonorrhea	0.45	(0.12–1.67)
Kelaghan (1982) US Hospitals* Diaphragm	Pelvic Inflammatory Disease	0.40	(0.20–0.70)
Berger (1975) Louisiana Family Planning Clinic** Diaphragm or Condom, with foam	Gonorrhea	0.53	(0.18–1.59)

Source: adapted from Cates, et al., (1992b)

*Case-control study; **Cross-sectional study, ***Randomized study, ***Subjects volunteered to use female condom after initial treatment and did so with 100% compliance
[a]Full reference listed in original article by Cates.

Table 18-4 Contraceptive method and cervical neoplasia risk

Study and Method	Risk Estimate
Parazzini (1989)	Relative Risk (RR) / Use of Barrier Method (Condom or Diaphragm)
Never Used Barrier	1.0
Used Less Than 2 Years	0.86
Used 2 Years or More	0.57
Celentano (1987)	Odds Ratio/ Ever Used Method
Oral Contraceptives	0.48
Diaphragm	0.29
Vaginal Spermicides	0.28
Peters (1986)	Matched Risk / Duration of Use (Use Less Than 2 Years = RR 1.0)
Oral Contraceptives, 2–9 Years	1.0
Oral Contraceptives, 10 Years or More	1.1
Diaphragm, 2–9 Years	0.7
Diaphragm, 10 Years or More	0.3
Spermicide Alone, 2–9 Years	0.7
Spermicide Alone, 10 Years or More	0.2
Condoms, 2–9 Years	0.5
Condoms,10 Years or More	0.4
Vessey (1978)	Neoplasia Incidence / 1,000 Woman–Years
All Women	0.73
Oral Contraceptives	0.95
IUD Users	0.87
Diaphragm Users	0.17

Source: Celentano, et al., (1987); Parazzini, et al., (1989); Peters, et al., (1986); Vessey (1978).

using spermicide along with a mechanical barrier had lower risks for PID and ectopic pregnancy than did women who chose to use condoms alone or spermicide alone.[6]

Some studies that have compared STI risks for women who rely on condom use with the risks for vaginal barrier users have found lower risk among barrier users,[47] concluding that these methods can in some circumstances be more effective than condoms because they are managed entirely by the woman.[4] The variation in the observed risks, however, could also be explained by other differences between women who choose to use barrier methods and those who choose to rely on condoms.

Cervical neoplasia risk. A lower risk of cervical dysplasia and cancer has been reported for women using the diaphragm as well as for condom users and spermicide users in several studies (Table 18-4). Because cervical infection with certain strains of human papilloma virus (HPV) has been implicated as an important factor in cervical neoplasia, the role of diaphragm use here may be similar to the reduced risk observed for other STIs; alternatively, women who choose to use the diaphragm may be at lower risk for HPV for reasons unrelated to effects of the diaphragm itself.

D ISADVANTAGES AND CAUTIONS

Few serious medical problems are associated with use of vaginal barriers, and most women are medically appropriate candidates for their use. Both TSS and pregnancy complications (following method failure) are potentially life-threatening, but rare. An increased susceptibility to acquiring HIV infection also would be a serious disadvantage, if this proves to be a consequence of spermicide-induced irritation (see the section on Special Issues).[31] Using vaginal barrier methods with spermicide also increases the risk for urinary tract infection (UTI), bacterial vaginosis, and vaginal candidiasis.

Common minor problems. Problems are not common with use of the female condom. Among 360 women in the efficacy study, one discontinued using the method because of vaginal discomfort and one because her partner experienced penile irritation.

The most common problem associated with vaginal barriers used with spermicide is local skin irritation. Some patients are allergic or sensitive to nonoxynol-9, and some women have cramps, bladder pain, or rectal pain when wearing a diaphragm or cap. Rare cases of vaginal trauma, including abrasion and laceration, have been reported with use of the Prentif cap and the diaphragm.[3] Partners occasionally report penile pain during intercourse. For diaphragm users, refitting with an alternative size or rim type resolves the problem in some cases.

Problems with sponge removal are fairly common. Some sponge users have difficulty with vaginal dryness. Foul odor and vaginal discharge are likely to occur if a diaphragm, cap, or sponge is inadvertently left in the vagina for more than a few days. Symptoms abate promptly when the device is removed.

Latex allergy. Latex allergy is an increasingly common and potentially serious problem that requires clinical alertness. In most cases allergy causes local cutaneous symptoms such as erythema, pruritis, and rash. For some individuals, however, latex allergy triggers serious systemic hypersensitivity with the potential for anaphylaxis that can be fatal. The incidence of latex allergy is especially high among health care workers repeatedly exposed to use of latex gloves, and among individuals who have had multiple surgeries, especially those involving latex medical equipment such as ostomy devices. Anyone who has a confirmed or suspected latex allergy should avoid exposure to latex vaginal barrier devices including latex diaphragms and caps as well as latex male condoms. Plastic female or male condoms are appropriate alternatives.

Vaginal and urinary tract infections. Both sexual intercourse itself and sexual intercourse with use of a diaphragm and spermicide are followed by increased vaginal colonization with *Escherichia coli.*[27] The shift in vaginal flora is prolonged among women who use spermicide alone or in combination with condoms, and even more prolonged among diaphragm users, when compared with women using oral contraceptives.[27,48] This finding is of concern because bacterial vaginosis (BV) may be associated with increased risk for upper genital tract infection[5] and serious perinatal morbidity and because it may account for the increased risk of UTI observed among diaphragm users.[22,24,64] A study of UTIs among women exposed to condoms lubricated with spermicide challenges the hypothesis that diaphragm rim pressure on the urethra accounts for UTI risk among diaphragm users. Researchers documented a significantly increased frequency of UTIs among women using spermicide-coated condoms more than once weekly (relative odds 2.11) compared with age-matched controls, and increasing risk with increased exposure (relative odds 5.65 for those using the method more than twice weekly). Women exposed to use of plain condoms did not have an increased risk of UTI.[21] These results indicate that spermicide exposure is an important risk factor for UTI, although it is possible mechanical factors in diaphragm use also may contribute to the risk of developing UTI for some women.

Toxic shock syndrome. TSS is a rare but serious disorder caused by toxin(s) released by some strains of *Staphylococcus aureus.* Most TSS occurs in association with tampon use during menses; nonmenstrual TSS risk is increased for women who use vaginal barrier methods.[51] The overall health risks attributable to TSS, however, are very low. Two or three cases of TSS per year can be expected for every 100,000 women using vaginal barrier methods.[51] These cases would result in less than 1 death (0.18) annually for every 100,000 vaginal barrier users, while complications of pregnancy that occur as a result of method failure would cause almost seven times this many deaths (1.2 deaths per 100,000 users).

Nevertheless, patients using vaginal barriers need to be aware of the TSS danger signs and receive user instructions consistent with recommended TSS precautions.

Systemic effects and pregnancy exposure. No serious systemic side effects have been reported in association with human use of spermicides; safety concerns have centered on the issue of fetal exposure related to their accidental use during early pregnancy. Although studies in 1981 and 1982 suggested a possible link between spermicides and birth defects,[28,29,49] subsequent studies have not confirmed this finding. Experts in the field have concluded no true association exists between spermicide use and fetal defects.[14,23,53,60]

CAUTIONS

The following conditions may preclude satisfactory use or make use of one or more of the vaginal barrier methods inadvisable:

1. Allergy to spermicide, rubber, latex, or polyurethane
2. Abnormalities in vaginal anatomy that interfere with a satisfactory fit or stable placement of a female condom, diaphragm, cap or sponge
3. Inability to learn correct insertion technique
4. (For all vaginal barriers except female condom) History of TSS
5. (For all vaginal barriers except female condom) Repeated UTIs
6. (For all vaginal barriers except female condom) Need for HIV protection
7. (For the diaphragm and cap) Lack of trained personnel to fit the device or lack of clinical time to provide instruction
8. (For the cap and sponges) Full-term delivery within the past 6 weeks, recent spontaneous or induced abortion, or vaginal bleeding from any cause, including menstrual flow
9. (For the cap) Known or suspected cervical or uterine malignancy, an abnormal Pap smear result, or vaginal or cervical infection.

SPECIAL ISSUES
VAGINAL BARRIER INFLUENCE ON HIV TRANSMISSION

Human research to determine whether use of spermicides or vaginal barrier methods with spermicide reduces risks for transmission of HIV is limited, and results are not clear or consistent.[20,46,66] Concern that spermicide use could have an adverse effect on HIV transmission risk is based on the fact that nonoxynol-9 is a detergent and can irritate the surface of exposed vaginal and cervical tissue.[38,44] Irritation could adversely affect transmission risk.

The results of some studies are worrisome. The rate of HIV seroconversion in a group of Nairobi prostitutes who used nonoxynol-9 sponges was higher than the rate for a comparison group using placebo suppositories.[31] Genital ulcers were also more common among the nonoxynol-9 users. In another study, vaginal irritation was observed among prostitutes in Vancouver who used nonoxynol-9 lubricated condoms.[44] Subjects in both of these studies had unusually high exposure to spermicide and to the trauma of intercourse. Other studies, however, have not found adverse effects for nonoxynol-9 suppositories,[20,66] and some evidence suggests the occurrence of vaginal irritation may depend on the dose and/or frequency of exposure to spermicide.[15,19,67]

It is possible nonoxynol-9 might be helpful rather than harmful in regard to HIV susceptibility when used under less extreme circumstances.[56] The presence of a mechanical barrier, to reduce exposure of the fragile cervical epithelium to semen and microbes, could also potentially affect infection risk.[57] Because of the synergy between common STIs such as chlamydia, gonorrhea, trichomoniasis, genital herpes, syphilis, and chancroid in facilitating the transmission of HIV, researchers estimate that heterosexual transmission of HIV infection could be substantially, perhaps even mostly, prevented by reducing the prevalence of other underlying STIs.[16] Any public health steps, such as use of vaginal barriers, that can reduce the prevalence of ordinary STIs would have the indirect effect of helping to prevent heterosexual transmission of HIV.[18]

Nevertheless, further research is needed before it will be possible to determine how spermicide use, or use of vaginal barrier methods that involve spermicide, affect HIV risk.[59] Until the HIV risk issue is clarified, be cautious in making recommendations about using vaginal barrier methods that involve spermicide whenever STI risk is a concern.

PROVIDING VAGINAL BARRIER METHODS

Help the woman choose which of the available barrier options is most likely to meet her needs. Women who plan to use female condoms or sponges do not require a fitting, or even a pelvic exam. If you perform a routine exam, however, you can make sure the woman does not have an unusual anatomic anomaly such as a septate vagina or duplicate cervices. For a woman who wishes to use a diaphragm or cervical cap, select a device that fits well, or determine that a satisfactory fit is not possible so the patient can choose another contraceptive method.

Be sure each patient has an opportunity to practice inserting and removing her device. After the patient has inserted her device, verify that its position is correct and that the fit is good. Most patients find inserting a cap somewhat more difficult than inserting a diaphragm, and removal can be tricky. New cap users should try the cap initially while still using another method of birth control, such as condoms or oral contraceptives, to be sure the cap remains in position after intercourse.

Barrier method differences. Vaginal barriers differ in both efficacy (Table 18-1) and in rules for their use (Table 18-5). These differences may make one option or another easier or more appealing for a specific woman. For parous women, the diaphragm and female condom provide more effective contraceptive protection than do the cervical cap or contraceptive sponge. For nulliparous women, the difference in efficacy is less striking. Because consistent use is so important, a match between the method's characteristics and the woman's personal needs and sexual patterns may improve efficacy. For example, a woman who is sexually intimate only on weekends may find the diaphragm cumbersome because of the need for extra spermicide with repeated intercourse and the 24-hour limit for wear. For her, a cap that can be left in place without additional spermicide may be easier to use correctly. Similarly, washing and storing a diaphragm or cap and having spermicide available may be awkward for a woman who is not at her own home.

A woman who finds spermicide irritating or does not like the messiness of other vaginal barriers may prefer the female condom. Unlike other vaginal barrier methods, the female condom prevents semen from contacting the vagina. Its use does not require the precise timing in relation to erection and intercourse that is necessary with male condoms, so some couples may find the female condom easier to use or that it involves less interruption in lovemaking.

Origins of barrier use rules. Rules for using vaginal barrier methods (Table 18-5) are based on decisions by U.S. Food and Drug Administration (FDA) and device manufacturers that balance concerns about possible TSS risk, spermicide efficacy, and making the method convenient for users. The scientific basis for these rules is woefully inadequate. For example, no evidence exists for specifying a safe or an unsafe duration of wear to minimize TSS risk. Similarly, optimal spermicide dose and concentration, as well as duration of spermicide efficacy, are unknown. Whether an extra application of spermicide for repeated intercourse improves efficacy for diaphragm users is not known.

The official rules also do not necessarily replicate the protocols used in efficacy studies conducted for FDA approval. Women in the cap and diaphragm study, for example, were allowed cap wear for as long as 3 days (72 hours).[3] Most women in the study, however, reported wear of less than 40 hours, so the reviewers decided that cap efficacy with longer wear had not been documented, and a 48-hour maximum was chosen for the labeling.

Table 18-5 Vaginal barrier methods–rules for use

	Diaphragm	Cap	Sponge	Female Condom
Pelvic Exam Required for Fitting	Yes	Yes	No	No
Spermicide Needed	Yes	Yes	Yes	No
Spermicide Supplies Needed for Insertion	Yes	Yes	No	No
Additional Spermicide Needed for Repeated Intercourse	Yes	No	No	No
Supplies Needed to Add Spermicide After Initial Insertion	Yes	No	No	No
Equipment Needed For Storage After Use	Yes	Yes	No	No
Can Be Used During Menses	Yes	No	No	Yes
Duration of Protection After Insertion	6 hours	48 hours	24 hours	8 hours
Longest Wear Recommended	24 hours	48 hours	30 hours	8 hours

CLINICIAN'S ROLE IN BARRIER SUCCESS

You play an important role in helping women make wise decisions about vaginal barrier methods and use them successfully:

1. Help the woman *assess her own risk of failure.* If her risk is low, do not discourage her confidence in vaginal barriers. If her risk is high, however, a vaginal barrier may not be a wise solo method choice. Characteristics that may be associated with higher than average risk of failure include:

- Frequent intercourse (three times or more weekly)
- Age less than 30 years
- Personal style or sexual patterns that make consistent use difficult
- Previous contraceptive failure (any method)
- Ambivalent feelings (patient or partner) about the current desirability of pregnancy
- Intention to delay (rather than prevent) next pregnancy[50]

2. Help the woman *assess her risk of STI exposure.* If the risk is high, she needs to know abstinence is the safest option. Encourage her to use condoms along with her diaphragm, sponge, or cap. (Female condoms should not be used simultaneously with male condoms because the two condoms may stick together.)

3. If unintended pregnancy would be devastating for the woman, or if she is at high risk for vaginal barrier failure, encourage her to *consider using a combination of methods* such as a diaphragm, sponge, or cap plus male condoms or oral contraceptives.

4. Be sure every vaginal barrier user has an *accurate understanding of ovulation timing* and knows high-risk days for conception begin about 4 days before ovulation.

5. Be sure every vaginal barrier user is *aware of emergency contraception (postcoital treatment)* and knows how to obtain it if a contraceptive emergency arises. If possible, provide her with a kit containing an instruction sheet and a supply of oral contraceptive pills sufficient for one or more emergency treatment regimens. (See Chapter 12 on Emergency Contraception.)

6. If a user becomes pregnant, help her determine whether incorrect use or method failure was the culprit. In many cases women assume incorrect use was responsible when in fact it was not (i.e., estimated gestation does not match the date of unprotected intercourse). A woman who has one method failure (any method) is probably at high risk for another method failure and would be wise to consider using two methods simultaneously.

PRACTICAL CAUTION: AVOID OIL-BASED LUBRICANTS AND MEDICATIONS

Lubricants such as mineral oil, baby oil, suntan oil, vegetable oil, and butter; and vaginal medications such as Femstat cream, Monistat cream, estrogen cream, and Vagisil have a rapid, deleterious effect on latex.[2] Their effect on diaphragm or cap integrity has not been studied, but it is reasonable to warn vaginal barrier users to avoid oil products. If additional lubrication is needed, a vaginal spermicide or a product intended for use with latex condoms would be reasonable options.

FITTING A DIAPHRAGM

Choosing a style to try. The first step in fitting a diaphragm is to select an initial diaphragm style (rim type) to try. Most women find the arcing rim style is easier to insert correctly than are the other rim styles; it is quite difficult to insert an arcing style incorrectly. The gentle spring strength of the coil and flat spring types, however, is often more comfortable, and these styles can be inserted with a diaphragm introducer (Figure 18-5).

Diaphragm manufacturers produce sets of fitting rings—sample diaphragm rims with no dome. Whole diaphragms, however, are preferable for fitting so the patient can practice insertion and removal with the sample diaphragm. Fitting rings are not adequate for patient practice. The various products differ in rim spring strength, so prescribe precisely the same brand and rim type as was used in fitting. Although flat spring diaphragms may not be stocked in all drugstores, coil and arcing diaphragms are widely available; wide-seal diaphragms are distributed directly to physicians and clinics.

Flat spring rim. This diaphragm has a thin, delicate rim with gentle spring strength and is intended for a woman with a very firm vaginal muscle tone (nulliparous) or a shallow notch behind the pubic bone. The flat spring folds flat for insertion. Products available: Ortho-White Diaphragm, sizes 55 to 95, latex.

Coil spring rim. The coil spring has a sturdy rim with a firm spring strength intended for women with average vaginal muscle tone and an average pubic arch notch. It folds flat for insertion. Products available:

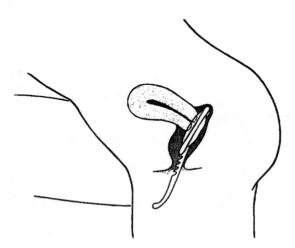

Figure 18-5 Some women prefer to use a plastic introducer for diaphragm insertion

Koromex Diaphragm, sizes 50 to 95, latex; Ortho Diaphragm (coil spring), sizes 50 to 100, latex; and Ramses Flexible Cushioned Diaphragm (coil spring), sizes 50 to 95, gum rubber.

Arcing spring rim. This diaphragm has a very sturdy rim with firm spring strength. Most women are able to use the arcing rim comfortably. It can often be used despite a rectocele or a cystocele or lax vaginal muscle tone. Products available: Koroflex Diaphragm, sizes 60 to 95, latex; Allflex Diaphragm (Ortho), sizes 55 to 95, latex; and Ramses Bendex Diaphragm, sizes 65 to 95, gum rubber.

The Allflex (Ortho) arcing diaphragm folds at any point along its rim and is slightly less rigid than the Koroflex (Holland Rantos) or the Ramses Bendex (Schmid) products. The Koroflex and Bendex fold at two points only (a hinge or bow-bend construction). Many women find the bow-bend rim is easier to insert because the fold compresses to a narrow leading edge and the two stiff halves of the arc can be held in the folded position close to either end of the arc, whereas the Allflex must be held in the middle.

Wide-seal rim. The wide-seal rim has a flexible flange about 1.5 cm wide attached to the inner edge of the rim. The flange is intended to hold spermicide in place inside the diaphragm and to create a better seal between the diaphragm and the vaginal wall. Wide-seal diaphragms are available in two different rim styles, arcing and coil spring. The arcing model folds at two points (bow-bend) but is similar in rigidity to the lighter Allflex arcing spring. The coil spring model folds at any point on the rim, but because of the inner flange, assumes a slight arc shape unlike other coil spring diaphragms that are flat when folded. Products available: Milex Wide-seal arcing diaphragm, sizes 60 to 95, latex; and Milex Wide-seal Omniflex coil spring diaphragm, sizes 60 to 95, latex.

Choosing a diaphragm size.   Estimate the diaphragm size that will be needed:

1. Insert your index and middle fingers into the vagina until your middle finger reaches the posterior wall of the vagina.
2. Use the tip of your thumb to mark the point at which your index finger touches the pubic bone.
3. Extract your fingers.
4. Place the diaphragm rim on the tip of your middle finger. The opposite rim should lie just in front of your thumb.

Insert a sample diaphragm of the size you have selected into the patient's vagina. The device should rest snugly in the vagina, but without tension against the vaginal walls. Its rim should be in contact with the lateral walls and posterior fornix, and there should be just enough space to insert one finger tip comfortably between the inside of the pubic arch and the anterior edge of the diaphragm rim.

Choose the largest rim size that is comfortable for the patient. Try more than one rim size or type before making a final selection. Do not choose a size that is too small; vaginal depth increases during sexual arousal (3 to 5 cm in nulliparous women), and a too-small diaphragm may fail to maintain its position covering the cervix. A diaphragm that is too large, however, may cause vaginal pressure, abdominal pain or cramping, or vaginal ulceration, and may be a factor in recurrent UTI.

Disinfecting Diaphragms and Rings Used for Fitting

Scrupulously attend to universal precautions when fitting diaphragms, as well as when cleaning and disinfecting them after fitting. Use gloves during fitting and eye splash protection and gloves during cleaning. Because they come into contact with intact mucous membrane, diaphragms and rings used for fitting are classified as semi-critical devices that require processing with a high-level disinfectant according to OSHA guidelines. After thorough scrubbing with a liquid detergent and water, three disinfection options are recommended (although some experts believe that autoclave sterilization is the only safe option[68]):[39]

- Autoclave at 121 degrees Centigrade, 15 pounds per square inch (psi) for 20 minutes unwrapped or 30 minutes wrapped.
- Soak in a solution of one part Clorox to nine parts water (results in a solution of sodium hypochlorite 5,000 ppm) for 30 minutes at room temperature; rinse with tap water; then soak in 70% ethyl or isopropyl alcohol for 15 minutes. Discard all solutions.
- Immerse in Cidex (2% glutaraldehyde) for 20 minutes at room temperature; then rinse and place in boiling water for 30 minutes. Follow manufacturer's instructions concerning preparation and disposal or reuse of Cidex solution.

After disinfection, allow the diaphragms or rings to air dry, then store them in a disinfected container until later use.

FITTING A CERVICAL CAP

Prentif Cavity-Rim cervical caps are available in sizes 22 mm, 25 mm, 28 mm, and 31 mm (internal rim diameter). They are manufactured by Lamberts (Dalston) Ltd. in Luton, England, and can be purchased from the U.S. distributor: Cervical Cap Ltd., P.O. Box 38003-292, Los Gatos, California 95031.

Because of normal variations in women's cervical anatomy and the limited number of cap sizes available, it will not be possible to fit every patient properly. Factors such as average parity in each patient population affect the frequency of fitting problems; 6% to 10% of subjects could not be fitted in the large U.S. cap studies.[3,45]

When a Prentif cap is fitted correctly, the inner diameter of the cap rim must be almost identical to the diameter of the base of the cervix, or just a few millimeters larger. The rim forms a seal with the cervical surface to maintain the cap's position. The rim should rest at the base of the cervix so the vaginal walls surround the outer side of the rim. The cervix should be completely covered. The dome of the cap should be deep enough so that it does not rest on the cervical os.

A Prentif cap that is too tight can cause cervical trauma, and one that is too loose or fails to make a secure seal over the entire circumference of the cervix will be more likely to dislodge. Dislodgement during intercourse is also more likely if, during thrusting, the penis bumps the cap's side or rim rather than the dome. For this reason, a woman whose uterus is acutely anteflexed, so her cervical portio faces downward toward the back of her vagina, may find that her cap dislodges.

Estimating cap size. Perform a bimanual exam to determine the position and size of the uterus and cervix. Next, inspect the woman's cervix to estimate the proper cap size. The cervix must be fairly symmetrical, without extensive laceration or scarring that could interfere with uniform contact around its full diameter between the cap rim and cervix. The cervix must also be long enough to accommodate the height of the cap. A cervix that is flush or partially flush with the vaginal vault cannot be fit with the Prentif cap. Try two or more cap sizes to determine the fit.

Inserting, checking, and removing a cap. To insert the cap, fold the rim and compress the cap dome so when it is released in place over the cervix, the unfolding dome can create suction between the rim of the cap and the cervix. After inserting the cap, check it with one finger around its entire circumference to be sure no gaps occur between the cap rim and the cervix. Next the check stability by noting its resistance to dislodgement when the cap and cervix are probed with a finger tip.

Check for evidence of suction after the cap has been in place for a minute or two. Pinch the cap dome and tug gently. The dome should remain collapsed, and the cap should resist the tug and not slide off easily. Finally, try to rotate the cap in place on the cervix. If it does not rotate at all, it is too tight; if it rotates too easily or comes off the cervix, it is too large. To be considered a good fit, the cap must cover the cervix completely, with no gaps between the rim and the cervix. It must have good suction and not dislodge easily when the dome is probed with a finger tip.[9]

To remove the cap, probe the rim with the end of your index finger; tip the cap rim to break the seal, then gently pull the cap down and out.

Disinfecting Caps Used for Fitting

Scrupulously attend to universal precautions when fitting caps, as well as when cleaning and disinfecting them after fitting. Use gloves during fitting, and eye splash protection and gloves during cleaning. Because they come into contact with intact mucous membrane, caps used for fitting are classified as semi-critical devices that require processing with a high-level disinfectant according to OSHA guidelines. After a thorough scrubbing with a liquid detergent and water, three disinfection options are recommended (although some experts believe that autoclave sterilization is the only safe option[68]):[39]

- Autoclave at 121 degrees Centigrade, 15 psi for 20 minutes unwrapped or 30 minutes wrapped.
- Soak in a solution of one part Clorox to nine parts water (results in a solution of sodium hypochlorite 5,000 ppm) for 30 minutes at room temperature; rinse with tap water; then soak in 70% ethyl or isopropyl alcohol for 15 minutes. Discard all solutions.
- Immerse in Cidex (2% glutaraldehyde) for 20 minutes at room temperature; then rinse and place in boiling water for 30 minutes. Follow manufacturer's instructions concerning preparation and disposal or reuse of Cidex solution.

After disinfection, allow the caps to air dry, then store them in a disinfected container until use.

MANAGING PROBLEMS AND FOLLOW-UP

Women using vaginal barriers need no special follow-up. Pap smear abnormalities were a special concern in the FDA's initial review of data for the Prentif cap. For this reason, a Pap smear before providing a cap and a repeat Pap smear after 3 months of cap use were specified in the initial product labeling, with a recommendation to discontinue cap use if the Pap smear results are not benign or indicate likely HPV infection.[43] A subsequent reanalysis of the data from this study found no statistically significant differences in Pap smear results between women wearing the cap and women wearing the diaphragm either after 3 months of use or throughout the first year of use.[25] Other cap research has not found any increase in Pap smear abnormalities with cap use.[45] Protection against cervical neoplasia is an important benefit for diaphragm users (see the section on Advantages and Indications).

Labeling for the diaphragm recommends refitting annually, after a weight gain or loss of 10 pounds or more, after an abortion, or after a full-term pregnancy.[40] Weight change does not commonly require a new diaphragm size, nor does an abortion.[32] Remind women to avoid wearing vaginal barriers for the last 2 or 3 days before routine exams, if possible, to provide optimal conditions for Pap screening.

When a barrier user returns for a routine exam, ask open-ended questions about how the method is working out. If the woman finds it inconvenient or uncomfortable, offer her an opportunity to consider an alternative method. Refitting her with a different size or rim style may also be helpful.

Problems caused by vaginal barrier methods may require clinical intervention. Recurrent vaginal or introital irritation, with no evidence of vaginal infection, may indicate an allergy or sensitivity to spermicide or to latex. Recurrent UTI, recurrent yeast infection, and bacterial vaginosis may be associated with use of contraceptive sponges or a diaphragm.

If a diaphragm user experiences recurring UTIs, consider refitting her with a smaller diaphragm size, alternative rim style, or with a cervical cap. If her UTI problems persist despite these measures, changing to an alternative method of contraception that does not involve spermicide may be advisable.

A vaginal barrier user who develops signs or symptoms of TSS requires urgent and intensive evaluation and treatment. A vaginal culture can confirm the presence of *Staphylococcus aureus*. Treat the patient with antibiotics, and follow her carefully. If her symptoms are severe, she may need hospitalization for surveillance. Because TSS risk is increased for a woman who has had TSS in the past, the woman should avoid use of vaginal barrier methods in the future.

INSTRUCTIONS FOR USING VAGINAL BARRIERS

1. Use your method every time you have intercourse. Be sure your vaginal barrier method (female condom, diaphragm or cap with spermicidal cream or jelly, or sponge) is in place before your partner's penis enters your vagina.

2. If you are using a diaphragm, cap, or sponges, learn the danger signs for toxic shock syndrome and watch for them. If you have a high fever and one or more of the danger signs, you may have early toxic shock syndrome. Remove the sponge, diaphragm, or cap and contact your clinician.

3. Wash your hands carefully with soap and water before inserting, checking, or removing your vaginal barrier method. This precaution may reduce your risk for toxic shock syndrome and for other infections as well.

4. If you are having problems with vaginal or penile irritation, try a different spermicide product. If you have problems with recurring bladder infections or vaginal yeast infections, discuss these with your clinician.

5. If you feel unsure about the proper fit or placement of your diaphragm, cap, or sponge use male condoms until you see your clinician to be sure your insertion technique is correct.

6. Douching after intercourse is not recommended. If you are using a diaphragm, sponge, or cap and choose to use a douche, wait at least 6 hours after intercourse to avoid washing away essential spermicide.

7. You can use male condoms along with your diaphragm, sponge, or cap if you wish. Using this combination, you will have extremely effective protection against both pregnancy and sexually transmitted infection. Do not use a male condom along with a female condom; the two may adhere and increase the chance your female condom will dislodge or male condom will slip off.

8. No conclusive studies show just how long spermicide is fully active or exactly how long the diaphragm, cap, or sponge must be left in place after intercourse. The most important thing is having your device in place, protecting your cervix—not in your drawer. So, if you need to vary the length of time you leave the device in place, do that rather than "take a chance" just once.

BEFORE INTERCOURSE

1. Check that you have all the supplies you need.

   - *Female condoms.* You need enough new, unopened condoms to last until you can obtain more.
   - *Sponges.* You need clean water and enough fresh, unopened sponges to last until you can obtain more. You may also need a supply of condoms to use instead of sponges if you have intercourse while you are having a menstrual period.
   - *Diaphragm.* You need fresh spermicidal cream or jelly, a plastic applicator for inserting additional spermicide, and a diaphragm. Check your diaphragm to be sure it has no holes, cracks, or tears.
   - *Cap.* You need fresh spermicidal cream or jelly and a cap. Check your cap to be sure it has no holes, cracks, or tears. You may also need a supply of condoms to use instead of your cap while you are having a menstrual period.

2. Plan ahead about when to insert your method. Try to find a routine that is comfortable for you.

- *Female condoms.* You can insert the female condom for immediate protection just before intercourse or as long as 8 hours ahead of time if you prefer. It provides effective contraceptive protection for just one act of intercourse.
- *Sponges.* You can insert the sponge for immediate protection just before intercourse, or ahead of time. It provides effective contraceptive protection for 24 hours, no matter how many times you have intercourse.
- *Diaphragm.* The diaphragm may be inserted just before intercourse, or up to 6 hours beforehand.
- *Cap.* The cap can be inserted just before intercourse, or ahead of time if you wish. Some cap experts recommend that you allow 30 minutes between insertion and intercourse, if possible, so a good suction develops. The cap provides effective contraceptive protection for 48 hours, no matter how many times you have intercourse.

INSERTION

1. Wash your hands carefully with soap and water.

2. Insert your method carefully; it must be in the proper location in your vagina to be maximally effective.

- *Female condom.* Remove the Reality condom from its package and check to be sure the inner ring is at the bottom, closed end of the pouch. Follow the directions for insertion in the package; the illustrations can help you. Hold the pouch with the open end hanging down. Use the thumb and middle finger of one hand to squeeze the inner ring into a narrow oval for insertion; place your index finger between your thumb and middle finger to guide the Reality during insertion. With your other hand, spread the lips of your vagina. Insert the inner ring and the pouch of Reality into the vaginal opening and with your index finger, push the inner ring with the pouch the rest of the way up into the vagina. The outside ring lies against the outer lips when Reality is in place; about 1 inch of the open end will stay outside your body. Once the penis enters, the vagina will expand and the slack will decrease.

- *Sponges*. Remove the sponge from its package, moisten it with about 2 tablespoons of clean water, and squeeze it once. Then insert the sponge into the vagina and slide it along the back wall of the vagina until it rests against your cervix. The dimple side should face your cervix, with the loop away from your cervix. Check with your finger to be sure you can feel your cervix covered by the sponge.

- *Diaphragm*. First apply spermicidal jelly or cream. Hold the diaphragm with the dome down (like a cup). Squeeze the jelly or cream from the tube into the dome (use about 1 teaspoon); spread a little bit around the rim of the diaphragm with your finger. To insert the diaphragm hold it with the dome down (spermicide in the dome) and squeeze opposite sides of the rim together so the diaphragm folds. Hold it folded in one hand between your thumb and fingers. Spread the opening of your vagina with your other hand, and insert the folded diaphragm into your vaginal canal. This can be done standing with one foot propped up (on the edge of a chair, a bathtub, or a toilet), squatting, or lying on your back.

  Push the diaphragm downward and along the back wall of your vagina as far as it will go. Then tuck the front rim up along the roof of your vagina behind your pubic bone. Once it is in place properly, you should not be able to feel the diaphragm except, of course, with your fingers. If it is uncomfortable, then most likely it is not in the correct position; take it out and reinsert it.

  After insertion, check placement. When correctly placed, the back rim of the diaphragm is below and behind the cervix, and the front edge of the rim is tucked up behind the pubic bone. Often you may not be able to feel the back rim. You should check to be sure you can feel that your cervix is covered by the soft rubber dome of the diaphragm and the front rim is snugly in place behind your pubic bone. The spermicidal cream (inside the dome of the diaphragm) should be next to your cervix.

- *Cap*. Before insertion, fill the dome of the cap 1/3 full with spermicidal cream or jelly. Next, find your cervix with your finger. It feels like a short, firm nose projecting into the vagina. This can be done standing, with one foot propped up (on the edge of a chair, a bathtub, or a toilet), squatting, or lying on your back. Separate the lips of your vagina with one hand. With the other hand, squeeze (fold) the rim of the cap between your thumb and index finger. Slide the cap into your vagina, and push it along the rear wall of the vagina as far as it will go. Using your finger to locate your cervix, press the rim of the cap around the cervix until it is completely covered. Finally, check the cap position by pressing the dome of the cap to make sure your cervix is covered. Sweep your finger around the cap rim. The cervix should not be felt outside the cap.

REPEATED INTERCOURSE

- *Female condoms.* Use a new Reality condom for each act of intercourse.
- *Sponges.* One sponge provides continuous protection for up to 24 hours, no matter how many times you have intercourse.
- *Diaphragm.* If you have intercourse more than once within the 6 hour time your diaphragm must remain in place, an additional dose of spermicidal cream or jelly is recommended. Do not remove your diaphragm; use the plastic applicator to insert fresh jelly or cream into your vagina in front of the diaphragm.
- *Cap.* Use of additional spermicide for repeated intercourse with the cap is optional. Do not remove your cap. If you wish to add spermicide, use the plastic introducer to insert fresh cream or jelly into your vagina in front of the cap.

AFTER INTERCOURSE

1. Remove your female condom immediately after intercourse, before you stand up. Squeeze and twist the outer ring to keep semen inside the pouch. Pull Reality out gently and discard it in a trash can. Do not try to flush a used Reality down the toilet. Do not try to reuse the Reality condom.
2. Leave the cap, diaphragm, or sponge in place for at least 6 hours after intercourse. After that time, remove the device as soon as is practical. Douching is not recommended, but if you choose to douche, wait at least 6 hours.
3. Your sponge, diaphragm, or cap should not interfere with normal activities. Urination or a bowel movement should not affect its position, but you can check its placement afterward if you wish. It is fine to shower or bathe with a sponge, diaphragm, or cap in place.
4. Before removing a cap, diaphragm, or sponge, wash your hands carefully with soap and water.

5. Check the position of the device. If it is dislodged, or seems not to be in correct position, you may want to contact your clinician about emergency postcoital contraception.

- *Sponges.* Grasp the loop on the sponge with one finger and pull it gently to remove the sponge. Check to be sure the sponge is intact, then throw it away. If it is torn, remove all the pieces from the vagina.
- *Diaphragm.* Locate the front rim of the diaphragm with your finger. Hook your finger over the rim or behind it, then pull the diaphragm down and out. Wash the diaphragm with plain soap and water, and dry it. Hold it up to the light to check for holes, tears, or cracks.
- *Cap.* Locate the cap rim on your cervix. Press on the cap rim until the seal against your cervix is broken, then tilt the cap off the cervix. Hook your finger around the rim and pull it sideways out of the vagina. Wash the cap with plain soap and water, and dry it. Check the cap for holes, tears or cracks.

TAKING CARE OF YOUR VAGINAL BARRIER METHOD

1. Store your supplies in a convenient location that is clean, cool, and dark.
2. Wash your spermicide inserter, diaphragm, or cap after each use. Plain soap is best; avoid deodorant soap or perfumed soap. Do not use talcum powder on your diaphragm or cap, or in the case.
3. Contact with oil-based products can deteriorate a diaphragm or cap. Do not use oil-based vaginal medications or lubricants when you are using a diaphragm or cap. Some examples include petroleum jelly (Vaseline), mineral oil, hand lotion, vegetable oil, cold cream, and cocoa butter as well as common vaginal yeast creams and vaginal hormone creams. If you need extra lubrication for intercourse, contraceptive jelly is a good choice, or you can try a water-soluble lubricant specifically intended for use with condoms.

Toxic Shock Syndrome Danger Signs

Caution

- ■ Sudden high fever
- ■ Vomiting, diarrhea
- ■ Dizziness, faintness, weakness
- ■ Sore throat, aching muscles and joints
- ■ Rash (like a sunburn)

REFERENCES

1. Alexander NJ. Barriers to sexually transmitted diseases. Scientific American 1996;3:31-41.
2. Anonymous. Tests show commonly used substances harm latex condoms. Contraceptive Technology Update 1980;10:20-21.
3. Bernstein GS, Clark V, Coulson AH, Frezieres RG, Kilzer L, Moyer D, Nakamura RM, Walsh T. Use effectiveness of cervical caps. Final report. Washington DC: National Institute of Child Health and Human Development, Contract No. 1-HD-1-2804, July, 1986.
4. Cates W Jr, Stewart FH, Trussell J. Commentary: the quest for women's prophylactic methods—hopes vs. science. Am J Publ Health 1992;82:1479-1482.
5. Cates W Jr, Stone KM. Family planning, sexually transmitted diseases and contraceptive choice: a literature update—Part I. Fam Plann Persp 1992;24:75-84.
6. Cates W Jr., Tubal infertility: an ounce of (more specific) prevention. JAMA 1987;257:2480.
7. Cattanach JF. Letter. Intravaginal barriers: reliable protection against pregnancy and STDs? Fam Plann Perspect 1995;27:176.
8. Celentano DD, Klassen AC, Weisman CS, Rosenshein NB. The role of contraceptive use in cervical cancer: the Maryland cervical cancer case-control study. Am J Epidemiology 1987;126:592-604.
9. Chalker R. The complete cervical cap guide. New York: Harper & Row Publishers, 1987.
10. Cramer DW, Goldman MB, Schiff I, Belisle S, Albrecht B, Stadel B, Gibson M, Wilson E, Stillman R, Thompson I. The relationship of tubal infertility to barrier method and oral contraceptive use. JAMA 1987;257:2446-2450.
11. d'Oro LC, Parazzini F, Naldi L, LaVecchia C. Barrier methods of contraception, spermicides, and sexually transmitted diseases: a review. Genitourin Med 1994;70:410-417.
12. Drew WL, Blair M, Miner RC, Conant M. Evaluation of the virus permeability of a new condom for women. Sex Transm Dis 1990;17:110-112.
13. Edelman DA, McIntyre SL, Harper J. A comparative trial of the Today contraceptive sponge and diaphragm. Am J Obstet Gynecol 1984;150:869-876.
14. Einarson TR, Koren G, Mattice D, Schechter-Tsafriri O. Maternal spermicide use and adverse reproductive outcome: a meta-analysis. Am J Obstet Gynecol 1990;162:655-660.
15. Elias CJ, Heise L. The development of microbicides: a new method of HIV prevention for women. The Population Council, Working Papers, No.6, 1993. The Population Council, One Dag Hammarskjold Plaza, New York 10017.
16. Eng TR, Butler WT (eds). The hidden epidemic: confronting sexually transmitted diseases. Washington DC: National Academy Press, 1996.
17. Farr G, Gabelnick H, Sturgen K, Dorflinger L. Contraceptive efficacy and acceptability of the female condom. Am J Publ Health 1994;84:1960-1964.
18. Faundes A, Elias C, Coggins C. Spermicides and barrier contraception. Current Opin Obstet Gynecol 1994;6:552-558.
19. Feldblum PJ, Fortney JA. Condoms, spermicides, and the transmission of human immunodeficiency virus: a review of the literature. Am J Publ Health 1988;78:52-54.

20. Feldblum PJ, Weir SS. Letter. The protective effect of nonoxynol-9 against HIV infection. Am J Publ Health 1994;84:1032-1034.
21. Fihn SD, Boyko EJ, Normand EH, Chen C-L, Grafton JR, Hunt M, Yarbro P, Scholes D, Stergachis A. Association between use of spermicide-coated condoms and Escherichia coli urinary tract infection in young women. Am J Epidmiol 1996;144:512-520.
22. Fihn SD, Latham RH, Roberts P, Running K, Stamm WE. Association between diaphragm use and urinary tract infection. JAMA 1985;254:240-245.
23. Food and Drug Administration. Data do not support association between spermicides, birth defects. FDA Drug Bulletin 1986;11:21.
24. Foxman B. Recurring urinary tract infection: incidence and risk factors. Am J Publ Health 1990;80:331-333.
25. Gollub EL, Sivin I. The Prentif cervical cap and Pap smear results: a critical appraisal. Contraception 1989;40:343-349.
26. Hooton TM, Roberts PL, Stamm WE. Effects of recent sexual activity and use of a diaphragm on the vaginal microflora. Clinical Infectious Diseases 1994;19:274-278.
27. Hooten TM, Hillier S, Johnson C, Roberts PL, Stamm WE. Escherichia coli bacteriuria and contraceptive method. JAMA 1991;265:64-69.
28. Huggins G, Vessey M, Flavel R, Yeates D, McPherson K. Vaginal spermicides and outcome of pregnancy: findings in a large cohort study. Contraception 1982;25:219-230.
29. Jick H, Walker AM, Rothman KJ, Hunter JK, Holmes LB, Watkins RN, D'Ewart DC, Danford A, Madsen S. Vaginal spermicides and congenital disorders. JAMA 1981;245:1329-1332.
30. Kelaghan J, Rubin GL, Ory HW, Layde PM. Barrier-method contraceptives and pelvic inflammatory disease. JAMA 1982;248:185.
31. Kreiss J, Ngugi E, Holmes K, Ndinya-Achola J, Waiyaki P, Roberts PL, Ruminjo I, Sajabi R, Kimata J, Fleming TR, Anzala A, Holton D, Plummer F. Efficacy of nonoxynol-9 contraceptive sponge use in preventing heterosexual acquisition of HIV in Nairobi prostitutes. JAMA 1992;268:477-482.
32. Kugel C, Verson H. Relationship between weight change and diaphragm size change. J Ob Gyn Nursing 1986;15:123-129.
33. Lane M, Arceo R, Sobrero AJ. Successful use of the diaphragm and jelly by a young population: report of a clinical study. Fam Plann Perspect 1976; 8:81-86.
34. Leeper MA, Conrardy M. Preliminary evaluation of Reality, a condom for women to wear. Adv Contracept 1989;5:229-235.
35. Lettau LA, Bond WW, McDougal JS. Hepatitis and diaphragm fitting [letter to editor]. JAMA 1985;254:752.
36. Louv WC, Austin H, Alexander WJ, Stagno S, Cheeks J. A clinical trial of nonoxynol-9 for preventing gonococcal and chlamydial infections. J Infect Dis 1988;158:518-523.
37. Mauck C, Glover LH, Miller E, Allen S, Archer DF, Blumenthal P, Rosenzweig BA, Dominik R, Sturgen K, Cooper J, Fingerhut F, Peacock L, Gabelnick HL. Lea's Shield: a study of the safety and efficacy of a new vaginal barrier contraceptive used with and without spermicide. Contraception 1996;53:329-335.
38. Niruthisard S, Roddy RE, Chutivongse S. The effects of frequent nonoxynol-9 use on the vaginal and cervical mucosa. Sex Transm Dis 1991;18:176-179.

39. Ortho-McNeil Pharmaceutical, personal communication, April 1997.
40. Ortho Diaphragm. FDA-approved product literature, 1996 in Physician's Desk Reference, 51st Edition, Montvale NJ: Medical Economics Co, 1997.
41. Parazzini F, Negri E, LaVecchia C, Fedele L. Barrier methods of contraception and the risk of cervical neoplasia. Contraception 1989;40:519-530.
42. Peters RK, Thomas D, Hagan DG, Mack TM, Henderson BE. Risk factors for invasive cervical cancer among Latinas and non-Latinas in Los Angeles County. JNCI 1986;77:1063-1077.
43. Prentif cavity-rim cervical cap. FDA-approved product literature, 1988.
44. Rekart ML. The toxicity and local effects of the spermicide nonoxynol-9. J AIDS 1992;5:425-526.
45. Richwald GA, Greenland S, Gerber MM, Potik R, Kersey L, Comas MA. Effectiveness of the cavity-rim cervical cap: results of a large clinical study. Obstet Gynecol 1989;74:143-148.
46. Roddy RE, Zekeng L, Ryan KA, Tamoufe U, Weir SS, Din E, Wong E, Dominik R, Taylor D, Wheeless A. A randomized controlled trial of the effect of non-oxynol-9 film on male-to-female transmission of HIV-1. Presented at National Institute of Allergy and Infectious Disease Ad Hoc Meeting, Bethesda, Maryland, April 9, 1997.
47. Rosenberg MJ, Gollub EL. Commentary: methods women can use that may prevent sexually transmitted disease, including HIV. Am J Publ Health 1992;82:1473-1478.
48. Rosenberg MJ, Rojanapithayakorn W, Feldblum PJ, Higgins JE. Effect of contraceptive sponge on chlamydial infection, gonorrhea, and candidiasis. JAMA 1987;257:2308-2312.
49. Rothman M. Spermicide use and Down's syndrome. Am J Publ Health 1982;72:329-401.
50. Schirm AL, Trussell J, Menken J, Grady WR. Contraceptive failure in the United States: the impact of social, economic and demographic factors. Fam Plann Perspect 1982;14:68-75.
51. Schwartz B, Gaventa S, Broome CV, Reingold AL, Hightower AW, Perlman JA, Wolf PH. Nonmenstrual toxic shock syndrome associated with barrier contraceptives: report of a case-control study. Rev Infect Dis 1989;2:S43-S49.
52. Shiata AA, Trussell J. New female intravaginal barrier contraceptive device: preliminary clinical trial. Contraception 1991; 44:11-19.
53. Simpson JL, Phillips OP. Spermicides, hormonal contraception and congenital malformations. Adv Contracept 1990;6:141-167.
54. Smith C, Farr G, Feldblum PJ, Spence A. Effectiveness of the non-spermicidal fit-free diaphragm. Contraception 1995;51:289-291.
55. Soper DE, Shoupe D, Shangold GA, Shangold MM, Gutmann J, Mercer L. Prevention of vaginal trichomoniasis by compliant use of the female condom. Sex Transm Dis 1993;20:137-139.
56. Stein Z. Editorial: the double bind in science policy and the protection of women from HIV infection. Am J Publ Health 1992;82:1471-1472.
57. Stein Z. Editorial: more on women and the prevention of HIV infection. Am J Publ Health 1995;85:1485-1486.
58. Stim EM. The nonspermicide fit-free diaphragm: a new contraceptive method. Adv Plann Parenthood 1980;15:88-98.

59. Stone KM, Peterson HB. Spermicides, HIV, and the vaginal sponge [editorial]. JAMA 1992;268:521-523.
60. Strobino B, Kline J, Warburton D. Spermicide use and pregnancy outcome. Am J Publ Health 1988;78:260-263.
61. Trussell J, Strickler J, Vaughan B. Contraceptive efficacy of the diaphragm, sponge and cervical cap. Fam Plann Persp 1993;25:101-105,135.
62. Trussell J, Sturgen K, Strickler J, Dominik R. Contraceptive efficacy of the Reality female condom: comparison with other barrier methods. Fam Plann Perspect 1994;26:66-72.
63. Vessey MP. Contraceptive methods: risks and benefits. Brit Med J 1978;2(6139):721-722.
64. Vessey MP, Metcalfe MA, McPherson K, Yeates D. Urinary tract infection in relation to diaphragm use and obesity. Intl J Epiderm 1987;16:441-444.
65. Weir SS, Feldblum PJ, Zekeng L, Roddy RE. The use of nonoxynol-9 for protection against cervical gonorrhea. Am J Publ Health 1994;84:910-914.
66. Weir SS, Roddy RE, Zekeng L, Feldblum PJ. Nonoxynol-9 use, genital ulcers, and HIV infection in a cohort of sex workers. Genitourin Med 1995;71:78-81.
67. Zekeng L, Feldblum PJ, Oliver RM, Capt L. Barrier contraceptive use and HIV infection among high risk women in Cameroon. JAIDS 1993;7:725-731.

LATE REFERENCE

68. Bounds W, Hoffman P. Decontamination of contraceptive practice diaphragms and caps. Br J Fam Plann 1995;21:30.

The Pill: Combined Oral Contraceptives

Robert A. Hatcher, MD, MPH
John Guillebaud, MA, FRCSE, FRCOG, MFFP

- Oral contraceptive pills (OCs) effectively prevent pregnancy. Of 1,000 women taking pills *perfectly*, only 1 will become pregnant within a year. Of 1,000 women taking pills *typically*, however, 50 women will become pregnant. Some women may find it reassuring to use a back-up contraceptive consistently.
- A woman who uses condoms concurrently with OCs will protect herself against reproductive tract infection as well as pregnancy.

- A woman who misses hormonal pills, or is late starting a new cycle of pills, should strongly consider using a back-up contraceptive until she has taken 7 consecutive pills. Emergency contraceptive pills are an option in some circumstances.

The combined oral contraceptive (OC) pill is safe and effective. It is one of the most extensively studied medications ever prescribed. The overall risks and benefits of OCs suggest that it may be appropriate to make them available without a prescription; many countries already do so.[46,102] In this text, we use the terms pills or OCs when referring to oral contraceptive pills containing both an estrogen and a progestin.

MECHANISM OF ACTION

Oral contraceptives prevent pregnancy primarily by suppressing ovulation through the combined actions of an estrogen and a progestin. Estrogens and progestins act upon many different organ systems and produce a broad range of effects, both contraceptive and other.

Estrogenic effects.   Each woman taking OCs is affected by estrogen in the pill as well as by her endogenous estrogen:[49,94]

- Ovulation is inhibited in part by the suppression of follicle stimulating hormone (FSH) and luteinizing hormone (LH). This suppression mimics the changes that occur during pregnancy, so the pituitary gland does not release hormones to stimulate the ovary.[49]
- Secretions and the cellular structure of the endometrium within the uterus are altered, leading to areas of edema alternating with areas of dense cellularity.
- Luteolysis, the degeneration of the corpus luteum, may occur when high levels of estrogen (higher than levels found in current OCs) alter local prostaglandins. This effect may help explain how estrogens work as postcoital pills.[94]

Progestational effects.   The potential contraceptive effects of progestins are as follows:[49,94]

- Ovulation is inhibited by suppression of luteinizing hormone (LH).
- Cervical mucus is thickened, hampering the transport of sperm (although this is probably not an important contraceptive effect).
- Capacitation of sperm may be inhibited.
- Implantation is hampered by production of a decidualized endometrial bed with exhausted and atrophied glands.

COMBINED PILL OPTIONS

In pharmacologic terms, the power of a drug is a combination of its dose and its potency (the amount of a substance required to produce a biological effect). Figure 19-1 depicts estimates of the power of the hormones in many of the OCs currently on the U.S. market. (OCs containing the new progestins are not included.) Statements about the overall power of an estrogen or a progestin tend to be oversimplifications.[32,55]

Estrogens.   Only two estrogenic compounds are used in current U.S. OCs: ethinyl estradiol (EE) and mestranol. EE is pharmacologically active, whereas mestranol must be converted into EE by the liver before it is pharmacologically active, and conversion is not complete. All OCs with 35 micrograms (mcg) of estrogen or less contain EE.

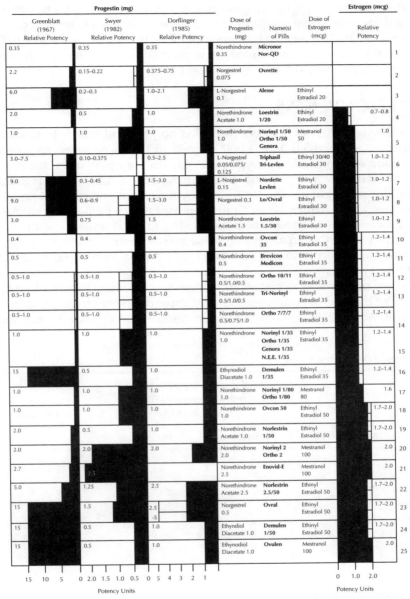

Sources: Dorflinger (1985).
Greenblatt (1967).
Swyer (1982).
Heinen (1971).

Figure 19-1 Relative potency of estrogens and progestins in currently available oral contraceptives reflecting the debate about the strength of the progestins

Progestins. Several progestins are found in OCs: norethindrone, norethindrone acetate, ethynodiol diacetate, norgestrel, levonorgestrel, norethynodrel, desogestrel, norgestimate, and gestodene. The final 3 progestins are sometimes called "new progestins," and the brands using them are often called "third-generation pills."

EFFECTIVENESS

Among *perfect* users (users who miss no pills and follow instructions perfectly), only about 1 in 1,000 women (0.1%) is expected to become pregnant within the first year (Table 19-1). Among *typical* users, about 1 in 20 women (5%) will become pregnant during the first year. Pregnancy rates during *typical* use are determined by the extent and type of imperfect use. (See also Chapter 31 on Contraceptive Efficacy.) Pill-taking mistakes that increase the length of the hormone-free interval undermine the pill's effectiveness. OCs can always be made more effective by eliminating or shortening this interval (pill-free days for 21-day packs or placebo pill days for 28-day packs).

Many pregnancies occur when women discontinue OCs, fail to begin another method of contraception, and therefore have unprotected intercourse. About 25% to 50% of women discontinue OCs by 1 year. Most

Table 19-1 First-year probability of pregnancy* of combined pills compared with other hormonal contraceptives

Method	% of Women Experiencing an Unintended Pregnancy Within the First Year of Use		% of Women Continuing Use at One Year
	Typical Use	Perfect Use	
Pill	5		71
Progestin Only		0.5	
Combined		0.1	
IUD			
Progesterone T	2.0	1.5	81
Copper T 380A	0.8	0.6	78
LNg 20	0.1	0.1	81
Depo-Provera	0.3	0.3	70
Norplant and Norplant-2	0.05	0.05	88

*See Table 9-2 for pregnancy year failure rates of all methods.

Emergency Contraceptive Pills: Treatment initiated within 72 hours after unprotected intercourse reduces the risk of pregnancy by at least 75%. (See Chapter 12 for more information.)

women who discontinue OCs do so for personal nonmedical reasons. Because of these high discontinuation rates, recommend that women starting OCs have on hand a second method of contraception. Instruct them how to use this back-up method and encourage them to practice using it. Inform women about the availability of emergency hormonal contraception. (See the section on Instructions for Using Combined Pills.)

COST

On an annual basis, generic OCs cost a woman $100 to $130, and nongeneric OCs cost $200 to $300. In a managed care setting, OCs cost about $21.00 per cycle. In a public payer system, OCs cost about $17.60 per cycle (see Chapter 9 on The Essentials of Contraception).[101] Public clinics may pay as little as 30 cents to $1 per cycle of OCs and pass these low prices to clients.

ADVANTAGES AND INDICATIONS

Unfortunately, most women are *unaware* of the pill's many beneficial effects. In a recent survey of women at Yale University, 80% to 95% were unaware of the major noncontraceptive benefits: protective effects against endometrial cancer, ovarian cancer, benign breast disease, ovarian cysts, ectopic pregnancy, pelvic inflammatory disease (PID), and anemia. In contrast, most were aware of the pill's positive effects on menstrual bleeding and cramping.[78] The advantages conferred by pill use are listed here; some advantages are also discussed in the section on Special Issues:

1. **Effectiveness.** When taken consistently and correctly, OCs are very effective contraceptives that give women control over their own fertility.

2. **Safety.** Women are reassured to learn that although some questions remain, OCs are one of the best-studied medications ever prescribed. OCs are very safe for most women. In the United States, it is safer to use OCs than to deliver a baby. The risk of death from taking OCs is exceedingly low and would be even lower if heavy smokers over 35 years of age did not take OCs.[54]

3. **Option throughout reproductive years.** Most women can safely use OCs throughout their reproductive years as long as they have no specific reason to avoid OCs. Age in itself is not a reason to avoid OCs. Women do *not* need a "rest" period every few years.

4. **Reversibility.** Although a woman may take several months longer to become pregnant after taking OCs than after using some other contraceptives, she does not suffer a loss in fertility.[15]

5. Menstrual benefits. OCs cause a number of positive effects on the menstrual cycle:

- OCs tend to decrease menstrual cramps and pain, including symptoms that have been resistant to therapy with prostaglandin inhibitors.
- By preventing ovulation, OCs can eliminate the midcycle pain some women experience at the time of ovulation (mittelschmerz).
- OCs decrease the number of days of bleeding and the amount of blood loss. Menstrual flow decreases by 60% or more.[94]
- Women can avoid menstrual periods on weekends or vacations by extending the number of days they take "active" hormonal pills or by simply skipping the pill-free week.
- Women who wish to have fewer menstrual cycles (e.g., travelers; women with dysmenorrhea, PMS, or migraine headaches during menses; or retarded women with severe hygienic problems) can *tricycle*: they can take three consecutive packages of 21 pills; after 63 consecutive days of taking a pill, they take no pill for 7 days before beginning another package. (Four packs of pills can be used for 84 consecutive days.)
- Some women note a reduction in premenstrual symptoms such as anxiety, depression, headaches, and fluid retention.[73] For other women, these symptoms become worse. Tricycling or eliminating the pill-free interval leads to less frequent or no PMS symptoms.

6. Improvement in hirsutism. Because OCs raise sex hormone binding globulin (SHBG) levels and suppress the androgens produced by the ovaries, they are a standard part of the management of hirsutism.[30,64,82,103]

7. Prevention of ovarian and endometrial cancer.[21,22,47,86] When compared with never-users, women who have used OCs for 4 years or less are 30% less likely to develop ovarian cancer; for 5-11 years, 60% less likely; and for 12 or more years, 80% less likely.[54] The risk of endometrial cancer among women who have used OCs for at least 2 years is about 40% less than among women who have never used OCs. This protective effect increases to 60% in women who have used OCs for 4 or more years.[54] The protective effect against ovarian and endometrial cancer is even greater in nulliparous women and appears to persist long after use is discontinued.

8. **Prevention of functional ovarian cysts.** Because OCs suppress stimulation of the ovaries by FSH and LH, the incidence of functional ovarian cysts among women using OCs is reduced.[17,33] (Triphasic and other low-dose OCs provide less, if any, protection against functional ovarian cysts than do earlier, higher potency OCs.[48,49])

9. **Decreased risk for benign breast disease.** OC users are less likely to develop benign breast tumors than are women who are not using the pill.[114] OCs do not appear to protect against breast lesions caused by ductal atypia (thought to be premalignant).

10. **Ectopic pregnancy prevention.** By stopping ovulation, OCs prevent almost all ectopic pregnancies.[38,67]

11. **Acne improvement.** OCs lower serum testosterone levels through a number of mechanisms, thereby improving acne.[49,93]

12. **Enhanced sexual enjoyment.** Probably because the fear of pregnancy is diminished, many couples enjoy sexual intimacy more.

13. **Improvement of other medical conditions.** OCs may protect against osteoporosis,[29,37] endometriosis,[50,93] and rheumatoid arthritis. OC use prevents 1,614 hospitalizations per 100,000 current OC users while only 133 hospitalizations per 100,000 women are a result of a condition that occurs more commonly in OC users (Figure 19-2).[54]

14. **Emergency hormonal contraception.** An emergency contraceptive pill regimen used just after unprotected intercourse could prevent as many as 2.3 million unintended pregnancies and 1 million induced abortions annually in the United States.[100] (See Chapter 12 on Emergency Contraception.)

15. **Prevention of atherogenesis.** Estrogens tend to have desirable effects on lipids: increasing high-density lipoproteins (HDLs) and decreasing low-density lipoproteins (LDLs).[108] Estrogens also relax arterial smooth muscle and may have a direct anti-atherogenic effect on the vessel wall.

16. Decreased risk of symptomatic PID. (See the section on Special Issues.)

INDICATIONS

OCs are an attractive contraceptive option for women with the following conditions:

- Heavy, painful, or irregular menstrual periods
- Recurrent ovarian cysts
- Premenstrual symptoms, cyclic headaches, or cyclic depression (*tricycling* may help)

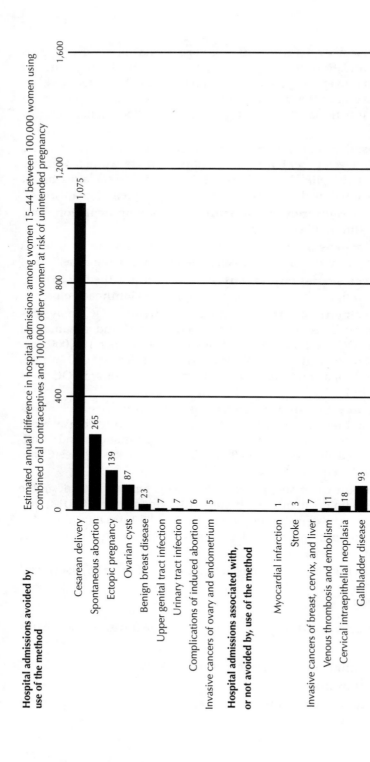

Hospital admissions avoided by use of the method

Estimated annual difference in hospital admissions among women 15–44 between 100,000 women using combined oral contraceptives and 100,000 other women at risk of unintended pregnancy

- Cesarean delivery — 1,075
- Spontaneous abortion — 265
- Ectopic pregnancy — 139
- Ovarian cysts — 87
- Benign breast disease — 23
- Upper genital tract infection — 7
- Urinary tract infection — 7
- Complications of induced abortion — 6
- Invasive cancers of ovary and endometrium — 5

Hospital admissions associated with, or not avoided by, use of the method

- Myocardial infarction — 1
- Stroke — 3
- Invasive cancers of breast, cervix, and liver — 7
- Venous thrombosis and embolism — 11
- Cervical intraepithelial neoplasia — 18
- Gallbladder disease — 93

Source: Harlap et al. (1991) with permission of the Alan Guttmacher Institute.

Figure 19-2 Use of combined oral contraceptives prevents many more hospital admissions than it causes

- Family history of ovarian cancer
- Desire for reversible contraception
- Recent delivery (3 weeks) and not breastfeeding
- Endometriosis and not ready to get pregnant
- Need for contraception immediately following an abortion
- Acne, hirsutism, or chronic anovulation
- Past experience using OCs correctly
- Need for emergency contraception

DISADVANTAGES AND CAUTIONS

Inform women that OC use may be associated with some disadvantages, many of which can be overcome or managed. Consult the section on Managing Problems and Follow-Up to learn more about some of these disadvantages. Some disadvantages are also discussed in the section on Special Issues.

1. **Lack of protection against sexually transmitted infections (STIs).** OCs provide no known protection against STIs, such as infection with the human immunodeficiency virus (HIV). Persons at risk of HIV or other STIs should use condoms. Abstinence and a long-term mutually faithful relationship are the safest approaches to avoiding STIs.

2. **Daily administration.** Pills must be taken every day. Inconsistent or incorrect use raises the risk of pregnancy.

3. **Expense.** The high cost of OCs may prompt some women to discontinue them. (See Chapter 9 on The Essentials of Contraception.)

4. **Unwanted menstrual cycle changes.** OCs may be associated with some negative menstrual changes including missed periods, very scanty bleeding, spotting, or breakthrough bleeding.

5. **Nausea or vomiting.** During the first several cycles, OCs may cause nausea.

6. **Headaches.** Some women may begin to suffer headaches or their headaches may worsen. In rare cases, headaches may be accompanied by changes in vision. Focal (asymmetrical) neurologic symptoms, whether preexisting or pill-associated, indicate that OCs not be used.[53] It is possible migraine headaches indicate a small increased risk for stroke.[65]

7. **Effect on depression.** Depression may decrease or increase under the influence of OCs. However, depression is more likely to improve than to worsen.[42] In some cases, OCs produce a deficiency of pyridoxine (vitamin B_6). Premenstrual irritability and depression

tend to decrease in women taking low-dose OCs, although on occasion a woman may have more severe premenstrual symptoms.

8. **Decreased libido.** In some women, the pill alters vaginal secretions and decreases levels of free testosterone, which may decrease libido.[44]

9. **Increased cervical ectopy and chlamydia infection.** Chlamydial cervicitis is more common in women on OCs.[109] OCs can cause cervical ectopy,[26] a condition in which part of the cervical surface near the opening of the canal becomes covered by the delicate mucus-secreting columnar cells that normally line the cervical canal. With an ectropion, the cervix of the OC user is more vulnerable to *Chlamydia trachomatis* infection,[68] although no evidence exists that this increased risk places women using OCs at greater risk for pelvic inflammatory disease (PID) and many studies show a decreased risk.

10. **Risk of cardiovascular disease.** Although the attributable risk is small, the most serious complications attributable to oral contraceptive use have been circulatory system diseases (Table 19-2 and Table 19-3).[53] In general, however, women's habits are more important than the use of OCs in determining their risk for cardiovascular system disease. Cardiovascular disease, including deep vein thrombosis (DVT), is most likely to occur in women with the following characteristics:

   - Sedentary, overweight, and over 50 years of age
   - Hypertensive or with a history of heart or vascular disease
   - Diabetic or with a family history of diabetes or heart attack in a person under the age of 50 years (particularly a heart attack in a female relative)
   - Hypercholesterolemic or with a high LDL/HDL cholesterol ratio
   - Smoker (smoking is a risk factor for atherosclerotic cardiovascular disease but not DVT)

Table 19-2 Hospitalizations for cardiovascular conditions

Condition	Incidence per 100,000 Women on Pills
Myocardial infarction	1
Stroke	3
Venous thrombosis/embolism	11

Source: Harlap, et al. (1991).

Table 19-3 Circulatory diseases attributable to pills

Diagnosis	Location of Pathology	Symptoms
Thrombophlebitis	Lower leg	Calf pains, swelling, heat or tenderness
Thrombophlebitis	Thigh	Pain, heat, or redness
Pulmonary embolism	Lung	Cough, including coughing up blood, chest pains; shortness of breath
Myocardial infarction	Heart	Chest pains, left arm and shoulder pain, shortness of breath, weakness
Thrombotic stroke	Brain	Headache, weakness or numbness, visual problem, sudden intellectual impairment
Hemorrhagic stroke, including subarach-noid hemorrhage	Brain	Headache, weakness or numbness, visual problem, sudden intellectual impairment
Retinal vein thrombosis	Eye	Headache, complete or partial loss of vision
Mesenteric vein thrombosis	Intestines	Abdominal pain, vomiting, weakness
Pelvic vein thrombosis	Pelvis	Lower abdominal pain, cramps

Source: Stewart F, et al. (1987).

Hypercoagulability. The estrogen component of OCs appears to be capable of activating blood clotting mechanisms. Low-dose OCs appear to have fewer deleterious effects on blood clotting than did earlier higher-dose OCs. In addition, recent studies suggest that second-generation progestins are less likely to increase DVT than previously believed.[61,97] Some risk factors place women at risk for arterial thrombosis: heavy smoking; high or abnormal blood lipids; severe diabetes with damage to arteries or kidneys or with ophthalmologic complications; consistently elevated blood pressure; and obesity (50% above ideal body weight).[11,88] Women with polycythemia vera should not take OCs because of their increased risk of DVT. Traditionally, it has been recommended that women should discontinue OCs for 1 month prior to surgery; however, minor small surgical procedures such as tubal sterilization are not linked with an excess risk of venous thrombosis in women who take OCs and therefore do not merit discontinuing the pill and exposing them to the risk of pregnancy. Women who are anticoagulated and women who bleed heavily because of a bleeding disorder are considered excellent candidates for OC use; indeed, some clinicians consider these to be *indications for the use of OCs.*

Hypertension. Both estrogens and progestins may affect blood pressure. Rarely, an individual has an idiosyncratic reaction to the hormones in OCs and becomes hypertensive. A WHO collaborative study found that OC users with current hypertension or a history of hypertension had a greater increase in the risk of ischemic stroke and myocardial infarcts.[80,110] The risk was lowest in young women who did not smoke, took low-dose OCs (of any generation of progestins), and had their blood pressure measured at the time OCs were initiated. One large study of African-American women in the southeastern United States did not find blood pressure changes in OC users that differed significantly from changes in nonusers.[13] Although some have recommended that women who start OCs may not need to return for 12 months,[2] we favor a blood pressure check in 3 months. If a woman's blood pressure rises from normal levels to over 90 mm Hg (confirmed on several visits), discontinue her OCs. It may be appropriate to switch to a progestin-only pill.

Atherogenesis. Androgens and some progestins decrease HDLs and increase LDLs. Recent changes in OC formulations have involved efforts to lower the progestins in OCs and to find new formulations capable of producing a more favorable lipoprotein pattern. Desogen, Ortho-Cept, Ortho Cyclen, Ortho Tricyclen, Ovcon-35, Modicon, and Brevicon all produce a favorable HDL and LDL cholesterol pattern.[40,59]

11. **Possible effects on glucose intolerance**. Some evidence suggests that progestins and progesterone increase tissue resistance to insulin by decreasing the number of insulin receptors.[116] The early literature on high-dose OCs demonstrated increased glucose levels, increased plasma insulin levels, and a slightly decreased glucose tolerance, which rapidly returned to normal after OC discontinuation. More recent studies of lower dose OCs have shown minimal or no change in glucose tolerance, plasma insulin, or insulin binding to erythrocytes and monocytes.[34,90,92,116] In summary, carbohydrate metabolism is *not* affected to an important degree in most women using low-dose OCs.[34] (See the discussion on Women with Diabetes under the section on Providing Combined Pills.)

12. **Gallbladder disease acceleration**. Recent studies conclude that OCs are not an important risk factor for the development of gallstones or gallbladder cancer, although they may accelerate the

development of gallbladder disease for women who are already susceptible (Figure 19-2).[93,114] The World Health Organization recommends that combined pills usually not be used if a woman has symptomatic gallbladder disease (Table 19-2).[110] OCs do not increase the risk for gallbladder cancer.[71]

13. **Hepatocellular adenoma**. Benign liver tumors have been associated with use of combined pills. Although histologically benign, these tumors may lead to rupture of the capsule of the liver, extensive bleeding, and death. Abdominal pain often continues for months before this rare tumor is diagnosed.[83] With the current low-dose OCs, the risk for liver tumors is much lower than with higher dose OCs.[107] As of 1995, no major prospective study (Walnut Creek, Puget Sound, Boston Nurses' Health Study, Royal College of General Practitioners) reported cases of hepatocellular carcinoma or adenoma.[42,43]

14. **Reproductive tract cancer questions**. Because of the long latency period between exposure to a carcinogen and the subsequent clinical manifestations of cancer, the final word is still not in on OCs and cancer. Taking all cancers as a single group, a recent model estimated that for every 100,000 women, 44 fewer OC users would develop reproductive cancers in their lifetime than would non-pill users. This model assumed that 5 years or more of OC use was associated with a 20% increase in breast cancer diagnosed before age 50, a 20% increase in cervical cancer, and a 50% decrease in ovarian and endometrial cancer.[24]

Breast cancer. The present consensus is that OCs can lead to breast cancer, but the risk is small and resulting tumors spread less aggressively than usual. OCs may be a co-factor that interacts with another primary cause to stimulate the cancer. It remains to be seen whether an increased risk for breast cancer can be shown repeatedly for any specific subgroup of women.[23,25] A 1996 re-analysis of more than 54 studies showed *current* OC users at a 24% increased risk for having breast cancer diagnosed. One to 4 years after discontinuing OCs, women were at a 16% increased risk. Five to 9 years after discontinuation, the risk fell to 7%. Women who had stopped taking OCs 10 or more years previously were at no significant increased risk.[25] The risk of breast cancer was not influenced by OC initiation during adolescence, use prior to having a first baby, the duration of OC use, the dose or type of hormone in the pill, or a family history of breast cancer.

ORAL CONTRACEPTIVES AND BREAST CANCER

Imagine two halls, each holding 1,000 women who are 45 years of age. In one hall, the women never used the pill. In the other hall, the women used the pill until 10 years ago, when they were 35 years old. What would be the difference in the women's risk of breast cancer? In the hall of women who had never used oral contraceptives (OCs), 10 women would be diagnosed with breast cancer. In the other hall, 11 women, only 1 more, would be diagnosed with it. Moreover, the remaining 989 (past pill-using) women in the second hall will from this time on have only the *same risk of breast cancer* as never-users, meaning no ongoing extra pill-connected risk.[49]

Why? Because more than 10 years have passed since they last used OCs. This is reassuring to millions of women who took the pill in the past. In addition, the cancers diagnosed in women who use or have ever used OCs *are less advanced* than those who have never used the pill and are less likely to have spread beyond the breast. This raises the possibility that OC use is not *causing* breast cancer but rather is leading to an *earlier diagnosis* of existing cancers.

Cervical cancer. The risk of cervical cancer appears to be increased slightly in women using oral contraceptives, particularly long-term users.[99,117] Whether this is a biologic effect or not remains controversial. OCs may affect the later stages of carcino-genesis. Another confounding variable is that OC users tend to have more sexual partners. OC use may also affect cervical cancer by altering susceptibility to infection with human papilloma virus (HPV), a known risk factor. Epidemiological studies indicate that excess risk persists even after adjusting for potential confounding factors such as cigarette smoking, age at first intercourse, number of sexual partners, sexual behavior of male partners, and Pap smear screening history.[16] In a large British study, the risk increased as duration of OC use increased.[106] OCs may be used by women with cervical intraepithelial neoplasia.

15. **Other side effects.** In any given woman, synthetic hormones may stimulate end-organs differently than do endogenous hormones. Side effects may be due to the estrogenic, progestogenic, or androgenic properties of OCs (Table 19-4).

Table 19-4 Estrogenic, progestogenic, and androgenic effects of oral contraceptive pills

Estrogenic effects	Progestogenic effects	Androgenic effects
• Nausea • Increased breast size (ductal and fatty tissue) • Cyclic weight gain due to fluid retention • Leukorrhea • Cervical eversion or ectopy • Hypertension • Rise in cholesterol concentration in gallbladder bile • Growth of leiomyomata • Telangiectasia • Hepatocellular adenomas or hepatocellular cancer (rare) • Cerebrovascular accidents (rare) • Thromboembolic complications including pulmonary emboli (rare) • Stimulation of breast neoplasia (exceedingly rare) (Most pills with less than 50 mcg of ethinyl estradiol do not produce troublesome estrogen-mediated side effects or complications.)	Both the estrogenic and the progestational components of oral contraceptives may contribute to the development of the following adverse effects: • Breast tenderness • Headaches • Hypertension • Myocardial infarction (rare)	All low-dose combined pills suppress a woman's production of testosterone, which has a beneficial effect on acne, oily skin and hirsutism. The progestin component may have androgenic as well as progestational effects: • Increased appetite and weight gain • Depression, fatigue, tiredness • Decreased libido and/or enjoyment of intercourse • Acne, oily skin • Increased breast tenderness or breast size • Increased LDL cholesterol levels • Decreased HDL cholesterol levels • Decreased carbohydrate tolerance; increased insulin resistance • Pruritus

PRECAUTIONS

The World Health Organization (WHO) has developed a list of precautions in providing OCs (Table 19-5).[113] Historically OCs have been denied to women with a number of the conditions the WHO considers *not* to be restrictions against OC use (WHO classification "1").

For example, OCs have been denied to women with a history of gestational diabetes, benign breast disease, obesity, or fibroids. These are common conditions; withholding OCs from women with these conditions exposes them to the risk of unintended pregnancy.

Table 19-5 Precautions in the provision of combined oral contraceptives (OCs)

Refrain from providing combined oral contraceptives for women with the following diagnoses (World Health Organization [WHO] category # 4):

Precautions	Rationale/Discussion
Deep vein thrombosis or pulmonary embolism, or a history thereof	Estrogens promote blood clotting. Thromboembolic events related to known trauma or an intravenous needle are not necessarily a reason to avoid use of pills.
Cerebrovascular accident (stroke), coronary artery or ischemic heart disease, or a history thereof	Estrogens promote blood clotting.
Structural heart disease, complicated by pulmonary hypertension, atrial fibrillation, or history of subacute bacterial endocarditis	Estrogens promote blood clotting.
Diabetes with nephropathy, retinopathy, neuropathy or other vascular disease; diabetes of more than 20 years duration	Estrogens promote blood clotting.
Breast cancer	Breast cancer is a hormonally sensitive tumor. In theory, the hormones in OCs might cause some masses to grow.
Pregnancy	Current data do *not* show that hormonal contraceptives taken during pregnancy cause any significant risk of birth defects. However, hormonal contraceptives should not be given to pregnant women.
Lactation (<6 weeks postpartum)	There is some theoretical concern that the neonate may be at risk due to exposure to steroid hormones during the first 6 weeks postpartum. OCs can diminish the volume of breast milk.
Liver problems: benign hepatic adenoma or liver cancer, or a history thereof; active viral hepatitis; severe cirrhosis	OCs are metabolized by the liver and their use may adversely affect prognosis of existing disease.
Headaches, including migraine, with focal neurologic symptoms	Focal neurologic symptoms such as blurred vision, seeing flashing lights or zigzag lines, or trouble speaking or moving may be an indication of an increased risk of stroke.
Major surgery with prolonged immobilization or any surgery on the legs	Increased risk for DVTs and PE
Over 35 years old and currently a heavy smoker (20 or more cigarettes a day)	Smoking increases the risk for cardiovascular disease.
Hypertension, 160+/100+ or with vascular disease	Hypertension is an important risk factor for cardiovascular disease.

(continued)

Table 19-5 Precautions in the provision of combined oral contraceptives (OCs) *(cont.)*

Precautions	Rationale/Discussion
Exercise caution if combined oral contraceptives are used or considered in the following situations and carefully monitor for adverse effects (WHO category #3):	
Postpartum <21 days	There is some theoretical concern regarding the association between OC use up to 3 weeks postpartum and risk of thrombosis.
Lactation (6 weeks to 6 months)	In the first 6 months postpartum, use of OCs during breast-feeding diminishes the quantity of breast milk and may adversely affect the health of the infant.
Undiagnosed abnormal vaginal/uterine bleeding	Although oral contraceptives are often used to manage heavy bleeding, clinicians should be sure that the cause of the bleeding is known before prescribing oral contraceptives.
Over 35 years of age and light smoker (less than 20 cigarettes/day)	Smoking increases the risk for cardiovascular disease. All smokers should be warned of this risk and should be encouraged and advised to stop smoking.
Past history of breast cancer but no evidence of recurrence for 5 years	Breast cancer is a hormonally sensitive tumor.
Use of drugs that affect liver enzymes: rifampicin, rifabutin and griseofulvin; anticonvulsants such as phenytoin, carbamazepine, barbiturates, topiramate and primidone	OCs are metabolized by the liver. Drugs that affect liver enzymes could reduce the contraceptive effectiveness of OCs.
Gallbladder disease: medically treated and current biliary tract disease and history of OC-related cholestasis	Recent reports show that OCs may be weakly associated with gallbladder disease. There is also concern that OCs may worsen existing gallbladder disease.
Advantages generally outweigh theoretical or proven disadvantages and generally can be provided without restrictions in these conditions (WHO category # 2):	
Severe headaches that definitely start *after* initiation of oral contraceptives; migraine headaches without focal neurological symptoms	Migraine headaches with focal neurologic symptoms have been associated with an increased risk of stroke; any headaches clearly starting after initiation of pills may be related to pill use.
Diabetes mellitus: gestational diabetes or diabetes without vascular disease	Women with diabetes are at increased risk of heart disease and stroke, particularly if the woman smokes. Estrogens and progestins may slightly decrease glucose tolerance but this is unlikely to happen with low-dose OCs.

(continued)

Table 19-5 Precautions in the provision of combined oral contraceptives (OCs) *(cont.)*

Precautions	Rationale/Discussion
Advantages generally outweigh theoretical or proven disadvantages and generally can be provided without restrictions in these conditions (WHO category # 2): (Continued)	
Major surgery *without* prolonged immobilization	With the current low-dose pills, the problems associated with pill use and elective surgery have decreased.
Sickle cell disease or sickle C disease	Women with sickle cell disease are predisposed to occlusion of the microvasculature (due to abnormal, inflexible red blood cells). Studies of women with sickle cell disease have shown no significant differences between OC users and non-users with regard to coagulation studies, blood viscosity measurements, or incidence or severity of painful sickle cell crises.
Moderate blood pressure: 140-159/100-109	Monitor blood pressure periodically. Hypertension is an important risk factor for cardiovascular disease.
Undiagnosed breast mass	Some clinicians and some clinical protocols suggest that women found to have a breast mass should not be provided combined OCs until cancer of the breast has been ruled out. Other clinicians are comfortable prescribing pills while the cause of the breast mass is being evaluated.
Cervical cancer awaiting treatment and cervical intraepithelial neoplasia	The risk of cervical cancer appears to be increased slightly in OC users. OC users may get Pap smears more regularly so that early dysplasia is more likely to be recognized. They also tend to have more sexual partners. Pill use may also alter susceptibility to infection with HPV, a known risk factor for cancer of the cervix.
Over 50 years of age	Women over 50 are at increased risk for heart and cerebrovascular disease.
Conditions likely to make it very difficult for a woman to take OCs consistently and correctly	Mental retardation, major psychiatric illness, alcoholism, or other chemical abuse, and/or a history of repeatedly taking oral contraception or other medications incorrectly, make compliance with taking OCs difficult.

(continued)

Table 19-5 Precautions in the provision of combined oral contraceptives (OCs) *(cont.)*

Precautions	Rationale/Discussion
Advantages generally outweigh theoretical or proven disadvantages and generally can be provided without restrictions in these conditions (WHO category # 2): (Continued)	
Family history of hyperlipidemia	Some types of hyperlipidemia increase a woman's risk for heart disease. Routine screening is not recommended by WHO because of the rarity of the conditions and the high cost of screening.
Family history of death of a parent or sibling due to myocardial infarction before age 50	Myocardial infarction in a mother or sister is especially significant and suggests a need for lipid evaluation.

Do not restrict use of combined oral contraceptives for the following conditions (WHO category # 1):

- Postpartum ≥ 21 days
- Postabortion after first or second trimester or immediately after post-septic abortion
- History of gestational diabetes
- Varicose veins
- Mild headaches
- Irregular vaginal bleeding patterns, *without* or *with* heavy or prolonged bleeding and no anemia
- Past history of pelvic inflammatory disease (PID)
- Current or recent history of (within last 3 months) PID
- Current or recent history of (within last 3 months) sexually transmitted infection (STI)
- Vaginitis without purulent cervicitis
- Increased risk of STI (e.g., multiple partners or partner who has multiple partners)
- HIV-positive, high risk of HIV, or AIDS
- Benign breast disease
- Family history of breast cancer
- Cervical ectropion
- Endometrial or ovarian cancer
- Viral hepatitis carrier
- Uterine fibroids
- Past ectopic pregnancy
- Obesity
- Thyroid conditions: simple goiter, hyperthyroidism, hypothyroidism

(continued)

Table 19-5 Precautions in the provision of combined oral contraceptives (OCs) *(cont.)*

Precautions	Rationale/Discussion

Do not restrict use of combined oral contraceptives for the following conditions (WHO category # 1): (Continued)

- Benign or malignant gestational trophoblastic disease
- Iron deficiency anemia
- Epilepsy
- Schistosomiasis (uncomplicated or with fibrosis of the liver)
- Malaria
- Current use of antibiotics
- Nulliparity or parity
- Severe dysmenorrhea
- Tuberculosis, including pelvic
- Endometriosis
- Benign ovarian tumors
- Prior pelvic surgery

SPECIAL ISSUES
NEW PROGESTINS

Deep vein thrombosis. In 1995-1996, three epidemiologic studies reported that women using third-generation OCs containing a new progestin (gestodene and desogestrel) were at increased risk for venous thromboembolic complications when compared with women using second-generation OCs.[12,58,95,111,112] A "Dear Doctor" letter warning of the DVT risk was sent to British physicians. This letter led to Britain's biggest "pill scare" since 1983 and resulted in an increase of abortion due to unintended pregnancy. Norgestimate was not implicated in the initial studies demonstrating an increased risk for DVT, but it was implicated in the transnational study published subsequently.[61] The data also demonstrated that women using older progestins are at *less of an increased risk for blood clotting complications than had previously been documented.*

Reanalyses questioned the epidemiologic studies of new progestins and DVT.[35,51,87,97] The evidence that third-generation OCs were associated with the increased risk may have been due at least in some measure to prescribing patterns. Clinicians apparently choose to use newer products (third-generation OCs and 20-microgram OCs) for women at higher risk for venous thrombosis.[35,57,61] The Food and Drug Administration concluded in a letter to U.S. clinicians that the additional risk of DVT due to third-generation OCs "is not great enough to justify switching to other products."[36] As a consequence, some clinicians have elected not to prescribe third-generation OCs for new users but have maintained current users on third-generation OCs, especially if the patients have had adverse experiences with other OCs.

It was also suggested that third-generation OCs and the factor V Leiden mutation each independently increases the risk of DVT by about the same amount. Women who have the mutation *and* use third-generation OCs were thought to have a 30-fold to 50-fold risk.[84,104,105] The results of this study have been questioned due to study design, lack of validation for the methodology used, and failure to replicate the data. The factor V mutation, which occurs in 3% to 5% of caucasians, is responsible for the majority of cases of venous thrombosis in which a prothrombotic mechanism is identifiable. It causes resistance to a plasma protein, called activated protein C, which prevents clotting.[104] Perhaps the day will come when women can be screened easily for this mutation.

Myocardial infarction. · An international case-control study found that third-generation OCs may be associated with a reduced risk (30% to 50%) of myocardial infarction or with no difference when compared with second-generation progestins. The authors suggested that "the excess risk of venous thromboembolism associated with the use of third-generation oral contraceptives may be offset by the reduced risk of acute myocardial infarction when compared with second-generation products."[62] Third-generation pills do not reduce a woman's risk of acute myocardial infarction below the background risk; rather they probably do not carry the significantly increased risk that is associated with second-generation pills.[20] If this beneficial effect of third-generation OCs compared with second-generation OCs is confirmed, it could shift the benefit/risk equation in the direction of third-generation OCs since more women die of myocardial infarcts than of venous thromboembolic events.

PELVIC INFLAMMATORY DISEASE

OCs are associated with a decreased risk of symptomatic PID.[115] When OC users do develop PID, the cases generally are less severe. The following reasons have been postulated:

- The average amount of menstrual blood a woman loses each month is decreased. Menstrual blood may act as culture medium, facilitating the development of PID.
- Scanty and thick cervical mucus produced by OC use is difficult to penetrate, thereby discouraging the ascent of sperm from the vagina. Bacteria attached to the surface of sperm gain entry to the upper genital tract through the ascent of sperm.

- The cervical canal is less dilated, principally because the volume of cervical secretions and menstrual blood diminishes.
- Uterine contractions are decreased in strength, thereby decreasing the likelihood of spreading an infection from the uterine cavity into the fallopian tubes.

However, epidemiologic and biologic evidence indicate that OC users more frequently have unrecognized PID and cervical infections with *C. trachomatis*, which possibly offsets the pill's protective effect against PID.[75,109] (See Chapter 8 on Reproductive Tract Infections.) This finding of more frequent infections may be due to a greater exposure to infection among women using OCs.

FETAL EFFECTS

Extensive research has found no significant effects on fetal development associated with long-term use of oral contraceptive steroids taken before pregnancy[14,54] or during early pregnancy.[3,15,28] The few studies of long-term growth and development of infants born to women who used OCs during pregnancy do not show significant adverse effects.[66,77] One recent study reported that infants born to mothers who took OCs during pregnancy had more urinary tract problems.[63] It is prudent to rule out suspected pregnancy before initiating any hormonal contraceptive use or when an OC user has missed two consecutive menstrual periods.

URINARY TRACT INFECTION

Although urinary tract infections occurred at an increased rate in women using OCs in the Royal College of General Practitioners Study, this link was not found in the Oxford/FPA Study.[85,93] Because women using OCs tend to have intercourse more frequently than do women who are not using OCs as their contraceptive, it is difficult to know if the infections are due to intercourse-induced cystitis or to the effect of the OCs.

PROVIDING COMBINED PILLS

Often, exam and laboratory requirements are hurdles clients must cross prior to receiving oral contraceptives. Although it is desirable to measure weight and blood pressure, take a Pap smear, and perform a pelvic examination at the time of the initial examination and at each annual exam, a pelvic exam is *not* necessary, because it does not detect problems that would suggest OCs not be used.[118] The reason for annual pelvic exams is primarily "well woman care" and the early detection of cervical cancer. Similarly, measuring lipid profiles and fasting blood sugar and ordering mammography may be recommended, but they are not prerequisites for using OCs, unless a woman has noted risk factors. Provide OC instructions in writing as well as orally (see Chapter 11 on Selected Reproductive Health Resources).

- Measure the woman's blood pressure and use a checklist to evaluate whether she has reasons not to initiate or continue OCs.
- Avoid prescribing OCs for women who have important reasons to avoid OC use (Table 19-5).
- Avoid (in most cases) prescribing OCs with more than 35 mcg of estrogen, and prescribe OCs with low doses of progestin. Encourage all smokers to stop smoking.
- Give clear instructions on how to use OCs, what side effects to expect, and what to do if problems should occur. Explain what to do if the client misses pills, vomits, or uses drugs that decrease the effectiveness of OCs. Inform her of the noncontraceptive benefits of the pill.
- Encourage women at risk for HIV infection to consider using condoms in addition to OCs. In one national survey, approximately 21% of OC users were also using condoms.[76]
- At each visit, teach women to recognize the pill warning signals. Encourage clients to return on a regular basis and whenever they have any questions or problems.
- Encourage women to inform other clinicians that they are taking OCs.
- Explain use of one of the emergency contraceptive options if a woman misses pills.

Because side effects can appear in the first few months of OC use, a follow-up visit at 3 or 6 months is quite commonly recommended. A woman who has used the pill for 3 to 6 months, has no problems, and wants to continue the pill, may be given 7 to 13 packets (a 6-month to 1-year supply). One author of this chapter strongly recommends providing only 3 cycles of pills at the first visit and then giving only a year supply at maximum. Recent suggestions that it may be appropriate to provide OCs over-the-counter also suggest that new OC users may not need such frequent reassessment.[2,46] An alternative approach is to prescribe or give a woman *a full year's supply of pills the very first visit* and then encourage a revisit or two in the first year for a blood pressure and headache check. After a woman has used OCs for 1 year (a cumulative year of OC use), you could consider prescribing a full year's supply of pills (or even 18 cycles) in an effort to decrease OC discontinuation rates.

Women Over 35 Years of Age

Healthy women who do not smoke and who have no cardiovascular disease may continue using OCs through their 40s.[48,72,93] It is primarily smoking, not OCs, that increases the risk of cardiovascular complications among older women taking low-dose OCs. If a woman wants to use OCs until she is 50, has no risk factors other than age for the use of combined oral contraceptives, is not a smoker, and experiences no side effects, OCs may be an appropriate option for her. The noncontraceptive benefits for mature women are important: prevention of ovarian and endometrial cancers, osteoporosis, and perimenopausal symptoms. In prescribing OCs to women over 35, the following steps may be helpful.

- Check for any reasons to refrain from using OCs (Table 19-5).
- Ask about a history of headaches, hypertension, and diabetes. Ask about a family history of premature cardiovascular disease.
- Measure her blood pressure and obtain blood to measure levels of cholesterol, HDL/LDL, triglycerides, and fasting blood sugar.
- Record her height and weight and perform a breast exam and discuss mammography.

When is a woman menopausal and no longer in need of pregnancy protection? If at the end of the 7-day hormone-free interval (or at the end of the 7 days of placebo pills) her FSH level is 30 or above, she can be considered menopausal. In some women, however, the FSH level does not rise as quickly as 1 week.[20] If a woman is not sexually active or will have no difficulty using a back-up contraceptive for 2 weeks, draw the FSH after she has not taken active pills for 2 weeks. (She can then restart the pills and use a back-up method until she has taken 7 pills.) Some clinicians repeat the FSH after 6 weeks and caution women that pregnancy is still possible because late ovulation can occur despite the presence of high levels of FSH.

At the Margaret Pyke Center in London, women continue taking pills until age 50 and are advised to discontinue contraception *only* if they meet the four criteria for infertility:

- Two FSH levels above 30 while off OCs
- Vasomotor symptoms
- Older than age 50
- No period-like bleeding since the OC withdrawal bleed

Smokers

Inform all OC users, regardless of their age, that smoking increases the risk of myocardial infarction, thrombotic stroke, and hemorrhagic stroke. However, it is not rational to withhold OCs from young women who are heavy smokers but who have no other reasons to avoid using the pill. Strongly consider prescribing a 20-mcg pill. Teach her to recognize the pill warning signals and advise that she stop smoking (provide information on smoking cessation programs).

Teenagers and College Students

If a young teenager is already sexually active, the medical and social risks of pregnancy exceed the risks of taking OCs, even if she has not started having menstrual periods. However, it is unusual to prescribe OCs to someone who has not had a first menses. If a teenager senses that she may become sexually active in the near future, she can start taking OCs before she has intercourse. A teenager who has had irregular periods or late onset of menses will have regular menses while taking OCs; however, when she stops taking her OCs, her periods may again become irregular. We have no evidence that the estrogen in our current low-dose OCs can limit height due to premature closure of the epiphyses, even in premenarchal teens. In menstruating teens, epiphyseal closure is well under way. Teens may be more likely to abandon OCs because of minor side effects such as nausea or spotting, so take all minor side effects in teenagers seriously. If acne is a particular problem, try one of the new progestin OCs (see the discussion on Acne in the section Managing Problems and Follow-up). Continuation rates are higher if potential side effects have been explained before teenagers experience them.

Postpartum and Lactating Women

Because of the elevated risk of thrombosis in the early postpartum period, women should not take estrogen-containing OCs in the 2 to 3 weeks following delivery. (See Chapter 23 on Postpartum Contraception and Lactation.) Breastmilk production has been shown to decline in women who use the combined pill formulations.[49] A better hormonal choice than the combined pill is a progestin-only pill, Norplant, or Depo-Provera. (See Chapter 20 on Progestin-Only Contraceptives.) If a woman still wants to use OCs while she is breastfeeding, then delay OC initiation until the milk supply is well established (provide a back-up contraceptive method until she is protected by the pill). Milk production generally reaches a plateau at about 6 weeks postpartum, so this is considered by some to be the absolutely earliest time to start the method.[53] Other experts urge delaying initiation until 8 to 12 weeks at the very earliest. The WHO argues that until 6 months postpartum, the risks of OC use outweigh the benefits.[113] The WHO guidance reflects the fact that milk volume increases through the sixth postpartum month, at which time it can also be said that the milk supply is "established." If the woman wants to wean her child in the near future, then the initiation of OCs would appear to be acceptable.

Women with Diabetes

Low-dose OCs (including the new progestin OCs), both triphasics and monophasics, may be provided to some gestational diabetics, to some women with a family history of diabetes, and to some women with insulin-dependent diabetes who have no evidence of diabetic tissue damage (Table 19-5). Some clinicians maintain that any increase in the amount of insulin a diabetic might require as a result of using OCs is far outweighed by the potential adverse effects of a pregnancy. Of the progestins, norgestrel appears to have the greatest insulin-antagonizing activity.[92,116] A 1986 study found significantly less effect on carbohydrate metabolism in women taking OCs with 20 mcg of EE and 1 mg of norethindrone acetate (Loestrin 1/20).[116] A 1988 study found no impairment in carbohydrate metabolism in women with postpartum gestational diabetes who took 0.4 mg of norethindrone and 35 mcg of EE (Ovcon-35); in contrast, women taking Triphasil had significantly elevated levels at 3 and 6 months.[89]

CHOOSING A COMBINED OC: WHICH PILL TO PRESCRIBE?

Clinicians in the United States have numerous OCs from which to choose (Table 19-6). Choose an OC based on the hormonal dose and on the woman's clinical picture (Figure 19-3).

Table 19-6 Equivalent brand names for sub-50 mcg combined pills available world-wide

As people travel and move their residence from place to place around the globe, it becomes more and more important for clinicians in Indiana or Idaho to know the estrogen and progestin prescribed for women in India or Indonesia. The following list gives details of some sub-50 mcg OCs used world-wide that are similar to U.S. brands. U.S. brands are shown in italics and boldface.

| Group, progestin | Dose | | Brand Name |
	Ethinyl Estradiol (mcg)	Progestin (mcg)	
Group A: norgestimate	35	250	***Ortho-Cyclen,*** Cilest, Effiprev, Effiprev 35
Triphasic formula	35	180	***Ortho Tri-Cyclen,*** Pramino, Tricilest
	35	215	
	35	250	
Group B: desogestrel	30	150	***Desogen, Ortho-Cept,*** Cycleane-30, Desolett, Frilavon, Marvelon, Marvelon 30, Marviol, Microdiol, Novelon, Planum, Practil, Prevenon, Varnoline
	20	150	Cycleane-20, Lovelle, Marvelon 20, Mercilon, Microdosis, Myralon, Securgin, Segurin

(continued)

Group, progestin	Dose		Brand Name
	Ethinyl Estradiol (mcg)	Progestin (mcg)	
Biphasic formula	40	25	Gracial
	30	125	
Group C: gestodene (not available in United States)	30	75	Ciclomex, Evacin, Femodeen, Femoden, Femodene, Femovan, Ginera, Ginoden, Gynera, Gynovin, Minulet, Minulette, Moneva, Myvlar
	20	75	Harmonet, Meliane
Triphasic formula	30	50	Milvane, Phaeva, Triadene, Triciclomex, Tri-Femoden, Trigynera, Tri-Gynera, Trigynovin, Triminulet, Triodeen
	40	70	Trioden, Triodena, Triodene
	30	100	
Group D (second generation): levonorgestrel	30	150	***Levlen, Levora, Lo-Ovral*, Nordette, Nordette 150/30,*** Ciclo, Ciclon, Combination 3, Contraceptive LD, Duofem, Egogyn 30, Femigoa, Femranette mikro, Follimin, Gynatrol, Levonorgestrel Pill, Lo-Femenal*, Lo-Gentrol*, Lo/Ovral*, Lo-Rondal*, Lorsax, Mala D, Microgest, Microginon, Microgyn, Microgyn 30, Microgynon, Microgynon 30, Microvlar, Minibora, Minidril, Minigynon, Minigynon 30, Minivlar, Min-Ovral*, Mithuri, Neo-Gentrol 150/30, Neomonovar, Neovletta, Nordet, Norgestrel, Norgylene, Norvetal, Ologyn-micro, Ovoplex 30/150, Ovral L*, Ovranet, Ovranette, Riget, Rigevidon, Sexcon, Stediril-30, Stediril-d 150/30, Stediril-M, Suginor
	30	125	Minisiston, Mene Step
	20	100	***Alesse,*** Loette, Leios, Miranova
Triphasic formula	30	50	***Tri-Levlen, Triphasil,*** Fironetta, Levordiol, Logynon
	40	75	Triagynon, Triciclor, Triette, Trigoa, Trigynon
	30	125	Trikvilar, Trinordiol, Trionetta, Triovlar, Triquilar, Tri-Regol, Trisisten, Tri-Stediril, Trolit

(continued)

Table 19-6 Equivalent brand names for sub-50 mcg combined pills available world-wide *(cont.)*

Group, progestin	Dose		Brand Name
	Ethinyl Estradiol (mcg)	Progestin (mcg)	
Group E (first generation): norethisterone (NET) norethindrone (NEA) ethynodiol diacetate (EDDA)	20	NEA 1000**	*Loestrin 1/20,* Loestrin, Loestrin 20, Minestril 20, Minestrin 1/20
	30	NEA 1500**	*Loestrin 1.5/30,* Minestril 30
	35	NET 500	*Brevicon, Genora 0.5/35, Modicon, Nelova 0.5/35E,* Brevinor, Gynex O.5/35E, Intercon 5/35, Mikro Plan, Nilocan, Norminest, Orthonett Novum, Ovacon, Ovysmen 0.5/35, Perle LD
	35	EDDA 1000**	Demulen 1/35
	35	NET 1000	*Genora 1/35, Jenest (biphasic pill), NEE/35, Norcept-E 1/35, Norethin 1/35E, Norinyl 1/35, Ortho-Novum 1/35,* Brevicon 1, Brevinor -1, Gynex 1/35 E, Intercon 1/35, Kanchan, Nelova 1+35, Neocon, Noremin, Noremin -1, Norquest, Ovysmen 1/35, Secure
	35	NET 400	*Ovcon 35,* Micropil, Norquen, Oviprem
Triphasic formula	35	NET 500	*Ortho Novum 7/7/7*
	35	NET 750	Triella, Trinovum
	35	NET 1000	
	35	NET 500	*Tri-Norinyl*
	35	NET 1000	
	35	NET 500	
	20	NEA 1000	*Estrostep*
	30		
	35		

Source: Kleinman RL (1996).

*These pills also contain dextronorgestrel (non-contraceptive).
**Converted to norethindrone as the active metabolite.

Figure 19-3 is designed to assist you in deciding which OC to prescribe.

Step 1: Avoiding Combined Pills Completely

Some women (but not many) should avoid using combined pills. See also Table 19-5.

Step 2: Selecting Alternatives to Estrogenic Pills

Women unable to use combined pills may be able to use a contraceptive listed in Step 2.

Step 3: Selecting a Combined Pill

Select any sub-50 mcg OC based on its availability, cost, or the woman's prior experience. No single OC is clearly better than all the rest.

Price. It is appropriate to consider price in choosing a pill. In many public-funded family planning settings, decisions about which OC to provide are influenced by the cost of OCs to that program. It is appropriate for the clinician in private practice to decide which low-dose combined pill to prescribe a new patient on the basis of the availability of free samples.

Dose. Any of the sub-50 mcg OCs may be used by most women. One approach is to prescribe the lowest dose:

Ethinyl estradiol: Loestrin 1/20 or Alesse both provide a woman with 33.3% less EE than she would receive in a 30 mcg OC and 43% less EE than in all the 35 mcg OCs. Two potential problems occur with 20 mcg OCs: spotting and a smaller margin of error for missed pills. Missed pills are associated with a higher pregnancy rate.

Norethindrone: Ovcon-35 has a total of 8.4 mg norethindrone, and Modicon or Brevicon have a cycle total of 10.5 mg norethindrone compared with Ortho-Novum 7/7/7 having 15.75 mg, Tri-Norinyl having 15 mg, or the higher-dose OCs such as Norinyl 1+35 or Ortho-Novum 1+35 having 21 mg.

Levonorgestrel: Triphasil or Tri-Levlen have a total of 1.925 mg of levonorgestrel per cycle, 39% less than the amount in Nordette (Levlen).

No OCs containing more than 35 mcg of estrogen are included in this flow sheet. Even if a woman is a satisfied user of a higher-dose pill, she generally should be switched to a lower-dose pill. (Most OCs containing 80 to 100 mcg estrogen have been removed from the market in the United States.) However, several clinical situations may call for a 50 mcg pill:

- Managing spotting or the absence of withdrawal bleeding that cannot be controlled on a lower-dose pill.
- Treating acne, dysfunctional uterine bleeding, ovarian cysts, and endometriosis. (Dysfunctional bleeding has been treated in the

Figure 19-3 Choosing a combined oral contraceptive with less than 50 micrograms of estrogen

Start by determining if the woman can safely use estrogen

Step 1	Step 2

Is this person a good ————————————→ YES, she can use ————————————→
candidate for a pill with estrogen? an estrogen.

In general, avoid prescribing ————————————→ NO, it would be best if she
a pill with estrogen to women with: did not use an estrogen.
Therefore, you can consider:

Step 1

- Current or a history of circulatory diseases due to blood clots (including heart attack, stroke, or blood clots in deep veins) or cardiovascular disease due to diabetes.
- Structural heart disease with complications such as atrial fibrillation or subacute bacterial endocarditis.
- Blood pressure of 160/100 or greater
- Age of 35 or more who are smokers.
- Breast cancer or history thereof (exceptions may be made if no evidence of disease in past 5 years)
- Active hepatic disease including symptomatic viral hepatitis, severe or mild cirrhosis; or benign or malignant liver tumors.
- Past history of jaundice (cholestasis) related to oral contraceptives.
- Migraine headaches with neurologic impairment such as blurred or lost vision, seeing flashing lights or zigzag lines, trouble speaking or moving.
- Diabetes and damaged vision (retinopathy), kidneys (nephropathy) or nervous system (neuropathy), or women who have diabetes for 20 years or longer.
- Plan to undergo major surgery or any leg surgery requiring immobilization for several days or more. Estrogen-containing pills should be discontinued 4 weeks before major surgery.

Step 2

- Progestin-only pills, such as:
  - Micronor (0.35 mg norethindrone daily) NOR QD (0.35 mg nonrethindrone daily)
  - Ovrette (0.075 mg nogestrel daily)
- Norplant (5-year levonorgestrel implants)
- Depo-Provera (150 mg medroxyprogestrone acetate injection every 3 months)
- Intrauterine device
  - Copper T 380-A
  - Levonorgestrel IUD
  - Progestasert System
- Condoms (male or female)
- Diaphragm, cervical cap, Reality female condom
- Foam, VCF Film, suppository
- Fertility awareness
- Male or female sterilization

Breastfeeding women, in general, should avoid estrogen until they start weaning the baby from breastfeeding.

Exceptions may be made in specific cases and occasionally pills may be prescribed for women in the above categories, provided that the specialized (individualized) grounds are well documented in the record. For a fuller list of precautions see Table 19-5.

© Robert A. Hatcher, MD, MPH
April 1993

The following individuals assisted in the develpment of this flow chart:
Marcia Angle, MD, MPH, Program for International Training and Health (INTRAH)
James Bellinger, PAC, Emory University School of Medicine
Willard Cates, Jr., MD, MPH, Family Health International (FHI)
John Guillebaud, MA, FRSCE, FRCOG, MFFP, Margaret Pyke Center, London
Robert A. Hatcher, MD, MPH, Emory University School of Medicine
Michael Policar, MD, MPH, Solano Partnership Health Plan
Sharon Schnare, CNM, MSN, FNP, DHHS/PHS – Region 10
Gary S. Stewart, MD, MPH, Plamnned Parenhood of Sacramento Valley
Susan Wysocki, RNC, BSN, NP, National Association of Nurse Practitioners in Reproductive Health

Most woman may use any of the sub-50 microgram pills

Step 3	Step 4

Step 3

If there is no reason to avoid estrogen, you may choose between any of the following OCs based on:
- Number of micrograms of ethinyl estradiol
- Availability of pill
- Ease of understanding packaging of pills
- Price of pills to clinic**
- Price of pills to client**
- Prior experience of this individual woman or the clinician caring for this woman with a special pill

Pills are listed from the lowest to the highest number of micrograms of ethinyl estradiol:

Combined Pill	Estrogen (mcg)	Availability/Cost In Your Clinic	Company
Loestrin 1/20	20		Parke-Davis
Alesse	20		Wyeth
Estrostep 21	20/30/35		Parke-Davis
Loestrin 1.5/30	30		Parke-Davis
*Desogen	30		Organon
Lo-Ovral	30		Wyeth
Nordette	30		Wyeth
Levlen	30		Berlex
*Ortho-Cept	30		Ortho
Tri-Levlen	30/40/30		Berlex
Triphasil	30/40/30		Wyeth
Ovcon 35	35		Mead Johnson
Demulen 1/35	35		Searle
Ortho-Cyclen	35		Ortho
Ortho Tri-Cyclen	35		Ortho
Ortho Novum 777	35		Ortho
Ortho-Novum 1/35	35		Ortho
Modicon	35		Ortho
Brevicon	35		Syntex
Norinyl 1/35	35		Syntex
Tri-Norinyl	35		Syntex
**Norcept-E 1/35	35		Syntex
**Nelova 0.5/35	35		GynoPharma
**Nelova 1/35	35		Warner-Chilcott
NEE 0.5/35	35		Lexis
NEE 1/35	35		Lexis
**Genora 0.5/35	35		Rugby
Genora 1/35	35		Rugby
Jenest	35		Organon
NEE 10/11	35		Lexes
Norethin 1/35E	35		Schiaparelli-Searle

*Women using pills containing desogestrel may have an increased risk of venous thombosis.

** The four pills costing pharmacists less than $10.00 per cycle: Norcept E ($5.72); Nelova 0.5/35; Nelova 1/35 ($6.25); and Genora 0.5/35 ($8.23). Cost of most pills to pharmacists was $17.00 to $22.33 per cycle. In some clinics, pills may be purchased at prices as low as $0.50 to $1.00 per cycle. [Source: Anonymous. Drug Topics Red Book. Average wholesale price listing. The Medical Letter 1992; December 11.

Step 4

Other clinical considerations that might help in OC choice

A. To minimize the risk potential for *thrombosis* due to estrogen in a woman 40–50 years of age, or any woman at increased risk for thrombosis due to another cause (e.g., diabetic, very overweight woman or a young woman who is a heavy smoker), prescribe:
- Loestrin 1/20
- Alesse

B. To minimize *nausea, breast tenderness, vascular headaches*, and estrogen-mediated side effects, prescribe:
- Loestrin 1/20
- Alesse
- Estrostep

Or a 30 mcg pill, such as:
- Levlen
- Loestrin 1.5–30
- Lo-Ovral
- Nordette

C. To minimize *spotting and/or break-through bleeding*, prescribe:
- Low-Ovral, Nordette or Levlen
- Estrostep
- Ortho-Cyclen or Ortho Tri-Cyclen
- Desogen or Ortho-Cept

D. To minimize androgen effects such as *acne, hirsutism, oily skin, sebaceous cysts, pilonidal cysts, or weight gain*, prescribe:
- Ortho-Cyclen or Ortho Tri-Cyclen
- Desogen or Ortho-Cept
- Ovcon-35, Brevicon or Modicon
- Demulen-35

E. To produce the most *favorable lipid profile*, prescribe:
- Ortho-Cyclen or Ortho Tri-Cyclen
- Desogen or Ortho-Cept
- Ovcon-35, Brevicon or Modicon

F. To use a combined pill as an emergency contraceptive:
- Ovral (2 within 72 hours, repeat in 12 hours)
- Lo-Ovral (4 within 72 hours, repeat in 12 hours)
- Levlen, Nordette (4 within 72 hours, repeat in 12 hours)
- Triphasil, Tri-Levlen (4 yellow pills within 72 hours, repeat in 12 hours)

following regimen: 1 pill four times a day for 5 to 7 days, subsequently a pill a day for 21 days, followed by 7 pill-free days for several months. Ovarian cysts have been treated with 50 mcg combined monophasic OCs.)

- Improving contraceptive effectiveness for women who become pregnant despite perfect use of a 30 to 35 mcg pill. Prescribe a 50 mcg pill such as Ovcon-50, Demulen 50, or Ovral. A second approach is to decrease the number of pill-free days from 7 to 4 days (21 active pills followed by only 4 days of no oral contraceptives). A third approach is to *tricycle.* Only active pills, with no pill-free break, are taken for 3 consecutive cycles to gain greater effectiveness.
- Increasing the dose for women using enzyme-inducing drugs. (Rifampin and Dilantin [phenytoin] both accelerate the breakdown of estrogens in OCs.[7] Women can improve OC effectiveness by taking 50 mcg OCs or by *tricycling* with a pill-free interval of just 4 days after the third cycle. Rifampin is such a potent enzyme-inducer that clinicians in the United Kingdom do not prescribe OCs for women using this drug.)

Step 4. Clinical Considerations

The estrogenic, progestational, and androgenic effects of OCs affect a number of organs and tissues throughout the body. A specific OC may suppress hormone production or affect one organ system or tissue differently in two different women. There are ways to minimize a woman's risk of specific side effects or metabolic changes brought about by OCs:

Thrombosis.   The clinician faced with a client already at an increased risk for thrombophlebitis may want to use the 20-mcg pill.[10,19,39]

Estrogenic side effects.   A low-estrogen OC may minimize the likelihood of side effects or complications associated with either the estrogen or the progestin in a pill. When the estrogen in an OC is diminished, the progestin is as well.

Spotting or breakthrough bleeding.   Spotting and breakthrough bleeding (BTB) are trade-offs for lower-dose OCs. Several OCs minimize spotting and BTB. If one pill does not lead to an acceptable pattern of bleeding, another pill may. Spotting and BTB tend to diminish over the first few months of OC use. *Always keep in mind that spotting and BTB may be due to chlamydia, endometriosis, or other pathology, including cancer of the cervix.*

Androgenic effects.   New progestin OCs may help in treating hirsutism, chronic anovulation associated with the syndrome of polycystic ovarian disease, and acne.[30,82] Long before the entry of the new progestins, it was known that the pill with the lowest dose of norethindrone (Ovcon 35) was associated with a 270% increase in SHBG and with a decrease in free testosterone levels. Clinical evidence from several trials also confirms that SHBG levels increase and plasma androgen levels decrease, albeit to a lesser extent, in women taking levonorgestrel OCs.[64,103] When combined with a given dose of estrogen, desogestrel raises SHBG and therefore lowers free testosterone levels to a greater extent than does levonorgestrel.[25,52] New progestin OCs also appear to have as good or better patterns of weight gain as do low-dose OCs. This may be related to greater suppression of free testosterone levels.

Lipid changes.   The new progestin OCs tend to increase HDL cholesterol and decrease LDL cholesterol. When prescribing a pill containing norethindrone, choose one with 0.4 mg, Ovcon-35, or one of the 0.5-mg norethindrone OCs.

Emergency contraception.   Combined pills with levonorgestrel and EE are effective emergency contraceptives. Although other combined pills may be effective, no data support their use as emergency contraceptives. (See Chapter 12 on Emergency Contraception.)

M ANAGING PROBLEMS AND FOLLOW-UP
(The following problems are listed in alphabetical order.)

Absence of Withdrawal Bleeding While Taking OCs

With sub-50 mcg OCs, the amount of vaginal bleeding in the 7 hormone-free days may be minimal, or no bleeding at all may occur. The most important differential diagnoses of missed periods or prolonged amenorrhea are pregnancy (intrauterine or ectopic) and inadequate buildup of endometrium due to use of a low-dose OC.

Has the patient had any bleeding, spotting (while taking pills), or staining of underwear? Ask about missing pills, patterns of sexual intercourse, date of last sexual intercourse, the symptoms of pregnancy (including enlarging breasts, breast tenderness, and nausea), breast discharge, vigorous exercise, increased stress, weight changes, major life changes, recreational drug use, and use of drugs causing rapid clearance of estrogens from the blood stream, such as rifampin or phenobarbital.

Determine whether the patient is pregnant by checking for uterine enlargement, softening of the cervix, and other signs of pregnancy. An elevated basal body temperature may indicate the possibility of pregnancy. (See the discussion of Pregnancy in this section.)

Manage the absence of withdrawal bleeding by using the following approaches:

- **Rule out pregnancy.** Consider having the client check her basal body temperature on three consecutive mornings when she is not taking active hormone pills. A temperature below 98° F on three consecutive mornings during these days suggests that ovulation and pregnancy have not occurred. If the patient has missed a period after missing pills and has been sexually active without a back-up method, order a sensitive beta-hCG test. Also rule out pregnancy in any woman who has missed two or more periods.
- **Switch pills.** Because women using the new progestin OCs virtually never miss two consecutive menstrual periods, it may now be possible to manage amenorrhea in women on *other* OCs by switching them to one of the new progestin preparations. Triphasic OCs may lead to dependable withdrawal bleeding when other approaches have not worked.
- **Inform women in advance.** Warn women using low-dose OCs that they may have scanty or no bleeding.

Androgenic Effects (Acne, Oily Skin, Hirsutism)

The differential diagnoses of acne or oily skin while using OCs may include high endogenous ovarian or adrenal androgenic production; dietary, allergic, hygienic, familial, or other factors; polycystic ovarian syndrome; an androgen-producing ovarian or adrenal tumor; or use of an OC with high androgenic potency.

Ask when acne erupts: age of onset, duration and progression of symptoms, association with stress or dietary intake, and relationship to taking OCs. Family history, any pre-pill history of oligomenorrhea, acne, hirsutism, and inability to become pregnant may suggest chronic anovulation associated with polycystic ovarian syndrome.

Assess the lesions (location, size, number, and color), hair growth (amount, thickness, and distribution), and ovaries (enlargement or cysts). Consider ordering serum levels of testosterone, DHAS, and 170HP only if there has been sudden onset of hirsutism or rapidly progressive hirsutism.

Manage androgenic effects as follows:

- **Decrease androgenic effects.** Provide a low-androgen OC that suppresses ovarian androgenic production while providing the least exogenous androgen: any of the new progestin OCs, Ovcon-35, Brevicon, Modicon, or Demulen-35. All OCs *may* have a beneficial effect on acne. Ortho Tricyclen is now formally approved by the FDA for the treatment of acne.
- **Increase estrogenic effects.** Increase the estrogen dose of the OC to increase SHBG, thus decreasing free serum testosterone levels.

- **Treat the acne.** Advise use of a broad spectrum of antibiotic such as tetracycline, good hygiene, use of special soaps or skin cleansers, or the vitamin A analogue, Accutane. *Women taking Accutane must use a reliable contraceptive.* A high percentage of infants born to mothers using Accutane in early pregnancy have severe neurological defects. Contraception should continue for at least 30 days after Accutane is discontinued. Discontinue the pill if acne clearly became worse since starting OCs.
- **Refer.** Refer the patient to a dermatologist or endocrinologist for further assessment if the previous measures do not improve the androgenic conditions.

Breakthrough Bleeding and Spotting Between Periods

The lower the dose of pill, the more common the spotting and breakthrough bleeding. Although annoying, breakthrough bleeding is not harmful. The differential diagnoses of breakthrough bleeding or spotting include the following:

- Inadequate estrogenic or progestogenic stimulation of endometrial activity
- Missing pill(s) or altering the time of taking them
- Impaired absorption of hormones because the woman takes an enzyme-inducing antiseizure drug or antibiotic or has had severe diarrhea or vomiting
- Threatened or spontaneous abortion (If OCs were started just after an abortion or miscarriage, the bleeding should be evaluated right away.)
- Ectopic pregnancy
- Trophoblastic disease
- Infection, such as pelvic inflammatory disease, cervical inflammation, or condylomata *(Remember the possibility of chlamydia as the cause of spotting or breakthrough bleeding, particularly following a recent change in sexual partners.)*
- Endometriosis
- Endometrial or cervical growth such as leiomyomata (particularly submucous myoma), cancer, or polyp

Ask about pill use patterns (duration, dosage, regularity of taking OCs), bleeding patterns (duration and amount of spotting, most recent period), symptoms of pregnancy, past history of gynecologic problems, symptoms of infection (pelvic pain, chills, fever, malaise, pain during intercourse, vaginal discharge), use of other drugs that may interact with oral contraceptives (such as rifampin, phenytoin, phenobarbital, carbamazepine; very little data suggest ampicillin or tetracycline alter OC effectiveness[74]), or the possibility of impaired absorption of hormones (nausea and vomiting, diarrhea, or other intestinal or liver problems).

Assess for signs of pregnancy (intrauterine, ectopic, or trophoblastic disease), pelvic infection (consider obtaining cultures for chlamydia and gonorrhea), myomata, cervical inflammation, dysplasia or polyp, or endometriosis. Obtain a hematocrit in women as appropriate.

After other gynecologic causes of bleeding have been eliminated, manage spotting and breakthrough bleeding as follows:

- **Inform the patient.** Tell her that breakthrough bleeding decreases dramatically over the first 4 months of OC use. Tell her that lower dose OCs are safer, but they also are associated with more breakthrough bleeding.

- **Alter progestin dose.** Switch to a new progestin pill or increase the progestin potency of the pill. Lo/Ovral may be more powerful than Nordette and less likely to result in spotting.

- **Increase the estrogenic potency.** While leaving the progestin unchanged, switch to a pill with less estrogen. Estrostep is a triphasic pill designed to minimize spotting by increasing the amount of EE from 20 mcg to 30 or 35 mcg as the cycle progresses. An alternative is to supplement the active hormonal pills for 1 to 3 cycles with exogenous estrogen in the form of 17-beta estradiol, such as Estrace 1 mg or 2 mg daily, ethinyl estradiol (20 mcg per day), or conjugated estrogen (Premarin 0.625 mg daily).

- **Try a prostaglandin inhibitor.** Prostaglandin inhibitors decrease menstrual bleeding, menstrual cramps, and pain.

Breastfeeding Problems

Certified lactation consultants can help diagnose and treat problems with breastfeeding mechanics that could be responsible for a diminishing milk volume. (Call 1-919-787-5185 to find a local consultant.) Because the estrogen in combined pills can diminish milk volume, avoid combined pills during lactation whenever possible. If, through informed choice, the breastfeeding woman decides to use combined oral pills, she should do so only after an adequate milk supply has been established (after at least 6 weeks, but preferably after 6 months) or if the woman decides to accept the decline in milk volume or if she plans to wean her infant soon. Progestin-only OCs, Depo-Provera, or Norplant represent better hormonal contraceptive alternatives for breastfeeding women once lactation has been established. (See Chapter 23 on Postpartum Contraception and Lactation.)

Breast Fullness, Tenderness (Mastalgia) or Tingling

Lowering the amount of estrogen provided in each pill tends to reduce breast tenderness. The differential diagnoses include actual growth of breast tissue; cyclic edema due to either the estrogen or the progestin; early pregnancy; masses or tenderness due to benign breast disease, fibroadenomata, or breast cancer; or an elevated prolactin level.

Ask about duration and severity, when during the cycle discomfort occurs, severity prior to use of OCs, symptoms of pregnancy, progression of symptoms, cyclic changes in weight, change in bra size, breast discharge, past history of benign breast disease, biopsies or mammography, and family history of breast cancer.

Look for local or generalized tenderness, difference in fullness, nodularity or masses, and nipple fluid. Note the comparative size of the two breasts. Look for signs of early pregnancy. Even if a breast mass is not palpable, order baseline mammography if the woman is 35 to 40 years of age or older, has a family history of breast cancer, or simply expresses a desire to have a mammogram. Further tests may include microscopic or cytologic evaluation of breast discharge, fine-needle aspiration of masses for cytologic study, biopsy, urine or serum pregnancy tests, or prolactin level. *Draw blood to obtain a prolactin level before examining the breast, because breast stimulation immediately raises the serum prolactin level.*

After ruling out the possibility of pregnancy and breast cancer, try the following approaches:

- **Try a lower-dose pill.** Recommend that the client switch to a 20 mcg or progestin-only pill.
- **Recommend good bra support for symptomatic relief.**
- **Avoid jostling of breasts.** Inform her that her symptoms may improve if she avoids vigorous exercise during times of most discomfort.
- **Watch diet.** Some women have benefitted from decreasing intake of methylxanthines found in coffee, tea, chocolate, and soft drinks.
- **Suggest vitamin E.** Vitamin E, 400 IU two times a day, may help relieve the symptoms of fibrocystic breast tenderness.
- **Prescribe medication.** Bromocriptine or Danocrine may benefit some women who have severe tenderness. Bromocriptine should not be used with diuretics or hypotensive drugs.

Chloasma or the Mask of Pregnancy

Chloasma may occur in pregnancy or in women on the pill. Darkening of skin pigment usually occurs on the upper lip, under the eyes, in front of the ears, and on the forehead. It is usually noted in women with frequent exposure to the sun. Although not dangerous, chloasma may cause a woman a great deal of concern. The increased pigmentation may be slow to fade when OCs are discontinued and occasionally may be permanent. Other skin conditions that may occur in OC users include telangiectasia, neurodermatitis, erythema multiforme, erythema nodosum, eczema, photosensitivity, and loss of hair. Use of special sunscreens may help prevent this problem, as may discontinuing OCs or switching to a progestin-only pill.

Depression and Other Mood Changes

Accurately diagnosing the cause of depression in an OC user may be extremely difficult. The onset of depression may be quite insidious. It may be diagnosed by a person's acquaintances before it is recognized by the patient herself. OCs are more likely to improve depression and premenstrual irritability, although they may make these conditions worse.[42] In some instances, OCs produce a deficiency of pyridoxine (vitamin B_6).

Ask about the association between OC use and depression (relative to initiating the current pill, while using the other OCs, and prior to OC use), severity of depression (changes in appetite, weight change, ability to sleep, past history of suicide attempts, or thoughts of suicide), use of alcohol, and other possible causes (changes in life situation, postpartum depression, fear of contracting HIV and other sexually transmitted infections, relationship with partner, physical abuse, job dissatisfaction, or illness). Ask about changes in the frequency of intercourse, libido, and the ability to have orgasm, and use of diazepam and other mood-altering drugs that may interact with OCs.

Assess the woman's level of depression including lethargy, depressed mood, and expressions of inability to cope. Determine whether the depression began or became worse after starting OCs. Pill-induced depression has the following mechanisms:

- Progestogenic effects
- Decreased pyridoxine (B_6) levels
- Cyclic fluid retention caused by the estrogen or the progestin
- Interaction with diazepam. (Because the OC increases the half-life of diazepam [Valium] from 47 to 60 hours, the dose of diazepam may need to be lowered for the woman on OCs.[1])

If the depression is severe, discuss immediate sources of psychiatric help. Take severe depression seriously, regardless of its etiology. Leave the patient with the clear message that severe depression can be effectively treated in most individuals. If the depression is clearly temporally related to OC use and bothersome to the patient, try the following approaches:

- **Discontinue OCs.** The easiest approach is to provide an alternative method and discontinue OCs completely for 3 to 6 cycles to see what happens.
- **Tricycle.** Taking active pills continuously for 3 cycles, without a pill-free interval or using placebo pills, may help avoid cyclic depression and premenstrual-like symptoms.
- **Lower hormone levels in the pill.** Lowering the estrogen or the progestin (or both) may benefit pill-induced depression. Switching to a progestin-only pill eliminates estrogen and lowers the progestin-dose provided to a woman.
- **Increase intake of vitamin B_6.** Consider supplementing the patient diet with no more than 50 mg of vitamin B_6 daily. Foods rich in pyridoxine include wheat germ, liver, meats, fish, milk, bananas and peanuts.

Eye Problems (Blurred or Loss of Vision)

Women using OCs may be at an increased risk of retinal artery and retinal vein thrombosis. Pill-related fluid retention may cause edema of the optic nerve with loss of vision, double vision, or swelling or pain in one or both eyes. The fluid retention may also cause corneal edema, leading to an increased likelihood of discomfort or even corneal damage among contact lens users. Thanks to soft contact lenses and low-dose OCs, most contact lens wearers can continue wearing their lenses.[79] Eye problems may accompany headaches that may or may not be induced by OCs. No evidence suggests that OCs cause or aggravate glaucoma.

When strokes occur in women on OCs, they are often preceded for weeks or months by either visual symptoms or headaches or both. *Visual symptoms and severe headaches are important early danger signals of a potentially serious problem.* If a patient has experienced transient, total, or partial loss of vision, discontinue OCs immediately and refer her to a neurologist. If visual impairment accompanies migraine headaches that have become worse, discontinue OCs immediately.

Galactorrhea

Galactorrhea associated with excessive estrogen in OCs may be most noticeable in the pill-free week. Galactorrhea caused by excessive estrogen is less common now with lower-dose OCs. However, if galactorrhea is due to OCs, it will disappear within 3 to 6 months after discontinuing OCs.[93] The differential diagnoses include OC suppression of prolactin-inhibiting factor, galactorrhea secondary to breast suckling, prolactin-secreting tumor, or drug treatment, especially with phenothiazines, haloperidol, or metoclopramide.

If an OC user has milk flow that is excessive or that occurs when she is not breastfeeding, ask whether her breasts have been stimulated by suckling or breast manipulation. Ask about the characteristics of her milk flow (duration and amount of discharge), any past history of galactorrhea, symptoms of pregnancy (nausea, breast fullness or tenderness, change in appetite, missed menses, and weight gain), and symptoms of pituitary tumor (headaches or changes in vision). There is little evidence of an increase in the incidence of pituitary tumors in women, either in case control or cohort studies.[71]

Determine if the secretions can be expressed. If so, send the discharge sample to the cytology laboratory. Fix the sample as you would fix a Pap smear of the cervix (unless galactorrhea is felt to be due to breast suckling). Look at the discharge under a microscope (fat globules, white blood cells, etc.) Draw blood to measure the serum prolactin level. Breasts cannot have been examined before blood is drawn because this immediately raises serum prolactin levels; wait until the next day if breast examination has already been performed. If an elevated level is found, consider whether a breast examination occurred immediately prior to obtaining blood or whether breasts were stimulated the previous night. Perform a sensitive pregnancy test if pregnancy is a possibilty.

Once serious causes of galactorrhea have been excluded, manage the galactorrhea as follows:

- **Continue the OCs.** Explain that OCs can simply be continued if the galactorrhea is something she can live with.
- **Discontinue the OCs.** Consider discontinuing OCs if the galactorrhea is of concern to the woman. Initiate alternative contraception if she is sexually active. But reassurance is otherwise all that is necessary.[93]
- **Advise less stimulation.** If galactorrhea is felt to be due to breast suckling during lovemaking, discuss how much the galactorrhea is bothering the patient and consider recommending less intense breast stimulation.

Headaches

Headaches may be mild, severe, recurrent, or persistent. Women may note an increase (or a decrease) in the severity of migrane headaches. Pill-induced headaches are sometimes associated with blurred vision, loss of vision, or weakness in an extremity. These symptoms are more significant if they are asymmetric. *Take headaches in an OC user seriously, because they are the major warning signal that precedes cerebrovascular accidents.*

The differential diagnoses of headaches in a patient using OCs may include the following:

- Transient ischemic attacks, migraine headaches, vascular headaches associated with using OCs or a cerebrovascular accident
- Hypertension
- Cyclic fluid retention induced by the estrogen or progestin component in OCs
- Anxiety, tension, or stress
- Caffeine withdrawal; use of alcohol, drugs, or specific foods
- Sinusitis, viremia, sepsis, or seasonal allergies
- Temporomandibular joint (TMJ) disorder or dental problems
- Central nervous system tumor

Ask about age at onset of headaches and their severity, duration, character (throbbing or constant), cyclicity, and location (including asymmetry). Ask about associated symptoms such as nausea, vomiting, dizziness, scotomata or blurred vision, watering of the eyes, loss of vision or speech, and weakness or numbness in a limb. Can the patient function when the headaches are most severe? Ask about a history of sinusitis or postnasal drip. Ask about alcohol use, caffeine intake, drug history, and any relationship to taking OCs. The patient's or her family's history of migraines is important.

Measure the patient's blood pressure, and perform a funduscopic exam. Check for localized tenderness at sites on the face, head, and neck. A complete neurological exam may be indicated.

Immediately refer the patient to a neurologist if her headaches are severe or accompanied by an elevated blood pressure or neurological symptoms such as asymmetry or loss of vision. Have the patient discontinue her OCs. If the headaches are not serious and are related to OC use, consider the following approaches:

- **Discontinue the OCs.**
- **Lower the dose of estrogen.**
- **Lower the dose of progestin.**
- **Tricycle.** Eliminate the pill-free interval for 3 consecutive cycles of pills. This recommendation is helpful if a woman's headaches occur during the pill-free interval.

Decreased Libido or Sex Drive

Some women experience decreased libido, possibly due to decreased androgen production by the ovary. Some women also experience decreased vaginal lubrication, making sexual intercourse less comfortable and, occasionally, painful; this is possibly an estrogen deficiency effect. Free testosterone levels fall dramatically in women taking OCs, most strikingly in women on the new progestin OCs. If the initiation of OCs is accompanied by a clear loss of interest in sex or inability to have orgasms, discontinue the OCs while evaluating other potential causes of the decreased libido or anorgasmia, including depression. More often OC users enjoy sex *more* because fear of pregnancy is removed by OCs. (See the discussion on Depression in this section.)

Nausea, Queasiness, or Dizziness

Nausea most often occurs during the first cycle of pills or during the first few pills of each new package. It is more common in underweight women.[49] More severe nausea or vomiting may occur when a woman doubles up after missing 2 or 3 pills. Vomiting is rare.

The differential diagnoses include pregnancy (nausea, especially early morning nausea, occurs for the first time after months or years of taking OCs), influenza, or acute gastrointestinal infection. Further tests in the evaluation of nausea may include sensitive urine or serum pregnancy tests and diagnostic tests for HIV, hepatitis, mononucleosis, or gallbladder disease.

If nausea is related to taking the pill, try the following approaches:

- **Inform the client.** Nausea often decreases after the first few cycles or becomes limited to the first day or so of each cycle.
- **Recommend consistent pill taking.** Have the patient consistently take the pill at the time of the evening meal. Taking the pill at bedtime has proven helpful for some women.
- **Avoid double dosing.** Counsel the patient to "catch up" any pills she forgets by taking pills at 12-hour intervals, rather than 2 pills at one time, which increases the likelihood of nausea.
- **Watch the 2-hour mark.** Inform the patient that should she vomit, she need not take a "replacement" pill if the vomiting began after 2 hours of taking the pill. If she vomited within 2 hours of taking the pill, she should take an extra pill from a separate pack to replace the pill she just vomited. (See the section on Instructions.)
- **Decrease hormone dose.** Change to a combined pill with less estrogen or to a progestin-only pill containing no estrogen. A 20 mcg OC dramatically decreases nausea for many women although it may also lead to more spotting and breakthrough bleeding.

Pregnancy

Although uncommon, pregnancy may occur even if pills have been taken perfectly. Ask about whether the patient has missed taking any pills in the past two cycles, taken medications that may have reduced the effectiveness of the OCs, or missed any menstrual periods. Determine whether she has signs of being pregnant, such as nausea or vomiting, breast tenderness, or enlarged breasts. Ask the patient if she has performed a home pregnancy test. Look for signs of pregnancy on physical exam. Perform a sensitive pregnancy test. (See the discussion on Absence of Withdrawal Bleeding, in this section.)

Consider discontinuing OCs if the patient would not want an abortion and an early gestation cannot be ruled out. Offer alternative contraception, such as condoms, a spermicide, or a diaphragm. If the patient is pregnant, ask the patient what she wishes to do: carry pregnancy to term or seek an abortion:

- **Carry the pregnancy.** If she wishes to continue the pregnancy, inform her that little if any increased risk of birth defects exists as a result of OC use during pregnancy. Discontinue the OCs. Refer her for prenatal care. Have her immediately begin prenatal vitamins including folic acid. Counsel her about the fetal effects from alcohol and tobacco. Ask about alcohol use during the time of the pregnancy; history of miscarriages, abortions, and abnormalities in previous pregnancies; and risk of HIV infection.

- **Seek an abortion.** Refer the patient for an abortion if she does not wish to be pregnant and wants to have the pregnancy termination procedure. Discuss future plans for contraception.

Weight Change

In most instances, weight change is minimal and unrelated to OC use. Approximately as many women lose weight as gain weight while taking OCs. In some women, however, weight gain is definitely caused by oral contraceptives. Rarely, OCs can cause a gain of 10 to 20 pounds or more. The differential diagnoses include the following:

- Fluid retention due to either the progestin or the estrogen in an oral contraceptive (This pattern of weight gain occurs in the month or so after initiating OCs.)

- Estrogen-induced weight gain due to increased subcutaneous fat, particularly in the hips, thighs, and breasts (This type of weight gain is noted after several months on OCs.)

- Increased appetite and increased intake of food (anabolic effect). (This type of weight gain occurs over several years.)
- Depression, anxiety, or stress, which may be accompanied by increased caloric intake
- Increased availability of high-caloric foods and a change in pattern of eating
- Decreased exercise

Ask about the relationship of weight gain to the initiation of current OCs, weight changes while taking any other OCs, change in appetite, cyclicity of weight gain, symptoms of early pregnancy, and patient recall of previous weights. Current work, sleep, and exercise habits; signs of depression; and any changes in lifestyle may be significant factors in weight gain. In young teens, weight gain is to be expected.

Check for edema, the amount and distribution of fat, uterine enlargement, and signs of pregnancy. Consider ordering sensitive urine or serum pregnancy tests, or a 2-hour postprandial glucose test. Record the woman's weight and note her previous weights in the chart.

Weight gain usually responds to decreasing caloric intake and increasing exercise. Inform the patient who has experienced weight gain that using OCs is a possible cause. Therapy for weight gain believed to be related to using OCs may include one of the following interventions:

- **Decrease androgenic effects.** Switch to an OC with decreased androgenic potency if the patient has experienced an anabolic effect and persistent weight increase over time. It may be necessary to discontinue OCs.
- **Decrease dose of OCs.** Decrease the estrogen, progestin, or both, or discontinue the OCs if the patient has clearly been experiencing cyclic weight change.
- **Decrease estrogen in OCs.** Switch to an OC with decreased estrogenic potency if the patient has had weight gain due to increased breast tissue and subcutaneous fat, particularly in the thighs or hips.

Young obese women can be started on low-dose OCs, just as one would prescribe them for women of normal weight. In women over 35 who are very overweight, obesity may be a reason to avoid using OCs. On the other hand, the pill's protective effect against endometrial cancer may be particularly desirable in overweight women, whose risk of endometrial cancer is increased. There is no evidence that overweight women need to be prescribed a higher-dose OC for oral contraceptives to be effective. Strongly consider performing a lipid profile and 2-hour postprandial glucose test, particularly if the patient has a family history of diabetes or of heart disease at a young age. Some experts would not give OCs to morbidly obese women, even if they were young and had no other risk factors. *One of the new progestin OCs, Ovcon-35, Modicon, or Brevicon may improve the lipid profile of a young obese women who will be on OCs for a number of years.*

PILL INTERACTIONS

A number of drugs can alter the metabolism of OCs. The lower the dose of the estrogen or the progestin provided to a woman as a contraceptive, the greater the risk that a medication may decrease effectiveness. Educate OC users about the possibility of certain medications decreasing effectiveness and suggest they use a back-up contraceptive such as condoms, a higher dose pill, or tricycling. The effectiveness of low-dose OCs may be lowered by the following OC interaction mechanisms:

- A second medication may induce liver enzymes that cause breakdown of an estrogen or progestin (microsomal liver enzyme induction). The anticonvulsants most likely to have this effect are phenobarbital, phenytoin, topirimate, carbamazepine, and primidone. The anticonvulsants sodium valproate and ethosuximide do not have this effect nor do some of the new anticonvulsant drugs such as vigabatrin and lamotrigine.[5,7,50] Several investigators have suggested that pregnancy may occur more often in low-dose OC users on anticonvulsants.[31,49] The contraceptive efficacy can be restored by using a higher-dose pill.[31] Women receiving long-term phenobarbital therapy may initially be placed on a pill containing 50 mcg of EE and the dose increased should breakthrough bleeding occur. Rifampin also has potent enzyme-inducing effects,[6,8] so potent that some clinicians avoid prescribing OCs completely. The antifungal drug griseofulvin has similar but less powerful enzyme-inducing properties.

- A second medication may increase plasma SHBG levels, thereby decreasing the amount of biologically active free steroid.

- A second medication may decrease the amount of hormone absorbed initially or reabsorbed following passage through the liver. Despite anecdotal case reports of contraceptive failure in OC users on antibiotics, no firm pharmacokinetic evidence exists linking antibiotic use to altered steroid blood levels.[9,74] If broad spectrum antibiotics have any effect on the bioavailability of EE, it is probably in the first 2 weeks. The International Planned Parenthood Federation recommends that women taking short-term broad spectrum antibiotics use back-up contraceptive precautions for 2 weeks. After 2 weeks, the initial bacterial flora recover because they develop resistance to the antibiotic.[60] (See the section on Instructions for Using Combined Pills.)

- Side effects of medication may cause nausea, diarrhea, or drowsiness that may prompt a woman to stop taking her contraceptive pills. Women who miss a low-dose pill may compromise contraceptive protection more than women who miss a higher-dose pill.
- Spotting or breakthrough bleeding may lead to patient concern and either several missed pills or discontinuation of the method, both of which could lead to unplanned pregnancy.

Oral contraceptive pills may also affect the pharmacokinetics of other drugs a woman is taking. Studies have suggested that OCs can decrease clearance of benzodiazepines such as diazepine, nitrazepine, chlordiazepoxide, and alprazolam, which suggests the need for lower doses of these medications.[1,9] OCs may increase the effects of anti-inflammatory corticosteroids by decreasing their clearance and increasing their half-life. Lower doses of steroids may be indicated. Clearance of bronchodilating drugs such as theophylline and aminophylline, as well as the closely related drug, caffeine, may be reduced by 30% to 40% in OC users. Theophylline may have a greater effect in pill-takers.[81] More rapid clearance of acetaminophen and aspirin may necessitate higher doses of these drugs in women on OCs.[81]

OCs can also alter the results of several laboratory tests.[69,70] (See Table 10-7 of the 16th edition of *Contraceptive Technology*). Notify the laboratory that a patient is taking contraceptive OCs.

INSTRUCTIONS FOR USING COMBINED PILLS

Pills work primarily by stopping ovulation (release of an egg). Although pills are *not 100% effective* even if taken *perfectly,* they are close to 100% effective if you take them every day on schedule. If women take pills perfectly, only 1 woman in 1,000 becomes pregnant in the course of an entire year. In addition to preventing pregnancy, pills lower your risk of ovarian cancer, cancer of the lining of the uterus (endometrium), benign breast masses, and ovarian cysts. Pills decrease menstrual blood loss, cramps, and pain. Pills tend to make acne and oily skin better. Pills also decrease your chance of having a dangerous ectopic pregnancy—a pregnancy outside of the uterus. Remember: pills do *not* protect you from AIDS (acquired immunodeficiency syndrome) or other sexually transmitted infections. *Use a latex or plastic male condom or a female condom every time sexual intercourse may expose you or your partner to infection.*

Starting Pills

1. **Choose a back-up method of birth control** (such as condoms or foam) to use with your first 7 days of pills, because the pills may not fully protect you from pregnancy during this first cycle. A back-up method is probably not necessary if you start taking pills on the first day of bleeding (see instruction #2 below). Keep this back-up method handy all the time and learn to use it correctly in case you:

   - Run out of pills
   - Forget to swallow pills for 2 or more days in a row
   - Have a serious pill warning signal and stop taking your pills
   - Want protection from AIDS or other infections

2. You may start taking your pills according to one of several different schedules:

   - Start on the first day of menstrual bleeding.
   - Start on the first Sunday after your menstrual bleeding begins.
   - Start *today* if you are sure you are not pregnant and have had no unprotected sex since your last period.

3. Read the most recent pill package insert for the brand of pills you use.
4. Be sure you know your clinician's telephone number if you have questions or problems.

Daily Pill Routine

1. Take 1 pill a day until you finish the pack. Then:

   - If you are using a 28-day pack, begin a new pack immediately. Skip no days between packages.
   - If you are using a 21-day pack, stop taking pills for 1 week and then start your new pack.

2. **Associate taking your pill with something else that you do at about the same time every day,** like going to bed, eating a meal, or brushing your teeth.
3. Mark your calendar to remind yourself of the days you will begin a new pack of pills. Some women mark their calendar each day as they take their pill.
4. **Check your pack of pills each morning** to make sure you took your pill the day before.

5. Many women have nausea the first month they take pills. This tends to go away in the next cycle or so. If nausea continues, see your clinician.

6. **Use a back-up contraceptive method** if you suspect your pills may be less effective: you missed taking pills, were late starting your new pill pack, had severe vomiting or diarrhea, or are taking medications that lower the ability of the body to absorb contraceptive hormones (see the instructions on these specific problems). If you think you may have had sexual intercourse that was not adequately protected, consider *emergency contraception*. Call *1-888-NOT-2-LATE* for more information.

7. **Use condoms** if you suspect, even a little, that you or your partner may be exposed to a sexually transmitted infection.

8. If you see a clinician for any reason or are hospitalized, be sure to mention that you are taking pills.

MISSED PILLS

Oral contraceptive pills should be taken every day at about the same time. Missing a pill means taking it late or not at all (**completely** missing a pill).

Oral contraceptives are packaged in either 21-day packs or 28-day packs. All pills in 21-pill packs and the first 21 pills in a 28-pill package contain hormones. Taking these hormonal pills is essential for pregnancy protection. In a 28-pill pack the final 7 pills are reminder pills, containing no hormones.

If you miss any of the 7 reminder pills, you are not at an increased risk of pregnancy and you do not need any back-up contraception:

- Throw out the reminder pills you missed.
- Keep taking 1 pill each day until you finish the pack.
- Start your next pack on your usual day.

If you miss any of the 21 hormonal pills, there are three things to think about:

1. **Back-up contraception.** Completely missing a pill, or even taking a pill as much as 12 hours late, may decrease your protection against pregnancy. Use a back-up contraceptive such as condoms for 7 days or abstain from sex for 7 days.

2. **Getting back on schedule.** Your answers to the following two questions will guide you in getting back to your daily pill-taking routine:

- *How late are you in taking your pill?*

Less than 24 hours	• Take the missed pill right away. • Return to your daily pill-taking routine; take your next pill at the usual time.
24 hours	Take *both* the missed pill and today's pill at the same time.
More than 24 hours (you completely missed 1 pill and are late for or completely missed a second pill, too)	• Take the last pill you missed right away. • Take the next pill on time. • Throw out the other missed pills. • Take the rest of the pills in the package right on schedule.

- *Did you completely miss a pill during the third week of pills (pills 15-21)?*

  — Finish the rest of the hormonal pills in the pack.

  — *Do not* take a week off pills if you use a 21-day pill pack or *do not* take the reminder pills (the last 7 pills) if you use a 28-day pill pack.

  — Start taking a new pack of pills *as soon as you finish* the hormonal pills in your current pack. You may not have a period until the end of your second pack of pills, but missing a period does you no harm.

3. **Emergency contraception**. If you have not taken your pills on schedule and have had unprotected sex in the past 72 hours, you may want to use emergency contraceptive pills (or rarely an IUD) to reduce the risk of pregnancy.

   - *When to consider emergency contraception.* There is much debate about the situations that may call for emergency contraception. Even the authors of this chapter (RAH and JG) are divided on the issue. One author (RAH) suggests emergency contraception be *considered* if a woman completely misses *any* hormonal pills. The other author (JG) suggests that emergency contraception be advised only if a woman completely misses 2 or more of the first 7 hormonal pills—because they come just after the 7 pill-free days—or completely misses 4 or more pills during the second week (pills 8-14). Call your clinician for advice.

   - *How to get back on schedule.* If you do use emergency contraceptive pills, ignore the instructions above about getting back on schedule.

     — The day after you take the second dose of emergency contraceptive pills, get back on your regular pill-taking schedule.

     — Discard all the missed pills in your current pill pack.

VOMITING OR DIARRHEA

1. **If you vomit within 2 hours** of taking a pill, take another pill from a separate pill pack as soon as you feel better. Make sure you always have extra pills on hand for situations like this.

2. **If you have severe diarrhea or vomiting for more than 24 hours**, keep taking your pills on schedule, if you can. During the time you are ill and for 7 days after you feel better, use a back-up contraceptive or abstain from sexual intercourse.

If your illness caused you to miss any pills from the third week (pills 15-21), do not take your usual week off hormonal pills (do not take the reminder pills in the 28-day pack). Start a new pack of pills immediately. (See the instructions under Missed Pills.)

PILLS AND YOUR PERIODS

1. Women taking pills note that their periods tend to be short and scanty, and they may see no fresh blood at all. **A drop of blood, or a brown smudge on your tampon, pad or on your underwear during the week you are taking no hormonal pills, is counted as a period when you are on the pills.**

2. **Spotting (very light bleeding between periods)** is very likely to occur the first few months you are on pills. If you have bleeding between periods, try to take your pills at the same time every day. Spotting is generally not a sign of any serious problem. Your clinician may suggest a "continue pills but watch carefully" approach. If you suddenly begin to have bleeding between periods or have not missed pills or taken pills late, consider having your clinician check you for an infection. Spotting between periods may also signal decreased pill effectiveness. It is particularly important to start each new package of pills on time. Some clinicians recommend a back-up contraceptive for women who have spotting on pills, especially if the woman is taking a medication that may make the pill less effective.

3. **If you have not missed any pills and you miss one period** without any other signs of pregnancy, pregnancy is very unlikely. Many women miss one period now and then. Call the clinic if you are worried. You are fairly safe and can start a new pack of pills on your regular day.

4. **If you missed 2 or more pills and miss a period,** you may need to stop taking pills and use another method of contraception. Contact your clinic for a pelvic exam or a sensitive pregnancy test. Ordinary 2-minute urine tests available in drug stores are very sensitive and will diagnose pregnancy 12 to 14 days after ovulation.

5. **If you miss 2 periods in a row,** come to the clinic for a pregnancy test right away (or do a home pregnancy test), even if you took your pills every day. Bring a sample of your first morning urine in a clean container.

HERE IS A SIMPLE WAY TO CONFIRM THAT YOU ARE NOT PREGNANT:

If your period does not start during the last few days on "reminder" pills or during the first 3 days of the pill-free interval, take your temperature with a special kind of thermometer. The basal body temperature (BBT) thermometer measures your lowest temperature, generally in the morning before you get out of bed. If your BBT is 98° F for 3 days in a row during the pill-free week, you are probably not pregnant.

PILLS AND PREGNANCY

1. **If you become pregnant** while taking oral contraceptive pills, decide whether you want to keep the pregnancy or have an abortion. Getting pregnant while taking the pill does not seem to increase the risk of having a baby with birth defects,[3,14,18] although there is a chance the baby could have urinary tract problems.[63]

2. **If you decide you want to become pregnant,** stop taking pills. It is safe to become pregnant immediately. The pill does not decrease your fertility; however, after you stop taking pills, you may have a 1 to 2 month delay before your periods become regular.[4] You may wish to use another contraceptive method until you have 2 or 3 normal menstrual periods off the pill. That way, when you become pregnant, your date of delivery can be calculated more easily.

PILLS AND MOOD CHANGES

1. **If you notice mood changes**—depression, irritability, change in sex drive—see your clinician. Switching pill brands may help if your mood changes are related to the pill.
2. Depression and premenstrual symptoms (PMS) tend to *improve* on pills. But in some women they become worse. So if these symptoms change for the better or for the worse, the pills may be the reason.

PILLS AND DRUG INTERACTIONS

1. The effectiveness of oral contraceptive pills may be decreased by a number of drugs that change how the liver works or lower the ability of the body to absorb the hormones. Be sure to tell your clinician if you are using these enzyme-inducing drugs, which include **rifampin, rifabutin griseofulvin, Dilantin (phenytoin), phenobarbital, topirimate, or Tegretol (carbamazepine).** If you are using these drugs for a **short time,** use a back-up contraceptive such as condoms and the instructions below in #2. If you are using these drugs for a **long time,** follow one of these three options to improve the pill's protection:

   - Use a higher dose pill with 50 mcg of estrogen.
   - Take the 21 active pills and then begin a new pack of pills immediately and skip completely the interval you would

ordinarily have a period. You will not have a period. After you have taken 3 packs in this manner, stop taking pills for 4 days. Continue this pattern of pill taking as long as you are taking one of the medications listed above. This pattern is called *tricycling.*

- *Tricycle* (see the explanation above) in addition to using a higher-dose pill with 50 mcg of estrogen.

2. **If for a short time you are taking *any* drugs** that could possibly interact with your oral contraceptive pills and decrease their effectiveness, use your back-up contraceptive. **Antibiotics** such as *ampicillin, doxycycline, or tetracycline* also may decrease the effectiveness of oral contraceptive pills, although their effect is less and of more limited duration than that caused by the enzyme-inducing drugs mentioned above in #1.

Type of Drug	Use of Back-up Contraceptive
Enzyme-inducing drug (such as the ones listed in #1)	• Entire duration of treatment • *Plus* 7 days, or longer if advised by your clinician
Nonenzyme-inducing drug (such as broad-spectrum antibiotics listed in #2)	• Entire duration of treatment or 14 days, whichever is shorter • *Plus* 7 days

If by following these schedules you need back-up contraception into the **third week of pills** (pills 15-21), do not take a week off hormonal pills (do not take the reminder pills in a 28-day pack). Start a new pack immediately. See the instructions under Missed Pills.

PILL WARNING SIGNALS

1. Learn the pill warning signals. Any one of these symptoms could mean that you are in serious trouble. Note that the first letters of each symptom spell out the word **ACHES.**

Early Pill Warning Signs

Caution

A ■ Abdominal pain (severe)

C ■ Chest pain (severe, cough, shortness of breath or sharp pain on breathing in)

H ■ Headache (severe), dizziness, weakness, or numbness, especially if one-sided

E ■ Eye problems (vision loss or blurring), speech problems

S ■ Severe leg pain (calf or thigh)

See your clinician if you have any of these problems or if you develop depression, yellow jaundice, a breast lump, a bad fainting attack or collapse, a seizure (epilepsy), difficulty speaking, a blood pressure above 160/95, a severe allergic skin rash, or if you are immobilized after an accident or major surgery. If major surgery is planned, switch your contraceptive method 4 weeks before your operation. The risk of a blood clot in a vein is greatest if any of the following apply to you: if you are overweight, are immobile (in a wheelchair or bedridden), have severe varicose veins, or if a member of your family had a blood clot in a vein before they were 45. Usually these warning signs have an explanation other than pills, but you should be checked out to be sure. Do not ignore these problems or wait to see if they disappear. Contact your clinician right away.

2. **If you smoke, stop smoking. This is the single most important thing you can do for your health.** If you can't stop, it is all the more important that you watch for the pill warning signals. If you smoke, you should probably STOP taking pills at age 35, and definitely by age 40.

THE MOST COMMONLY ASKED QUESTION ABOUT PILLS

Do birth control pills cause cancer? Although the final word is still not in, we continue to learn more.

Good news. Pills make women *less likely* to develop some cancers and tumors:

- Ovarian cancer
- Endometrial cancer
- Benign breast masses (fibroadenomas and cysts)
- Fibroids (leiomyomata)
- Ovarian cysts
- Endometriomas (from endometriosis)
- Abscesses from pelvic inflammatory disease

Pills probably have no effect on a woman's likelihood of developing a malignant melanoma; kidney, colon, or gallbladder cancer; or pituitary tumors.

Bad news. While there is no type of cancer (malignant tumor) definitely known to be caused by pill use, one benign tumor of the liver called a hepatic adenoma is *more likely* to develop in women using pills. The increased risk for this tumor is one of the reasons why women using pills are encouraged to contact their clinicians if they develop upper abdominal pain. Fortunately, benign liver tumors are very rare.

(Continued)

Uncertain news. The jury is still out on the pill's effect on these cancers:

Breast cancer. By age 55, women who have used pills are equally likely to be diagnosed with breast cancer as women who have not used pills. However, women face a slightly increased risk of having breast cancer diagnosed while they are using oral contraceptives and until 10 years after stopping pills. Cancers diagnosed in these women are *less* advanced than are the cancers diagnosed in women of the same age who have never used pills. It is uncertain whether the pill increases the risk of breast cancer in current and recent users or whether users are just more likely to have existing tumors detected.

Cervical cancer. Barrier contraceptives and spermicides protect women against cervical cancer caused by the human papilloma virus. Pills do not have this protective effect. Some studies have shown an increased risk for cervical cancer among pill users; others have not. Women taking pills should have a Pap smear once a year.

Cancer of the liver. Some studies have shown an increased risk for hepatocellular cancer. Others, including a large World Health Organization study, have not.

If we add up all the good news, the bad news, and the uncertain news, we can say that by age 55, a woman is less likely to be diagnosed with cancer if she has used pills than if she has used no method of contraception.

REFERENCES

1. Abernathy DR, Greenblatt DJ, Divoll M, Arendt R, Ochs HR, Shader RI. Impairment of diazepam metabolism by low-dose estrogen-containing oral contraceptive steroids. N Engl J Med 1982;306:791-792.
2. Adesanya O, Colie CF. Evaluating oral contraceptive use at 6 and 12 months. J Reprod Med 1996;41:431-434.
3. American College of Obstetricians and Gynecologists. Contraceptives and congenital anomalies. Int J Gynaecol Obstet 1993;42:316-317.
4. American College of Obstetricians and Gynecologists. Oral contraceptives. ACOG Bulletin No. 106, 1987.
5. Anderson GD, Graves NM. Drug interactions with antiepileptic agents: prevention and management. CNS Drugs 1994;2:268-79.
6. Baciewicz AM, Self TH, Bekemeer WB. Update on rifampin drug interactions. Arch Intern Med 1987;147:565-568.
7. Back DJ. Can the pill be given to women with particular needs? Epilepsy and drug interactions. In: Hannaford PC, Webb AMC (eds). New York: Parthenon Publishing Group 1996;273-81.
8. Back DJ, Orme ML'E. Drug interactions. In: Goldzieher JW, Fotherby K (eds). Pharmacology of the contraceptive steroids. New York: Raven Press, 1994:407-426.
9. Back DJ, Orme ML'E. Pharmacokinetic drug interactions with oral contraceptives. Clin Pharmacokinet 1990;18:472-484.

10. Basdevant A, Conard J, Pelissier C. Hemostatic and metabolic effects of lowering the ethinyl-estradiol dose from 30 mg to 20 mg in oral contraceptives containing desogestrel. Contraception 1993;48:193.

11. Beller FK. Coagulation, thrombosis and contraceptive steroids—Is there a link? In: Goldzhieher JW, Fotherby K (eds). Pharmacology of the contraceptive steroids. New York: Raven Press, 1994;309-333.

12. Bloemenkamp KWM, Rosendaal FR, Helmerhorst FM, Buller HR, Vandenbroucke JP. Enhancement by factor V Leiden mutation of deep-vein thrombosis associated with oral contraceptives containing a third-generation progestagen. Lancet 1995;346:1593-1596.

13. Blumenstein BA, Douglas MB, Hall WD. Blood pressure changes and oral contraceptive use: a study of 2,676 black women in the southeastern United States. Am J Epidemiol 1980;112:539-552.

14. Bracken MB. Oral contraception and congenital malformations in offspring: a review and meta-analysis of the prospective studies. Obstet Gynecol 1990;76:552-557.

15. Bracken MB, Hellenbrand KG, Holford TR. Conception delay after oral contraceptive use: the effect of estrogen dose. Fertil Steril 1990;53:21-27.

16. Brinton LA. Oral contraceptives and cervical neoplasia. Contraception 1991;43:581-595.

17. Broome M, Clayton J, Fotherby K. Enlarged follicles in women using oral contraceptives. Contraception 1995;52:13-16.

18. Cardy GC. Outcomes of pregancies after failed hormonal postcoital contraception—an interim report. Brit J Fam Plann 1995;21:112-115.

19. Castelli WP. Reducing risk in OC users who smoke. Contemp Obstet/Gynecol 1996;:116-126.

20. Castracane VD, Gimpel T, Goldzieher JW. When is it safe to switch from oral contraceptives to hormonal replacement therapy? Contraception 1995;52:371-376.

21. Centers for Disease Control and Prevention. Oral contraceptive use and the risk of endometrial cancer. The Centers for Disease Control Cancer and Steroid Hormone (CASH) study. JAMA 1983;249(12):1600-1604.

22. Centers for Disease Control and Prevention. Oral contraceptive use and the risk of ovarian cancer. The Centers for Disease Control Cancer and Steroid Hormone (CASH) study. JAMA 1983;249(12):1596-1599.

23. Centers for Disease Control and Prevention. The Cancer and Steroid Hormone (CASH) study of the Centers for Disease Control and the National Institute of Child Health and Human Development: oral contraceptive use and the risk of breast cancer. N Engl J Med 1986;315:405-411.

24. Coker AL, Harlap S, Fortney JA. Oral contraceptives and reproductive cancers: weighing the risks and benefits. Fam Plann Perspect 1993;25:17-22,36.

25. Collaborative Group on Hormonal Factors in Breast Cancer. Breast cancer and hormonal contraceptives: collaborative reanalysis of individual data on 53,297 women with breast cancer and 100,239 women without breast cancer from 54 epidemiological studies. Lancet 1996;347:1713-1727.

26. Critchlow CW, Wölner-Hanssen P, Eschenbach DA, Kiviat NB, Koutsky LA, Stevens CE, Holmes KK. Determinants of cervical ectopia and of cervicitis: age, oral contraception, specific cervical infection, smoking, and douching. Am J Obstet Gynecol 1995;173:534-543.

27. Crona N, Silfverstolpe G, Samsioe G. Changes in serum apo-lipoprotein AI and sex-hormone-binding globulin levels after treatment with two different progestins administered alone and in combination with ethinyl estradiol. Contraception 1984;29:261-270.

28. Czeizel AE, Kodaj I. A changing pattern in the association of oral contraceptives and the different groups of congenital limb deficiencies. Contraception 1995;51:19-24.

29. DeCherney A. Bone-sparing properties of oral contraceptives. Am J Obstet Gynecol 1996;174:15-20.

30. Dewis P, Petsos M, Anderson DC. The treatment of hirsutism with a combination of desogestrel and ethinyl oestradiol. Clin Endocrin 1985;22:29-36.

31. Diamond MP, Greene JW, Thompson JM, Van Hooydonk JE, Wentz AC. Interaction of anticonvulsants and oral contraceptives in epileptic adolescents. Contraception 1985;31(6):623-632.

32. Dorflinger LJ. Relative potency of progestins used in oral contraceptives. Contraception 1985;31:557-570.

33. Egarter CH, Putz M, Strohmer H, Speiser P, Wenzl R, Huber J. Ovarian function during low-dose oral contraceptive use. Contraception 1995;51:329-333.

34. Elkind-Hirsch K, Goldzieher JW. Carbohydrate metabolism. In: Goldzieher JW, Fotherby K (eds). Pharmacology of the Contraceptive Steroids. New York: Raven Press, 1994:345-356.

35. Farmer RDT, Lawrenson RA, Thompson CR, Kennedy JG, Hambleton IR. Population-based study of risk of venous thromboembolism associated with various oral contraceptives. Lancet 1997;349:83-88.

36. Food and Drug Administration. Oral contraceptives and risk of blood clots. FDA Talk Paper Nov. 14, 1995.

37. Fortney JA, Feldblum PJ, Talmage RV, Zhang J, Godwin SE. Bone mineral density and history of oral contraceptive use. J Reprod Med 1994;39:105-109.

38. Franks AL, Beral V, Cates W, Hogue CJR. Contraception and ectopic pregnancy risk. Am J Obstet Gynecol 1990;163:1120-1123.

39. Fruzzetti F, Ricci C, Fioretti P. Haemostasis profile in smoking and nonsmoking women taking low-dose oral contraceptives. Contraception 1994;49:579.

40. Godsland IF, Wynn V. Does the new progestagen desogestrel have metabolic advantages? Lancet 1984;2:359-360.

41. Godsland IF, Crook D, Simpson R, Proudler T, Felton C, Lees B, Anyaoku V, Devenport M, Wynn V. The effects of different formulations of oral contraceptive agents on lipid and carbohydrate metabolism. N Engl J Med 1990;323:1375-1381.

42. Goldzieher JW, Zamah NM. Oral contraceptive side effects: where's the beef? Contraception 1995;52:327-335.

43. Goodman ZD, Ishak KG. Hepatocellular carcinoma in women probable lack of etiologic association with oral contraceptive steroids. Hepatology 1982;2:440-444.

44. Graham CA, Ramos R, Bancroft J, Maglaya C, Farley TMM. The effects of steroidal contraceptives on the well-being and sexuality of women: A double-blind, placebo-controlled, two-centre study of combined and progestogen-only methods. Contraception 1995;52:363-369.

45. Greenblatt RB. Progestational agents in clinical practice. Med Science 1967;18:37-49.

46. Grimes DA. Editorial: Over the counter oral contraceptives—an immodest proposal? Amer J Public Health 1993;83:1092-103.

47. Grimes DA, Economy KE. Primary prevention of gynecologic cancers. Am J Obstet Gynecol 1995;172:227-235.

48. Grimes DA, Godwin AJ, Rubin A, Smith JA, Lacarra M. Ovulation and follicular development associated with three low-dose oral contraceptives: a randomized controlled trial. Obstet Gynecol 1994;83:29-34.

49. Guillebaud J. The pill and other hormones for contraception, 5th ed. Oxford: Oxford University Press, 1997.

50. Guillebaud J. Contraception Today: A pocket book for general practitioners. 3rd ed. London: Martin Dunitz, 1997.

51. Guillebaud J, Lidegaard O, Skouby SO. Oral contraceptives and thrombotic diseases. FIGO 1997 Press Release. August 7, 1997.

52. Hammond GL, Langley MS, Robinson PA, Nummi S, Lund L. Serum steroid binding protein concentrations, distribution of progestogens, and bioavailability of testosterone during treatment with contraceptives containing desogestrel or levonorgestrel. Fertil Steril 1984;42:44-51.

53. Hannaford PC, Webb AMC. Evidence-guided prescribing of combined oral contraceptives: Consensus Statement. Contraception 1996;54:125-129.

54. Harlap S, Kost K, Forrest JD, Preventing pregnancy, protesting health: a new look at birth control choices in the United States. New York and Washington DC: The Alan Guttmacher Institute, 1991.

55. Heinen G. The discriminating use of combination and sequential preparations in hormonal inhibition of ovulation. Contraception 1971;4:393-400.

56. Helmrich SP, Rosenberg L, Kaufman DW, Miller DR, Schottenfeld MD, Stolley PD, Shapiro S. Lack of an elevated risk of malignant melanoma in relation to oral contraceptive use. J Natl Cancer Inst 1984;72:617-620.

57. Jamin C, deMouzon J. Selective prescribing of third-generation oral contraceptives (OCs). Contraception 1996;54:55-56.

58. Jick H, Jick SS, Gurewich V, Myers MW, Vasilakis C. Risk of idiopathic cardiovascular death and nonfatal venous thromboembolism in women using oral contraceptives with differing progestagen components. Lancet 1995; 346:1589-1593.

59. Krauss RM. The effects of oral contraceptives on plasma lipids and lipoproteins. Int J Fertil 1988;33 (Suppl 2):35-42.

60. Kubba Ali. Drug interactions with hormonal contraceptives. IPPF Medical Bulletin. 1996;30(3):3-4.

61. Lewis MA, Heinemann LAJ, MacRae KD, Bruppacher R, Spitzer WO (Transnational Research Group on Oral Contraceptives and the Health of Young Women). The increased risk of venous thromboembolism and the use of third generation progestogens: role of bias in observational research. Contraception 1996;54:5-13.

62. Lewis MA, Spitzer WO, Heinemann LAJ, MacRae KD, Bruppacher R, Thorogood M (Transnational Research Group on Oral Contraceptives and the Health of Young Women). Third generation oral contraceptives and risk of myocardial infarction: an international case-control study. Br Med J 1996;312:88-90.

63. Li De-Kun, Daling JR, Mueller BA, Hickok DE, Fantel AG, Weiss NS. Oral contraceptive use after conception in relation to the risk of cogenital urinary tract anomalies. Teratology 1995;51:30-36.
64. Lobo RA. The androgenicity of progestational agents. Int J Fertil 1988;33 (Suppl 2):6-12.
65. MacGregor EA. Migraine and combined oral contraceptives—a response to the joint statement. Brit J Family Planning 1995;21:15-17.
66. Magidor S, Palti H, Harlap S, Baras M. Long-term follow-up of children whose mother used oral contraceptives prior to conception. Contraception 1984;29:203-214.
67. Marchbanks P, Annegers JF, Coulam CB, Strathy JH, Kurland LT. Risk factors for ectopic pregnancy: a population-based study. JAMA 1988;259:1823-1827.
68. McGregor JA, Hammill HA. Contraception and sexually transmitted disease: interactions and opportunities. Am J Obstet Gynecol 1993;168:2033-2041.
69. The Medical Letter. Effects of oral contraceptives on laboratory test results. Med Lett Drugs Ther 1979;21:54-56.
70. Miale JB, Kent JW. The effects of oral contraceptives on the results of laboratory tests. Am J Obstet Gynecol 1974;120:264-272.
71. Milne R, Vessey M. The association of oral contraception with kidney cancer, colon cancer, gallbladder cancer (including extrahepatic bile duct cancer) and pituitary tumours. Contraception 1991;43:667-693.
72. Mishell DR. Use of oral contraceptives in women of older reproductive age. Am J Obstet Gynecol 1988;158:1652-1657.
73. Mortola JF. A risk-benefit appraisal of drugs used in the management of premenstrual syndrome. Drug Safety 1994;10:160-169.
74. Murphy AA, Zacur HA, Charache P, Burkman R. The effect of tetracycline on levels of oral contraceptives. Am Jour Obstet Gynecol 1991;164:28-33.
75. Ness RA, Keder LM, Soper DF, Amortegui AJ, Gluck J, Wiesenfeld H, Sweet RL, Rice PA, Peipert JF, Donegan SP, Kanbour-Shakir A. Oral contraception and the recognition of endometritis. Am J Obstet Gynecol 1997;176:580-585.
76. Ortho Pharmaceutical Laboratories. The Ortho Annual Birth Control Study. Raritan NJ, 1991.
77. Pardthaisong T, Yenchit C, Gray R. The long-term growth and development of children exposed to Depo-Provera during pregnancy or lactation. Contraception 1992;45:313-324.
78. Peipert JF, Gutman J. Oral contraceptive risk assessment: a survey of 247 educated women. Obstet & Gynecol 1993;82:112-117.
79. Petursson GJ, Fraunfelder FT, Meyer SM. Oral contraceptives. Ophthalmology 1981;88:368-371.
80. Poulter N. The pill and acute myocardial infarction (heart attack). IPPF Medical Bulletin 1997;31:3-4.
81. Rizack MA, Hillman CDM. The Medical Letter handbook of adverse drug interactions. New Rochell NY: The Medical Letter, 1985.
82. Rojanasakul A, Chailurkit L, Sirimongkolkasem R, Chaturachinda K. Effects of combined desogestrel-ethinylestradiol treatment on lipid profiles in women with polycystic ovarian disease. Fertil Steril 1987;48:581-585.

83. Rooks JB, Ory HW, Ishak KG, Strauss LT, Greenspan JR, Hill AP, Tyler CW. Epidemiology of hepatocellular adenoma. The role of oral contraceptive use. JAMA 1979;242:644-648.

84. Rosing J, Tans G, Nicolaes GAF, Thomassen MCLGD, Van Oerle R, Van Der Ploeq PMEN, Heinen P, Hamulyak K, Hemker HC. Oral contraceptives and venous thrombosis: different sensitivities to activated protein C in women using second- and third-generation oral contraceptives. Br J Haematology 1997;97:233-238.

85. Royal College of General Practitioners. Oral contraceptives and health: report of Royal College of General Practitioners. New York NY: Pitman Publishing Corporation, 1974.

86. Schlesselman JJ. Net effect of oral contraceptive use on the risk of cancer in women in the United States. Obstet Gynecol 1995;85:793-801.

87. Schwingl PJ, Shelton J. Modeled estimates of myocardial infarction and venous thromboembolic disease in users of second- and third-generation oral contraceptives. Contraception 1997;55:125-129.

88. The Second European Conference on Sex Steroids and Metabolism. Consensus Statement: Consensus development meeting 1995: Combined oral contraceptives and cardiovascular disease. Amsterdam, November 1995. Gynecol Endocrinol 1996;10:1-5.

89. Shoupe D, Bopp B. Contraceptive options for the gestational diabetic woman. Int J Fertil 1991;(Suppl 2):80-86.

90. Skouby SO, Anderson O, Kuhl C. Oral contraceptives and insulin receptor binding in normal women and those with previous gestational diabetes. Am J Obstet Gynecol 1986,155:802-807.

91. Skouby SO (Committee chairman). Consensus development meeting: metabolic aspects of oral contraceptives of relevance for cardiovascular diseases. Am J Obstet Gynecol 1990;162:1335-1337.

92. Spellacy WN, Buhi WC, Birk SA. Prospective studies of carbohydrate metabolism in "normal" women using norgestrel for 18 months. Fertil Steril 1981;35:167-171.

93. Speroff L, Darney P. A clinical guide for contraception. Baltimore MD: Williams & Wilkins, 1996.

94. Speroff L, Glass RH, Kase NG. Clinical gynecologic endocrinology and infertility 4th ed. Baltimore MD: Williams & Wilkins, 1994.

95. Spitzer WO, Lewis MA, Heinemann LA, Thorogood M, McCrae KD. Third generation oral contraceptives and risk of venous thromboembolic disorders: an international case study. Brit Med J 1996;312:83-88.

96. Stewart FH, Guest F, Stewart G, Hatcher RA. Understanding your body. New York NY: Bantam, 1987.

97. Suissa S. Risk profiles of venous thromboembolism and the use of newer oral contraceptives. FIGO 1997 Abstract;August 7, 1997.

98. Swyer GI. Potency of progestogens in oral contraceptives—further delay of menses data. Contraception 1982;26:23-27.

99. Thomas DB, Ray RM and the World Health Organization Collaborative Study of Neoplasia and Steroid Contraceptives. Oral contraceptives and invasive adenocarcinomas and adenosquamous carcinomas of the uterine cervix. Am J Epidemiol 1996;144:281-289.

100. Trussell J, Stewart F, Guest F, Hatcher RA. Emergency contraceptive pills (ECPs): a simple proposal to reduce unintended pregnancies. Fam Plann Perspect 1992;24:269-273.
101. Trussell J, Leveque JA, Koenig JD, Lenden R, Bordem S, Henneberry J, LaGuardia KD, Stewart F, Wilson G, Wysocki S, Strauss M. The economic value of contraception: a comparison of 15 methods. Am J Public Health 1995;85:494-503.
102. Trussell J, Stewart F, Potts M, Guest F, Ellertson C. Should oral contraceptives be available without a prescription? Am J Public Health 1993;83:1094-1099.
103. Upton GV, Corbin A. The relevance of the pharmacologic properties of a progestational agent to its clinical effects as a combination oral contraceptive. Yale J Bio Med 1989;62:445-457.
104. Vandenbrouke JP, Koster T, Briet E, Reitsma PH, Bertina RM, Rosendaal FR. Increased risk of venous thrombosis in oral-contraceptive users who are carriers of factor V Leiden mutation. Lancet 1994;344:1453-1457.
105. Vandenbrouke JP, Rosendaal FR. End of the line for "third-generation pill" controversy? Lancet 1997;349:1114-1115.
106. Vessey MP, Lawless M, McPherson K, Yeates D. Neoplasia of the cervix uteri and contraception: a possible adverse effect of the pill. Lancet 1983;2:930-934.
107. Waetjen LE, Grimes DA. Oral contraceptives and primary liver cancer: Temporal trends in three countries. Obstet Gynecol 1996;88:945-949.
108. Washburn SA, Wagner JD, Adams MR, Clarkson TB. Cardiovascular system: contraceptive steroids, plasma lipoprotein levels, and coronary artery aterosclerosis. In: Goldzieher JW, Fotherby K (eds). Pharmacology of the contraceptive steroids. New York: Raven Press, 1994:335-344.
109. Washington AE, Gove S, Schachter J, Sweet RL. Oral contraceptives, *Chlamydia trachomatis* infection, and pelvic inflammatory disease. A word of caution about protection. JAMA 1985;253:2246-2250.
110. WHO. Collaborative Study of Cardiovascular Disease and Steroid Hormone Contraception. Ischaemic stroke and combined oral contraceptives: results of an international, multicentre, case-control study. Lancet 1996;348:498-505.
111. WHO. Collaborative Study of Cardiovascular Disease and Steroid Hormone Contraception. Effect of different progestagens in low oestrogen oral contraceptives on venous thromboembolic disease. Lancet 1995;346:1582-1588.
112. WHO. Collaborative Study of Cardiovascular Diseases and Steroid Hormone Contraception. Venous thromboembolic disease and combined oral contraceptives: results of international multicentre case-control study. Lancet 1995;346:1575-1582.
113. WHO. Improving access to quality care in family planning: medical eligibility criteria for contraceptive use. World Health Organization, 1996:13-26.
114. WHO. Scientific Group. Oral contraceptives and neoplasia. Technical Report Series, No. 817. Geneva: WHO, 1992.
115. Wolner-Hanssen P, Eschenbach DA, Paavonen J, Kiviat N, Stevens CE, Critchlow C, DeRouen T, Holmes KK. Decreased risk of symptomatic chlamydial pelvic inflammatory disease associated with oral contraceptive use. JAMA 1990;263:54-59.
116. Wynn V, Godsland I. Effects of oral contraceptives on carbohydrate metabolism. J Repro Med 1986;31(Suppl 9):892-897.

117. Zondervan KT, Carpenter LM, Painter R, Vessey MP. Oral contraceptives and cervical cancer—further findings from the Oxford Family Planning Association Contraceptive Study. Brit J Cancer 1996;73:1291-1297.

LATE REFERENCES

118. Hatcher RA, Rinchart W, Blackburn R, Geller JS. The essentials of contraception technology. Baltimore MD: Population Information Program, 1997.
119. Kleinman RL. Directory of hormonal contraceptives. London: International Planned Parenthood Federation, 1996.
120. Lewis MA, Heinemann LA, MacRae KD, Bruppacher R, Spitzer WO. The increased risk of venous thromboembolism and the use of third generation progestagens: role of bias in observational research. The Transnational Research Group on Oral Contraceptives and the Health of Young Women. Contraception 1996;54:5-13.

Depo-Provera, Norplant, and Progestin-Only Pills (Minipills)

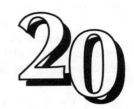

Robert A. Hatcher, MD, MPH

- Progestin-only contraceptives offer several highly effective options, especially to women who cannot use a contraceptive that contains estrogen.
- Counsel clients about menstrual cycle changes associated with progestin-only methods; counseling contributes substantially to successful use.
- Lactating women may use progestin-only contraceptives. Just how soon after delivery they should start remains a debatable point.

- Progestin-only methods provide no protection against sexually transmitted infections (STIs). Condoms should be used consistently and correctly if intercourse poses any risk of transmitting STIs, including infection with the human immunodeficiency virus (HIV).

Depo-Provera (DMPA). The most commonly used injectable contraceptive is Depo-Provera, given in a deep intramuscular injection of 150 milligrams (mg) every 12 weeks. Depo-Provera is extremely effective, in part because it is forgiving if a woman returns late for an injection.[18,35]

Norplant implants. With a single decision, a woman can elect to have 5 years of effective contraception. Each set of Norplant implants contains 36 mg of levonorgestrel, which is released at a low, steady rate of 85 micrograms (mcg) daily initially, decreasing to 50 mcg at 9 months, 35 mcg at 18 months, and to 30 mcg per day thereafter. The method can be reversed at any time by removing the capsules.

Progestin-only pills (minipills).   Minipills containing levonorgestrel only may also be used as emergency contraceptive pills (ECPs); minipill preparations cause far less vomiting or nausea than do ECP regimens using combined oral contraceptive (OC) pills. (See Chapter 12 on Emergency Contraception.)

Intrauterine devices (IUD).   The Levonorgestrel IUD and the Progestasert System elaborate a progestin. These are discussed in Chapter 21 on Intrauterine Devices.

M ECHANISM OF ACTION

Progestin-only contraceptives may be administered via different routes: by mouth, injection, implants, intrauterine devices, and vaginal rings. The mechanisms of action are summarized in Table 20-1. Progestins may prevent pregnancy by causing the following conditions:

- Inhibition of ovulation
- Thickened and decreased cervical mucus (preventing sperm penetration)
- Suppression of midcycle peaks of LH and FSH
- Inhibition of progesterone receptor synthesis
- Reduction in number and size of endometrial glands associated with a thin, atrophic endometrium
- Reduction in the activity of the cilia in the fallopian tube
- Premature luteolysis (diminished functioning of corpus luteum)

Depo-Provera.   Depo-Provera inhibits ovulation by suppressing levels of follicle stimulating hormone (FSH) and luteinizing hormone (LH) and by eliminating the LH surge. The pituitary gland remains responsive to gonadotropin releasing hormone, which suggests that the site of action of Depo-Provera is the hypothalamus.[37]

Norplant.   The levonorgestrel in Norplant suppresses ovulation in at least half the cycles. Even if ovulation were to occur, fertilization would be prevented by the endocrine dysfunction.[34]

Minipills.   The effectiveness of minipills may be highest when ovulation is inhibited consistently, causing amenorrhea or prolonged periods of time between menstrual bleeding episodes. When ovulation is not suppressed, menstrual bleeding occurs as it had before the woman initiated minipills.

Table 20-1 Delivery systems for progestin-only contraceptives and combined pills

	Injectable	Implant	Oral	
	Depo-Provera	Norplant	Progestin-only Pill	Combined OC
Administration				
Frequency	Every 3 months	5 years	Daily	Daily
Progestin dose	High	Ultra-low	Ultra-low	Low
Blood levels	Initial peak then decline	Constant	Rapidly fluctuating	
1st pass through liver	No	No	Yes	Yes
Major Mechanisms of Action				
Ovary: ↓ovulation	+++	++	+	+++
Cervical mucus: ↓sperm penetrability	Yes	Yes	Yes	Yes
Endometrium: ↓receptivity to blastocyst	Yes	Yes	Yes	Yes
First-year failure rate (perfect use)	0.3	0.05	0.5	0.1
Menstrual pattern	Very irregular	Very irregular	Often irregular	Regular
Amenorrhea during use	Very common	Common	Occasional	Rare
Reversibility				
Immediate termination possible	No	Yes	Yes	Yes
By woman herself at any time	No	No	Yes	Yes
Median time to conception from first omitted dose, removal	6 months	c.1 month	<3 months	3 months

Adapted from Guilleband (1985).

*By several mechanisms—LH and FSH surges suppressed; preovulatory follicles suppressed

EFFECTIVENESS

DEPO-PROVERA

Depo-Provera is an extremely effective contraceptive option (Table 20-2). In the first year of use, the probability of pregnancy is only 0.3%. This estimate applies to a 12-week regimen with each injection providing 150 mg of DMPA per 1 cc. Although some women may miss a scheduled injection, each 150 mg dose probably provides more than 3 months of contraceptive protection. Because we have no information concerning pregnancies that may have resulted from late injections, we estimate that the probability of pregnancy among typical users is equal to the rate for perfect users. (See also Chapter 31 on Contraceptive Efficacy.)

Questions have been raised about the effectiveness of much less expensive solutions that provide 400 mg of DMPA per 1 cc. This volume of DMPA in solution (0.37 cc) is difficult to provide exactly, and the injection and absorption of DMPA from this very concentrated solution is not approved as a contraceptive. An unpublished Upjohn-sponsored trial of 400 mg/milliliter (ml), administered as 1 ml every 6 months did not demonstrate suitable contraceptive efficacy; failures occurred throughout the 6-month treatment period.[5] This concentrated form of DMPA is also more painful.

Table 20-2 First-year probability of pregnancy* for women using progestin-containing contraceptives

Method	% of Women Experiencing an Unintended Pregnancy Within the First Year of Use		% of Women Continuing Use at One Year
	Typical Use	Perfect Use	
Pill	5		71
Progestin Only		0.5	
Combined		0.1	
IUD			
Progesterone T	2.0	1.5	81
Copper T 380A	0.8	0.6	78
LNg 20	0.1	0.1	81
Depo-Provera	0.3	0.3	70**
Norplant and Norplant-2	0.05	0.05	88

*See Table 9-2 for first-year pregnancy rates of all methods.
**Recent U.S. studies reported lower continuation rates.

Continuation rate. In the largest U.S. study, continuation rates for women on Depo-Provera were 59.4% at 1 year, 41.5% at 2 years, 30.2% at 3 years, and 24.1% at 4 years.[47] At one year, about 70% of women were still using Depo-Provera. Recent studies report lower continuation rates: from 42% to 53%.[26,41,43] One of these studies found a continuation rate of 62% among teenagers.[26]

NORPLANT

An extremely effective contraceptive, Norplant has a perfect-use probability of pregnancy of 0.05%. Because there is no scope for user error, the typical-use and perfect-use estimates are the same. Although studies of currently used versions of Norplant recorded no pregnancies, it is highly implausible that the new versions of these implants never fail.[53,54] (See Chapter 31 on Contraceptive Efficacy.) Earlier studies included implants with an elastomer core and a hard tubing, both of which are no longer used.[54] Cumulative pregnancy rates through the end of 5 years were three times higher among women with the hard capsules (4.9%) than among women with soft ones (1.6%).[52] The Finnish company that produces all the Norplant implants used throughout the world, Leiras Oy, now produces implants only with the new soft tubing.[34] Even with soft tubing, Norplant has a higher rate of pregnancy among heavy women: 2.4% after 5 years among women weighing more than 154 pounds and 1.5% among women weighing 131 to 153 pounds.[53]

Because failures increase in the sixth year, it is generally recommended that Norplant capsules be removed at the end of the fifth year. In a study in Chile, 11 of the 19 pregnancies occurred during years 6 through 8 of treatment. The failure rate during years 6 through 8 was six times that during the first 5 years.[14] An Indonesian study found a net cumulative pregnancy rate at 5 years of 1.8%. However, 6 of the 8 pregnancies occurred in the last month of the fifth year.[1]

In Colorado, almost one-third (30%) of teens covered by Medicaid in 1992 chose the implant as their contraceptive. The repeat birth rate for Medicaid-covered teens choosing the implant in 1992 was 2.5% after 24 months; the repeat birth rate for teens not using the implant was 22.1% (a rate almost 10 times higher, and the same rate found among all teens prior to the availability of the implant).[45]

Continuation rate. Approximately 88% of women continue to use Norplant implants at one year. About half of the women continue Norplant use for 3 years.[27] In five international studies, 76% to 90% of users completed 1 year of use, and 33% to 78% completed 5 years.[34] In a recent study of the current versions of Norplant and Norplant-2, the proportion of women continuing use of at the end of 1 year was 95%.[54]

MINIPILL

Progestin-only pills are generally less effective than combined OCs. In the first-year of use, the probability of pregnancy among typical users is 5%. Under conditions of perfect use, only 0.5% women would become pregnant in the first year. A multicenter, double-blind study compared progestin-only pills (containing levonorgestrel [0.03 mg] or norethindrone [0.35 mg]) with two combined OCs (containing mestranol [50 mcg] and norethindrone [1 mg] or ethinyl estradiol [30 mcg] and levonorgestrel [0.15 mg]). The pregnancy rates for the progestin-only pills were only slightly higher than the rates for combined OCs; at 670 days, the pregnancy rate for progestin-only pills containing levonorgestrel was actually lower than the rate for OCs containing mestranol and norethindrone (9.5% vs. 12.9%).[50]

In lactating women, the progestin-only pill is nearly 100% effective because of the added contraceptive effect of breastfeeding.[38] Moreover, progestin-only pills do not alter the quantity of milk, so they represent an effective form of contraception for the lactating woman.[33]

Cost

Depo-Provera.   Each vial containing 150 mg of DMPA in a 1 cc injection will cost the provider $29. If the client is charged $35 per injection, then her annual cost will be $140 plus the cost of her annual examination, routine laboratory tests, transportation, and the loss of work necessitated by repeat visits for injections. No laboratory tests are specifically indicated unless a woman is more than 1 to 2 weeks late for her shot and may need a pregnancy test.

Norplant.   In the United States, each set of Norplant implants costs the health care provider from $365 to $375. (Programs in developing countries pay US $23 per set of six implants.[34]) The client's cost of insertion ranges from $500 to $700 (this cost may include a physical exam and some laboratory tests, such as a sensitive pregnancy test). Removal generally costs more because it takes more time. While the initial cost of Norplant is high, over 5 years' time this can be a cost-effective method.[57]

Some health plans cover the cost of insertion and removal. Medicaid covers costs of eligible women living in any of the 50 states. The Norplant Foundation (1-800-760-9030) provides free sets of Norplant implants and removal certificates to women who do not qualify for Medicaid but who cannot afford the cost of Norplant insertion or removal. *If a woman wants her implants removed, removal must be done regardless of her ability to pay.*

Minipills. Minipills cost women between $100 and $300 per year, depending on whether they are generic or brand name. Public clinics and college health services usually charge lower prices.

A DVANTAGES AND INDICATIONS

Progestin-only contraceptives in general offer users several advantages. In addition, each specific progestin-only method offers advantages:

Advantages of All Progestin-Only Methods

1. **No estrogen.** Because progestin-only contraceptives contain no estrogen, they do not appear to cause the rare but serious complications attributable to estrogenic agents (including thrombophlebitis and pulmonary embolism). Studies thus far have not shown serious cardiovascular effects associated with use of progestin-only contraceptives.[33,37]

2. **Noncontraceptive benefits.** Norplant, Depo-Provera, and minipills may lead to several noncontraceptive benefits, including the following:

   - Scanty menses or no menses; less anemia
   - Decreased menstrual cramps and pain
   - Suppression of pain associated with ovulation (mittelschmerz)
   - Decreased risk of endometrial cancer, ovarian cancer, and pelvic inflammatory disease (PID)
   - Management of pain associated with endometriosis

3. **Reversibility.** Minipills are immediately reversible. Although the contraceptive effect of Norplant implants ends immediately when the implants are removed, some women find it takes a long time to find a clinician who will surgically remove their implants. Contraception must be initiated the same day that the Norplant implants are removed. Depo-Provera is reversible once the effect of the last shot wears off. Depo-Provera does not cause long-term loss of fertility; however, ovulation may not return until 9 to 10 months after the last shot.[35]

4. **Long-term effective contraception.** Norplant implants and Depo-Provera are extremely effective long-term contraceptives. Minipills provide contraception only as long as they are taken.

5. **Low risk of ectopic pregnancy.** Norplant and Depo-Provera reduce a woman's risk for having an ectopic pregnancy compared with women using no contraceptive at all. The risk of ectopic

pregnancy may be greater in heavier women or in long-term Norplant users (which reinforces the importance of removal after 5 years of use).[34] The overall incidence of ectopic pregnancy in women taking minipills is similar to that for women using no contraceptive.[33] While the overall risk of ectopic pregnancy is lowered by these contraceptive methods, any pregnancy that does occur is more likely to be ectopic. As many as 10% of pregnancies among women taking minipills are ectopic.[33]

6. **Absence of menstrual bleeding.** Progestin-only contraceptives cause women to miss periods, which is considered by many women to be an advantage. Depo-Provera is especially likely to cause amenorrhea. During the first year of Depo-Provera use, for example, 30% to 50% of women are amenorrheic; by the end of the second year, 70%; and by the end of the fifth year, 80% are amenorrheic.[36] In a study of teenagers, nearly two-thirds of Depo-Provera users and one-third of Norplant users reported amenorrhea at 6 months.[10] Over time, Norplant users are less likely to miss periods. Amenorrhea is least common among minipill users.[33]

Advantages of Depo-Provera

7. **Culturally acceptable.** In some cultures, a woman may consider medication by injection desirable. In others, a woman may wish to use a contraceptive without the knowledge of her partner. Many couples find Depo-Provera use attractive because it is not coitally dependent.

8. **No drug interaction.** There has been no demonstrated interaction between Depo-Provera and antibiotics or enzyme-inducing drugs.[60] The only drug that decreases the effectiveness of Depo-Provera is aminoglutethimide (Cytadren), which is usually used to suppress adrenal function in selected cases of Cushings syndrome.

9. **Fewer seizures.** Depo-Provera has been found to decrease the frequency of seizures.[29,30] Improvement in seizure control is probably due to the sedative properties of progestins. Taking anti seizure medicine has no impact on the efficacy of Depo-Provera.

Advantages of Norplant

10. **Continuation rates.** Norplant has higher continuation rates than do other hormonal contraceptives.[13]

11. **Not coitus dependent.** Norplant is an excellent contraceptive option for women who have difficulty remembering to use a contraceptive at the time of intercourse or on a daily basis. Norplant may be a particularly attractive option for adolescents or for women who are injection drug users.[13,22,45]

Advantages of Minipills

12. **Not confusing.** Users take the same type of pill every day (same color and hormone content) and do not have a pill-free week (reminder pills are the same color as the other pills). Many women find it less confusing to take minipills than to take combined OCs.

13. **Health benefits.** Most of the health benefits of progestin-only pills are similar to combined OCs: decreased menstrual cramps or pain, less heavy bleeding, decreased premenstrual syndrome symptoms, and decreased breast tenderness. In theory, the thick, less penetrable cervical mucus in women on progestin-only pills should decrease the risk of PID.

INDICATIONS

Breastfeeding women. Although non-hormonal methods are generally preferable during breastfeeding, progestin-only hormonal methods may be quite appropriate if care is taken in the timing of initiation so as to avoid fetal effects or a diminution in the production of breast milk. (See the discussion in the section on Special Issues.)

Older women. The absence of thrombotic complications makes Depo-Provera, Norplant, and progestin-only pills advantageous for older women. A woman may have Norplant inserted when she is fairly certain she wants no more children but is not ready to undergo sterilization. For a woman who may choose sterilization in the next 3 to 12 months, Depo-Provera may be a better option than Norplant. Progestin-only pills may also be an excellent option for women who are late in their reproductive years.[7]

Young women. For younger women, Norplant is desirable because of its extremely low failure rate and its rapid reversibility (although some women have great difficulty finding a clinician to remove their implants). The production of a thick cervical mucus throughout the time a progestin-only method is used may cause them to have a protective effect against PID. Because teenage women are still building bone mass, the suppressive effect of Depo-Provera on serum estradiol levels needs further study.[9,10]

Women who cannot take estrogen. Progestin-only methods may be desirable for women who want to use an OC but who have contraindications to combined pills. Women who have developed nausea, breast tenderness, severe headaches, or hypertension while taking combined OCs may be candidates for progestin-only pills. Advise lactating women who desire a hormonal contraceptive that progestin-only contraceptives can be an excellent option.

Women who need excellent temporary contraception. Depo-Provera provides excellent short-term contraception for women who require maximum protection following rubella immunization, while using Accutane, while awaiting sterilization, or at the time the partner is undergoing vasectomy.

D ISADVANTAGES AND PRECAUTIONS

1. **Lack of protection against sexually transmitted infections, including infection with the human immunodeficiency virus.** Progestin-only contraceptives provide no known protection against sexually transmitted infections including with the human immunodeficiency virus (HIV). It is possible that vaginal thinning caused by progestin-only contraceptives may increase a woman's risk of acquiring HIV.[4,15,28]

2. **Menstrual cycle disturbance.** Menstrual irregularity is the most common reason for discontinuation. Many women experience either an increased number of days of light bleeding or amenorrhea. *While amenorrhea becomes less common over time among women using Norplant, it becomes more common among Depo-Provera users* (Table 20-3).[51] Rarely do women using Norplant or Depo-Provera experience an increased number of days of heavy bleeding.

Table 20-3 Bleeding patterns over a 5-year period among women using Depo-Provera injections and Norplant implants

	DMPA Injections		Norplant Implants	
	1 Yr.	5 Yr.	1 Yr.	5 Yr.
Regular cycles*	30	17	27	67
Amenorrhea	25	80	5	9

Sources: Shoup et al. (1993).
Depo-Provera NDA 20-246

*Regular cycle—Norplant: 21–35 days
Regular cycle—DMPA: 25–34 days

3. **Weight gain.** Some women using progestin-only methods, particularly women receiving Depo-Provera injections, gain weight or complain of feeling bloated. The weight gain is probably due to increased appetite rather than fluid retention.[60] Weight gain is predictable in women using DMPA: 5.4 pounds (average) in the first year, 8.1 pounds after 2 years of use, and 13.8 pounds after 4 years of use (according to the Depo-Provera package insert). Over 5 years, the weight gain among Norplant users averages just under 5 pounds,

close to the average weight gain for women in their early to mid-reproductive years. Weight gain is not an important problem in women taking minipills.

4. **Breast tenderness.** Some women using Norplant, Depo-Provera, and minipills experience breast tenderness.

5. **Depression.** Some women experience depression when they use progestin-only contraceptives. Depression becomes a particular concern when it occurs in a woman following a Depo-Provera injection because it is not possible to discontinue Depo-Provera immediately.[6]

Disadvantages of Depo-Provera

6. **No immediate discontinuation.** Weight gain, depression, breast tenderness, and menstrual irregularities may continue until Depo-Provera is cleared from a woman's body, about 6 to 8 months after her last injection. After discontinuing Depo-Provera, women have a 6 to 12 month delay in return of fertility.[35,47,60]

7. **Return visits every 12 weeks.** For some women, the repeated injections of Depo-Provera are unacceptable. About 70% of women continue to use Depo-Provera at 1 year (Table 20-2).

8. **Lipid changes.** High density lipoprotein (HDL) cholesterol levels fall significantly in women using Depo-Provera.[37] These adverse changes in lipids do not occur in women using Norplant.

9. **Allergic reactions.** Although rare, allergic reactions may occur. Some programs encourage women to remain in the vicinity of the clinic for 20 minutes after an injection.

10. **Bone density decrease.** Long-term Depo-Provera users may develop decreased bone density.[12] Smoking may be a risk factor. *Very low serum estradiol levels below 20 picograms/ml have occurred in some DMPA users. Avoid falsely reassuring women about the possible long-term effects of amenorrhea in association with very low serum estradiol levels.* When the serum estradiol level falls below 30, confirmed by a second determination, women in the Grady Memorial Hospital Family Planning Program are encouraged to take exogenous estrogen if they want to continue using DMPA as a contraceptive.[9]

Disadvantages of Norplant

11. **Difficult removal.** Both insertion and removal require a minor surgical procedure. Removal is likely to be difficult if an implant was inserted too deeply. Norplant removal requires a clinic visit and occasionally more than one visit.

12. **Higher initial cost.** The initial cost of Norplant is high. If the implants are removed soon after insertion, then this method is extremely expensive per month of contraception provided. Over a 5-year period, the cost of Norplant compares favorably with the cost of most other hormonal contraceptives. Recently, Wyeth Laboratories made the decision to replace Norplant implants or refund the amount paid if a woman's implants were removed after fewer than 180 days. You can reduce the likelihood of removal by explaining in advance the menstrual cycle changes that are likely to occur, by avoiding Norplant insertion for the woman who may change her mind quickly and want to become pregnant in the near future, and by avoiding insertions in women who are already pregnant.

13. **Extremely low-dose contraceptive.** The average release rate of 35 mcg per day is less than 25% of the dose provided by a low-dose combination OC containing levonorgestrel. Because of its low dose, Norplant's effectiveness is more significantly lowered than other hormonal contraceptives by antiseizure medicines (except for valproic acid) and by rifampin. Norplant failure rates increase to unacceptable levels when a user takes certain drugs:[19,39]

carbamazepine	primidone
phenytoin (Dilantin)	phenylbutazone
phenobarbital	rifampin

Antiseizure medications are strong inducers of the hepatic enzymes that break down levonorgestrel. If a Norplant user begins one of these medications, she should use a back-up contraceptive.

14. **Local inflammation or infection at site of implants.** A pooled analysis of 2,674 first-year users in seven countries found that 0.8% experienced infection, 0.4% experienced expulsion of a capsule, and 4.7% had skin irritation at the insertion site. Complications did not always occur immediately after insertion. Some 35% of infections and 64% of expulsions occurred after the first 2 months of use.[24] Slightly increased pigmentation of the skin occasionally appears over the site of the implants.

15. **Ovarian cysts.** Norplant causes less suppression of the hypothalamic pituitary axis, particularity FSH, than do combined OCs. Most ovarian cysts regress spontaneously and so do not need to be evaluated sonographically or laparoscopically unless they become large and painful or fail to regress.[55]

Disadvantages of Minipills

16. **Vulnerable efficacy.** The primary disadvantage of minipills is the need for obsessive regularity in pill-taking.

17. **Less availability.** Minipills are less likely to be stocked by pharmacies, and clinicians are less likely to have had experience prescribing minipills.

18. **Extremely low-dose contraceptive.** Certain medications will affect the effectiveness of low-dose contraceptives such as minipills (see Disadvantage 13).

PRECAUTIONS

The World Health Organization (WHO) has developed a list of precautions in providing progestin-only contraceptives.[59] The listing is intended to be a checklist for known medical conditions and is not meant to replace counseling. Because studies have not shown any serious short- or long-term effects of Depo-Provera or norethindrone enanthate (NET-EN), the World Health Organization (WHO) has placed few precautions on the provision of these methods (Table 20-4).[59]

Table 20-4 Precautions in the provision of progestin-only contraceptives

Refrain from providing *combined oral contraceptives for women with the following diagnoses (World Health Organization [WHO] category # 4):*

Precautions	Rationale/Discussion
Pregnancy	Although current data do not show an increased risk for birth defects caused by taking hormones during pregnancy, it is best to avoid any exposure of the fetus to hormones.
Unexplained abnormal vaginal bleeding suspicious for a serious underlying condition	Progestin-only contraceptives usually lead to irregular menses, increased days of light bleeding, or amenorrhea. These changes may mask an underlying problem such as pelvic inflammatory disease, cancer of the reproductive tract, or pregnancy. Until a diagnosis of the cause of unexplained vaginal bleeding is reached, do not inject Depo-Provera or insert Norplant. (*Exercise caution [WHO #3] in providing minipills.*)
Breast cancer	Some breast cancers are sensitive to progestins. Suspicious masses should be evaluated as soon as possible.

(continued)

Table 20-4 Precautions in the provision of progestin-only contraceptives *(cont.)*

Exercise caution if combined oral contraceptives are used or considered in the following situations and carefully monitor for adverse effects (WHO category #3):

Precautions	Rationale/Discussion
Certain medications Antiseizure: phenytoin (Dilantin), carbamazepine, primidone, phenylbutazone Antibiotics: rifampin/rifampicin	Medications for epilepsy (except valproic acid) cause the liver to metabolize progestins more rapidly, decreasing already low blood levels of levonorgestrel, the hormone found in *Norplant* and *minipills*. *(Advantages generally outweigh theoretical or proven disadvantages [WHO #2] when providing Depo-Provera. See the next section.)*
Breast cancer with 5-year disease-free interval	Some breast cancers are sensitive to progestins. Evaluate suspicious masses as soon as possible.
Liver conditions such as severe decompensated cirrhosis, adenoma or cancer, active viral hepatitis	Progestin-only contraceptives are metabolized by the liver and their use may adversely affect prognosis of existing disease. There is a concern that progestin-only contraceptives may increase the risk of hepatoma, as combined oral contraceptives do.
Cardiovascular conditions such as hypertension with or without vascular disease, current or history of ischemic heart disease, history of cerebrovascular accident (stroke)	High density lipoprotein (HDL) cholesterol levels fall in women using progestin-only contraceptives, especially Depo-Provera. There is also some concern regarding their hypoestrogenic effect. Although Norplant patient package inserts warn of cardiovascular complications, these concerns are based on past experience with high dose combined oral contraceptives, not on data about Norplant. *(Advantages generally outweigh theoretical or proven disadvantages [WHO #2] when providing Norplant or minipills; see the next section.)*
Diabetes with nephropathy, retinopathy, and neuropathy	Exercise caution in providing Depo-Provera to women with diabetes complicated by other organic conditions. See the discussion on cardiovascular and liver conditions.

(continued)

Table 20-4 Precautions in the provision of progestin-only contraceptives *(cont.)*

Do not restrict use *of progestion-only contraceptives because of the following conditions (WHO category #1)* **or**

The advantages generally outweigh *theoretical or proven disadvantages and the method generally can be provided without restrictions in these conditions, although more use requires greater follow-up (WHO category # 2):*

	Depo-Provera	Norplant	Minipills
• Age: menarche to 16 years	2	2	2
• Age 16 or older	1	1	1
• Smokers, light or heavy, any age	1	1	1
• Over 16 years of age	1	1	1
• Obesity	1	1	1
Gynecologic or Obstetric Conditions			
• Breastfeeding: 6 weeks postpartum and thereafter	1	1	1
• Immediately postpartum, not breastfeeding	1	1	1
• Post-abortion: first or second trimester or septic	1	1	1
• History of pre-eclampsia or gestational diabetes	1	1	1
• Benign breast disease or family history of breast cancer	1	1	1
• Cervical ectropion	1	1	1
• Cholestasis of pregnancy	1	1	1
• Uterine fibroids or endometriosis	1	1	1
• Benign or malignant trophoblastic disease	1	1	1
• Nulliparous	1	1	1
• Benign ovarian tumors including cysts	1	1	1
• Prior pelvic surgery	1	1	1
• Past ectopic pregnancy	2	1	1
• Irregular, heavy, or prolonged vaginal bleeding	2	2	2
• Undiagnosed breast mass	2	2	2
• Cervical intraepithelial neoplasia (CIN) or cancer	2	2	2

(continued)

Table 20-4 Precautions in the provision of progestin-only contraceptives *(cont.)*

Do not restrict use of progestion-only contraceptives because of the following conditions (WHO category #1) *or*

The advantages generally outweigh theoretical or proven disadvantages and the method generally can be provided without restrictions in these conditions, although more use requires greater follow-up (WHO category # 2):

	Depo-Provera	Norplant	Minipills
Chronic Diseases or Other Conditions			
• Cholestasis while on combined pills	2	2	2
• History/current deep vein thrombosis or pulmonary embolism	1	1	1
• Major or minor surgery with or without immobilization	1	1	1
• Superficial venous thrombosis (varicose veins or other)	1	1	1
• Valvular heart disease: uncomplicated or complicated	1	1	1
• Mild headaches	1	1	1
• Severe headaches including migraine *without* focal neurologic symptoms	2	2	1
• Gallbladder disease of any kind	1	1	1
• Thyroid: goiter, hypothyroid, hyperthyroid	1	1	1
• Iron deficiency anemia	1	1	1
• Epilepsy	1	1	1
• BP 140-179/90-109	2	1	1
• Hypertension by history which cannot be evaluated (except hypertension in pregnancy)	2	2	2
• BP 180+/110+		2	2
• Diabetes *without* vascular disease (non-insulin dependent or insulin dependent)	2	2	2
• Past elevated blood sugar levels during pregnancy	1	1	1
• Diabetes *with* nephropathy/retinopathy/neuropathy	*	2	2
• Diabetes with other vascular disease or 20 years duration	*	2	2
• Current or history of ischemic heart disease	*	2	2

*See the previous section of this table.

(continued)

Table 20-4 Precautions in the provision of progestin-only contraceptives *(cont.)*

Do not restrict use of progestion-only contraceptives because of the following conditions (WHO category #1) or

The advantages generally outweigh theoretical or proven disadvantages and the method generally can be provided without restrictions in these conditions, although more use requires greater follow-up (WHO category # 2):

	Depo-Provera	Norplant	Minipills
Chronic Diseases or Other Conditions (Cont.)			
• History of cerebrovascular accident (stroke)	*	2	2
• Severe headaches, including migraine *with* focal neurologic symptoms	2	2	2
• Mild (compensated) cirrhosis	2	2	2
• Rifampicin, griseofulvin, phenytoin, carbamezapine, barbiturates, primadone	2	*	*
Infections: Sexually Transmissable (STI) and Other			
• Pelvic inflammatory disease (PID), past or present	1	1	1
• Any STI, HIV-positive or AIDS	1	1	1
• Viral hepatitis carrier	1	1	1
• Schistosomiasis: uncomplicated or with fibrosis of liver (if severe, see cirrhosis); or malaria	1	1	1
• Antibiotics other than rifampicin and griseofulvin	1	1	1
• Tuberculosis (but also see antibiotics)	1	1	1

*See the previous section of this table.

S PECIAL ISSUES
BREASTFEEDING WOMEN

In theory, progestin-only methods may thwart lactogenesis if they are initiated before the postpartum decline in natural progesterone after delivery, which functions as the trigger for milk synthesis.[23] A prudent approach may be to wait until breastfeeding is well established. Unlike the use of combined OCs, use of progestin-only contraceptives once breastfeeding has been established has not been shown to have an adverse effect on breast milk volume; in some studies, milk production has been enhanced. The quality of breast milk is not affected. Because of theoretical concerns over early neonatal exposure to exogenous steroids, several international organizations have urged that progestin-only methods not be initiated until at least 6 weeks postpartum.[21,56,59] It is unlikely that a lactating woman will conceive during this time. (See Chapter 23 on Postpartum Contraception and Lactation.)

Depo-Provera.   Studies of Depo-Provera initiated within 7 days postpartum[31] or within 6 weeks postpartum[25] have found no adverse effects. Because Depo-Provera confers less contraceptive benefit to the lactating woman than does Norplant, and because the theoretical risks of Depo-Provera use might be higher (hormonal levels are relatively high in the immediate post-injection days), a case would be less compelling for injecting Depo-Provera before breastfeeding is well established.

Norplant.   If a breastfeeding woman is unlikely to return for a postpartum visit and requests Norplant before leaving the hospital after delivery, the long-term contraceptive benefit of using this method seems likely to exceed the theoretical risks. In studies of Norplant, the method has not been started until at least 30 days postpartum. In one Egyptian study, Norplant was inserted between 30 and 42 days postpartum in 50 lactating women. There was no difference in lactational performance between the Norplant group and two control groups. In all three groups, infant growth was above average for Egyptian infants. Among exclusively breast-fed infants, weight gains in the early postpartum months were slightly but statistically significantly lower in the Norplant group.[49] In a second Egyptian study, Norplant was inserted between 30 and 49 days postpartum in 120 lactating women. There was no difference in breastfeeding performance between the women using Norplant and women in the control group. Moreover, there was no difference in growth or in mental development between infants of the Norplant users and infants of the women in the control group.[48]

Minipills.   When initiated in the first week postpartum but after withdrawal of natural progesterone, minipills have demonstrated no adverse effects on lactation or infant growth.[32,33,38]

BREAST CANCERS AND DEPO-PROVERA

Toxicologic studies of beagle dogs given DMPA that showed an increase in mammary gland tumors, some of which became malignant, raised the concern that humans may also be at risk.[16] Several international studies found no effect in humans (Table 20-5). In a New Zealand study, the overall relative risk associated with the use of DMPA was 1.0; however, among women aged 25 to 34 years, the relative risk was 2.0.[40] The risk was greatest among women who used the drug for 6 years or longer. This study suggests that Depo-Provera may accelerate the presentation of breast cancer in young women, perhaps acting as a promoter in the late

Table 20-5 Risks of 5 types of cancers in DMPA users

Site of Cancer	No. of Cases Who Used DMPA/ All Cases (%)	No. of Controls Who Used DMPA/All Controls (%)	Relative Risk for Women Who Have Ever Used DMPA*
Breast	39/427 (9)	557/5,951 (9)	1.0
Cervix	126/920 (14)	545/5,833 (9)	1.2
Ovary	7/105 (7)	74/637 (12)	0.7
Endometrium	1/52 (2)	30/316 (9)	0.3
Liver	7/57 (12)	34/920 (12)	1.0

Sources: WHO (1986).
Liskin (1987).

stages of carcinogenesis. The WHO Collaborative Study failed to demonstrate a significantly increased risk for either breast cancer or cervical cancer among women using Depo-Provera.[61,62]

DEPO-PROVERA

PROVIDING DEPO-PROVERA

Before Depo-Provera was approved by the Food and Drug Administration, it was used for adolescents who were mentally retarded or who had emotional or behavioral problems.[22] Take special care in making certain that a woman's use of Depo-Provera is *completely* voluntary.

Depo-Provera is usually provided from vials of 150 mg in each 1 cc. The label states a 2-year shelf-life (in Belgium, the label states a 5-year shelf-life). Using a sterile needle and syringe, inject the Depo-Provera deeply into the deltoid or the gluteus maximus muscles. Injections into the deltoid are less embarrassing but may be slightly more painful. The 21 to 23 gauge needle should be 2.5 to 4 cm long.[60] Do *not* massage the area over the injection because it could lower the effectiveness of Depo-Provera and also cause pain. Schedule injections every 12 weeks, although the contraceptive effect usually lasts longer. Some programs provide injections to women who are as much as 4 weeks late. These women are informed that they could have become pregnant during the time they were late, although this possibility is rare.

Some women are late for injections because of fear of cancer, changes in the pattern of menstrual bleeding or other side effects, cost of injections, time lost coming to the clinic, or partner or family disapproval of the method. At Grady Memorial Hospital in Atlanta, clinicians schedule injections at 11-week intervals so that for as long as 2 weeks beyond the appointment date a woman may return and receive her next shot without having to take a pregnancy test or recount her sexual activity during that time.

At each 12-week follow-up visit, ask about weight gain, any problems or concerns, the date of the last menstrual period, and any risk of HIV infection and other sexually transmissible infections (STIs). Record the patient's weight and blood pressure. At the time of the annual exam, perform a pelvic examination, take a Papanicolaou (Pap) smear, and order a mammogram. If the client is not gaining weight excessively or having any unacceptable symptoms or problems, she may continue getting Depo-Provera injections.

MANAGING DEPO-PROVERA PROBLEMS AND FOLLOW-UP

In one of the largest studies of Depo-Provera users, 17% of the 3,875 women complained of headaches, 11% of nervousness, 5% of decreased libido, 3% of breast discomfort, and 2% of depression.[47]

Menstrual changes.   Inform women in advance that changes will occur in their menstrual cycles. Do not belittle the impact of bleeding changes: they are the major reason that women discontinue this method. Spotting or breakthrough bleeding may be managed most easily in a family planning clinic by offering women one or more cycles of combined OCs. Five days of pills may be enough. Inform women that the irregular bleeding may return. Teenagers *can* manage the bleeding patterns occurring during Depo-Provera use. Amenorrhea will increase over time, but it is not harmful.

Allergic reactions.   The *Physicians' Desk Reference (PDR)* notes that anaphylactic and anaphylactoid reactions may occur immediately following Depo-Provera injection. Fortunately, severe anaphylactic reactions are rare. However, because Depo-Provera is irretrievable once injected, have on hand emergency supportive measures such as epinephrine, steroids, and diphenhydramine. At Grady Memorial Hospital, clients are encouraged to stay in the area for 20 minutes following an injection.

Common Questions About Depo-Provera

1. In what situations might Depo-Provera injections be a better choice than Norplant implants?

- Concern about the minor surgical procedure required to insert the implants
- History of sickle cell disease or of seizures, both of which may be improved by Depo-Provera[29,30]

- Use of a medication (such as phenobarbital, phenytoin [Dilantin], primidone, carbamazepine, and phenylbutazone) that markedly increases production of liver enzymes, which speeds the breakdown of the levonorgestrel in Norplant
- Need for highly effective contraception for just a *few months* prior to tubal sterilization or vasectomy, at the time of receiving rubella immunization, and during use of medications such as anticoagulants, valproic acid, or Accutane (for acne), which is known to produce severe fetal defects
- Need for *only a year* of extremely effective contraception, such as for a woman who has recently had a molar pregnancy and must not become pregnant for 1 year
- Preference for receiving medications by injection
- Desire to keep all information about contraceptive use from her partner (for example, from an abusive husband who does not want her to use contraception)

2. Can a woman who is breastfeeding her baby receive Depo-Provera injections?

Yes. Depo-Provera is a reasonable option for breastfeeding mothers, although non-hormonal methods are generally preferred. Breastfeeding in itself confers a contraceptive effect, so as long as the woman will return for her postpartum exam, she can wait until then to begin injections.

3. Why is a method that was "bad" 15 years ago now a good method?

Depo-Provera has always been a good method. The reason it was not approved by the Food and Drug Administration (FDA) had more to do with politics than science. By 1992, when Depo-Provera was approved in the United States, it was already being used by 8 million to 9 million women in over 90 countries.

4. What is the most important difference between Depo-Provera (DMPA) and norethindrone enanthate (NET-EN) injections?

Depo-Provera is given every 12 weeks from the first 150 mg injection on. NET-EN injections, which are not available in the United States, are given every 8 weeks for the first 6 months and then every 8 to 12 weeks thereafter. They deliver norethindrone in an oily base.[20] Women using NET-EN every 12 weeks *cannot be late* for the next injection. Depo-Provera is more forgiving of the woman who is late for her injection.

NORPLANT IMPLANTS

PROVIDING NORPLANT IMPLANTS

Each Norplant kit distributed in the United States comes with detailed step-by-step instructions and diagrams. Wyeth Laboratories also makes available at no cost two excellent videos—one for clinicians and one for clients. When available, a two-capsule Norplant system approved by the FDA will simplify both insertion and removal.

Consider scheduling a follow-up visit after 1 month to answer any questions or to check the incision and placement of implants. However, routine reappointment of Norplant users at 1 month appears to be neither cost-effective nor of clinical benefit.[11] Encourage women to call if they are bothered by the pattern of bleeding.

Suitability test. "Should I try a suitability test to see if this woman is going to tolerate Norplant?" In general, the answer is "no." Testing a woman's response to several injections of Depo-Provera makes no sense at all as a suitability test. The hormones in the two methods are completely different, as are the fluctuations in hormone levels in the serum. Prescribing a minipill containing levonorgestrel (Ovrette) to a woman for several months is generally not necessary. However, Ovrette may be useful to test suitability when patients have a history of or concern about the following conditions:

- Acne
- Weight gain
- Severe headaches
- Depression
- Allergy to levonorgestrel

Norplant Insertion: 20 Helpful Hints

Norplant implants are inserted during a minor surgical procedure done under local anesthesia. Using a trocar, the clinician places Norplant implants under the skin on the inside of a woman's upper arm in a fan-shaped configuration.

1. Practice insertion on the arm model if this is the first, second, or third time you have inserted Norplant implants.
2. The number one concern of women is whether insertion causes pain.[11] Have someone who has already had Norplant implants inserted reassure your client.
3. Raise the head of the exam table. Your patient will be more comfortable.

4. Locate the incision site by measuring the width of four fingers if you are a man, or five fingers if you are a woman, proximally from the crease of the elbow. Mark this site.

5. Use a template (Figure 20-1) and a pen every time you insert a set of Norplant implants. Using a template will show the precise site where you should place the trocar and inject local anesthetic. Removals will be easier because the template will be a guide. Do *not* insert implants directly over the brachial groove because the neurovascular structures underlie the surface (Figure 20-2).

6. To decrease the sting of local anesthetic, add 0.5 cc sodium bicarbonate to every 5 cc of 1% xylocaine (1:10 ratio). By adding 3 cc of $NaHCO_3$ to the 30 cc bottle of xylocaine, you will have enough local anesthetic for a number of insertions in a single session. Mix only as much of the 1:10 solution as you will need in a day.

7. The patient will feel less discomfort if you inject the local anesthetic slowly, especially if you are injecting xylocaine with no sodium bicarbonate. By the time the injection has been made for the sixth implant, the local anesthesia will have taken effect near the first incision site.

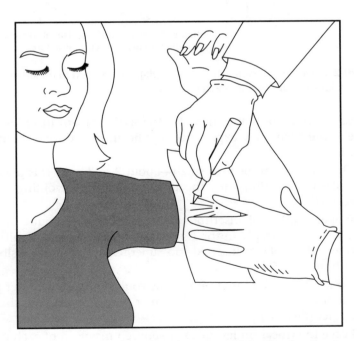

Figure 20-1 Template for fan-shaped configuration of Norplant implant insertion

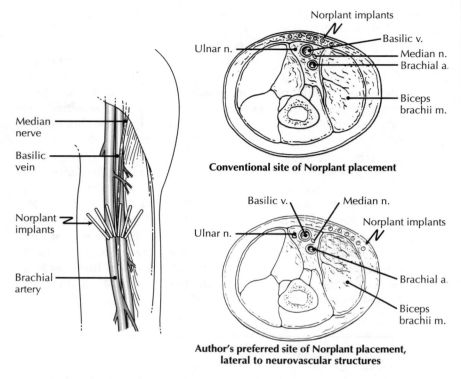

Figure 20-2 Location of inserted Norplant implants in relation to underlying neurovascular structures in the brachial groove

8. Save 1 cc of local anesthetic for the sixth implant insertion site or else the client may experience significant pain during insertion of the last implant.

9. The incision can be very small—about 2 to 3 mm. It is possible to make the incision with the trocar itself, thus avoiding use of a scalpel.

10. Proper subdermal insertion of implants is paramount. Implants inserted too deeply in the tissue layers cause more difficulty upon removal. Implants inserted too superficially are more visible and at times painful.

11. Do not move the inner plunger as you withdraw the outer part of the trocar. Do not push on the inner plunger with your thumb or retract the inner plunger.

12. Leave the trocar under the skin between insertion of each individual implant.

13. Once you have inserted an implant, hold it in place while you advance the trocar to insert the next implant (Figure 20-3).

14. Locate the distal tips of all six implants. If an implant is 5 mm to 1 cm further from the incision than the others, it is often possible to push the implant toward the incision.

15. Gently clean the area with an alcohol swab before bandaging.

16. Show the client the incision site before you put on the butterfly bandage or gauze. She will be reassured when she sees how small the incision is.

17. Roll the gauze bandage over a square 4" by 4" folded pad. Do not wrap it too tightly. Suggest that your client leave the gauze wrapping on her arm for 3 to 5 days to avoid having people touch the area while it is still tender.

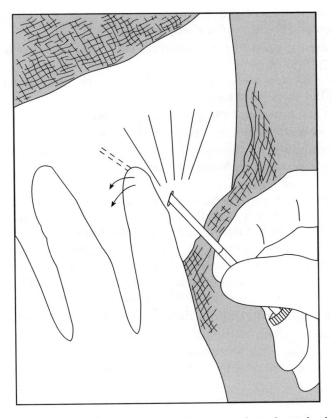

Figure 20-3 Technique of pulling inserted implant away from the path of the trocar as the next implant is inserted

18. Warn your client that she may have a large bruise when her bandage is removed.

19. Inform the client if any implant has been inserted too deeply or too far or if the proximal end of one implant was pulled distally.

20. Remind the client that Norplant will change her menstrual bleeding patterns. Give her your phone number and encourage her to call if she has questions or problems, including annoying patterns of menstual bleeding.

Norplant Removal: 20 Helpful Hints

1. Use the arm model to practice removal.

2. When you perform your first Norplant removal, try to have someone at your side who has experience. Initially, it make take you 45 to 60 minutes to remove the implants.

3. Remind the client that removal may be more difficult than insertion and could require a second visit.

4. Raise the head of the examining table. The patient will be more comfortable.

5. Be sure you are comfortable. You may be more at ease sitting rather than standing.

6. An assistant may be helpful during the removal procedure.

7. Mark both the proximal and distal ends of each of the six implants.

8. Add sodium bicarbonate to the local anesthetic to decrease stinging. (See #6 under Norplant Insertion.)

9. Inject the local anesthetic slowly under the proximal 1/3 of the implants. Wyeth instructions recommend that you initially inject approximately 3 cc of 1% xylocaine. Have an additional 3 to 5 cc of xylocaine available in case you need it later.

10. Rather than making your incision at exactly the same site as the location of the incision used to insert implants, you may want to make the incision as close as possible to the tips of all 6 implants. Some clinicians use the same incision so as to avoid a second scar.

11. Make an incision 4 to 10 mm long (see #17 for more discussion).

12. Make a second incision if one implant is far from the others.

13. Throughout the procedure, ask the client if she feels any pain and provide additional local anesthetic as needed.

14. With your finger, apply pressure to the distal end of each implant as you remove it. Push the implant toward the incision (Figure 20-4).

15. With a sharp blade, a gauze pad, or Adson's forceps remove the scar tissue covering the implants.

16. Do not pull an implant too hard. It may break.

17. The Emory method of Norplant removal can speed up the procedure. Some clinicians average less than 15 minutes per removal.[46]

- Use 6 to 8 cc of local anesthesia rather than 3 cc.
- Make a 8 mm to 1 cm incision rather than a 4 mm incision.
- Before attempting to remove the implants, gently disrupt adhesions for 30 seconds by repeatedly opening and closing a small curved hemostat in the tissue near the end of the implants.[46]

18. The "U" Technique can also facilitate Norplant removal.[8,44] The instrument is available through Wyeth Laboratories at no cost (see Figure 20-4).

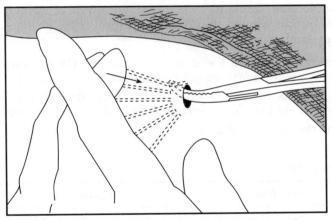

Use of hemostat to remove implant while clinician's finger pushes implant toward incision

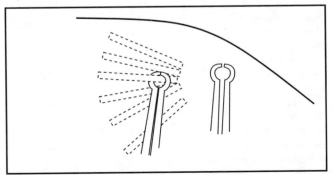

U-technique for removing Norplant implants (similar to use of forceps during a vasectomy)

Figure 20-4 Norplant removal techniques

19. Warn your client that she may develop a bruise after removal, but that it will go away completely. Prostaglandin inhibitors may ease any pain in her arm following removal.

20. Remind your client that she may become pregnant immediately following Norplant removal. If she does not want to become pregnant, discuss contraception.

MANAGING NORPLANT PROBLEMS AND FOLLOW-UP

A number of side effects may occur, especially during the first year of Norplant use (Table 20-6).[33,34] Occasionally, Norplant implants must be removed to eliminate these complications.

Menstrual disturbances. During years 1 and 2, changes in the pattern of menstrual bleeding are the most common reason women ask that their Norplant implants be removed. Over 80% of women will note a change. Inform women in advance to expect these changes. The following approaches may help:

- Several cycles of a low-dose combined OC (While low-dose pills usually work, a 50 mcg pill [Ovral] may also be used.[2])
- Exogenous estrogens such as oral 17-beta estradiol, (Estrace), ethinyl estradiol (Estinyl), or conjugated estrogens (Premarin)
- Prostaglandin inhibitors

Table 20-6 Norplant side effects during first year of use

Side Effect	Norplant Users	
	Study 1	*Study 2*
Headaches	16.7	18.5
Ovarian enlargement	3.1	11.6
Dizziness	5.6	8.1
Breast tenderness	6.2	6.8
Nervousness	6.2	6.8
Nausea	5.1	7.7
Acne	4.5	7.2
Dermatitis	3.8	8.2
Breast discharge	3.5	5.1
Change in appetite	3.5	6.2
Weight gain	3.3	6.2
Hair growth or loss	1.8	2.6

Source: McCauley (1992).

Headaches. If a Norplant user develops severe headaches associated with blurred vision and papilledema, remove the implants immediately. In December of 1992, Wyeth Laboratories sent a letter to physicians describing severe headaches, papilledema, and a pseudotumor cerebri-like syndrome in 14 women using Norplant implants. Whether Norplant is causally related to the development of these symptoms is not yet clear.

Breast tenderness. Treatments include Vitamin E (600 units/day), bromocriptine (2.5 mg/day), tamoxifen (20 mg/day), or danazol (200 mg/day).[55]

Weight gain. Although weight gain may accompany use of Norplant, it is usually due to other causes.

Common Questions About Norplant Implants

1. In what situations might Norplant implants be a better choice than the injectable contraceptive Depo-Provera?

Norplant is the preferable method for women who—

- Will have difficulty returning consistently for injections
- Are concerned about weight gain (although some Norplant users gain weight)
- Fear repeated shots
- Desire to become pregnant immediately after discontinuation (This most concerns women who are late in their reproductive years.)
- Need very effective reversible contraceptive for a long period of time (Women taking Accutane, Coumadin, and chemotherapeutic agents should not become pregnant because of the risk of severe birth defects.)
- Are concerned about decreased HDL cholesterol

2. Can anything be done for a woman who has persistent bleeding on Norplant?

The problem is usually an atrophic endometrium. Cycle your patient for several months. The additional hormones should not be a problem for most women if you use low-dose OCs or a low dose of conjugated estrogens, ethinyl estradiol, or estradiol. Explain that using these extra hormones would probably not be harmful, that the amount of blood loss she is experiencing is probably less not more, and that she can have sexual intercourse in spite of the spotting. Consider drawing blood to measure her hematocrit. Differential diagnoses include chlamydia infection, fibroids, or cervical inflammation.

3. **Can a woman using Norplant implants have ovarian cysts?**

Yes, the great majority of cysts disappear on their own without surgery. If you discover an ovarian cyst, re-examine the woman again in about 3 weeks to make sure it is decreasing in size and not becoming painful.

4. **Should heavy women avoid Norplant implants?**

No, changes in the capsules that hold the levonorgestrel were made in 1991. All women receiving the new implants receive excellent protection from pregnancy.

5. **What if a woman decides she wants to have her capsules removed before 5 years?**

Ask her why she wants the capsules removed; you may be able to reassure her that her problems or concerns are not serious. Answer her questions clearly and accurately. After counseling, ask if she wants to keep the implants or have them removed. Make certain that she does not feel pressured to respond in any given way. If she wants them removed, no matter what her reason, do so immediately or arrange for their prompt removal.[18]

PROGESTIN-ONLY PILLS (MINIPILLS)

PROVIDING MINIPILLS

Because of the small number of women who use minipills, large-scale studies that document benefits and side effects are unavailable. In general, progestin-only pills have lower effectiveness, more breakthrough bleeding, fewer noncontraceptive benefits than combined OCs, and fewer serious complications.[33]

Minipills must be taken on time. Figure 20-5 illustrates how more sperm penetrate cervical mucus if the interval between progestin-only pills is longer than 24 hours. Because minipills must be taken at close to the same hour each day, they may not be the best choice for women who are disorganized. However, an advantage of minipills is that each day, whether or not she is bleeding, the woman takes exactly the same type of pill with no pill-free interval.

MANAGING MINIPILL PROBLEMS AND FOLLOW-UP

The approaches for managing increased days of light or heavy bleeding, spotting, or amenorrhea are the same as would be considered for the woman using implants or injectable contraceptives: switch to a combined OC, use supplemental estrogen, or use prostaglandin inhibitors. Rule out pregnancy and provide counseling.

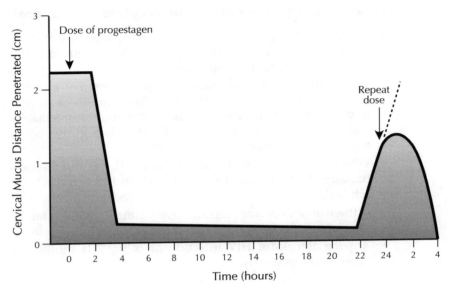

Note: Minimum reduction in sperm penetration between 4 hours and 22 hours after a single dose of megestrol acetate

(0.5 mg). Unlike the rest of the figure, the effect of a repeat dose is presumed, not experimental.

Source: Guillebaud (1985).

Figure 20-5 Sperm penetration test following progestin-only pill

As in the case with Norplant and IUD users, when a pregnancy occurs in a woman using minipills, it is more likely to be ectopic because of the contraceptive effect of minipills on the endometrial lining.

Minipills are theoretically safer than combined OCs. Minipills have not been shown to increase the risk of either cardiovascular complications or malignant disease and are less likely to cause headaches, blood pressure elevation, depression, and other side effects than are higher-dose combined OCs.[33,58]

Common Questions About Minipills

1. What effect do minipills have on ovulation?

- Users may ovulate every month. Women who have regular periods may be more likely to become pregnant using minipills.
- Users may never ovulate. A woman may go months without any bleeding.
- Users may ovulate some months and not others, in which case their periods are irregular.

2. When are back-up methods of contraception a good idea?

- Women with regular periods are ovulating regularly and are more likely to become pregnant, so a back-up method would enhance the efficacy of minipills.
- During the first cycle of taking minipills, a woman may forget pills or take them late. However, the minipills cause production of a thick cervical mucus that starts immediately and continues as long as minipills are taken every day at about the same time.
- When a woman is late in taking a minipill, she should use a back-up contraceptive for 48 hours until she is back on schedule.
- If the woman becomes anxious every time a period is late, a back-up method will allow her to feel more secure.
- Anyone at risk for HIV infection or other STIs should use condoms consistently.

INSTRUCTIONS FOR USING PROGESTIN-ONLY CONTRACEPTIVES

DEPO-PROVERA

Depo-Provera injections are very effective if you return every 12 weeks for a repeat injection. Of 1,000 women who consistently get repeat injections every 12 weeks, only 3 will become pregnant over a year's time. Depo-Provera injections confer a number of noncontraceptive benefits by decreasing the following:

- Menstrual blood flow
- Menstrual cramping
- Risk of anemia
- Risk of endometrial cancer
- Risk of pelvic infection
- Risk of ectopic pregnancy (a pregnancy outside of your uterus)
- Risk of a sickle cell crisis
- Frequency of grand mal seizures

On the other hand, you must be willing to accept unpredictable, even frequent or absent, bleeding to use Depo-Provera. About 50% of women using Depo-Provera will stop having any bleeding after a year of injections. *Depo-Provera injections do not protect you from sexually transmitted infections, including infection with the virus that causes AIDS (acquired immune deficiency syndrome).* If you decide to have intercourse, use a latex or plastic male or female condom every time that sexual intercourse may expose you or your partner to infection.

1. **Have on hand a back-up contraceptive method** such as foam, spermicidal tablets or suppositories, condoms, or a diaphragm. You will need to use your back-up method **for 1 week after your first injection.** (This precaution may not be necessary if the first shot is given during the first 5 days after the beginning of a normal menstrual period.)

2. Because of the rare possibility of an allergic reaction, some programs ask that women remain in the vicinity of the clinic for 20 minutes after having their Depo-Provera injections.

3. **Return to the clinic every 12 weeks for another injection.** Mark your calendar for your next Depo-Provera shot to be sure you will be on time. You may want to get your partner to mark his calendar, too. Some programs are beginning to offer women (who have been using Depo-Provera successfully), the opportunity to *take home* enough Depo-Provera and syringes to last for a full year. If you would like to learn to give yourself your injections of Depo-Provera, ask your clinician.

4. **Have a latex or plastic condom ready if you—**

   - Are late for your injection
   - May be at risk for a sexually transmitted infection, including infection with the virus that causes AIDS

5. See your clinician regularly for routine checkups. Be sure to have a blood pressure check, Pap smear, breast exam, and pelvic exam.

6. Depression and premenstrual symptoms may improve or become worse. If you become severely depressed, see your clinician immediately.

7. There are still some unanswered questions about the long-term effects of Depo-Provera injections on women's estrogen levels and on their bones. This is very important because estrogen is important in preventing heart disease and osteoporosis. Exercise and take in adequate amounts of calcium from foods like milk, cheese, yogurt, or ice cream or from several tablets of Tums a day.

8. Depo-Provera users may gain weight due to an increased appetite. Pay close attention to what you eat and exercise regularly.

Late for Injection

1. **If you realize after intercourse that you have missed your injection or are late for it,** use another contraceptive or do not have intercourse. Return as soon as possible for your shot.

2. If you have already had intercourse without being protected by a contraceptive, come to the clinic or call your clinician immediately to discuss options, including *emergency contraception*, which will keep you from getting pregnant. You can also call *1-888-NOT- 2-LATE* to find the phone numbers of 5 providers of emergency contraception nearest to you.

Depo-Provera and Your Periods

1. Depo-Provera tends to make a woman's periods less regular, and spotting between periods is fairly common. Some women stop having periods completely. This is not harmful, and many women like not having periods.

2. If your pattern of bleeding concerns you, return to the clinic to get a blood test for anemia and to rule out the possibility of pregnancy or infection.

3. If the pattern of bleeding you experience is annoying, contact your clinician. There are medications you can take to make you have a more acceptable pattern of bleeding.

4. When you discontinue taking Depo-Provera, it may be a number of months before your periods return to normal after your last Depo-Provera injection.

Discontinuing Depo-Provera

1. If you are more than 1 week late for your injection, **use a back-up method of contraception.** Visit your clinician right away for your injection. You will need to continue using a back-up method until you get your injection and for a week *after* your next injection. Many clinicians will give you a pregnancy test make sure you are not pregnant.

2. If you discontinue Depo-Provera and do not want to become pregnant, start using a new contraceptive 13 weeks after your last shot.

3. If you are discontinuing Depo-Provera because you *want* to become pregnant, remember that the contraceptive effect may take a number of months to go away. Be patient.

Depo-Provera and Pregnancy

1. Depo-Provera injections may keep you from getting pregnant for more than 12 weeks after your last shot. The average delay in return

of fertility is 10 months from the last injection. Depo-Provera does not decrease your fertility in the long run.

2. If you are 35 to 45 years old and want to become pregnant in the future, you may want to use a contraceptive that has minimal or no delay in return of fertility after you stop using that other method.

Depo-Provera Warning Signals

1. See your clinician if you develop any of the warning signals or any other symptoms that concern you.

Depo-Provera® (The Shot) Warning Signals

Caution

■ Repeated, very painful headaches

■ Heavy bleeding

■ Depression

■ Severe, lower abdominal pain (may be a sign of pregnancy)

■ Pus, prolonged pain, or bleeding at injection site

NORPLANT IMPLANTS

Norplant implants offer very effective contraception. Only 1 in 2,000 women will become pregnant during their first year of Norplant use. Norplant implants have a number of noncontraceptive benefits by decreasing the following:

- Menstrual blood flow
- Menstrual cramping
- Risk of anemia
- Risk of endometrial cancer
- Risk of pelvic infection
- Risk of ectopic pregnancy (a pregnancy outside of your uterus)

On the other hand, you must be willing to accept unpredictable, even frequent or absent, bleeding to use Norplant. *Norplant implants do not protect you from sexually transmitted infections, including infection with the virus that causes AIDS (acquired immune deficiency syndrome).* If you decide to have intercourse, use a latex or plastic male or female condom every time that sexual intercourse may expose you or your partner to infection.

1. **Have on hand a back-up contraceptive method** such as foam, spermicidal tablets or suppositories, condoms, or a diaphragm. You will need to use your back-up method on the first day

after your implants have been inserted. A back-up contraceptive probably is not necessary for more than 3 days, but it will do no harm if you use it for a week.

2. If you have pain after insertion, return to see your clinician. You might need antibiotics for an infection. Try to avoid direct pressure on the insertion area for a few days. After the incision has healed, you may touch the skin over the implants. The soft, flexible implants cannot break inside your body, so you should not be concerned about putting pressure on the area.

3. Be sure you know the telephone number to call if you have questions or if you develop a problem.

4. Depression and premenstrual symptoms may improve or they may become worse. If you become severely depressed, see your clinician immediately.

5. Return after one month to have your arm checked and your questions answered.

6. See your clinician regularly for routine checkups. Be sure to have a blood pressure check, Pap smear, breast exam, and pelvic exam.

7. Your implants should be removed in 5 years.

Norplant and Your Periods

1. Norplant tends to make a woman's periods less regular, and spotting between periods is fairly common. Some women stop having periods completely. This is not harmful, and many women like not having periods. As time goes by, menstrual bleeding tends to become more regular.

2. If your pattern of bleeding concerns you, return to the clinic to get a blood test for anemia and to rule out the possibility of pregnancy or infection.

3. If the pattern of bleeding you experience is annoying, contact your clinician. There are medications you can take to make you have a more acceptable pattern of bleeding.

4. Your periods will return to normal (and you will be able to get pregnant) very quickly after your implants are removed.

Discontinuing Norplant Implants

1. Removal of Norplant implants is more difficult than insertion. In general, the implants can be removed in a matter of minutes (5 to 30 minutes) without causing you much discomfort or pain. Find out in advance if your health care provider has had experience removing Norplant implants.

2. Replace your implants after 5 years or have them removed and start using another method. Norplant's effectiveness drops after 5 years. It is not dangerous to leave the implants in your arm, although they will not provide contraception you can count on.

3. A new set of implants may be inserted the day your old set is removed.

4. You will be able to become pregnant right away after your implants are removed.

Norplant Warning Signals

1. Return to your clinician if you have any questions. Watch for the following signs of potential problems:

Norplant Warning Signs

Caution

- ■ Severe lower abdominal pain (ectopic pregnancy is rare but can occur)
- ■ Heavy vaginal bleeding
- ■ Arm pain
- ■ Pus or bleeding at the insertion site (these may be signs of infection)
- ■ Expulsion of an implant
- ■ Delayed menstrual periods after a long interval of regular periods
- ■ Migraine headaches, repeated very painful headaches, or blurred vision

Avoid bumping the area where your Norplant implants were inserted and keep this area dry for several days after insertion.

MINIPILLS

Minipills are contraceptive pills that do not contain estrogen. When they are taken about the same time every day, only 1 out of 200 women will become pregnant over a year's time.

Minipills have a number of noncontraceptive benefits by decreasing the following:

- • Menstrual blood flow
- • Menstrual cramping
- • Risk of anemia
- • Risk of endometrial cancer
- • Risk of pelvic infection

On the other hand, you must be willing to accept unpredictable, even frequent or absent bleeding, to use minipills. *Minipills do not protect you from sexually transmitted infections, including infection with the virus that causes AIDS (acquired immune deficiency syndrome).* If you decide to have intercourse, use a latex or plastic male or female condom every time that sexual intercourse may expose you or your partner to infection.

1. **Have on hand a back-up contraceptive method** such as foam, spermicidal tablets or suppositories, condoms, or a diaphragm. You will need to use your back-up method:

   - While you are waiting to start your first pack of minipills
   - During your first 7 to 28 days on minipills
   - If you miss a minipill (See the instructions for Late or Missed Pills.)

2. You may be able to take your first pill today or on the first day of your next period. Be sure you know when your clinician wants you to take your first pill.

3. **Swallow one pill each day until you finish your pill pack.** Then start your new pack the next day. Never miss a day and try to take pills at about the same time each day. The evening meal may be the best time to take minipills.

4. Minipills are very low-dose contraceptives. You have a very narrow margin of error, so do not count on minipills unless you will be able to take pills every single day. *Some women use a back-up method at all times to increase the effectiveness of minipills.*

5. **Have a latex or plastic condom ready if you—**

   - Have missed pills
   - May be at risk for a sexually transmitted infection, including infection with the virus that causes AIDS

6. Depression and premenstrual symptoms may improve or become worse. If you become severely depressed, see your clinician immediately.

7. See your clinician regularly for routine checkups. Be sure to have a blood pressure check, Pap smear, breast exam, and pelvic exam.

Late or Missed Minipills

1. Start taking your minipills as soon as possible.

2. **If you miss one minipill,** take it (yesterday's minipill) as soon as you remember. Also take today's minipill at the regular time, even if that means taking two pills in 1 day. If you are more than 3 hours late taking a minipill, use your back-up birth control method for the next 48 hours (2 days).

3. **If you miss two or more minipills in a row,** there is an increased chance you could become pregnant. Immediately start using your back-up method. Restart your minipills right away and take 2 pills a day for 2 days. If your menstrual period does not begin within 4 to 6 weeks, see your clinician for an exam and a pregnancy test.

4. If you have already had intercourse *without adequate protection* because you missed pills, call your clinician immediately. You may be able to use an emergency contraceptive. Call *1-888-NOT-2-LATE* to find the phone numbers of 5 providers of emergency contraception nearest to you.

Minipills and Your Periods

1. Minipills tend to make a woman's periods less regular, and spotting between periods is fairly common. Some women stop having periods completely. This is not harmful, and many women like not having periods.

2. If your pattern of bleeding concerns you, return to the clinic to get a blood test for anemia and to rule out the possibility of pregnancy or infection.

3. If the pattern of bleeding you experience is annoying, contact your clinician. There are medications you can take to make you have a more acceptable pattern of bleeding.

4. Your periods will return to normal (and you will be able to get pregnant) very quickly after your minipills are discontinued.

Discontinuing Minipills

1. If you discontinue minipills and do not want to become pregnant, start using another contraceptive immediately. Your ability to become pregnant returns right away after stopping minipills.

Minipill Warning Signals

1. See your clinician right away if you have severe lower abdominal pain while using minipills.

2. Return to see your clinician if you develop any of the following warning signals:

Progestin-Only Pills (Minipills) Warning Signs	
Caution	■ Abdominal pain—May be due to an ovarian cyst or an ectopic pregnancy (Don't stop pills but contact us right away.)
	■ Delayed period after several months of regular cycles may be a sign of pregnancy
	■ Repeated, very severe headaches
	■ Pill taken too late—Even if only 3 hours late use a back-up contraceptive for the next 2 days. Be careful to use minipill ON TIME.

REFERENCES

1. Affandi B, Santoso SS, Djajadilaga W, Hedispura W, Moelock FA, Prihartono J, Lubis F, Samil RS. Five-year experience with Norplant. Contraception 1987;36(4):417-428.
2. Alvarez-Sanchez F, Brache V, Thevenin F, Cochon L, Faundes A. Hormonal treatment for bleeding irregularities in Norplant implant users. Am J Obstet Gynecol; 1996(174):919-922.
3. Angle M, Murphy C. Guidelines for clinical procedures in family planning. A reference for trainers. Program for International Training in Health (INTRAH); Chapel Hill NC; 1992.
4. Anonymous. More research needed in link between progesterone and HIV infection: clinical recommendations unchanged by monkey study. Contraceptive Technology Update 1996;178:89-92 and Counseling Supplement.
5. Antal EG. Personal communication from Drug Information Clinical Pharmacist at the Upjohn Company to Robert A. Hatcher; March 18, 1993.
6. Archer B, Irwin D, Jensen K, Johnson ME, Rorie JA. Depo medroxyprogesterone: management of side-effects commonly associated with its contraceptive use. J Nurse Midwifery 1997;42;2:104-111.
7. Bertrabet SS, Shikary ZK, Toddywalla VS, Toddywalla SP, Patel D, Saxena BN. Transfer of norethisterone (NET) and levonorgestrel (LNG) from a single tablet into the infant's circulation through the mother's milk. Contraception 1987;35(6):517-522.
8. Blumenthal PD, Gafikin L, Affandi B, Bongiovanni A, McGrath J, Glew G. Training for Norplant removal: assessment of learning curves and competency. Obstet Gynecol 1997;89:174-178.
9. Canterbury C, Hatcher, RA, McGrann M. Serum estradiol levels in women using Depo-Provera for more than a year. Resident Research Day Paper; 1996.
10. Cromer BA, Smith RD, Blair JM, Dwyer J, Brown RT. A prospective study of adolescents who choose among levonorgestrel implants (Norplant), medroxyprogesterone acetate (Depo-Provera), or the combined oral contraceptive pill as contraception. Pediatrics 1994;94:687-694.
11. Cullins VE, Blumenthal PD, Remsburg RE, Huggins GR. Preliminary experience with Norplant in an inner city population. Contraception 1993;47:193-203.
12. Cundy T, Evans M, Roberts H, Wattie D, Ames R, Reid IR. Bone density in women receiving depo medroxyprogesterone acetate for contraception. BMJ 1991;303(6793):13-16.

13. Darney PD, Atkinson E, Tanner ST, MacPherson S, Hellerstein S, Alvarado AM. Acceptance and perceptions of Norplant among users in San Francisco, USA. Stud Fam Plann 1990;21(3):152-160.

14. Diaz S, Pavez M, Miranda P, Johannson EDB, Croxatto HB. Long-term follow-up of women treated with Norplant implants. Contraception 1987;35:551-567.

15. Duerr A, Warren D, Smith D, Nagachinta T, Marx PA. Contraceptives and HIV transmission [letter]. Nature Medicine 1997;3:124.

16. Finkel MJ, Berliner VR. The extrapolation of experimental findings (animal to man): the dilemma of the systemically administered contraceptives. Bulletin of the Society of Pharmacological and Environmental Pathologists, December 1973.

17. Guillebaud J. Contraception: your questions answered. New York NY: Pitman, 1985.

18. Hatcher RA, Rinehart W, Blackburn R, Geller JS. The Essentials of Contraceptive Technology. Baltimore, Johns Hopkins School of Public Health, Population Information Program, 1997.

19. Haukkamaa M. Contraception by Norplant subdermal capsules is not reliable in epileptic patients on anticonvulsant treatment. Contraception 1986;33(6):559-565.

20. Huezo CM, Briggs C. Medical and service delivery guidelines for family planning. London: International Planned Parenthood Federation Medical Department, 1992.

21. International Planned Parenthood Federation. IMAP statement on breast feeding, fertility and postpartum contraception. IPPF Medical Bulletin 1996;30(3)1-3.

22. Isart F, Weber FT, Merrick CL, Rowe S. Use of injectable progestin (medroxyprogesterone acetate) in adolescent health care. Contraception 1992;46(1):41-48.

23. Kennedy KL, Short RV, Tully MR. Premature introduction of progestin-only contraceptive methods during lactation. Contraception 1997;55:347-350.

24. Klavon SL, Grubb G. Insertion site complications during the first year of Norplant use. Contraception 1990;41(1):27-37.

25. Koetsawang S, Boonyaprakob V, Suvanichati S, Paipeekul S. Long term study of growth and development of children breast-fed by mothers receiving Depo-Provera (medroxyprogesterone acetate) during lactation. In: Zatuchni GI, Goldsmith A, Shelton JD, Sciarra JJ (eds). Long-acting contraceptive delivery systems: proceedings from an international workshop on long-acting contraceptive delivery systems, May 31-June 3, 1983, New Orleans LA. Philadelphia PA: Harper & Row, 1983:378-387.

26. Koo HP, Griffith JD, Nennstiel M. Adolescents' use of Norplant and Depo-Provera: how do they do? Poster session at the 1996 APHA meeting.

27. Liskin L, Blackburn R. Hormonal contraception: new long-acting methods. Popul Rep 1987;Series K(3).

28. Marx PA, Spira AI, Gettie A, Dailey PJ, Veazey RS, Lackner AA, Mahoney CJ, Miller CJ, Claypool LE, Ho DD, Alexander NJ. Progesterone implants enhance SIV vaginal transmission and early virus load. Nature Medicine 1996;2:1084-1089.

29. Mattson RH, Cramer JA, Darney PD, Naftolin F. Use of oral contraceptives by women with epilepsy. JAMA 1986;256(2):238-240.

30. Mattson RH, Rebar RN. Contraceptive methods for women with neurologic disorders. Am J Obstet Gynecol 1993; 168: 2027-2032.
31. McCann MF, Liskin LS, Piotrow PT, Rinehart W, Fox G. Breastfeeding, fertility and family planning. Popul Reports 1984;12(2),Series J(24):525-575.
32. McCann MF, Moggia AV, Higgins JE, Potts M, Becker C. The effects of a progestin-only oral contraceptive (levonorgestrel 0.03 mg) on breast-feeding. Contraception 1989;40(6):635-648.
33. McCann MF, Potter LS. Progestin-only oral contraception: a comprehensive review. Contraception 1994;Suppl 50:S1-S195.
34. McCauley AP, Geller JS. Decisions for Norplant programs. Popul Rep 1992; Series K(4).
35. Mishell DR. Pharmacokinetics of depot medroxyprogesterone acetate contraception. J. Reprod Med [suppl] 1996;41:381-390.
36. Mishell DR, Kletzky OA, Brenner PF, Roy S, Nicoloff J. The effect of contraceptive steroids on hypothalamic-pituitary function. Am J Obstet Gynecol 1977: 128(1):60-74.
37. Mishell DR. Long-acting contraceptive steroids. Postcoital contraceptives and antiprogestins. In: Mishell DR, Davajan V, Lobo RA (eds). Infertility, contraception, and reproductive endocrinology. Cambridge: Blackwell Scientific Publications, 1991.
38. Moggia AV, Harris GS, Dunson TR, Diaz R, Moggia MS, Ferrer MA, McMullen SL. A comparative study of a progestin-only oral contraceptive versus non-hormonal methods in lactating women in Buenos Aires, Argentina. Contraception 1991;44(1):31-43.
39. Norplant Consensus Background Paper. July 3, 1997.
40. Paul C, Skegg DCG, Spears GFS. Depot medroxyprogesterone (Depo-Provera) and risk of breast cancer. Br Med J 1989;299(6702):759-762.
41. Polaneczky M, Guarnaccia M, Alon J, Wiley J. Early experience with the contraceptive use of depo-medroxyprogesterone acetate in an inner-city population. Family Planning Perspectives 1996;28:174-178.
42. Population Council. Norplant levonorgestrel implants: a summary of scientific data. Monograph. New York: Population Council, 1990.
43. Potter L, Dalberth B, Canamar R, Betts M. DMPA acceptors: a retrospective study at a North Carolina health department (forthcoming).
44. Praptohardjo U, Wibowo S. The "U" technique: a new method for Norplant implants removal. Contraception 1993;48(6):526-536.
45. Ricketts, SA. Repeat fertility and contraceptive implant use among medicaid recipients in Colorado. Family Planning Perspectives 1996;28(6):278-280, 284.
46. Sarma SP, Hatcher RA. The Emory method for rapid removal of Norplant implants. Contraception 1994;49:J 551-556.
47. Schwallie PC, Assenzo JR. Contraceptive use-efficacy study utilizing medroxyprogesterone acetate administered as an intramuscular injection once every 90 days. Fertil Steril 1973;24(5):331-339.
48. Shaaban MM. Contraception with progestogens and progesterone during lactation. J Steroid Biochem Mol Biol 1991;40(4-6):705-710.
49. Shaaban MM, Salem HT, Abdullah KA. Influence of levonorgestrel contraceptive implants, Norplant, initiated early postpartum upon lactation and infant growth. Contraception 1985;32(6):623-635.
50. Sheth A, Jain U, Sharma S, Adatia A, Patankar S, Andolsek L, Pretnar-Darovec A, Blesey MA, Hall PE, Parker RA, Ayeni S, Pinol A, Li-Hoi-Foo C. A randomized,

double-blind study of two combined and two progestogen-only oral contraceptives. Contraception 1982;25(3):243-252.

51. Shoup D, Mishell DR, Bopp B, Fielding M. The significance of bleeding patterns in Norplant implant users. Obstet Gynecol 1993;77:256-265.

52. Sivin I. Internation experience with Norplant and Norplant II. Contraception 1988;19(2):81-94.

53. Sivin I, Lähteenmäki P, Ranta S, Darney P, Klaisle C, Wan L, Mishell DR, Lacarra M, Viegas OAC, Bilhareus P, Koetsawang S, Piya-Anant M, Diaz S, Pavez M, Alvarez F, Brache V, LaGuardia K, Nash H, Stern J. Levonorgestrel concentrations during use of levonorgestrel rod (LNG ROD) implants. Contraception 1997;55:81-85.

54. Sivin I, Viegas O, Campodonico I, Diaz S, Pavez M, Wan L, Koetsawang S, Kiriwat O, Anant MP, Holma P, el din Abdalla K, Stern J. Clinical performance of a new two-rod levonorgestrel contraceptive implant: a three-year randomized study with Norplant implants as controls. Contraception 1997;55:73-80.

55. Speroff L, Darney P. A clinical guide for contraception. Baltimore MD: Williams & Wilkins, 1992.

56. Technical Guidance/Competence Working Group and the World Health Organization/Family Planning and Population Unit. Family planning methods: New guidance. Population Reports, Series J, No. 44. Baltimore, Johns Hopkins School of Public Health, Population Information Program, October 1996.

57. Trussell J, Leveque JA, Koenig JD, London R, Borden S, Henneberry J, LaGuardia KD, Steward F, Wilson G, Wysocki S, Strauss M. The economic value of contraception: a comparison of 15 methods. Am J Public Health 1995;85:494-503.

58. Vessey MP, Lawless M, Yeates D, McPherson K. Progestin-only oral contraception: findings in a large prospective study with special reference to effectiveness. Br J Fam Plann 1985;10:117-121.

59. World Health Organization. Improving access to quality care in family planning: medical eligibility criteria for contraceptive use. World Health Organization, 1996.

60. World Health Organization. Injectable contraceptives: their role in family planning, monograph. Geneva, 1990.

61. World Health Organization Collaborative Study of Neoplasia and Steroid Contraceptives. Breast cancer and depo-medroxyprogesterone acetate: a multinational study. Lancet 1991;338(8771):833-838.

62. World Health Organization Collaborative Study of Neoplasia and Steroid Contraceptives. Depo-medroxyprogesterone acetate (DMPA) and risk of invasive squamous cell cervical cancer. Contraception 1992;45(4):299-312.

63. Wyeth Laboratories. Norplant system prescribing information. Philadelphia PA: Wyeth Laboratories, December 10, 1990.

Intrauterine Devices (IUDs)

Gary K. Stewart, MD, MPH

- The intrauterine device (IUD) requires only a single decision to use. It is easily inserted and removed.
- The Cu T 380A (Paragard) has a probability of pregnancy of only 2.6% over 10 years of use.
- Among women screened to assure they are appropriate users, the IUD is extremely safe.
- Patients at risk of acquiring a sexually transmitted infection (STI) should use another contraceptive method because having an STI while using an IUD increases their risk of developing a serious pelvic infection.
- The IUD is the most cost-effective contraceptive method when used for at least 2 years.

Worldwide in 1995, an estimated 106 million women used an intrauterine device (IUD), about 12% of married women of reproductive age.[40] In the United States, according to the 1995 National Survey of Family Growth, fewer than 1% of women at risk of pregnancy use the IUD.[1] In the 1970s, IUDs had been used by as many as 10% of U.S. women using contraception; however, problems led to a negative perception of IUDs among women and providers and to the eventual removal of some devices from the market.[8,16] A major task is to provide correct information to consumers and professionals and thus increase the availability and use of this excellent method. Most IUD users in the United States are over the age of 35, and nearly 90% are in their 30s and 40s.[29]

M ECHANISM OF ACTION

Current evidence does not support the common belief that the IUD is an abortifacient.[35,40] The IUD appears to work primarily by preventing sperm from fertilizing ova. The copper IUD (Cu T 380A) causes an increase in uterine and tubal fluids containing copper ions, enzymes, prostaglandins, and white blood cells (macrophages) that alters tubal and uterine transport and affects the sperm and ovum so fertilization does not occur. In two studies, researchers recovered ova from 14 women using four types of copper IUDs and from a control group of 20 women not using any contraception.[3,30] All women had intercourse close to the time of ovulation. Clear signs of fertilization were apparent in half of the ova recovered from the controls but none of the ova recovered from IUD users. In addition, several studies of IUD users showed a marked *decrease* in the risk of ectopic pregnancies, which implied that IUDs inhibit fertilization. Other enzymatic and biochemical processes, as well as local effects on the endometrium, have been identified; however, their contribution to the IUD function are unclear.[39]

Progestin IUDs (the Levonorgestrel 20 IUD and the Progestasert) have a primarily hormonal method of action: the cervical mucous is thickened, ovulatory patterns disrupted, endometrial lining altered, and uterine and tubal motility impaired. The Levonorgestrel IUD (LNg 20) and the Progestasert IUD probably interfere with fertilization, although more data are needed to confirm this.

IUD OPTIONS

Only two IUDs are available in the United States as this edition goes to press; the LNg 20 may be approved for use before the year 2000 (Figure 21-1).

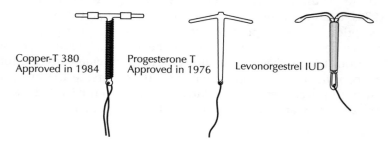

Copper-T 380
Approved in 1984

Progesterone T
Approved in 1976

Levonorgestrel IUD

Figure 21-1 Two currently used IUDs and the Levonorgestrel-IUD, which is not used in the U.S. but is anticipated to be approved by the Food and Drug Administration.

Cu T 380A (Paragard by the Ortho Pharmaceutical Corporation). Approved for at least 10 years of use, the Cu T 380A is made of polyethylene; added barium sulfate creates x-ray visibility. Fine copper wire (314 square millimeters [mm²]) is wound around the vertical stem of the T. Each of the two horizontal arms has a sleeve of copper measuring 33 mm². The bottom of the T has a knotted loop of polyethylene string (clear or white). Of women in North America using an IUD, more than 90% use the Cu T 380A.[40] Throughout the world, more than 25 million Cu T 380A IUDs have been distributed in 70 countries.[25]

Progesterone T (Progestasert System by the Alza Corporation). Approved for 1 year of contraceptive protection, the progesterone T releases 65 micrograms (mcg) of progesterone a day. The T consists of ethylene vinyl acetate copolymer. The vertical stem contains progesterone (38 milligrams) and barium sulphate (for visibility on x-rays) in a silicone oil base. The IUD is 36 mm long, 32 mm wide, and when placed in the inserter barrel, has a diameter of 8 mm. The blue-black double strings attach at a hole in the base of the T.

LNg 20-IUD (developed by Leiras). This IUD has been approved in a number of European and Asian-Pacific countries. The LNg 20 releases levonorgestrel directly into the uterus at a constant rate of 20 mcg per day for as long as 5 years. This dose minimizes the systemic hormonal effects. The LNg 20 is based on a NOVA T model polyethylene frame, with a cylinder of a polydimethylsiloxane-levonorgestrel mixture molded around its vertical arm. The cylinder is coated with a membrane that regulates the release of the hormone. The LNg 20 is visible on X-ray.

EFFECTIVENESS

The IUD's effectiveness is influenced both by its characteristics (size, shape, and presence of copper or progesterone) and the user's characteristics (age and parity). The risk of pregnancy tends to be lower under the following conditions:

- The IUD is medicated with copper, silver, progesterone, or another progestin.
- The IUD has a large surface area (especially important for non-medicated IUDs).
- The IUD is inserted all the way to the top of the fundus of the uterus (particularly important for non-medicated IUDs).
- The IUD was inserted easily.
- The user detects partial and complete expulsions quickly.

- The user has adequate access to medical services should complications appear.
- The clinician is experienced in IUD insertion.

Among women who use the IUD *perfectly* (checking strings regularly to detect expulsion), the probability of pregnancy during the first year of use is 0.6% for the Cu T 380A, 1.5% for the Progestasert, and 0.1% for the LNg 20. Among *typical* users, the corresponding probabilities of pregnancy are 0.8% for the Cu T 380A, 2.0% for the Progestasert, and 0.1% for the LNg 20 (Table 21-1). (See Chapter 31 on Contraceptive Efficacy.) Over the long run, the LNg 20 is the single most effective method of reversible contraceptive available in the world today, followed closely by the Cu T 380A. Over 7 years of wear, the cumulative probability of pregnancy is only 1.1% (the same as for Norplant after 5 years of use); for the Cu T 380A, it is 1.7%.[33]

COST

The Cu T 380A is the most cost-effective reversible contraceptive on the market today, provided that it is used for at least 2 years.[41] The initial costs for the device and its insertion are high; however, the ongoing costs

Table 21-1 First-year probability of pregnancy* for women using IUDs, pills, Depo-Provera, Norplant, and sterilization

Method	% of Women Experiencing Unintended Pregnancy in First Year of Use		% of Women Continuing Use at One Year
	Typical Use	Perfect Use	
Pill	5		71
Progestin Only		0.5	
Combined		0.1	
IUD			
Progesterone T	2.0	1.5	81
Copper T 380A	0.8	0.6	78
LNg 20	0.1	0.1	81
Depo-Provera	0.3	0.3	70
Norplant and Norplant 2	0.05	0.05	88
Female Sterilization	0.5	0.5	100

*See Table 9-2 for first-year probability of pregnancy of all methods.

are minimal. Although IUDs are cheap to manufacture, they are expensive because there are few competitive products, inserters require special training, and medical and legal fees affect the cost. The total cost of an IUD insertion in a public family planning clinic is between $150 to $200. In the private sector, costs are higher. (See Chapter 9 on Essentials of Contraception, Table 9-8).

A DVANTAGES AND INDICATIONS

With only a single decision, a woman who chooses the IUD has a contraceptive method that is highly effective, safe, long-acting, and reversible with a high degree of user satisfaction. Ideal candidates include women who are in a mutually faithful relationship; want a reversible, long-acting method; have had one (or more) children; and have received education and counseling necessary for informed consent, as discussed in Chapter 10. The IUD confers several advantages:

- Women who cannot use hormonal methods can use the copper IUD.
- The IUD does not interfere with lactation.
- The progestin or progesterone-releasing IUDs decrease menstrual blood loss and the incidence and intensity of dysmenorrhea.
- The LNg 20 appears to reduce a woman's risk of developing pelvic inflammatory disease (PID).[38]
- The LNg 20 is an effective treatment of menorrhagia.[4]
- IUDs can prevent and treat Asherman's syndrome (adherence of the two walls of the uterus by synechiae) that occurs after some uterine surgery.
- After the first year, the annual cost for using the IUD is less expensive per year.
- The IUD is easier than other contraceptive methods for patients to use.
- The IUD causes no systemic side-effects (except in patients with copper allergies or Wilson's disease).

D ISADVANTAGES AND CAUTIONS

Certain complications make screening critical for identifying women at risk for IUD-associated complications. Although IUD labeling states that nulliparous women should not receive an IUD, it can be an option as long as the risks are *carefully discussed* and alternative methods reviewed.

Table 21-2 PID risk after IUD insertion

Time After Insertion	PID Rate/1,000 Women-Years	Relative Risk
≤ 20 Days	9.66	6.36
≥ 20 Days	1.38	1.00

Source: Farley et al., (1992).

Pelvic inflammatory disease (PID). The risk of developing PID associated with IUD use is attributable to (1) insertion of the IUD and (2) subsequent exposure to sexually transmitted infection (STI). The greatest risk of PID occurs during the first few weeks following insertion,[14,22] possibly because of microbiological contamination of the endometrial cavity at the time of insertion[26] (Table 21-2). Strict asepsis at insertion and leaving the IUD in place for its lifespan can reduce the chance of developing PID. The LNg 20 provides a protective effect against PID as compared with a copper-releasing IUD.[38] Women who have more than one sexual partner or whose partner has other sexual partners are at high risk for acquiring an STI and are more likely to develop PID if they use an IUD instead of other barrier or hormonal methods of birth control.[22] Although the mechanism of infection due to STI exposure in IUD users is unclear, it has been hypothesized that nonbacterial inflammation of the fallopian tubes is more common in IUD users than nonusers. This inflammation may reduce resistance to disease-causing organisms.

Expulsions. Between 2% to 10% of IUD users spontaneously expel their IUD within the first year. An IUD expulsion can occur without the woman detecting it. Nulliparity, abnormal amount of menstrual flow, and severe dysmenorrhea are risk factors for Cu T 380A expulsion.[50] A woman who has expelled one IUD has a 30% chance of subsequent expulsions.[6]

Pregnancy complications. If a woman becomes pregnant with an IUD in place, remove the device immediately. If she wishes to continue the pregnancy or is undecided, and the IUD strings are visible, remove the IUD as soon as possible. If the woman desires an abortion, refer her immediately. The IUD should be removed during the abortion procedure. (See the section on Managing Problems and Follow-Up.) Although few data exist on current IUDs, data based on older IUD models suggest about 50% of intrauterine pregnancies occurring with the IUD in situ end in spontaneous abortion.[23,42,46] When the IUD is removed early in pregnancy, the rate of spontaneous abortion will be about 25%.[23] Severe PID resulting in death is more likely to occur if the IUD is left in place.[7]

About 5% of women pregnant with an IUD in place will have an ectopic pregnancy.[42] Progestasert System users have a rate of ectopic pregnancy six-fold to ten-fold higher than do copper IUD users.[2]

CAUTIONS

The eligibility guidelines drafted by the World Health Organization (WHO) increase access and reduce barriers to the use of the IUD.[47] These general recommendations encourage consideration of another contraceptive method in certain patient groups, careful patient assessment, and informed medical consent (Table 21-3).

Table 21-3 Precautions to use of copper-bearing intrauterine devices

Refrain from providing an IUD for women with the following diagnoses (World Health Organization [WHO] category #4):

Precautions	Rationale/Discussion
Active, recent (within past 3 months), or recurrent pelvic infection (acute or sub-acute): • Postpartum endometritis • Infection following an abortion • Active sexually transmitted infection (STI), including purulent cervicitis	IUD insertion will increase the risk of upper genital tract infection and infertility. The IUD is unique among all models of contraceptives in its failure to prevent upper genital tract infection.
Known or suspected pregnancy	IUD insertion can lead to a spontaneous abortion with the possibility of septic abortion.
Severely distorted uterine cavity caused by anatomical abnormalities of the uterus including: • Leiomyomata • Endometrial polyps • Cervical stenosis • Bicornuate uterus • Small uterus	Severe distortions of the uterine cavity could cause difficulties in insertion and increase the chance of expulsion.

Exercise caution if an IUD is used or considered in the following situations and carefully monitor for adverse effects (WHO category #3):

Risk factors for pelvic inflammatory disease (PID): • Purulent cervicitis, until treated • Any history of gonorrhea or chlamydia (especially recent infections)	During IUD insertion, bacteria from a preexisting STI can be introduced into the sterile uterine cavity, leading to PID. Most of the PID occurs in the initial 3 weeks following IUD insertion. A vaginal infection must be treated and resolved before an IUD is inserted. The woman and her partner(s) must be treated for STIs, if present, before considering IUD insertion.
Risk factors for an STI, including multiple sexual partners or a partner who has multiple sexual partners	IUDs fail to protect against STIs (in the vagina and cervix) that can ascend and cause an upper genital tract infection.

(continued)

Table 21-3 Precautions to use of copper-bearing intrauterine devices *(cont.)*

Precautions	Rationale/Discussion
Impaired response to infection: • Steroid treatment • Human immunodeficiency (HIV) infection and/or acquired immune deficiency syndrome (AIDS)	Women with impaired immune response may be at greater risk for severe PID.
Risk factors for infection with HIV and AIDS	IUDs cause increased menstrual flow and a sterile inflammatory reaction in the uterus with increased numbers of white blood cells. If the woman is HIV positive, the IUD may increase the risk of HIV transmission to her sexual partner(s). Recommend condoms instead. The decreased immune response may increase the risk of PID.
Undiagnosed, irregular, heavy or abnormal vaginal bleeding; cervical or uterine malignancy (known or suspected), including unresolved Pap smear	Gynecological problems should first be diagnosed before an IUD is inserted. Because IUDs may cause uterine bleeding between periods and may increase menstrual flow, bleeding abnormalities could be attributed to the IUD in error, and the woman's true problem of cervical or uterine malignancy may be missed.
Previous problems with IUD: • Pregnancies • Expulsion • Perforation • Pain • Heavy bleeding	Monitor patient carefully.
Past history of severe vasovagal reactivity or fainting	IUD use can occasionally cause a vasovagal reaction. This is most likely to occur in a nulliparous woman with a small uterus. Use of paracervical anesthesia (10 to 20 cc of 1% lidocaine) may decrease a woman's risk for severe pain or vasovagal reaction.
Difficulty obtaining emergency follow-up care and treatment for PID	PID with an IUD in place can be serious and, if untreated, can lead to hysterectomy or even death. Therefore, it is advisable to have a doctor nearby in case emergency care is needed.

Advantages generally outweigh *theoretical or proven disadvantages, and copper-bearing IUDs generally can be provided without restriction in these conditions (WHO category #2):*

Valvular heart disease such as aortic stenosis *without complications*	Valvular lesions may make women more susceptible to subacute bacterial endocarditis (SBE). Prophylactic antibiotics are recommended at time of IUD insertion. Mitral valve prolapse is generally not considered a reason to avoid IUD use.[13]

(continued)

Table 21-3 Precautions to use of copper-bearing intrauterine devices *(cont.)*

Precautions	Rationale/Discussion
Uterine fibroids, very narrow cervical canal, cervical lacerations, or other anatomical abnormality that does *not* distort the uterus	Severe distortions of the uterine cavity could cause difficulties in insertion and increased chance of expulsion of the IUD.
Heavy or prolonged menstrual bleeding *without clinical signs of anemia*	Increased menstrual blood loss from some IUDs can worsen anemia; however, the use of oral iron or nutritional counseling can reverse the effect.[4]
Woman who has never had a child	Other contraceptives (e.g., oral contraceptives, Depo-Provera, condoms) have a protective effect against PID and are better options for the woman who has never had a child and wants children in the future. Some studies demonstrate a slightly increased risk of infertility in women with a history of IUD use. Return of fertility, however, is excellent for most women following IUD use. Nulliparous women tend not to tolerate an IUD as well as women who have carried a pregnancy to term.[31]

Do not restrict use *of copper-bearing IUD because of these conditions (WHO category #1):*

- Previous pelvic inflammatory disease (PID), has been pregnant since, and is not now at risk of sexually transmitted infection (STI)
- Past ectopic pregnancy
- Irregular menstrual patterns *without* heavy bleeding
- IUD was removed because its period of effectiveness had ended
- IUD was expelled and client wants to try again
- Recent first-trimester abortion or miscarriage and no infection or risk of infection
- Breastfeeding
- Previous cesarean section
- Diabetes
- Current of past cardiovascular diseases or cardiovascular problems caused by diabetes; high blood pressure; stroke; deep or superficial venous thrombosis; pulmonary embolism; valvular heart disease without complications; ischemic heart disease; hyperlipidemia
- Headaches, including severe headaches and migraines
- Current or past breast cancer or benign breast disease
- Current or past liver or gallbladder disease
- Malaria; schistosomiasis; tuberculosis (other than pelvic tuberculosis); viral hepatitis
- Obesity
- Smoking
- Epilepsy
- Cervical intraepithelial neoplasia or cervical ectropion
- Thyroid conditions
- History of preeclampsia
- Benign ovarian tumors including cysts

IUDS in Nulliparous Women

Because of the slight increased risk of PID in IUD users, women who wish to bear children in the future should consider more suitable contraceptive methods. Exercise caution when inserting IUDs in nulliparous women, because they are more likely to experience vasovagal symptoms and postinsertion pain that might require immediate removal of the IUD. Gentleness, careful explanation, a warm and friendly environment, use of a small bivalve speculum, slow movement, and judicious use of paracervical anesthesia may prevent some of these problems.

SPECIAL ISSUES
INFECTION WITH HUMAN IMMUNODEFICIENCY VIRUS

Whether IUDs increase the risk of acquiring an infection with the human immunodeficiency virus (HIV) is unknown. One study showed that among women exposed to HIV, IUD users had a higher risk of infection compared with nonusers and users of other contraceptive methods.[27] The IUD may create an endometrial environment favorable to HIV transmission. The increased bleeding associated with some IUDs may increase the transmission of the virus (for HIV-positive women); however, further study is required. Under current guidelines,[47] copper-bearing IUDs are not recommended for women with acquired immune deficiency syndrome (AIDS) or HIV infection or women at high risk for HIV infection (Table 21-3). Carefully screen women to exclude most women at risk of HIV infection.

MENSTRUAL PROBLEMS

IUDs may be associated with dysmenorrhea or menstrual problems. About 10% to 15% of copper IUD users will have their IUD removed because of abnormal bleeding or spotting. However, the increase in blood loss is usually minor and of little consequence. One of the major indications for use of the LNg 20 is for the treatment of menstrual problems.[24] The use of this device is a more effective, cheaper, and considerably easier treatment than are most surgical methods such as endometrial ablation, surgical dilation and curettage (D&C), or hysterectomy.

PROVIDING THE IUD

A panel of experts at the Centers for Disease Control and Prevention has developed the following guidelines for counseling women about IUDs:[9]

- Foremost, allow the patient to choose her method. She must be an informed user.
- Make all presentations, counseling, and educational materials (handouts, flipcharts, and posters) compatible with the language, culture, and education of the patient.
- Make counseling a routine part of the clinic visit. During the initial visit, a woman needs counseling to help her select a method, then additional counseling after the IUD insertion to learn about IUD use.
- Be aware of the local myths and misconceptions about IUDs. Gaining this awareness may require background research. Address the misconceptions sensitively but directly. (See Myths and Misconceptions about IUDs.)
- Use a standard checklist to remember important information to tell the user.
- Ask the patient to repeat important information.
- Give each IUD user an identification card with the name and picture of the IUD, date of insertion, and date recommended for removal.
- If a patient is not accustomed to following a calendar, inform her about the recommended dates for checkups and IUD removal.
- Let women handle and examine sample IUDs.

The structural difference between one IUD and another is not as great a factor in successful IUD use as is the difference in the skill of the IUD inserter and the quality of counseling, selection, and follow-up.[5,39] However, because the Progestasert System must be replaced annually (thus subjecting the woman to an increased risk of infection), we believe it should be used only in indicated circumstances such as need for short-term contraception, heavy bleeding, dysmenorrhea, or at a patient's request. The Progestasert System may also be used as a starter IUD for women with anemia (to be followed a year later with a copper-bearing IUD).

With appropriate training, a broad range of trained personnel including nurses, nurse-midwives, physician assistants, and paramedical personnel can safely insert the IUD. Practice IUD insertions first on a model, then counsel women and insert an adequate number of IUDs under

Myths and Misconceptions about the IUD

Myth	Fact
IUDs are abortifacients.	This charge is *not true*. Copper IUDs prevent fertilization.
IUDs increase the risk of ectopic pregnancy.	This perception is *not true*. What is true is that IUDs are more efficient at preventing uterine than ectopic pregnancies, so that compared with other methods, a high fraction of the few pregnancies that do occur are ectopic.
IUDs expose the provider to a high degree of litigation.	Although there was a significant negative legal environment for manufacturers of IUDs (and, to a significantly lesser degree, for providers), recent emphasis on full informed consent, proper patient selection, documentation of advice and conversations, and full participation of the patient in the decision-making process, IUD litigation has nearly disappeared. There has only been one case since the Cu T 380A was introduced into the U.S. market in 1988. Litigation is no longer an important issue.
IUDs increase the long-term risk of developing PID.	In properly selected patients, the IUD does not increase PID risk in the long term. The small risk immediately following insertion disappears at about 20 days.

supervision to demonstrate your proficiency. Rather than an absolute number requirement, a level of proficiency in varying insertion situations (different uterine positions) should be the criterion for certification.

INSERTION TIMING

No scientific reason supports the common practice of inserting the IUD only during menstrual bleeding.[44,46,47] The inconvenience and cost to the patient caused by such a policy can impede an otherwise effective IUD program. Allowing insertion during the entire menstrual cycle gives the patient (and provider) options for more flexible appointment times. At midcycle the cervix is just as dilated as during menses and therefore the

Table 21-4 IUD termination rates (per 1,000 insertions) during the first and second post-insertion months, by menstrual cycle day of insertion

	Menstrual Cycle Days of Insertion				
Reason for Termination	**1–5**	**6–10**	**11–17**	**18+**	**All Cycle Days**
Expulsion	50.3	30.5	24.0	22.0	39.6
Pregnancy	3.0	4.1	4.8	6.1	3.7
Pain and Bleeding	20.9	20.6	27.2	36.7	22.7
Miscellaneous Medical	5.9	7.9	4.8	9.8	6.8
Personal	25.6	30.9	17.6	19.6	26.2
Pelvic Infection	3.0	3.1	3.2	1.2	2.9
Total	108.7	97.1	81.6	95.4	101.9

Source: White (1980).

IUD can be inserted easily.[44] Further, infection and expulsion rates may be higher when inserted during menses (Table 21-4).

Insert an IUD at any time during the menstrual cycle under the following conditions:

- She has been using a contraceptive method and is reasonably sure she is not pregnant.
- She has not had intercourse since her last menses.
- She is within 7 days of unprotected intercourse and desires emergency contraception (copper-bearing IUDs only). (See Chapter 12 on Emergency Contraception.)

The postpartum and postabortion periods also offer an excellent opportunity for IUD insertion:

Time period	**Condition**
Immediately following childbirth	Insert within the first 10 minutes of expelling the placenta (see the section on Immediate Postpartum Insertion of IUDs). An IUD inserted 1 or 2 days after childbirth is more likely to be expelled as the uterus contracts.[45]
Immediately after or within 3 weeks after abortion	Insert the IUD in a woman who has had an uncomplicated first-trimester spontaneous or legally induced abortion.
Up to 6 weeks postpartum	Insert if the woman has had no menses but is not breastfeeding.

(continued)

Time period	Condition
6 weeks or more postpartum	Insert if the woman has had no menses, has not had sexual intercourse since delivery of her baby, or has used condoms or vaginal spermicides or another contraceptive method each time she has had intercourse.
Within 6 months postpartum	Insert if the woman is breastfeeding and amenorrheic.

If you suspect the woman is pregnant, perform a pregnancy test or delay IUD insertion until the next menstrual flow, which usually indicates that the woman is not pregnant. *As a rule, trust the history given by a woman in a reproductive health clinic.* This basic principle contributes to thoughtful, dignified, and high-quality family planning services.

INSERTION TECHNIQUE

Prior to insertion, obtain a medical history and inform the patient about all available contraceptive methods. Assess and discuss safety and effectiveness. Explain the IUD insertion procedure to the patient. Answer questions, eliminate myths about the method, and create a comfortable, confident atmosphere for the patient. Consider administering an oral analgesic agent or non-steroidal anti-inflammatory drug (NSAID) at least 30 to 60 minutes before procedure to help reduce the discomfort some women feel.

Always insert an IUD slowly and gently. Insertion methods differ depending on the size and shape of the IUD, inserter barrel, plunger, packaging, and strings. Read and follow the manufacturer's instructions on insertion. Detailed handbooks and videos from manufacturers are available on insertion, withdrawal, and management techniques.[20]

The following instructions for insertion generally apply to all IUDs but refer specifically to the Cu T 380A and Progestasert System IUDs.[2,18] Figure 21-2 describes the equipment required for IUD insertion.

1. Perform a careful bimanual exam to rule out pregnancy and active pelvic infection and to identify the position and mobility of the uterus. The track of IUD perforations is usually at 90 degrees to the axis of the fundus. An unrecognized retroflexed uterus increases the possibility of uterine perforation at the time of the IUD insertion.

2. After you have inserted a warm speculum and viewed the cervix, apply an antiseptic solution, such as 1:2,500 iodine, in a motion of concentric circles beginning at the os and spiraling outward on the

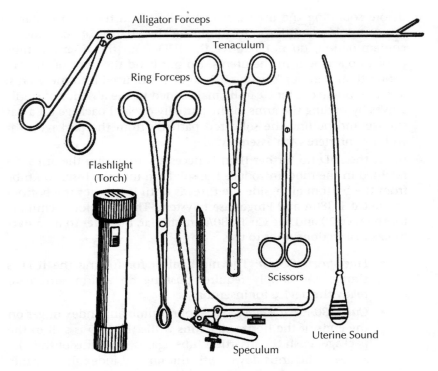

Alligator Forceps

Tenaculum

Ring Forceps

Flashlight
(Torch)

Scissors

Uterine Sound

Speculum

Figure 21-2 Minimal equipment for IUD insertion

cervix. (Some providers recommend also cleansing the internal cervical os.) If the patient is allergic to iodine, use a chlorhexidine (Hibiclens) solution.

3. If it is needed, inject intracervical local anesthesia. Most providers do not use local anesthesia, but the options include the following:

- Inject 1 to 2 cubic centimeters (cc) 1% lidocaine with a 22 to 26 gauge needle.
- Apply topical hurricane gel on cotton swab within cervical os.
- Place a paracervical block (see the section on Paracervical Anesthesia).

4. Grasp the anterior lip of the cervix with a tenaculum about 1.5 to 2.0 centimeters (cm) from the os. Close the single-tooth tenaculum slowly. (A small amount of local anesthesia may help decrease discomfort of tenaculum placement.) Before sounding the uterus, straighten the axis of the uterus by applying traction to the tenaculum.

5. Before sounding the uterus, load the IUD into the inserter barrel under sterile conditions. To minimize the chance of introducing contamination, do not remove the IUD from the insertion tube prior to placement in the uterus. Do not bend the arms of the "T" earlier than 5 minutes before it is to be introduced into the uterus. Strict aseptic technique can be maintained in the absence of sterile gloves by folding the arms in the partially opened package on a flat surface and pulling the solid rod partially from the package so it will not interfere with assembly.

6. Insert the IUD no further than is necessary to ensure the arms are retained in the tube. Introduce the solid rod into the insertion tube from the bottom alongside the threads until it touches the bottom of the Cu T 380A and Progestasert System. The insertion technique for the LNg 20 and the Cu T 380A are similar, but refer to manufacturer's instructions prior to use.

   - *Progestasert System:* The mechanism for folding the IUD is simple and simply requires pushing on a firm surface to ready the device for insertion.
   - *Cu T 380A (ParaGard):* Place your thumb and index finger on the ends of the horizontal arms while the IUD is still in the package. Push the insertion tube against the arms of the "T." Squeeze the arms down with thumb and index finger while using your other hand to maneuver the insertion tube to pick up the arms of the "T."

7. Sound the uterus slowly and gently. Place a cotton swab at the cervix when the sound is all the way in. Hold the sound and the swab together and remove them at the same time. The distance between the tip of the sound and the tip of the swab gives a measure of the depth of the fundus to within 0.25 cm. The Progestasert System has its own measuring device.

8. Adjust the movable flange on the tube so that it indicates the depth to which the IUD should be inserted and the direction in which the arms of the "T" will open. Make certain that the horizontal arms of the "T" and the long axis of the flange lie in the same horizontal plane.

9. Introduce the inserter tube through the cervical canal into the fundus. Apply steady, gentle traction on the tenaculum that is grasping the anterior lip of the cervix. Insert the tube only to the depth indicated by the flange. Do not force the insertion.

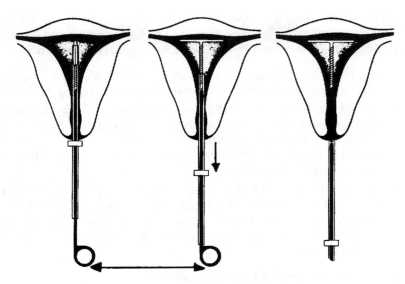

Source: Porter et al. (1983).

Figure 21-3 Withdrawal technique

10. Insert the IUD into the cavity of the uterus by withdrawing the outer barrel over the plunger (Figure 21-3). Insert the IUD slowly and without force. (This is the centerpiece of training, teaching clinicians the respect, feel, and confidence necessary to work with patients.)

11. Release the Cu T 380A or Progestasert System. Withdraw the insertion tube no more than 1/2 inch while holding the solid rod completely still. This releases the arms of the "T."

12. To guarantee the IUD is placed high in the fundus, gently push the inserter tube until you feel resistance.

13. Withdraw the solid rod while holding the insertion tube stationary.

14. Withdraw the insertion tube from the cervix.

15. Clip the strings. Leave a sufficient length of the strings (1 inch, or 2.5 cm) so the woman can easily check for the presence of the IUD. In the patient's record, note the length of the visible strings. *Have the patient feel for the strings of her IUD before she leaves the examining room.*

Prophylactic Antibiotics and IUD Insertion

No consensus exists on whether prophylactic antibiotics at the time of IUD insertion reduces the postinsertion PID syndrome.[21,34,43] If the IUD is inserted correctly under proper infection-control techniques, there is little risk of infection for healthy women. The following are the standard guidelines for the use of prophylactic antibiotics with IUD insertion:

- The patient must have no precautions to IUD insertion, no clinically acute infection, and no contraindications to taking antibiotics.
- The standard regimen is 200 mg of doxycycline orally at the time of insertion (some providers also give 100 mg 12 hours later). Doxycycline is cheap and well-tolerated, but other drugs or combinations of drugs may be more appropriate for the spectrum of coverage you wish to provide.
- Breastfeeding women may take 500 mg of erythromycin orally 1 hour before insertion or at the time of insertion, and then 500 mg orally 6 hours after insertion. (Doxycycline is contraindicated during pregnancy and lactation because of potential effects on the newborn's bone.)

Immediate Postpartum Insertion of IUDs

If labor and delivery were normal, the uterus is firm, and bleeding has subsided, a Cu T 380A may be inserted immediately postpartum. (The authors recommend only the ParaGard for immediate postpartum insertion because it has been shown to be the safest and most effective IUD model in postpartum women.) Post-placental IUD insertion immediately following delivery of the placenta and immediate postpartum insertion (during the first week after delivery) carry no increased risk of infection, perforation, or bleeding.[11,39] To minimize infection, use a sterile long-sleeved glove. Table 21-5 summarizes the major advantages and disadvantages of post-placental and immediate postpartum IUD insertion.

High expulsion rates are a major drawback to immediate postpartum insertion. Rates as low as 9% in a study in China,[49,51] 22% in a Family Health International multicenter trial,[12] and 31%–41% in a WHO multicenter trial[45] have been reported. The expulsion rate for copper-bearing IUDs appears to be lower than the expulsion rate for Lippes Loops.[37] The chance of expulsion can be minimized with post-placental IUD insertion if the individual inserting the IUD is experienced[28] and the following techniques are used:

- Administer an ergot preparation to enhance uterine contractility, but do not administer antibiotics, analgesia, or anesthesia.
- Massage the uterus until bleeding subsides.
- Insert the IUD within 10 minutes of delivery of the placenta.

Table 21-5 Advantages and disadvantages of post-placental/immediate postpartum IUD insertion

Advantages	Disadvantages
• Patient is already at health facility	• Expulsion rates are higher
• Contraindication of pregnancy is not present	• Continuation rates are slightly lower
• Fewer complaints of pain and bleeding	• Higher rates of missing strings
• Risk of perforation is same or lower	• Counseling postpartum is difficult
• Lower cost	• Special instructions are needed about expulsion
• Insertion technique is easier to master	

Sources: O'Hanley et al. (1992); Stewart (1993).

- Grasp the cervix with a pair of ring forceps.
- Grasp the IUD with a second pair of ring forceps. Place the IUD in the uterine cavity.
- Grasp abdomen and uterus with your hand.
- Place the IUD high in the fundus.
- Release the IUD and rotate the ring forceps 45 degrees.
- Move the forceps laterally and remove them.
- Inspect the vagina for strings. Cut the strings if they are visible.

Because of the potential problem of expulsion, fully inform the patient and encourage a post-insertion follow-up. In spite of the slightly higher expulsion rates, cumulative pregnancy rates for immediate postpartum IUD insertion are comparable to or lower than interval IUD insertions, perhaps because of lowered fertility during the postpartum period. With modern copper IUDs, proper insertion techniques, and adequate follow-up, 2.0% to 2.8% of women will become unintentionally pregnant within 24 months after postpartum IUD insertion.[28]

The strings of the Cu T 380A may lie entirely within the uterine cavity after post-placental insertion. If a postpartum woman is examined 1 month after delivery and the strings are not visible, determine the status of the Cu T 380A by sounding the uterine cavity (pregnancy at 4 weeks postpartum is very unlikely). Tease the strings down to the cervical os. Otherwise, leave the strings in the uterine cavity as long as the presence of the IUD was confirmed during sounding. If the strings are too long at the follow-up visit, they may need to be trimmed.

Paracervical Anesthesia or Paracervical Block

To prevent the pain from an IUD insertion or a difficult removal, place a paracervical block using no more than 10 to 20 cc of 1% lidocaine without epinephrine. Paracervical anesthesia is particularly beneficial for a woman who has never been pregnant or who has a history of vasovagal reactions. Ask the patient if she has any known allergies, especially to iodine or any local anesthetic. A suggested procedure for performing a paracervical block follows:

1. Perform a bimanual pelvic examination; insert a speculum into the vagina to obtain good visualization of the cervix.
2. Clean the cervix and paracervical area with antiseptic material.
3. Inject 2 cc of 1% lidocaine at the tenaculum site and then apply the tenaculum to the upper lip of the cervix. Ask the patient to inform you if she experiences nausea, dizziness, ringing of the ears, or tingling of the lips from the procedure. It is not uncommon for these symptoms to occur, and they will pass quickly. (A serious reaction will be extremely unlikely when using less than a total of 20 cc of 1% lidocaine.)
4. Varying sites around the cervix are suitable for injection. One technique is to inject 2 to 5 cc at sites corresponding to 5 o'clock and 7 o'clock on a clock face (a total of 10 cc).
5. Insert the needle just under the mucosa in the connective tissue. This method assures rapid and adequate distribution of the anesthetic because most of the smaller blood vessels and capillaries are in this region. Aspirate lightly with each injection to avoid direct intravenous injection. Anesthesia occurs in 2 to 5 minutes.

IUD REMOVAL

When removing an IUD, always apply gentle, steady traction and remove the IUD slowly. If you cannot remove the IUD with gentle traction, use a tenaculum to steady the cervix and straighten the anteversion or retroversion of the uterus. If this technique does not work, dilate the cervix with dilators. Dilators should always be available in a clinic managing IUD complications. For difficult removals, use a laminaria tent to dilate the cervix. A paracervical block may make the removal easier and less painful. Removing the IUD during menses or at midcycle may be easier than at other times during the cycle.

If you do not see the strings, probe for them in the cervical canal with narrow forceps (or the alligator forceps). When the IUD (with or without its strings) is in the uterus, probe the endometrial cavity with alligator forceps (with which the strings or the IUD itself may be grasped). The alligator forceps are a *must* for proper function of an IUD service. Proficiency in using this instrument for IUD removal when the strings are absent or entirely within the uterine cavity can prevent unnecessary hospitalizations.

MANAGING PROBLEMS AND FOLLOW-UP

Plan for a follow-up visit after the woman's next menses, about 3 to 6 weeks after insertion). Check that the IUD is still in place and that no signs of infection have developed. Further routine visits are not required;[19] however, encourage women to return at any time that they have problems, questions, or concerns. In particular, encourage revisits if they cannot feel the IUD strings or the strings seem to be too long.

Serious complications from IUDs are minimized when they are identified and treated early. Screening for appropriate candidates for IUD use and patient education also help prevent complications. Eight potential complications from IUDs are listed in order of increasing severity:

1. SPOTTING, BLEEDING, HEMORRHAGE, AND ANEMIA

Bleeding problems constitute one of the more common IUD complications. Abnormal bleeding may signal pregnancy, infection, or partial expulsion.

Condition	Action
1. Patient has a hemoglobin (Hgb) less than 11.5 gm at insertion:	• Prescribe FeSO$_4$ (300 mg) daily for 1 to 2 months. • Instruct in proper nutrition, including iron rich foods. • Repeat hemoglobin (Hgb) at 3-month follow-up.

2. Within 3 months of the IUD insertion user complains of excess bleeding:	• Reassure the patient that the bleeding will likely decline in subsequent cycles.
	• Perform Hgb and treat (as in conditions 1, 4, and 7).
	• Prescribe ibuprofen 400 mg t.i.d. for first 3 days of the cycle.
	• Prescribe FeSO$_4$ (as in condition 1).
	• Examine for other pathology or symptoms such as:
	  — Cancer of the cervix and uterus
	  — Cervical and uterine polyps
	  — Leiomyomata
	  — Postcoital bleeding
	  — Chronic cervicitis
	  — Dysfunctional uterine bleeding

3. Excess bleeding is associated with pain:	• Examine the patient to rule out a pelvic infection. • Consider obtaining a sensitive pregnancy test to rule out pregnancy (including ectopic pregnancy).

(continued)

Condition	Action
4. Hgb is less than 9 gm:	• Remove the IUD (if not a progestin-bearing IUD). • Prescribe $FeSO_4$ (300 mg) daily for 2 months. • Repeat Hgb at 1 month. • Provide alternative method of contraception.
5. Bleeding is thought to be associated with endometritis:	• Remove the IUD (pre-load patient with antibiotics). • Culture for gonorrhea and chlamydia. • Treat presumptively with antibiotics. (Doxycycline may not be adequate to cover anaerobes, consider adding ceftriazone 250 mg IM even if no gonorrhea is present, OR add metronidazole 500 mg b.i.d. for 10 days.) • Treat partner presumptively. • Provide alternative method of contraception.
6. Patient desires IUD removal because bleeding is not tolerable:	• Remove the IUD. • Provide alternative method of contraception.
7. Hgb falls >2 gm:	• Remove the IUD. • Treat as in condition 4.
8. Patient is over 40 and having prolonged menses:	• Remove the IUD. • If abnormal bleeding continues, refer the patient for diagnosis and treatment.

2. CRAMPING AND PAIN

Slight pain may be felt at the time of IUD insertion and may be followed by cramping pain over the next 10 to 15 minutes. Cramping and abdominal pain may be signs of pregnancy, infection, or perforation.

Condition	Action
1. Pain during sounding of uterus:	• Sound slowly and gently. • Consider using a smaller sound or smaller cervical dilators. • If the pain is severe, desist and check the alignment of the uterine cavity; if it is okay, use a paracervical block.
2. Cramping or pain immediately after insertion, for a day or so thereafter or with each menses:	
a. If severe:	• Rule out an IUD perforation. • Check the blood pressure and pulse.
b. If mild:	• Consider removing the IUD. • Prescribe mild analgesia such as acetaminophen 1 gm every 4 hours as needed or ibuprofen 400 mg p.o. every 4 hours as needed. (If necessary, use acetaminophen with codeine.)

(continued)

Condition	Action
3. Pain at time of insertion persists and increases, with signs of abdominal tenderness:	
a. If strings are present:	• Presume partial IUD perforation has occurred; remove the IUD and treat as per section 7 on PID.
b. If strings are present and IUD is not:	• Consider the possibility of perforation (see IUD Removal section). • Refer the patient for more specialized care.
4. Partial expulsion of an IUD:	
a. If no infection of cervix or uterus:	• Insert another IUD. • Prescribe 5 to 7 days of doxycycline 100 mg every 12 hours.
b. If infection of cervix or uterus or question of infection:	• Remove the IUD. • Provide alternative contraception. • Treat with antibiotic (as above) and insert another IUD after 3 cycles.
5. Pelvic inflammatory disease:	• Remove the IUD (ideally, pre-load patient with antibiotics). • Treat as per section 7 on PID.
6. Severe postinsertion pain, reaction, syncope or seizure:	• Give spirits of ammonia per nasal inhalation.
a. If question of improper placement:	• Remove the IUD, reevaluate the uterus, resound, and reinsert another IUD.
b. If IUD felt to be properly positioned and pulse less than 60 beats/minute:	• Consider giving atropine (0.4 to 0.6 mg intramuscularly [IM] or intravenously [IV]). • Consider placing a paracervical block. • Prescribe pain medication (e.g., acetaminophen or ibuprofen). • Remove the IUD if necessary.
7. Spontaneous abortion:	• Remove the IUD. • Treat the patient as per section 5 on Pregnancy.
8. Ectopic pregnancy:	• Treat the patient as per section 5 on Pregnancy.

3. EXPULSION OF THE IUD (PARTIAL OR COMPLETE)

The symptoms of an IUD expulsion include unusual vaginal discharge, cramping or pain, intermenstrual spotting, postcoital spotting, dyspareunia (for the man or the woman), absence or lengthening of the IUD string, and presence of the hard plastic of the IUD at the cervical os or in the vagina.[17] If the menstrual period is delayed, check for IUD strings. A missed period may be the first indication of a "silent" expulsion.

Condition	Action
1. Partial expulsion:	• Remove the IUD. • Evaluate the patient for pregnancy or infection. — If infection is present, treat as indicated. • If neither pregnancy nor infection is present, reinsert another IUD and give the patient 5 to 7 days of doxycycline 100 mg every 12 hours.
2. Complete expulsion:	• Evaluate the patient for a possible pregnancy. • Insert another IUD per insertion guidelines.

4. OTHER STRING PROBLEMS

Condition	Action
1. Partner is irritated by strings:	
a. Strings have short, sharp points coming from the cervix:	• Counsel the partner at the time of insertion that he may feel strings but they usually won't hurt him. • Cut the strings shorter, carefully record their length, and inform the patient. • Consider removing and replacing the IUD, leaving the strings longer.
b. Strings are long:	• Try cutting the strings shorter. • Consider removing the IUD.
2. Strings are too long:	• Rule out expulsion by exam and by sounding the cervix.
a. IUD seems in place:	• Trim the strings.
b. Any doubt:	• Remove the IUD and replace with a new IUD.
3. Strings are absent (either as determined by patient or examiner):	

a. Menses are missed:	• Rule out pregnancy by both physical exam and pregnancy test.
	  — If both are negative, evaluate as per 3b.
	  — If the patient is pregnant, manage as per next section 5 on Pregnancy.

b. Menses are not missed and no abdominal pain:	— *Either:* Advise use of another method of contraception and wait until next menses to reexamine. — *Or:* Prepare cervix (as per IUD insertion technique) and with alligator forceps gently explore the cervical canal (and if necessary, the uterus).

(continued)

Condition	Action
b. Menses are not missed… (*cont.*)	
I. IUD found:	• If the strings are brought to their appropriate place and the IUD appears to be in place, treat the patient with antibiotics and follow her routinely. • If you have any question of IUD dislodgement or abnormal position, remove the IUD, treat the patient with antibiotics, and reinsert another IUD.
II. IUD not found:	• Refer the patient for more specialized care if necessary. • Obtain an ultrasound (or x-ray).
c. No IUD seen on ultrasound:	• Obtain a pregnancy test. • Insert another IUD as per insertion guidelines.
d. IUD seen on ultrasound:	• Clarify the location of the IUD to determine whether or not it has perforated. — If the IUD is visualized in the uterus, nothing further need be done. • Consider placing another IUD; take another x-ray or ultrasound of pelvis. — If the IUD has perforated, treat the patient accordingly. — If the IUD has not perforated, then the x-ray should show two IUDs in the uterus (usually both will have to be removed and another inserted).

5. PREGNANCY

Determine whether the patient wishes to continue the pregnancy. If the IUD has completely perforated the uterus and is in the abdominal cavity, it may not pose any risk to the pregnancy. Because the degree of perforation is usually not known, treat the condition as though the IUD were in situ and the strings not seen. Approximately one-third or fewer of IUD-related pregnancies are attributable to undetected or partial expulsions. If the patient is pregnant with an IUD in place, inform her of the risk of spontaneous abortion.

Condition	Action
1. Patient is undergoing a spontaneous abortion:	• Empty the uterus. • Remove the IUD. • Prescribe doxycycline or ampicillin for 7 days.
a. Patient has severe pain:	• Prescribe analgesic medication.

(continued)

Condition	Action
1. Spontaneous abortion: … (*cont.*)	
b. Patient is anemic:	• Give the patient FeSO$_4$, as per section 1 on Spotting, Bleeding, and Hemorrhage.
2. Patient requests an abortion:	• Refer the patient for abortion (have IUD removed during the abortion).
3. Patient wishes to continue the pregnancy and the IUD strings are visible:	• Gently pull on the IUD strings and remove the IUD. • Warn the patient that an ectopic pregnancy is a possibility. • Refer the patient for prenatal care.
4. Patient wishes to continue the pregnancy and the IUD strings are not visible:	• Perform an ultrasound to determine if the IUD is in the uterus. • If the IUD is outside the uterus, deal with pregnancy first, then the perforation.
a. Signs of an intrauterine infection exist:	• Evacuate the uterus, and treat the infection with antibiotics. • Evaluate the tissue to rule out an ectopic pregnancy. • Refer the patient for more specialized care if necessary.
b. Signs of infection do not exist:	• Inform the patient to watch for signs of infection (such as pain, discharge, bleeding, fever, myalgia) and ectopic pregnancy; instruct her where to go for those complications. • Refer the patient for prenatal care. • Warn of possible perforation. • Recover the IUD at delivery.

6. Uterine Perforation, Embedding, and Cervical Perforation

The incidence of perforation is approximately 1 in 1,000 insertions. The IUD generally perforates the uterus at one of three sites: (1) uterine fundus, (2) body of the uterus and (3) cervical wall.

Condition	Action
1. IUD plastic device sticks through the cervix:	• Prescribe analgesia. • Perform a paracervical block, if needed, to perform the procedure. • Use alligator forceps to grasp IUD inside the cervix or lower uterine cavity and push the IUD back into uterus and then remove it through the cervical os. • Prescribe pain medication as needed. • Treat the patient with antibiotics. • Provide alternative contraception. • Reinsert the IUD.
2. IUD strings do not allow the IUD to be removed even with significant pressure:	• Try the recommendations in section 4 on other string problems. • Place a paracervical block.
a. IUD found in uterus:	• Use alligator forceps to grasp the IUD in cervix or uterus and remove it. • If the IUD cannot be removed, refer the patient for more specialized care.
b. IUD not found in uterus or cervix (and strings are seen):	• Refer the patient for more specialized care. • Provide alternative methods of contraception. • Prescribe an antibiotic.
3. IUD perforation is identified by x-ray or ultrasound; no strings are visible:	
a. Pain, evidence of bowel obstruction, or pelvic infection:	• Refer the patient for more specialized care (general surgery). • Treat the patient with antibiotics; surgery may be required.
b. No pain or evidence of obstruction, infection, or pregnancy:	• Provide the patient with alternative contraception. • Inform the patient to watch for signs of obstruction or pelvic infection.
c. Patient is pregnant and the IUD is extrauterine:	• Provide information as per condition b and as per section 5 on Pregnancy.

If the IUD has perforated the uterus, it is possible that the IUD strings could still hang outside of the cervix. In this case it would be difficult to detect that a perforation has occurred. This is one circumstance when expert help is truly required.

7. PELVIC INFLAMMATORY DISEASE

PID needs aggressive treatment and follow-up. *If in doubt, take the IUD out.* An IUD should not be reinserted in someone who is at high risk for developing another pelvic infection or who has had PID in the past 3 months. The accurate diagnosis of PID is difficult. The following signs suggest PID:

- Oral temperature of 38° C, or above
- Suprapubic tenderness and guarding
- Tenderness or pain associated with moving the cervix during pelvic exam
- Purulent discharge from the cervix
- Tenderness of the uterus upon palpation
- Adnexal tenderness or palpable mass or masses in the adnexae

Condition	Action
1. Patient is pregnant and has symptoms of PID:	• Confirm the diagnosis. • See section 5 on Pregnancy. • Remove the IUD. • Rule out ectopic pregnancy. • Aggressively treat the infection with parenteral antibiotics, as per PID regimen in Chapter 8 on Reproductive Tract Infections. • If the uterus is infected, terminate the pregnancy.
2. Patient has mild PID (oral temperature ≤38° C; no abdominal guarding; mild suprapubic, uterine, or adnexal tenderness; no adnexal mass:	• Consider removing the IUD. • Provide alternative contraception. • Prescribe treatment for PID (see Chapter 8 on Reproductive Tract Infections). • Reexamine the patient in 1 week. • Inform the patient to seek immediate care if her symptoms worsen.
3. Patient has moderate PID (fever ≤39° C, cervical motion tenderness, increased WBC count, abdominal guarding and no rebound, no adnexal masses, no vomiting):	• Manage the patient as per condition 2. • Treat the PID (see Chapter 8 on Reproductive Tract Infections). • Consider hospitalizing the patient.
4. Patient has severe PID (fever >39° C, abdominal guarding or rebound, pelvic masses or vomiting, or acutely ill appearance):	• Refer the patient for hospital care.

PID is a serious, life-threatening and life-changing problem that needs expert care.

8. Genital Actinomycosis

Several case reports in the past 20 years have described pelvic actinomycosis in patients with IUDs; in some cases, *Actinomyces* infection caused only endometritis, whereas in others, it caused PID and pelvic and abdominal abscesses.[15] The accurate diagnosis of genital actinomycosis is difficult. *Actinomyces* species are normal inhabitants of the human gastrointestinal tract, in both the oropharynx and the bowel. Under ordinary conditions, *Actinomyces* species do not cross mucosal barriers. *Actinomyces* on Papanicolaou (Pap) smears suggest genital actinomycosis in IUD users.

Condition	Action
1. Pap smear showing Actino-mycosis-like organisms:	

a. No symptoms:	• Repeat the Pap smear in 1 year.
	• If *Actinomyces* are present on the repeat Pap smear:
	  a. Remove the IUD, wait one menstrual cycle and re-insert another IUD (give the patient alternative contraception during this interval).
	  b. Treat the patient with the IUD in place: give doxycycline 100 mg b.i.d. for 14 days, then repeat the Pap smear.
	  c. Do nothing but have the patient return if she develops symptoms of PID.

b. Symptoms of PID:	• Remove the IUD after pre-loading the patient with antibiotic. • Treat the PID. • If the infection is severe, hospitalize the patient. • Consider ultrasound to rule out an abscess.

The diagnosis of Actinomyces on a Pap smear needs to be carefully discussed with the cytologist making the diagnosis. Manage the patient (or co-manage) with a provider knowledgeable about this condition.

Instructions For Using IUDs

Some women have a fair amount of pain or nausea immediately after IUD insertion. You may want to come to the clinic with your husband, partner, or friend in case you need someone to assist you home. Prior to arrival at the clinic, you can take an analgesic agent (such as ibuprofen) to help reduce discomfort during the procedure.

1. **Check your strings.** Before you leave the office or clinic, learn how to feel the strings that protrude 1 inch or so into your vagina. If you cannot feel the strings or if you can feel the plastic part, your

IUD may not protect you against pregnancy; use another method until you can return to the clinic to have your IUD checked. You can expel an IUD without knowing it. Check for the strings frequently during the first months you have the device, then after each period and any time you have abnormal cramping while menstruating.

2. **Beware of infection.** If at any time you have fever, pelvic pain or tenderness, severe cramping, or unusual vaginal bleeding, contact your clinician immediately because you may have an infection. Infections from IUDs can be serious and, if untreated, can lead to hysterectomy (removal of the uterus) or even death. When your IUD is inserted, find out where you can go to be treated for an infection. IUDs can occasionally cause internal pelvic infection (in contrast to vaginal infections) that can lead to chronic pain or infertility. Women in mutually monogamous relationships appear to have little increased risk of infection.

3. **Watch for your periods.** If you miss a menstrual period, contact your health care provider immediately. The most commonly reported nuisance side effects of the IUD are increased menstrual flow, menstrual cramping and spotting, and increased mucous discharge. Remember that if you cannot tolerate the IUD, you can always have it removed. Heavier menstrual bleeding may be serious if you are anemic. However, a small increase in the menstrual flow is normal with the IUD, especially during the first two to three periods. If you miss a period, you need to be sure that you are not pregnant. Though rare, pregnancies do occur with the IUD in place.

4. **Do not try to remove the IUD yourself.** Do not let your partner pull on the strings. The clinician will have a better idea of the angle at which the IUD went in. It should come out the same way.

5. **Learn and pay attention to the IUD Warning Signs.**

Early IUD Warning Signs

Caution

P ■ Period late (pregnancy), abnormal spotting or bleeding

A ■ Abdominal pain, pain with intercourse

I ■ Infection exposure (any STD), abnormal discharge

N ■ Not feeling well, fever, chills

S ■ String missing, shorter or longer

---

6. **And remember—if you have questions—ask them.** That is what we are here for.

REFERENCES

1. Abma JC, Chandra A, Mosher WD, Peterson LS, Piccinino LJ. Fertility, family planning, and women's health: new data from the 1995 National Survey of Family Growth. Vit Health Stat 1997;Series 12, Number 19.
2. Alza Corporation. Progestasert intrauterine progesterone contraceptive system. Alza Product Information, 1986.
3. Alvarez R, Brache V, Fernandez E, Guerrero B, Guiloff E, Hess R, Salvatierra AM, Zacharios S. New insights on the mode of action of intrauterine devices in women. Fertil Steril 1988;49:768-773.
4. Andersson K, Rybo G. Levonorgestrel-releasing intrauterine device in the treatment of menorrhagia. Br J Obstet Gynaecol 1990;97:690-694.
5. Arbab AAO, McNamara R, Lauro D, Aziz FA. Expanded services for intrauterine contraception in Sudan. East Afri Med J 1991;68:70-74.
6. Bahamondes L, Diaz J, Marchi NM, Petta CA, de Lourdes MC, Gomez G. Performance of copper intrauterine devices when inserted after an expulsion. Hum Reprod 1995; 10:2917-2918.
7. Bernstine RL. Review and analysis of the scientific and clinical data on the safety, efficacy, adverse reactions, biologic action, utilization, and design of intrauterine devices. Final report. Department of Health, Education, and Welfare/Food and Drug Administration, Technical Resources Development. Seattle WA: Batelle Memorial Institute, 1975.
8. Burnhill M. Intrauterine contraception. In: Corson SL, Derman RJ, Tyrer LB (eds). Fertility control. Boston: Little, Brown & Co., 1986.
9. Centers for Disease Control. IUDs: guidelines for informed decision making and uses. Atlanta GA: Centers for Disease Control, 1987.
10. Chi I-c. What we have learned from recent IUD studies: a researcher's perspective. Contraception 1993;48:81-108.
11. Chi I-c, Farr G. Postpartum IUD contraception—a review of an international experience. Adv Contracep 1989;5:127-146.
12. Cole LD, Edelman DA, Potts DM, Wheeler RG, Laufe LE. Postpartum insertion of modified intrauterine devices. J Repro Med 1984;29:677-682.
13. Dajani AS, Bisno AL, Chung KJ, et al. Prevention of bacterial endocarditis: recommendations by the American Heart Association. JAMA 1990;264: 2919-2922.
14. Farley TM, Rosenberg MS, Rowe PJ, Chen SH, Meirik O. Intrauterine devices and pelvic inflammatory disease: an international perspective. Lancet 1992; 339:785-788.
15. Fiorino A. Intrauterine contraceptive device-associated actinomycotic abscess and Actinomyces detection on cervical smear. Obstet and Gynecol 1996;87:142-149.
16. Forrest JD. Acceptability of IUD's in the United States. Presented at: A new look at IUD's—advancing contraceptive choices, March 27-28, 1992. New York.
17. Gruber A, Rabinerson D, Kaplan B, Pardo J, Neri A. The missing forgotten intrauterine contraceptive device. Contraception 1996;54:117-119.
18. GynoPharma. Prescribing information for the Copper T 380—an intrauterine copper contraceptive. Revised April 1994.

19. Janowitz B, Hubacher D, Petrick T, Dinghe N. Should the recommended number of IUD revisits be reduced? Stud Fam Plann 1994;25:362-367.
20. Johns Hopkins Program for International Education in Gynecology and Obstetrics. JHPIEGO IUD course handbook. November 1992.
21. Ladipo OA, Farr G, Otolorin E, Konje JC, Sturgen K, Cox P, Champion CB. Prevention of IUD-related pelvic infection: the efficacy of prophylactic doxycycline at IUD insertion. Adv Contracept 1991;7:43-54.
22. Lee NC, Rubin GL, Borucki R. The intrauterine device and pelvic inflammatory disease revisited: new results from the Women's Health Study. Obstet Gynecol 1988;72:1-6.
23. Lewit S. Outcome of pregnancy with intrauterine device. Contraception 1970;2:47-57.
24. Luukkainen T, Toivonen J. Levonorgestrel-releasing IUD as a method of contraception with therapeutic properties. Contraception 1995;52:269-276.
25. Mauldin WP, Segal SJ. IUD use throughout the world—past, present and future. In: Bardin CW, Mishell DR Jr. (eds). Proceedings from the Fourth International Conference on IUDs. Butterworth-Heinemann, Boston, 1994.
26. Mishell DR, Bell JH, Good RG, Moyer DL. The intrauterine device: a bacteriologic study of the endometrial cavity. Am J Obstet Gynecol 1966;96:119-126.
27. Musicco M, Nicolosi A, Saracco A, Lazzarin A. IUD use and man to woman sexual transmission of HIV-1. In: Bardin CW, Mishell DR Jr. (eds). Proceedings from the Fourth International Conference on IUDs. Butterworth-Heinemann, Boston, 1994.
28. O'Hanley K, Huber DH. Postpartum IUDs: keys for success. Contraception 1992;45:351-361.
29. Ortho Pharmaceutical Corporation. 1991 Ortho Annual Birth Control Survey. Raritan NJ.
30. Ortiz ME and Croxatto HB. The mode of action of IUDs. Contraception 1987;36:37-53.
31. Peterson KR, Brooks L, Jacobsen B, Skonsky SO. Intrauterine devices in nulliparous women. Adv Contraception 1991;7:333-338.
32. Porter CW, Waife RS, Holtrop HR. The health provider's guide to contraception. The international edition. Watertown MA: The Pathfinder Fund, 1983.
33. Rowe PJ. Research on intrauterine devices. Annual technical report 1991. Geneva, Switzerland: Special Programme of Research, Development and Research Training in Human Reproduction, World Health Organization, 1992:127-137.
34. Sinei SKA, Schulz KF, Lamptey PR, Grimes DA, Mati JKG, Rosenthal SM, Rosenberg MJ, Riara G, Njage PN, Bhullar VB, Ogembo HV. Preventing IUD-related pelvic infection: the efficacy of prophylactic doxycycline at insertion. Br J Obstet Gynaecol 1990;97:412-419.
35. Sivin I, Stern J, Coutinho E, Mattos CER, Diaz SEMS, Pavez M, Alvarez F, Brache V, Thevenin F, Diaz J, Foundes A, Diaz MM, McCarthy T, Mishell DR, Shoupe D. Proloned intrauterine contraception: a seven-year randomized study of the levonorgestrel 20 mcg/day (Lng 20) and the Copper T 380A IUS. Contraception 1991;44:473-480.
36. Stewart GK. Personal communication during Philippine Contraception Workshop, 1993.

37. Thiery M. Timing of IUD insertion. In: Zatuchni GI, Goldsmith A, Sciarra JJ, Osborn CK (eds). Intrauterine contraception: advances and future prospects. Philadelphia PA: Harper and Row, 1985; 365-374.

38. Toivonen J, Luukkainen T, Allonen H. Protective effect of intrauterine release of levonorgestrel on pelvic infections: three years' comparative experience of levonorgestrel and copper-releasing intrauterine devices. Obstet Gynecol 1991;77:261-264.

39. Treiman K, Liskin L. IUDs—a new look. Popul Rep 1988;Series B(5).

40. Treiman K, Liskin L, Kols A, Rinehart W. IUDs—an update. Popul Rep 1995;Series B(6).

41. Trussell J, Leveque JA, Koenig JD, London R, Borden S, Henneberry J, LaGuardia KD, Stewart F, Wilson TG, Wysocki S, Strauss M. The economic value of contraception: a comparison of 15 methods. Am J Public Health 1995; 85:494-503.

42. Vessey MP, Johnson B, Doll R, Peto R. Outcome of pregnancy in women using an intrauterine device. Lancet 1974;1:495-498.

43. Walsh TL, Bernstein GS, Grimes DA, et al. Effect of prophylactic antibiotics on morbidity associated with IUD insertion: results of a pilot randomized controlled trial. Contraception 1994;50:319-327.

44. White MK, Ory HW, Rooks JB, Rochat RW. Intrauterine device termination rates and the menstrual cycle day of insertion. Obstet Gynecol 1980;55: 220-224.

45. World Health Organization. Special programs on research, development and research training in human reproduction. Task force on intrauterine devices for fertility regulation. Comparative multicenter trial of three IUDs inserted immediately following delivery of the placenta. Contraception 1980;22:9-18.

46. World Health Organization. Mechanism of action, safety and efficacy of intrauterine devices. Technical Report Series 753. Geneva: WHO, 1987.

47. World Health Organization. Improving access to quality care in family planning: medical eligibility criteria for initiating and continuing use of contraceptive methods. Geneva: WHO, 1996.

48. Xiong X, Buekens P, Wollast E. IUD use and the risk of ectopic pregnancy: a meta- analysis of case-control studies. Contraception 1995;52:23-34.

49. Xu J-X, Rivera R, Dunson TR, Zhuang L-Q, Yang X-L, Ma G-T. Chi I-c. A comparative study of two techniques used in immediate postplacental insertion (IPPI) of the copper T-380A IUD in Shanghai, People's Republic of China. Contraception 1996;54:33-38.

50. Zhang J, Chi I-c, Feldblum PJ, Farr MG. Risk factors for copper T IUD expulsion: an epidemiologic analysis. Contraception 1992;46:427-433.

51. Zhou SW, Chi I-c. Immediate postpartum IUD insertions in a Chinese hospital—a two year follow-up. Inter J Gynaecol Obstet 1991;35:157-164.

Female and Male Sterilization

Gary K. Stewart, MD, MPH
Charles S. Carignan, MD

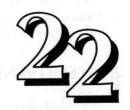

- A single decision and one simple surgical procedure provide permanent contraception.
- Sterilization is one of the safest, most effective, and most cost-effective contraceptive methods.
- Reversal of the sterilization procedure is expensive, not readily available, requires major surgery, and results are not guaranteed.
- Contraceptive sterilization (female sterilization and vasectomy) has become one of the most widely used methods of family planning in the world in both developed and developing countries.

Healthy women are fertile until about age 50 to 51; healthy men are fertile essentially throughout life. Because most couples have all the children they want well before the end of their reproductive lifespan, they will need effective contraception protection against unwanted pregnancies for many years.

Ideally, a couple should consider both vasectomy and female sterilization as options. They are comparable in effectiveness, and both are intended to be permanent. If both were equally acceptable, vasectomy would be recommended because it is simpler, safer, less expensive, and probably more effective than female sterilization. The acceptability of vasectomy depends on the effort of providers to make available high quality vasectomy services.

Better patient selection, improved anesthetic methods and patient monitoring, increased use of local anesthesia with light sedation, improved surgical techniques, better asepsis, and better trained personnel have contributed to the improved safety of sterilization over the past 20 years. Since 1970, more than 1 million sterilizations have been performed annually in the United States. Nearly 15 million women rely on sterilization as their contraceptive method: 10.7 million rely on female sterilization, and 4.2 million on vasectomy.[1]

M ECHANISM OF ACTION

Sterilization for women involves mechanically blocking the fallopian tubes to prevent the sperm and egg from uniting.

Vasectomy is the male sterilization operation that blocks the vasa deferentia to prevent the passage of sperm into the ejaculated seminal fluid.

E FFECTIVENESS

FEMALE STERILIZATION

The risk of pregnancy following sterilization is lower than the risks associated with use of most temporary contraceptive methods during the first year. It is similar to the risks associated with some of the long-term methods such as the Levonorgestrel 20 intrauterine system and Copper T 380A intrauterine device (IUD), Depo-Provera, and Norplant. The Collaborative Review of Sterilization (CREST) study points to a first-year probability of pregnancy of 5.5 for every 1,000 procedures (Table 22-1) and a 10-year

Table 22-1 First-year probability of pregnancy* for sterilization, condoms, pills, IUD, and Norplant

Method	% of Women Experiencing an Unintended Pregnancy Within the First Year of Use		% of Women Continuing Use at One Year
	Typical Use	Perfect Use	
Condom			
Male	14	3	61
Female (Reality)	21	5	56
Pill	5		72
Progestin Only		0.5	
Combined		0.1	
IUD			
Progesterone T	2.0	1.5	81
Copper T 380A	0.8	0.6	78
LNg 20	0.1	0.1	81
Norplant and Norplant 2	0.05	0.05	88
Female Sterilization	0.5	0.5	100
Male Sterilization	0.15	0.10	100

*See Table 9-2 for first-year probability of pregnancy for all methods.

cumulative probability of 18.5 pregnancies for every 1,000 procedures.[72] Luteal phase pregnancies were not reported as failures in the CREST studies. According to the CREST report, sterilization failure is more likely if the woman is relatively young when the procedure is performed, because young women are more fertile than older women. Although the bipolar method was associated with a high probability of pregnancy, the CREST study was initiated early in the use of the device and many technical issues had yet to be learned. There are many different reasons for failure, some of which can be prevented:[92]

- **Pregnancy at time of sterilization.** Perform female sterilization in the follicular phase of the menstrual cycle to prevent luteal phase pregnancies, assure that the patient uses effective contraception until after the sterilizing procedure, take a careful sexual history (use postcoital contraception when indicated), and use the dilation and curettage (D&C) procedure as indicated.
- **Occlusion method.** Fistula formation is associated with electrocautery and spontaneous reanastomosis with suture methods. Clips are not as occlusive as other methods.
- **Surgical error.** Error accounts for 30% to 50% of failures.[61] Training of surgeons, good care of instruments, and accurate identification of tubes and proper placement of devices are key to limiting this problem.
- **Equipment or device failure.** Laparoscopic procedures and electrical and clip methods can fail.

Because surgical skill can seldom be separated from the inherent effectiveness of the occlusion technique, current evidence makes it difficult to conclude one technique is superior to others. For surgeons well-trained in the techniques they perform, it is unlikely important differences in efficacy will occur among the recommended occlusion techniques described in this chapter. However, the literature does suggest guidance about which techniques will be more effective depending on pregnancy status and surgical approach. (See the section on Occlusion Techniques.)

VASECTOMY

Vasectomy is a very effective contraceptive method. Unfortunately, few studies of vasectomy clearly address the issue of pregnancy. Many studies report "failures," but these are failures to eliminate sperm from the ejaculate rather than to prevent pregnancies. The reported pregnancies may not always be attributable to the men who underwent the vasectomy. True failure of the technique can result from spontaneous recanalization of the vas, division or occlusion of the wrong structure during surgery, and (rarely) a congenital duplication of the vas that went unnoticed during the procedure. It is clear, nevertheless, that pregnancy can occur long after the vasectomy procedure.

We estimate vasectomy has a probability of pregnancy of about 0.1% in the first year. Studies that do report pregnancies are summarized in Chapter 31 on Contraceptive Efficacy, Table 31-16. These studies do not include pregnancies resulting from unprotected intercourse before the reproductive tract has been cleared of sperm. However, they probably are not representative of vasectomies actually performed in the United States, because clinicians are reluctant to publish studies calling attention to their failures. (See Chapter 9 on Essentials of Contraception.)

COST

The cost of sterilization procedures varies greatly. Nevertheless, in a recent study, vasectomy was found to be the most cost-effective contraceptive method among the 15 methods available in the United States.[98] Female sterilization ranked in the top one-third of the most cost-effective methods at 5 years of use. Unequivocally, however, female sterilization is much more expensive than male sterilization. Table 22-2 presents figures on the cost of sterilization in 1993 dollars.

Table 22-2 Cost of sterilization

	Female	Male
	Interval Laparoscopy or Minilaparotomy	Vasectomy
Public Sector*	± $1,200	$250–$400
Private Sector**	± $2,500	$500–$1,000

*Planned Parenthood of Sacramento Valley, CA, 1993.
**Compilation of Sacramento County Physician and Surgery Center fees, 1993.

ADVANTAGES AND INDICATIONS
FEMALE STERILIZATION

Sterilization for women is a safe operative procedure. Reported fatality rates for the U.S. are between 1 to 2 per 100,000.[28] By contrast, the maternal mortality rate is 7.9 deaths per 100,000 live births.[99] The risk of death from hysterectomy for benign disease is estimated to be 5/100,000 to 25/100,000 in women aged 35 to 44.[108] Laparoscopy is associated with a lower mortality than is minilaparotomy, although this difference may be related to biases of patient selection.[62]

Sterilization can be performed without increasing the health risks during the immediate postpartum or postabortion periods. When immediate postpartum sterilization is performed by trained personnel using local anesthesia, a small incision, and refined surgical technique, the normal postpartum stay is often 24 hours or less. Both laparoscopy and suprapubic minilaparotomy at 4 weeks or more after delivery can be performed on an outpatient basis using local anesthesia. (See Table 22-3 for a comparison of methods.)

Female sterilization is ideal for those persons who are certain they wish no further children and need a reliable contraceptive method. Other advantages include the following:

- Permanence
- High effectiveness
- Cost effectiveness
- Nothing to buy or remember
- Lack of significant long-term side effects
- No need for partner compliance
- No need to interrupt lovemaking
- Privacy of choice

VASECTOMY

Vasectomy continues to be simpler, safer, less expensive, and more effective than female sterilization. When both female and male sterilization are acceptable, vasectomy would be the preferred surgical contraceptive method. The main advantages of vasectomy are as follows:

- Permanence
- High effectiveness
- Cost effectiveness (most cost effective of all contraceptive methods)
- Removal of contraceptive burden from the woman
- Lack of significant long-term side effect
- High acceptability
- No need to interrupt lovemaking
- Safety
- Quick recovery

Table 22-3 Various occlusion methods and techniques (advantages and disadvantages)

Occlusion Method	Recommended Occlusion Techniques	Advantages	Disadvantages
Interval Female Sterilization			
Suprapubic Minilaparotomy	1. Pomeroy and Pritchard (Parkland) techniques 2. Silastic bands or Falope-rings 3. Hulka or Filshie clips	1. Local or general anesthesia 2. Incision site usually not visible (below pubic hairline)	1. Difficult technique if the woman is obese, the uterus immobile or the tubes have adhesions from infection or previous surgery 2. Recovery can be more painful than laparoscopy
Laparoscopy	1. Silastic bands or Falope-rings 2. Unipolar electrocoagulation 3. Bipolar coagulation 4. Hulka or Filshie clips	1. Small incision with either single- or double-puncture technique 2. Less pain than from mini-laparotomy 3. Low rate of complication 4. Short recovery time 5. Local or general anesthesia	1. Need for specialist with expensive and intense training 2. Other staff must be trained to technically adjust or use equipment 3. Necessary equipment is often difficult to obtain 4. Need a fully equipped operating and recovery room
Vaginal Approach (rarely used in 1997)	1. Pomeroy or Fimbriectomy technique	1. Direct visualization of the pelvic organs 2. Less pain after procedure	1. In several countries, this approach found to be less safe and less effective 2. Infection is more common 3. Technique is difficult to learn and perform

(continued)

Table 22-3 Various occlusion methods and techniques (advantages and disadvantages) *(cont.)*

Occlusion Method	Recommended Occlusion Techniques	Advantages	Disadvantages
Transcervical Approach (research method in 1997)	None are proven safe or effective. Method is under investigation: 1. Chemicals such as quinacrine or phenol 2. Devices such as S top	1. Nonsurgical approach 2. No scars 3. Able to be performed by lower-level staff	1. Still experimental techniques 2. Efficacy and safety rates unknown 3. Many questions yet to be answered
Postpartum Female Sterilization			
Subumbilical Minilaparotomy	1. Pomeroy technique 2. Pritchard (Parkland) technique	1. Convenience 2. Lower costs 3. Ease of surgery 4. Longer hospital stay (beyond that for a normal delivery) is not required	1. Use of occlusion rings or clips not indicated and more likely to fail if used 2. Electrocoagulation not indicated (Chi et al. 1995) 3. Counseling must be prior to labor to reduce risk of regret
Cesarean Section	1. Pomeroy technique 2. Pritchard technique 3. Irving technique	1. Convenience 2. Lower costs 3. Anatomy fully visible	1. Cesareans should not be performed solely to occlude the tubes 2. Counseling must be prior to labor to reduce risk of regret
Postabortion Sterilization	1. Pomeroy or Pritchard procedures with minilaparotomy 2. Silastic rings or spring clips	1. Convenience 2. Client motivation	1. Need for careful counseling (patients have a higher risk of regret following post-abortion sterilization) 2. May increase the amount of blood loss with abortion procedure

DISADVANTAGES AND CAUTIONS

FEMALE STERILIZATION

Female sterilization is not recommended for anyone who is not sure of her desire regarding future fertility. Other disadvantages include the following:

- Permanence
- Regret for decision high among some groups
- Reversibility difficult and expensive
- Technical difficulty of the procedure
- Need for surgeon, operating room (aseptic conditions), trained assistants, medications, surgical equipment
- Expense at the time of the procedure
- Probability of ectopic pregnancy if method fails
- Lack of protection against sexually transmitted infections (STIs), including infection with the human immunodeficiency virus (HIV)

VASECTOMY

Vasectomy is not effective until all sperm in the reproductive tract are ejaculated. Complications such as bleeding or infection, although infrequent, do occur. As a contraceptive method, vasectomy provides only indirect protection from pregnancy for women. The major disadvantages of vasectomy are as follows:

- Protection for the male (it is the female who is at risk for pregnancy)
- Surgical procedure, requiring surgical training, aseptic conditions, medications, and technical assistance
- Expense in the short term
- Potentially serious long-term effects, although unproven
- Permanence (although reversal is possible, it is expensive, requires a highly technical and major surgery, and its results cannot be guaranteed)
- Regret for decision high among some groups
- Lack of protection against STIs, including HIV

SPECIAL ISSUES

Sperm antibodies. About one-half to two-thirds of men will develop sperm antibodies following vasectomy. However, no physiological evidence of any pathologic complication arising from the condition has been noted.[59,75] Although two studies performed on vasectomized monkeys suggested the monkeys developed atherosclerotic plaques in the blood vessels at a greater rate than nonvasectomized monkeys,[2,18] extensive epidemiologic studies in men found no adverse effects or increase in heart disease.[32,63,73,74,75] Subsequent primate studies seemed to refute the earlier negative findings. One study found no association with an increase in mortality or morbidity from cardiovascular disease, but a slightly increased risk of cancer in men who had been sterilized for 20 or more years.[33]

Prostate cancer. As vasectomy becomes more prevalent, prostate cancer mortality rates are also increasing. Any relationship between vasectomy and prostate cancer would be important to know. Many studies show no increased risk of prostate cancer in vasectomized men.[65,67,89] Two recent studies were the first large cohort studies to show a weak but a statistically significant increased risk in a subgroup of men 20 years following vasectomy.[33,34] Though the studies were important, weakness in the study design and lack of support from previous studies left the issue unresolved. Subsequently, several additional studies have been published.[21,50] One comparing black and white men found a statistically significant difference in the risk of prostate cancer. The other, following over 10,000 matched pairs of vasectomized men and controls for up to 11 years, found no increase in risk for prostate cancer among vasectomized men. In one of the most recent studies, a large population-based investigation, vasectomy appears either not to cause prostate cancer or to have only a relatively weak relationship to the disease.[41] The reasons for differences with the previous positive studies are not evident.

The National Institutes of Health (NIH) convened a group of experts in 1993 to review the published reports. The committee found that although additional research was needed, a change in the current practice of vasectomy was not warranted. The NIH made the following recommendations:[42]

- Providers should continue to perform vasectomies.
- Vasectomy reversal is not warranted to prevent prostate cancer.
- Screening for prostate cancer should not be any different for men who have had a vasectomy than for those who have not.[101]

PROVIDING SURGICAL CONTRACEPTION FOR FEMALES

Female sterilization involves ligation, mechanical occlusion with clips or rings, or electrocoagulation (Figure 22-1). The fallopian tubes are usually approached through the abdomen via a minilaparotomy incision and laparoscopy or via a laparotomy at the time of a caesarean section or other abdominal surgery. The surgical approach through the vagina via a colpotomy has been largely abandoned because of increased risks of infection and failure.

Occlusion method. The choice of occlusion method depends upon the provider's training, personal experience, beliefs regarding effectiveness, and the availability of supplies. The differences in the risk of method failure depends upon a number of factors, only one of which is the occlusion method.

In September 1996, the U.S. Food and Drug Administration approved the Filshie clip for use as a new contraceptive device in the United States. The Filshie clip is a good option for patients and clinicians because it is easier to use than other occlusion devices, destroys a minimal amount of the fallopian tube, and has high efficacy.[6] Small and designed to occlude the tube with minimal destruction, the device is made of titanium with a silicone rubber lining, which expands to keep the tube compressed as it flattens.[6,7]

Family Health International (FHI) conducted 11 studies of the Filshie clip at 43 sites in 10 countries. In two studies, the 12-month cumulative rate of pregnancy was 0.1% for the Filshie clip and 0.7% for the Wolf clip. Two studies comparing the Filshie clip and the tubal ring found the same 12-month cumulative rate of pregnancy for both methods (0.2%).[7] The Filshie clip may be less effective when used postpartum than when applied during interval sterilizations. In the single postpartum study conducted by FHI, the pregnancy rate at 24 months was 1.7% for the Filshie clip and 0.4% for the Pomeroy method. The Filshie clip compared favorably with other occlusion devices on safety issues, although surgeons and clients should be aware of a low level of "migration" that can lead to a pregnancy.[7]

Timing. The timing of female sterilization, whether pregnancy-related or not, is very important for choosing the surgical approach, method of occlusion, presentation for counseling issues, use of staff and facilities, and organization of patient flow. Interval sterilization (at 4 or more weeks after delivery) is performed when the uterus is fully involuted.

The immediate postpartum period (within 48 hours of delivery) is the most common time for female sterilization in many countries and currently accounts for about 33% of female sterilizations in the United

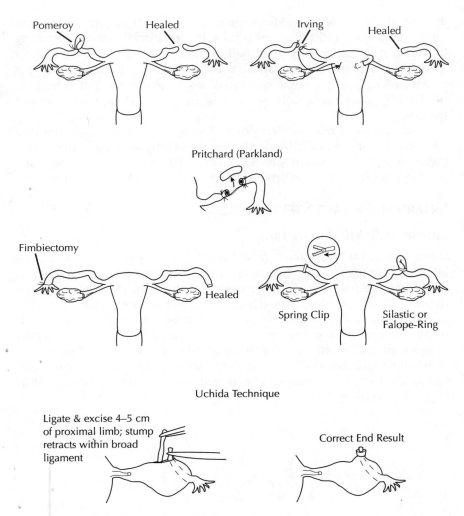

Figure 22-1 Tubal sterilization techniques

States.[85] This popularity is largely explained by the greater convenience, lower costs, ease of surgery, and more efficient use of health resources. A hospital stay beyond that for a normal delivery (24 hours or less in many hospitals) is usually not required. (See also Suprapubic Minilaparotomy.)

Immediate postpartum sterilization services should be an integral part of any maternity service. However, sterilization around the time of pregnancy is associated with an increased risk of regret[15,76,81] and therefore these patients should be counseled carefully. Informed consent before delivery is also important. Many hospitals use a simple procedure room for postpartum sterilization, although the delivery suite or operating theater is most commonly used. Following a procedure performed using local anesthesia and light sedation, the woman is often able to walk back to her bed with assistance. Preoperative assessment is facilitated because her health status can usually be assessed from the delivery and prenatal records.

Tubal occlusion may be performed immediately after a first-trimester spontaneous or medically induced abortion as long as careful attention is given to counseling (clients have a higher risk of regret following post-abortion sterilization[81]), informed choice, and medical contraindications.

INTERVAL FEMALE STERILIZATION

Suprapubic Minilaparotomy

Suprapubic minilaparotomy (also called microlaparotomy or Micro-Pfannenstiel) involves an 2 centimeter (cm) to 5 cm abdominal incision just above the pubic hairline. Through this incision, the surgeon grasps the tubes and occludes them (Figure 22-2.) For many women, the incision lies within the hairline and so will not be visible. If the woman is obese, the uterus immobile, or the tubes have adhesions from infection or previous surgery, the minilaparotomy technique may be difficult. This technique requires mobility of the pelvic structures so that by manipulation of the uterus the tubes can be moved into the incision site and thus be easily accessible.

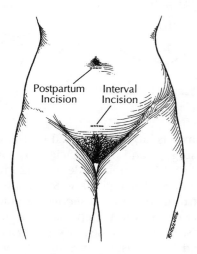

Figure 22-2 Minilaparotomy incision site and size

Ask about pelvic disease, previous abdominal or pelvic surgery, diabetes mellitus, heart or lung disease, bleeding problems, allergies, and recent infections. Ascertain the date of last menstrual period and make certain the woman is not pregnant. If the sterilization procedure is performed post-abortion or postpartum, make certain the client has no pregnancy-related problems, particularly anemia. Examine the heart, lungs, abdomen, and general condition of the patient. Perform a pelvic exam, paying special attention to uterine position and mobility and presence of pelvic infection or masses. Laboratory evaluations usually include at least a hemoglobin measurement.

Procedure. The patient should empty her bladder by voiding or by catheterization immediately before the operation. Place the woman in the lithotomy position with a slight Trendelenberg position to move the pelvic viscera toward the upper abdomen. If the uterus is not already anteverted, elevate the uterus manually or with a uterine manipulator, also termed an elevator (Figure 22-3).

Correct placement of the incision is essential to avoid injury. If the incision is too high, the tubes will be difficult to reach; if placed too low, the bladder may be incised. Significant anatomical variation occurs among patients; thus, take great care in entering the abdomen. Light sedation can be given preoperatively and local anesthesia used to infiltrate layer by

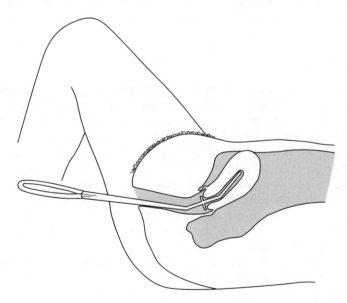

Source: Stewart et al. (1988).

Figure 22-3 A metal elevator raises the uterus and moves it from side to side so that the uterus and tubes will be closer to the incision.

layer (see the section on Anesthesia). When using local anesthesia, continue to communicate with the woman during the procedure to enhance the analgesic effect, reassure her, and when necessary, elicit her cooperation. Surgical manipulation should be slow and gentle. Be responsive to the patient's complaints. Avoid unnecessary trauma or manipulation. Often a tubal hook or small Babcock forceps facilitates lifting the fallopian tube from the abdomen. Identify the fimbria to ensure the structure is the tube and not the round ligament.

Use careful aseptic technique throughout. Achieve good hemostasis before closing the abdominal wound in layers. Growing evidence indicates it is unnecessary to suture the peritoneal layer because small peritoneal defects will heal without adhesions.[9] This principle applies as well to subumbilical minilaparotomy. AVSC International has published a training manual, *Minilaparotomy under Local Anaesthesia: A Curriculum for Doctors and Nurses*, that describes this technique in greater detail.[9]

Occlusion techniques. Occlusion options include the Pomeroy and Pritchard (Parkland) techniques, the Silastic or Falope-rings, the Spring clip (Hulka, Rocket or Wolf Clip), and the newly introduced Filshie clip. The rings and clips require special applicators. Fimbriectomy and the Madlener procedures have been associated with higher failure rates and have no advantages over the Pomeroy and Pritchard techniques for routine cases. The Irving technique cannot be done through a minilaparotomy incision and is essentially useful only after a caesarean section.

Laparoscopy

The laparoscopy approach to sterilization involves making a small incision and inserting an instrument to visualize the tubes so the surgeon can place rings (bands), apply clips, or electrocoagulate the oviducts. Use either a single- or double-puncture technique. With double puncture techniques, the second puncture is used for manipulating the organs and occluding the tubes (Figure 22-4). With single-puncture procedure, pass the operating instrument through an opening beside the fiberoptic channel.

Principally because the incision is smaller, this method is less painful than minilaparotomy, has a low rate of complications, a short recovery time, and leaves only a small scar. The same equipment and skills can be used for endoscopic diagnostic procedures.

One report, however, indicates a decline in numbers of laparoscopic sterilizations as newer diagnostic and therapeutic endoscopic procedures are performed.[47] Disadvantages of laparoscopic sterilizations include the need for a specialist with expensive and intense training, equipment that

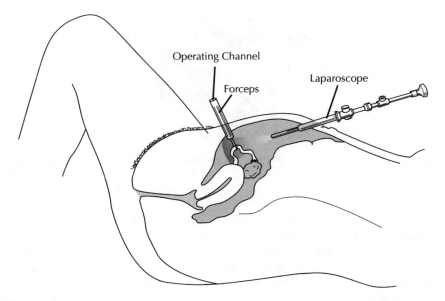

Figure 22-4 Laparoscopy

is difficult to maintain, and a fully equipped operating room. Laparoscopic sterilization is not recommended for the immediate postpartum period, and complications may be serious.

Procedure. Laparoscopic sterilizations can be performed using local or general anesthesia. (See the section on Anesthesia.) Clean the perineal area, the vagina, and the cervix. Scrub the abdominal site, especially the naval. Stabilize the cervix with a tenaculum and a uterine manipulator (Figure 22-5).

After making a small subumbilical incision, insert the Veress needle for insufflation. Apply upward traction on the abdomen. Advance the needle toward the pelvis, away from the great blood vessels. Place the patient in the Trendelenburg position and insufflate 1 to 3 liters of gas (the minimum needed for good visualization), nitrous oxide (N_2O), carbon dioxide (CO_2), or room air. Withdraw the needle and advance the trocar toward the pelvis, away from the great vessels, as the abdominal wall is firmly elevated. Remove the trocar from its sleeve (cannula) and insert the laparoscope. If you use the double-puncture procedure, make a second puncture under direct vision through the laparoscope. With single-puncture laparoscopy, insert the operating instruments through the operating channel of the laparoscope to grasp and occlude the oviducts. Variations

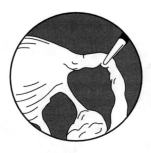

Figure 22-5 A laparoscopy instrument grasps one tube in preparation for cautery or application of a ring or clip.

from this description include "open laparoscopy," during which the peritoneal cavity is opened under visualization by the surgeon—similar to a subumbilical minilaparotomy. Then place a cannula for insertion of the laparoscope. In theory, this method avoids the blind entry of the sharp Veress needle and the trocar into the abdomen,[37,38,69] but it has gained little support for general use.

If clips are used, place them on the isthmic portion of the tube at 1 to 2 cm from the uterus. Place Silastic rings 3 cm from the uterus. Perform electrocoagulation in the midportion of the tube away from other structures (Figure 22-5).[113] After both tubes are occluded, inspect the pelvic organs to ensure no injury or bleeding has occurred, the laparoscope is removed, all the gas is carefully expelled from the abdomen; then remove the cannula, and suture the incision closed.

Occlusion techniques. Silastic bands, unipolar electrocoagulation, and Filshie clips appear to have similar short-term efficacy when correctly applied, although the ectopic pregnancy rate appears to be higher with electrocoagulation (bipolar and unipolar) in the longer term.[100] (See the section on Long-Term Complications). A 10-year follow-up of unipolar and bipolar sterilization cases found higher pregnancy rates with bipolar cautery than with unipolar cautery.[72] These high pregnancy rates appear to be related to training and to technical problems with the instrumentation (e.g., incorrect wattage).[52,110] The Spring clip (Hulka, Rocket, or Wolf Clip) has a lower force of compression than does the Filshie clip and requires precise placement at a 90-degree angle across the tube with the isthmic portion of the tube positioned at the hinged part of the jaws in order to avoid failures.

Vaginal Approach

The oviducts can be reached through an incision high in the vagina (called a colpotomy) posterior to the cervix. This allows direct visualization of the pelvic organs. The oviducts can also be reached and directly sutured and cut. In several countries, vaginal approaches have been found to be less safe and less effective than minilaparotomy and laparoscopic approaches. Infection has been more common, and the techniques are generally more difficult to learn and perform. Therefore, the vaginal approach should be used only for exceptional cases and performed in a well-equipped facility by a skilled surgeon.[109]

Uterine/Transcervical Approach

Most of the hysteroscopic techniques to inject occlusive materials into the tubes are still experimental. Hysteroscopic techniques are difficult to learn, equipment is expensive, and success rates for sterilization purposes have been generally disappointing.[82] However, new devices such as the S TOP device (Conceptus, Inc.) are currently under development.

Also considered experimental are nonsurgical sterilization techniques using a chemical or other material to occlude the tubes through the cervix.[25,93,114] These chemicals or other materials occlude the tubes by causing scarring at the cornual fallopian area in the upper uterus or by traveling into the proximal portion of the tube. Various agents, including quinacrine, methyl cyanoacrylate, and phenol have been used with varying success. However, despite enthusiastic supporters and several large field trials showing positive results, questions about the safety and effectiveness of quinacrine led the World Health Organization (WHO) to issue a statement saying quinacrine should not be used for sterilization purposes in human trials until questions about its safety had been answered.[12]

Hysterectomy

Hysterectomy, whether performed through a vaginal or abdominal approach, carries a much higher risk of morbidity and mortality than other sterilization procedures. Therefore, do not perform a hysterectomy for contraceptive purposes alone, but for a gynecologic disease or condition that justifies a hysterectomy.

POSTPARTUM AND POSTABORTION FEMALE STERILIZATION

Subumbilical Minilaparotomy

If minilaparotomy is performed at 10 or more hours after delivery, postpartum hemorrhage is unlikely to occur, and the status of the baby can be assessed more accurately.[78] (See Suprapubic Minilaparotomy for more on preoperative assessment.)

Procedure.   Immediately after delivery, the uterus and tubes are high in the abdomen. A small 1.5 to 3 cm incision just below the umbilicus is usually adequate to reach the tubes. Local anesthesia with light sedation or analgesia is frequently sufficient because several of the more painful aspects of minilaparotomy are reduced or eliminated:

- The incision is smaller.
- Intra-abdominal manipulation of the tubes is less extensive.
- The lithotomy position is not used.
- The cervical tenaculum or uterine elevator are not required.

The fallopian tubes are usually easier to reach if the incision is made over each tube by placing a hand on the side of the abdomen and moving the postpartum uterus. AVSC's training manual describes the postpartum procedure for minilaparotomy in greater detail.[9]

When a minilaparotomy is not feasible, perform a laparotomy (defined as an incision larger than 5 cm), usually with use of general, spinal, or epidural anesthesia. Laparotomy incisions carry higher morbidity,[54] however, and the anesthesia methods also increase the risk and prolong recovery times. The laparoscope is not used in the immediate postpartum period because of the risk of injury to the large vascular uterus. In addition, the edema and vascularity of the oviducts makes them larger, so laparoscopic occlusion methods are not appropriate.

Occlusion techniques (Figure 22-1).   The Pomeroy technique using plain catgut is an effective and safe approach and is the most widely used method to occlude the tubes in the immediate postpartum period. A loop of tube in the midportion is ligated with plain catgut and then excised. The Pritchard (Parkland) technique avoids the approximation of the cut ends and preserves more of the tube than the Pomeroy technique. The mesosalpinx is perforated in an avascular area; the tube is ligated in two places with one-zero chromic catgut; and the intervening segment is excised.[61,78]

A fimbriectomy has sometimes been performed since the ampullary and fimbrial portions of the tubes are more readily accessible than the isthmic and ampullary portions. However, the fimbriectomy method of sterilization has gained less favor because it is less reversible, removes more tissue, has been associated with high pregnancy rates, and may cause more postoperative complications.

The Falope-Ring, the Fishie clip, and the Spring clip (Hulka, Rocket, or Wolf clip) are not suitable or recommended for immediate postpartum application. Electrocoagulation is also not recommended as a postpartum method. It is usually delivered via laparoscopy.

Cesarean Section

Tubal occlusion can be readily accomplished during cesarean section. However, because of the greater risks involved with cesarean section, it should not be performed solely to occlude the tubes.

High pregnancy rates following simple ligature by silk suture has resulted in methods that excise a portion of the tube. Investigators using the Pomeroy technique (a single plain catgut ligature at midportion of tube with excision of around 2 cm of ligature portion) at the time of a cesarean section have reported a slightly higher pregnancy rate, but lack of surgical skill may be a factor.[49,51] However, this has not been born out by the CREST studies.[72] The Pritchard (Parkland) procedure (Figure 22-1) is the method now ideally favored. It involves two individual sutures, use of chronic catgut, and excision of a small central tubal portion. The Irving technique (which requires a wide surgical exposure for implanting the proximal end of the tube into the uterine wall and is thus possible with cesarean section) is one of the most effective methods and is unlikely to permit an ectopic pregnancy.[78]

Postabortion Sterilization

A minilaparotomy (incision somewhat higher than for a nonpregnant woman) or a laparoscopic approach may be used. The tubes will generally be less engorged and edematous than in the immediate postpartum period but will still require extra care during a minilaparotomy or a laparoscopy in which clips or Silastic rings are applied. (See the sections on Minilaparotomy and Laparoscopy Complications.)

Occlusion techniques may include the Pomeroy or Pritchard procedures with minilaparotomy. Failures with Silastic rings or Spring clips used in the postabortion period are of less concern than in the immediate postpartum period.

ANESTHESIA

General anesthesia provided by trained personnel in appropriate settings can be safe and is the most frequently used method for female sterilization procedures in the United States. A discussion of general anesthesia is beyond the scope of this text. Local anesthesia with light sedation is generally sufficient to minimize the pain caused by sterilization procedures and offers safety advantages over general anesthesia, which can lead to compromised cardiorespiratory function.[70,71] A higher level of training is required for administering general anesthesia than for administering local anesthesia. By not compromising the normal physiological control of vital functions, a high level of safety can be maintained. Both local and general anesthetic methods, however, need the attention of a trained professional who carefully monitors the patient and the drugs used. Avoid high doses of opioid (narcotic) analgesics and benzodiazepine (tranquilizer) sedatives that can compromise ventilation, sometimes dramatically, and may cause cardiovascular depression. The following regimen is suitable for minilaparotomy and, with modifications, laparoscopy. Doses given are for an adult with a body weight of 50 kilograms.

Premedication

Sedate the woman with diazepam (Valium) 10 milligrams (mg) about 30 to 60 minutes before the operation. Midazolam (Versed), a new short-acting parenteral benzodiazepine three to four times more potent than diazepam may be substituted. (Give 2.5 to 3 mg intramuscularly 1 hour preoperatively, or 1 to 2.5 mg intravenously in the operating room.)

Given in the Operating Room

1. Atropine 0.4 to 0.6 mg intravenously.
2. Meperidine (Demerol) 50 mg intravenously. Other opioid analgesics or ketamine can be substituted for meperidine. The intravenous doses, each of which give analgesia about equivalent to 50 mg meperidine, are listed in Table 22-4.[9]
3. Promethazine (Phenergan) 25 mg intravenously.
4. Lidocaine local anesthesia. Infiltrate the skin and subcutaneous tissues with 1% lidocaine (=lignocaine) (Xylocaine) 10 to 15 ml (without epinephrine). After opening the peritoneal cavity, 5 ml of 1% lidocaine may be flowed onto each tube and the uterus. During laparoscopy, this step is optional if the instrument does not permit

Table 22-4 Substitutes for meperedine anesthesia for female sterilization

Drug	Intravenous Dose	Analgesic Duration
Meperidine (Demerol)	50 mg	2–3 hours
Fentanyl (Sublimaze)	0.05–0.06 mg	30–60 minutes
Pentazocine (Talwin)	15–20 mg	2–3 hours
Butorphanol (Stadol)	1 mg	3–4 hours
Ketamine (Ketalar)	25–30 mg*	10–15 minutes

*Short acting—supplemental doses about one-third less than the initial ketamine dose may be given at 10-minute intervals as needed.

lidocaine application. During double-puncture laparoscopy, the second site will also be infiltrated. The maximum safe dose of 1% lidocaine (without epinephrine) is 5 mg/kg body weight; for a woman weighing 50 kg the maximum safe dose is 250 mg or 25 ml of 1% lidocaine. If only 2% lidocaine is available, dilute to 1% with 0.9% sodium chloride only in order to better obtain adequate volume for local infiltration and to avoid exceeding the safe dose. Some surgeons will use sodium bicarbonate (1 cc of 8.4% sodium bicarbonate with 25 cc of 1% lidocaine) to decrease the burning sensation caused by the anesthesia infiltration in the subcutaneous space.

Monitor vital signs regularly during the operation and postoperatively until the woman is fully recovered and alert. AVSC International publications as well the AVSC training manual, *Minilaparotomy under Local Anaesthesia: A Curriculum for Doctors and Nurses*,[9] describe anesthesia techniques in greater detail.

PROVIDING VASECTOMY

Strictly adhere to the technical guidelines on providing vasectomy.[111] During a preoperative history, take an inventory of past illnesses and surgeries, bleeding disorders, allergies (particularly to local anesthetics and pain medications), heart disease, kidney and bladder infection, diabetes, anemia, and STI. Evaluate the man's general health condition, including taking the pulse and blood pressure; assessing for local infections in the scrotal or inguinal area or inguinal hernia or previous surgery in the inguinal area; evaluating the scrotum for hydrocele or varicocele; and determining if the testicles are properly descended or are fixed in place. Assess the scrotal skin and subcutaneous tissues to see if there are factors that might affect a surgical procedure.

Laboratory examinations are not routinely performed, but should be available. If elements in the history or physical so indicate, obtain a lab test (e.g., liver function, bleeding and clotting time, etc.).

Conventional procedure. Clip the man's hair from around his scrotum and penis (if this was not already done at home). Wash the area with soap and water, just before surgery. Use an effective antiseptic (usually a water-based iodine or 4% chlorhexidine solution) to prep the scrotum, thighs, and perineum, then drape the area. Use sterile technique to perform the procedure. Anchor the vasa (two tubular structures, one in each side of the scrotum) with an atraumatic instrument or with your fingers. Infiltrate 1% lidocaine (lignocaine) without epinephrine into the area to be incised and then deeply into the perivasal tissue. Incise the skin and muscle overlying the vas, or open these with the no-scalpel

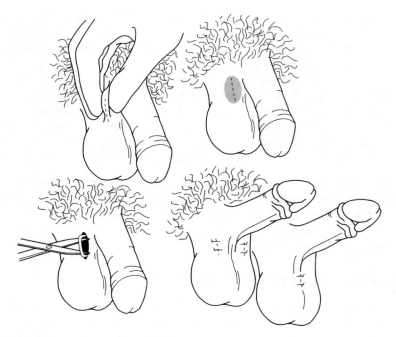

Figure 22-6 Sites of vasectomy incisions

method (see following section on No-Scalpel Vasectomy). Through this small incision, isolate the vas, occlude, and in most cases, resect a small portion (Figure 22-6). Perform the same procedure for the vas on the other side. Close the incisions with absorbable suture. Some surgeons use only a single midline incision, and some do not suture small skin incisions.[3,45,109] If possible, the patient should rest at least 15 minutes before he leaves.

Occlusion techniques. Once the vas is isolated, divide it. The cut ends may be fulgurated to a depth of 1 cm in each direction by inserting a needle electrode or hot wire cautery into the lumen. Alternatively, some surgeons tie each end with a simple ligature using absorbable or nonabsorbable suture, being careful not to cut through the vas. Sperm granulomas occur more often at the cut ends after the ligature technique, possibly contributing to a somewhat higher failure rate than when fulguration is used. A segment of the vas may be removed to obtain greater separation, although this procedure is not considered necessary. For either occlusion technique, create a fascial barrier between the ends by drawing the sheath over one end and suturing it.[3,109] This latter technique may decrease the failure rate.

A modification performed by a few surgeons is to leave the testicular end of the vas open ("open-ended vasectomy") and fulgurate the abdominal end to a depth of 1.5 cm. A fascial barrier may then be interposed. This method appears to reduce the frequency of postoperative congestive epididymitis without increasing the rate of painful sperm granulomas.[3,26,27] Some surgeons report increased failure rates, but open-ended vasectomy may reduce postoperative complaints. Success rates for reversal may also be higher than when both ends are fulgurated.

NO-SCALPEL VASECTOMY PROCEDURE

A "no-scalpel" procedure is currently being used in many programs around the world, including in the United States. The no-scalpel vasectomy technique was developed in 1974 in China, where more than 9 million men have had the procedure.[8] The surgical approach uses a different anesthetic technique and reaches the vas through a puncture in the scrotum rather than through a scalpel incision.[8] Thereafter, the surgical procedure is the same as the scalpel method. Compared with the scalpel method, the no-scalpel method appears to have lower complication rates.[45]

This procedure employs two unique instruments. After local anesthetic is injected, creating a perivasal block, a specially designed ring forceps encircles and firmly secures the vas without penetrating the skin. The second instrument, a sharp-tipped dissecting forceps, punctures and stretches a small opening in the skin and vas sheath. The vas is lifted out and occluded, as with other vasectomy techniques. The same midline puncture site is used to deliver and occlude the other vas in an almost bloodless procedure. No sutures are needed to close the small wound (Figure 22-7).

COUNSELING FOR FEMALE STERILIZATION AND VASECTOMY

The goal of counseling is to guide clients to help them select a contraceptive method that they will use, that will be effective, and that will not have adverse effects. The permanence of sterilization methods can be an advantage or a disadvantage. For some clients, reversals can be done but are expensive and require major surgery; results are not guaranteed. In the preoperative assessment, ensure the patient has been appropriately counseled and provided an informed consent for surgical sterilization. In addition, be certain she is selected and counseled regarding the anesthetic method to be used.

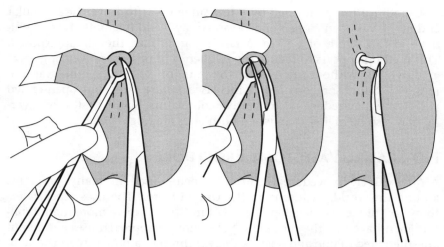

Reprinted with permission from the Population Information Program.

Figure 22-7 "No-scalpel vasectomy." The vas (dotted line) is grasped by special ring forceps and the skin and the vas sheath are pierced by sharp-tipped dissecting forceps (A). The forceps then stretch an opening (B) and the vas is lifted out (C).

FACTORS IN PATIENT REGRET AFTER STERILIZATION

A number of circumstances can lead to a high degree of regret among users.[14,43,105,106] Identifying these individuals prior to sterilization is helpful, but in many cases, unpredictable life changes are the cause of regret. Young age is the strongest pre-operative predictor of subsequent risk for regret. These individuals should receive special attention for consent prior to procedure. Persons who are recently divorced, whose life circumstances are changing, or whose reasons for being sterilized is because they are unhappy with a reversible method may benefit from professional counseling.

Strongly discourage sterilization in a client whose marriage is unstable. Sterilization around the time of pregnancy is associated with an increased incidence of regret in many studies.[15,76,81,106] People who are poor (e.g., Medicaid clients) or of Hispanic origin also make up a disproportionate group of those who would wish a reversal procedure.[43]

SPECIFIC COUNSELING GUIDELINES FOR FEMALE STERILIZATION

The factors in an individual's decision about female sterilization vary from woman to woman. Each woman needs to weigh the risks, benefits, effectiveness, and side effects of the various contraceptive options available to her, including sterilization, pills, the IUD, Norplant implants, injectables, and barrier methods such as condoms, the diaphragm, and spermicide.

1. **Provide choices.** The clear answer is to provide clients with choices. New and old long-term contraceptive methods (e.g., Depo-Provera, Copper T 380 A IUD, and Norplant) can be excellent methods for women who wish a highly effective, long-term method. In addition to providing contraceptive options, it is ethically and programmatically justifiable to provide resources for the surgical reversal of sterilization if the need arises.

2. **Assess client's understanding of the procedure.** In the United States, awareness of female sterilization is widespread, and one of the interviewer's tasks is to assure the individual correctly understands the procedure and has no misconceptions (Table 22-5).

3. **Facilitate the decision-making process.** Give the client sufficient time to make a thoughtful, informed decision about a permanent method of contraception, especially women having immediate postpartum or postabortion (spontaneous or induced) sterilization. Whenever possible, the woman should have decided she wants a permanent method well before delivery or a pregnancy-related event or procedure. Her decision may be unduly influenced by the emotional and physical stress produced by the pregnancy and related events. Postpartum and postabortion sterilization clients have a higher rate of regret following sterilization than interval sterilization clients.[105,106]

POSTPARTUM COUNSELING GUIDELINES

Women who come to the hospital for the first time during labor may be counseled after delivery when they are free of the immediate stresses

Table 22-5 Summary of medical complications of vasectomy

Complications	% of Procedures (N = 24,961)
Hematoma	1.6
Infection	1.5
Epididymitis	1.4
Granuloma	0.3
Failure	0.4

Source: Wortman (1975).

related to labor and delivery and are not under the influence of sedatives. If the baby is healthy and the woman clearly desires no more children, she may be a suitable candidate for sterilization. Husbands should also be brought into the discussion whenever possible; however, spousal consent should not be mandatory.

For postpartum clients, assure the patient has no medical problems such as eclampsia, postpartum hemorrhage, or endometritis that might contraindicate the sterilization surgical procedure.

Staff should be skilled in explaining and providing alternative postpartum methods, such as the IUD or Norplant, which may be inserted immediately postplacental or postpartum if the woman is not breastfeeding. Women should feel no pressure to decide upon sterilization because of the unavailability of alternative methods or lack of clinical skill to provide them. Moreover, delayed sterilization services should be available so if uncertainty or any medical contraindication exists at the time, the procedure can be comfortably scheduled at 4 weeks or later after delivery.

If the procedure is delayed beyond 6 months after delivery and she is not fully or nearly fully breastfeeding and not amenorrheic, advise the woman to use an effective contraceptive method until the sterilization procedure.

POLICY/LEGAL ISSUES

Laws and regulations regarding sterilization procedures have undergone many changes over the last few decades. Be aware of rulings in counseling sterilization candidates:

- Pragmatically, ethically, and legally, strict adherence to informed choice and consent procedures is critical prior to sterilization.[91]
- Partner or spousal consent in the United States is not legally required.[19]
- Clients using federal or state funds for sterilization must be age 21 or older, mentally competent, and must wait 30 days after signing a consent for performance of a sterilization procedure.[29]

Arbitrary decisions by health professionals to restrict access to sterilization have been judged by courts in the United States to violate a woman's basic rights. Although these rulings were set to address the concerns of women seeking sterilization, the laws and regulations set forth apply equally to men seeking services for vasectomy.

The policy and legal status of providing sterilization for mentally challenged women and men remains a problem. Clear guidelines need to be established. Health care providers, policy makers, and the public should be informed of the ethical and legal issues involved in providing voluntary sterilization to those who may not be able to provide informed consent.

INFORMED CONSENT

Informed consent is the voluntary decision made by a person who has been fully informed regarding the surgical procedure and its consequences. Provide the information in a language the client can understand. Most informed consent documents cover the following important points:

- Type of operation, including risks and benefits
- Availability of alternative methods of family planning
- Inability to have children once sterilized
- Intended permanence of sterilization
- Possibility of reversal
- Expense and major surgery required for reversal procedures that cannot be guaranteed
- Possibility of failure (pregnancy, including ectopic pregnancy) after the procedure
- Option to decline female sterilization without loss of medical or financial benefits
- For women, the high risk that any pregnancy would be ectopic

The client must always sign or mark the informed consent form. The surgeon or authorized representative must also sign the form. The authorized representative may be the person with the primary responsibility for counseling the client. Illiterate clients should mark the informed consent form with a thumbprint or "X"; a witness chosen by the client must also sign or mark the form. Preferably, the witness should be of the same sex as the client. The informed consent document should be readily understandable in the client's own language.

MANAGING PROBLEMS AND FOLLOW-UP
FEMALE STERILIZATION

Complications occur in less than 1% of all sterilization cases. The types of complications vary by the type of surgical procedure and anesthesia. Most of these complications can be prevented by careful screening, local anesthesia with light sedation, close monitoring of vital signs, good asepsis, and careful surgical technique. Infection prevention must always be a high priority.[97] The seriousness of complications can often be minimized by early recognition and aggressive management.

Anesthesia complications can be severe; therefore, use local anesthesia. (See the section on Anesthesia.) The abdominal wall is thin at the umbilicus and thus the dissection and entry into the peritoneal cavity must be cautious in order to avoid damaging the intestine.

- Brisk bleeding from the engorged postpartum vessels can be avoided by gentle handling of the tubes.
- Postoperative hemorrhage can be avoided if ligatures around the tubes are secure to prevent slipping.
- Infections are minimized by screening clients preoperatively and avoiding surgery on patients with prolonged ruptured membranes or evidence of current infection (with fever). Prophylactic antibiotics are usually given if the procedure is performed between the third and seventh postpartum day. If the procedure cannot be performed within 7 days after delivery, it is often advisable to wait until 4 to 6 weeks postpartum, primarily because of the technical difficulty of reaching the oviducts.[78,109]

Laparoscopy Complications

Although complications from laparoscopy are not more common than from minilaparotomy, some are more severe.[71] The rate of laparoscopic complications is highly dependent on the level of surgical skill. To reduce complications, the operator should receive special training in laparoscopy. Surgeons performing fewer than 100 procedures per year have a much higher complication rate than more experienced surgeons.

The insufflation needle should have a blunt obturator (as does the Veress needle), and correct placement should be verified by aspiration, hanging drop, or pressure test.[109] Keep equipment in good working order; keep the trocar sharp. When removing the cannula after all gas has been expelled, reinsert the laparoscope to the end of the cannula to prevent omentum or bowel from herniating into the abdominal wall defects as the cannula is removed.[109]

Anesthesia.   Anesthesia-related complications can be aggravated by the gas-filled abdomen and the Trendelenburg position, especially if general anesthesia is used.

Tears and transections.   Complications such as mesosalpingeal tears and transection of the tube can occur with ring application, which may require laparotomy to control bleeding. Sometimes an additional ring can be placed on each severed end of the tube for hemostasis.

Instrumental trauma.   Uterine perforation with the uterine elevator can usually be managed conservatively. Injuries to vessels, intestines, or other organs can occur with the insufflation needle or the trocar. General anesthesia back-up is necessary when doing laparoscopy sterilization procedures in order to manage rare complications of severe bleeding from a major vessel.

Burns.   Bowel burns can occur from electrocoagulation, resulting in late perforation and peritonitis. Although the bipolar cautery may carry less risk of burns than unipolar electrocoagulation, most international agencies discontinued support for electrocoagulation in the early 1980s. Most laparoscopic injuries are not related to the cautery (although electrical and technical changes can cause problems), but rather to the trocar or other surgical instruments.[24,57]

Minilaparotomy Complications

Wound infection.   As with all surgical procedures, careful aseptic technique, proper skin preparation, sterilization of instruments, appropriate operating room technique, and diligent postoperative wound care decrease the likelihood of infection.

Uterine perforation with uterine elevator.   Gentle use of all instruments on human tissues minimizes trauma. Determine the uterine position prior to inserting the elevator.

Bladder injury.   This common surgical complication occurs because of the proximity of the bladder at the lower incision. Careful dissection and attention to landmarks assist in prevention.

Intestinal injury.   Recognition of tissue layers and careful entry into the abdominal cavity help in prevention. If injury is unrecognized, serious complications arise; therefore, prompt recognition is paramount.

LONG-TERM COMPLICATIONS

Ectopic pregnancy. Rule out ectopic pregnancy any time a woman shows signs of pregnancy following tubal occlusion. Compared with an ectopic rate of 0.5% to 1.0% among pregnancies of nonsterilized women, the rate of ectopic pregnancies among pregnancies in sterilized women ranges from 4% to 73% of pregnancies, depending upon the procedure used.[61] The recent CREST study stated that 32% of subsequent pregnancies were ectopic.[72] A previous study preliminarily indicated 16% of clip pregnancies, 38% of ring pregnancies, 73% of unipolar pregnancies, 59% of bipolar pregnancies, and 44% of Pomeroy occlusion pregnancies were ectopic.[47]

A report from Korea of 4,361 ectopic pregnancies following sterilization suggests about a three-fold greater incidence of ectopic pregnancy associated with electrocoagulation than with the use of the Silastic ring. Ectopic pregnancies continued to occur at 6 and more years after sterilization. Ectopic pregnancy was most often related to the following:[104]

- Uteroperitoneal fistula after electrocoagulation (unipolar or bipolar)
- Inadequate coagulation after bipolar procedures
- Inadequate occlusion or fistula formation after the Pomeroy, clip, or ring procedure

Hormonal changes. The effect of tubal occlusion on hormonal feedback between the pituitary and ovaries has been extensively studied. While levels of luteinizing hormone (LH), follicular stimulating hormone (FSH), testosterone, and estrogen remain within the normal range, serum progesterone may decline,[65,79,80] different conclusions have been reached by other investigators.[5,20] No studies have evaluated presterilization and poststerilization levels.[46]

Menstrual changes. For many years there has been controversy over the existence of a post-tubal ligation syndrome, referring to symptoms such as dysmenorrhea, heavy bleeding or spotting, and changes in cycle length or regularity. It has also been suggested that those methods of occlusion resulting in more extensive damage to the fallopian tubes may be more likely to cause subsequent changes in menstrual function. To date, however, the evidence does not consistently support this hypothesis.

Some early criticism of studies on menstrual irregularities following sterilization were faulted for a failure to account for other factors leading to a change in menstrual function following sterilization such as presterilization use of oral contraceptives possibly masking underlying menstrual dysfunction. Recent prospective studies that accounted for these confounding factors have failed to find a significant difference in the change in menstrual function between sterilized and nonsterilized women over time.

Most studies of menstrual change following sterilization have had periods of follow-up for 1 to 2 years, and have found no increase in risk of menstrual change.[30,83] One well-designed prospective study did find sterilized women were more likely to experience adverse menstrual changes, but follow-up was for only 1 year.[87] Studies with longer follow-up periods have been less consistent in their findings. Data analyzed from the Walnut Creek Contraceptive Drug Study found no change in menstrual function among 719 subjects and 1,083 controls in the first 2 years of follow-up.[23] However, after 2 years, those having undergone sterilization were more likely to experience a change in menstrual symptoms. A later prospective study found no changes between sterilized women and control subjects up to 4.5 years following sterilization, after controlling for oral contraceptive use immediately prior to sterilization. Women who had a slight increase in dysmenorrhea at 6 to 10 months of follow-up did not have a progression of this symptom over the next 3 to 4.5 years.[84]

Two years following sterilization, women enrolled in the CREST study showed no increase in risk of menstrual changes.[22] The same cohort followed up at 5 years showed an increase in menstrual pain, menstrual bleeding, and spotting. However, the authors suggest these changes might be related to the aging of the study cohort; no control population was included in the analysis to address this issue.[64,107] This study also found the methods causing the most tissue destruction were more likely to be associated with menstrual dysfunction. No single method of occlusion was more likely to result in adverse menstrual changes.[23]

Two studies have evaluated the likelihood of hospitalization for menstrual disorders in women having undergone sterilization. One large study followed a large cohort of women in Britain for up to 6 years.[102] There was a slight, but not statistically significant, increased likelihood of hospitalization among the sterilization group. A second study carried out in the United States showed a statistically significant increased risk (1.6) of hospitalization for menstrual disorders in a group of sterilized women as compared with a control group of wives of vasectomized men.[88]

Laboratory studies of hormone levels have yielded little useful information on the post-ligation syndrome. Although many studies include control subjects, they do not measure the subject serum levels preoperatively in women undergoing sterilization. Studies that did measure such levels preoperatively found no changes following sterilization, but these involved only small numbers of women.[4,31] Further research needs to be conducted on this issue.

Psychological problems. Sterilized women have no more psychological problems than nonsterilized women.[13,102,107,110] A study of female marital sexuality found no detrimental long-term effects from female or male sterilization. Conversely, the study found an increase in coital frequency after 1 year among women who had undergone tubal sterilization as compared with women not planning sterilization.[86]

Hysterectomy and other surgery. The questionable hormonal and menstrual changes following sterilization procedures have prompted some surgeons to perform hysterectomies and D&Cs. One study found women who were sterilized while 20 to 29 years old were more likely to have a hysterectomy than were women sterilized after the age of 30.[94] There appeared to be no biological basis for these surgeries. If sterilization does increase the incidence of hysterectomy or D&C, this must be considered an adverse outcome associated with sterilization.[17]

VASECTOMY

Vasectomy is a minor surgical procedure. Mortality is extremely rare (Table 9-4).[36] Complications occur in fewer than 3% of cases.[58] Bleeding complications can be minimized by careful surgical technique and having men avoid strenuous activity for a day or two. Hemostasis (controlling any bleeding) during the operation can control the formation of hematomas (Table 22-6). Small noninfected hematomas may be managed with rest and analgesics; large, painful, or infected hematomas usually require surgical drainage. One of the main advantages of the no-scalpel method is a decreased rate of bleeding complications.[56]

Infections are prevented by strict aseptic practices, using sterilized equipment, and keeping the incision clean. An infection should be treated with antibiotics and wet heat applied locally. Leakage of sperm from the occluded end of the vas can cause an inflammatory nodule (granuloma) that generally subsides spontaneously, although pain medication may be required. The rare granuloma that increases in size, is painful, and does not recede can be treated surgically. Back pressure in the occluded vas can cause congestive epididymitis, which usually subsides in a week with heat treatment and scrotal support.

REVERSAL OF FEMALE STERILIZATION AND VASECTOMY

Sterilization should be considered permanent, but even with careful counseling, some women and men will request reversal following a divorce or remarriage, a child's death, or the desire for more children.[90,105] Emphasize the following points:

- Reversal requires major surgery and special skills.
- Some clients are not appropriate candidates because of the way the sterilization was performed, because of the client's or partner's advanced age, or because of the partner's infertility.

Table 22-6 Tubal damage and reversal pregnancy rate by tubal occlusion method

Technique	Tubal Damage (cm)	Reversal Pregnancy Rate (%)
Clip	1	88
Thermal Cautery	2	No Studies
Ring	3	75
Pomeroy	3–4	59
Electrocoagulation	3–6	43

Sources: Haber (1988), Liskin (1985).

- Success cannot be guaranteed, even when the patient is a good candidate and the surgery is performed by an experienced micro-surgeon.
- Reversal surgery is very expensive for both male and female procedures.
- Surgery, especially major abdominal surgery, carries operative risks as well as risks due to anesthesia.
- Ectopic pregnancy is more common among pregnancies occurring after reversal of female sterilization—about 5% for women who have an electrocoagulation procedure reversed and about 2% for women who have other occlusion techniques reversed.[61]

If the woman wishes to have a reversal even after counseling, perform a laparoscopy to determine the condition of the tubes. Perform infertility tests on her and her partner. Most surgeons will not operate if less than 4 cm of healthy tube remains.

SUCCESS RATES FOR REVERSAL OF FEMALE STERILIZATION

Success rates based on intrauterine pregnancies after reversal surgery are highest for occlusion techniques that damage the smallest segment of oviduct (Table 22-7).[61] Higher success rates are generally achieved through the use of microsurgical techniques:

- Use of magnification (loupe, hood, or operating microscope)
- Accurate alignment of the fallopian tube segments and placement of sutures
- Constant irrigation of tissues to prevent drying
- Use of very fine suture and needles
- Microsurgical electrocautery to minimize bleeding
- Care to keep foreign materials from being left in the wound.

Women must consider any sterilization technique as permanent, even clips, because reversal is not always successful and reversal surgery will not be available to all who want it. For women who are poor candidates for reversal surgery, in vitro fertilization (IVF) may be an option. (See Chapter 27 on Impaired Fertility.)

SUCCESS RATES FOR REVERSAL OF VASECTOMY

Microsurgical technique is important when restoring continuity of the vas. With an operating microscope using higher magnification (25 power), reported pregnancy rates range from 16% to 79%, with most rates approaching 50% or higher. The pregnancy rate depends on the skill of the surgeon/microsurgeon, the time since the vasectomy was performed,[10,11,55] presence of antisperm antibodies, age of the female, and the length and location of the removed vas segment. The percentage of men with sperm in the ejaculate ranges from 81% to 98%; presence of sperm should not be presented to men as the measure of success, since pregnancy is the desired outcome.

Attempts to develop a plug, valve, or simple reversible vasectomy have not been successful.[60] Men must accept vasectomy as a permanent procedure even though improved microsurgical techniques have increased the chances of restoring fertility.

INSTRUCTIONS FOR FEMALE STERILIZATION AND VASECTOMY

FEMALE STERILIZATION

Preoperative Instructions

1. Be completely comfortable with your decision to use a surgical method for contraception. You must be certain you understand sterilization is permanent and that you desire a permanent method of contraception. Be certain all of your questions have been asked and answered. You can change your mind at any time before the procedure or can postpone the operation if you need more time to think about it.

2. Shower or bathe just before surgery. Pay particular attention to the area around the umbilicus (navel) and the pubic hair.

3. **Do not eat or drink** in the 8 hours before surgery.

4. Have someone accompany you on the day of surgery, if at all possible. This person should accompany you when you go home. You should plan to have someone with you for the first 24 hours following surgery.

5. **Rest for at least 24 hours** after the procedure and avoid heavy lifting for 1 week.

6. Be prepared for pain over the incision and occasional pelvic aching or discomfort. The pain is usually not severe and can be relieved with mild pain medications provided to you.

7. Plan a flexible schedule for the week after the sterilization. Some women recover less quickly than others from the effects of anesthesia and surgery.

8. Be certain to ask questions if you have them.

Postoperative Instructions

1. **Rest for 24 hours following surgery.** Resume normal activities as you gradually become more comfortable.
2. **Avoid intercourse for 1 week** and when you resume having intercourse, stop if it is uncomfortable.
3. **Avoid strenuous lifting for 1 week** to allow the incisions to heal.
4. Return to the clinic or contact the clinic or doctor promptly if you develop:

Condition:	Action:
Temperature: 100+ degrees Fahrenheit	Immediate contact with M.D. either by phone or for exam.
Fainting: Fainting spells	Contact M.D. by phone.
Pain: Abdominal pain that is persistent, severe and/or increasing after 12 hours	Immediate contact with M.D. for exam.
Incision sites:	
Bleeding or spotting from incision sites	1. Put pressure and tape x 12 hours. 2. Keep clean with betadine or peroxide. 3. If condition continues or worsens, contact M.D.
Pus or discharge from incision sites	1. Clean with betadine or peroxide 2 times/day. 2. If condition continues or worsens, contact M.D.
Stitch in wound	It will eventually fall out (unless a permanent suture was put in place).

Postoperative Warning Signs

Caution

- Fever (greater than 100.4° F, 39° C)
- Dizziness with fainting
- Abdominal pain that is persistent or increasing
- Bleeding or fluid coming from the incision
- If you should ever get pregnant, you must be seen immediately

5. Take one or two analgesic tablets at 4- to 6-hour intervals if you need them for pain. (Do not use aspirin since it may promote bleeding.)

6. You may bathe 48 hours after surgery but avoid putting tension on the incision and do not rub or irritate the incision for 1 week. Dry the incision site after bathing.

7. Stitches will dissolve and do not require removal. (Note to provider: this instruction must be modified if nonabsorbable sutures such as silk are used.)

8. **Return to the clinic 1 week after the procedure** to make sure the healing process is normal.

9. If you think you are pregnant at any time in the future, return to the clinic immediately. Although pregnancy after female sterilization is rare, when it does occur, chances are increased that it will be outside the uterus (an ectopic pregnancy). This is a dangerous life-threatening condition and must be treated immediately.

10. You should know this method of birth control is permanent. Reversal surgery is possible under certain conditions, but it is expensive, requires highly technical and major surgery, and its results cannot be guaranteed.

VASECTOMY

Preoperative Instructions

1. Become completely sure of your decision to have a vasectomy. You must be certain you understand and desire the permanence of vasectomy. You can change your mind at any time before the operation.

2. Before surgery while you are home, use scissors to cut all hair from around the penis and scrotum to about 1/4-in. in length.

3. Shower or bathe, washing the penis and scrotum thoroughly to remove all loose hairs.

4. If possible, have someone accompany you home when you have the procedure done. Do not ride a bicycle and avoid walking long distances or using other transportation that may rub or put pressure on the scrotum.

5. **Plan to remain quiet for about 48 hours** following the vasectomy. A 48-hour "rest" is important to decrease the risk of complications.

Postoperative Instructions

1. Following the surgery, return home and rest for about 2 days. If possible, **keep an ice pack on the scrotum for at least 4 hours** to reduce the chances of swelling, bleeding, and discomfort. Wear a scrotal support for 2 days. (Jockey shorts will be adequate.) You may be able to resume your normal activities after 2 or 3 days.

2. **Avoid strenuous physical exercise for 1 week.** Strenuous exercise means hard physical exertion or lifting or straining that could bring pressure to the groin or scrotum.

3. Do not shower or bathe for the first 2 days after the vasectomy.

4. The stitches will dissolve and do not have to be removed. (Note to provider: this instruction must be modified if nonabsorbable skin sutures, such as silk, are used or if no skin sutures are used.)

5. **You may resume sexual intercourse after 2 or 3 days** if you feel it would be comfortable; but remember, **you are not sterile immediately.** For many men, sperm will not be cleared from the tubes until after about 20 ejaculations. Until then, use condoms or another method of birth control to prevent pregnancy. The best way of finding out if you are sterile is to have the doctor look at your semen under a microscope after you have 20 ejaculations.

6. If you have pain or discomfort, simple analgesics taken at intervals of 4 to 6 hours usually give adequate relief. (Note to provider: name and dose should be specified.)

7. It is important for you to know what is normal and what is abnormal following your surgery. You will probably have some pain and swelling in the scrotal region; the scrotum may be somewhat discolored. These conditions are normal and should not worry you. Occasionally, blood from a tiny blood vessel may escape into the scrotum at the time of surgery, and bleeding may continue. Notify your doctor or health worker if you have any of the following danger signals or if you notice any other unusual body changes:

Condition:	Action:
Temperature: 100 degrees + Fahrenheit	Contact with M.D. either by phone or for exam.
Pain: Unable to sleep or work	If unrelieved by analgesic, see a clinician.
Discharge: Pus or inflammation at incision site	Clean with betadine or peroxide. If redness in skin increases, contact M.D.
Bleeding: Bleeding from incision site	If after placing pressure on area for 10 minutes the bleeding continues, contact clinician for further assessment.
Swelling: Greater than twice normal size	Contact M.D. by phone.
Nodules: Larger than a nickel (5 cent piece), pain and tenderness	Contact M.D. by phone.
Stitches: Extreme pulling sensation	Contact M.D. by phone.

8. You should know this method of birth control is permanent. Reversal surgery is possible under certain conditions, but it is expensive, requires highly technical and major surgery, and its results cannot be guaranteed.

REFERENCES

1. Abma JC, Chandra A, Mosher WD, Peterson LS, Piccinino LJ. Fertility, family planning, and women's health: new data from the 1995 National Survey of Family Growth. Vital Health Stat 1997;Series 23, Number 19.
2. Alexander NJ, Clarkson TB. Vasectomy increases the severity of diet-induced atherosclerosis in Macaca fascicularis. Science 1978;201(4355):538-541.
3. Alderman P. The lurking sperm: a review of failures in 8879 vasectomies performed by one physician. JAMA 1988;259:3142-3144.
4. Alvarez F, Faundes A, Brache V, Tejada AS, Segal S. Prospective study of the pituitary-ovarian function after tubal sterilization by the Pomeroy or Uchida techniques. Fertil Steril 1989;51:604-608.
5. Alvarez-Sanchez F, Segal SJ, Brache V, Adejuwan CA, Leon P, Faundes A. Pituitary-ovarian function after tubal ligation. Fertil Steril 1981;36:606-609.
6. Anonymous. Sterilization device to offer ease of use. Contraceptive Technology Update 1996;17:53-64.
7. Anonymous. Update on female sterilization. The Contraception Report 1996;7(3):13-14.
8. AVSC International. 2nd edition. No-scalpel vasectomy: an illustrated guide for surgeons. New York NY: AVSC International, 1997.
9. AVSC International. Training manual. Minilaparotomy under local anaesthesia: a curriculum for doctors and nurses. New York: AVSC International, 1993.
10. Bagshaw HA, Masters JRW, Pryor JP. Factors influencing the outcome of vasectomy reversal. Br J Urol 1990;52:57-60.
11. Belker AM, Konnak JW, Sharlip ID, Thomas AJ. Intraoperative observations during vasovasotomy in 334 patients. J Urol 1993;149:524-527.
12. Benagiano G. Sterilisation by quinacrine. The Lancet 1994;344:689.
13. Bledin KD, Cooper JE, Mackenzie S, Brice B. Psychological sequelae of female sterilization: short-term outcome in a prospective controlled study. Psychol Med 1984;14:379-390.
14. Boring CC, Rochat RW, Becerra J. Sterilization regret among Puerto Rican women. Fertil Steril 1988;49:973-981.
15. Chi I-c, Gates D, Thapa S. Performing tubal sterilizations during a women's postpartum hospitalization: a review of the United States and international experiences. Obstet Gynecol Surv 1992;47:71-79.
16. Chi I-c, Petta CA, McPheeters M. A review of safety, efficacy, pros and cons, and issues of puerperal tubal sterilization—an update. Adv Contracept 1995;11:187-206.
17. Chi I-c. Is tubal sterilization associated with an increased risk of subsequent hysterectomy but a decreased risk of ovarian cancer? A review of recent literature. Adv Contr 1996;12:77-99.

18. Clarkson TB, Alexander NJ. Long-term vasectomy: effects on the occurrence and extent of atherosclerosis in rhesus monkeys. J Clin Invest 1980;65(1): 15-25.
19. Coe vs. Bolton. United States District Court, Civil Action No. C-76-785-A. September 29, 1976 (N.D. Georgia).
20. Corson SL, Levinson CJ, Batzer FR, Otis C. Hormonal levels following sterilization and hysterectomy. J Repro Med 1981;26(7):363-370.
21. Coulson AH, Crozier R, Massey FJ, O'Fallon WM, Schuman LM, Spivey GH. Health status of American men - a study of post-vasectomy sequelae: results. J Clin Epidemiol 1993;46:857-920.
22. DeStefano F, Huezo CM, Peterson HB, Rubin GL, Layde PM, Ory HW. Menstrual changes after sterilization. Obstet Gynecol 1983;62(6):673-681.
23. DeStefano F, Perlman JA, Peterson HB, Diamond EL. Long-term risk of menstrual disturbances after tubal sterilization. Am J Obstet Gynecol 1985;152: 835-841.
24. DiGiovanni M, Vasilenko P, Belsky D. Laparoscopic tubal sterilization. The potential for thermal bowel injury. J Repro Med 1990;35(10):951-954.
25. El Kady AA, Nagib HS, Kessel E. Efficacy and safety of repeated transcervical quinacrine pellet insertions for female sterilization. Fertil Steril 1993;59(2): 301-304.
26. Errey BB. Follow-up of 6014 open-ended vasectomy cases. Personal communication with Gary Stewart, Sept. 4, 1987.
27. Errey BB, Edwards IS. Open-ended vasectomy: an assessment. Fertil Steril 1986; 45(6):843- 846.
28. Escobedo LG, Peterson HB, Grubb GS, Franks AL. Case-fatality rates for tubal sterilization in U.S. hospitals, 1979 to 1980. Am J Obstet Gynecol 1989; 160(1):147-150.
29. Federal Register 1978;43 Nov. 8:52146-52175.
30. Foulkes J, Chamberlain G. Effects of sterilization on menstruation. South Med J 1985;78:544-547.
31. Garza-Flores J et al. Assessment of luteal function after surgical tubal sterilization. Adv Contracept 1991;7:371-377.
32. Goldacre MJ, Holford TR, Vessey MP. Cardiovascular disease and vasectomy: findings from two epidemiologic studies. N Engl J Med 1983;308(14): 805-808.
33. Giovannucci E, Tosteson TD, Speizer FE, Vessey MP, Colditz GA. A long-term study of mortality in men who have undergone vasectomy. N Engl J Med 1992;326(21):1392-1398.
34. Giovannucci E, Ascherio A, Rimm EB, Colditz GA, Stampfer MJ, Willett WC. A prospective study of vasectomy and prostate cancer in U.S. men. JAMA 1993;269(7):873-877.
35. Giovannucci E, Tosteson TD, Speizer FE, Ascherio A, Vessey MP, Colditz GA. A retrospective cohort study of vasectomy and prostate cancer in U.S. men. JAMA 1993;269(7):878-882.
36. Harlap S, Kost K, Forrest JD. Preventing pregnancy, protecting health: a new look at birth control choices in the United States. New York NY: The Alan Guttmacher Institute, 1991.
37. Hasson HM. Open laparoscopy. Biomedical Bulletin, Association for Voluntary Surgical Contraception 1984;5(1).

38. Hasson HM. Open laparoscopy. In: Sciarra JJ (ed). Gynecology and obstetrics. Philadelphia PA: Harper & Row, 1982:44.
39. Hatcher RA, Dalmat ME, Delano GE, Fadhel SB, Kowal D, Mandara NA, Mati JK, Sai FT, Stewart FH, Stewart GK. Family planning methods and practice: Africa. DHHS, Atlanta GA: Centers for Disease Control, 1983.
40. Hayes RB, Pottern LM, Greenberg R, Schoenberg J, Swanson GM, Liff J, Schwartz AG, Brown LM, Hoover RN. Vasectomy and prostate cancer in U.S. blacks and whites. Am J Epidemiol 1993;137:263-269.
41. Hayes RB. Are dietary fat and vasectomy risk factors for prostate cancer? J Nat Cancer Inst 1995;87:629-630.
42. Healy B. From the National Institutes of Health: does vasectomy cause prostate cancer? JAMA 1993;269:2620.
43. Henshaw SK, Singh S. Sterilization regret among U.S. couples. Fam Plann Perspect 1986:18:238-240.
44. Huber DH. Advances in voluntary surgical contraception. Outlook 1988;6(1).
45. Huber D. (Association for Voluntary Sterilization) Trip report, The People's Republic of China. June 19-30, 1985.
46. Hulka JF, Peterson HB, Phillips JM. American Association of Gynecologic Laparoscopist's 1988 Membership Survey on Laparoscopic Sterilization. J Repro Med 1990;35:584-586.
47. Hulka JF. The spring clip: current clinical experience. In: Phillips JM. Endoscopic female sterilization. Downey CA: The American Association of Gynecologic Laparoscopists, 1983.
48. Husband ME Jr., Pritchard JA, Pritchard SA. Failure of tubal sterilization accompanying cesarean section. Am J Obstet Gynecol 1970:107(6):966-967.
49. Indian Council of Medical Research. Collaborative study on sequelae of tubal sterilization. New Delhi, India, 1982.
50. John EM, Whittemore AS, Wu AH, Kolonel LN, Hislop TG, Howe GR, West DW, Hankin J, Dreon DM, The C-Z, Burch JD, Paffenbarger RS. Vasectomy and prostate cancer: results from a multiethnic case-control study. J Nat Cancer Inst 1995;87:662-669.
51. Kleppinger RK. An analysis of 7,000 laparoscopic sterilizations: unipolar, bipolar and mechanical occlusive. In: Phillips JM. Endoscopic female sterilization. Downey CA: The American Association of Gynecologic Laparoscopists, 1983.
52. Kwak Hyon-Mo. Laparoscopic sterilization: Korean experience, particularly ectopic pregnancy subsequent to female sterilization. Proceedings of the Pre-Congress Seminar of the XIth AUFOG Congress, Bangkok, Thailand, Dec. 1-4, 1987.
53. Layde PM, Peterson HB, Dicker RC, DeStefano F, Rubin GL. Risk factors for complications of interval tubal sterilization by laparotomy. Obstet Gynecol 1983;62:180-184.
54. Lee HY. Twenty-year experience with vasovasotomy. J Urol 1986;136: 413-415.
55. Levy BS, Soderstrom RM, Dail DH. Bowel injuries during laparoscopy. Gross anatomy and histology. J Repro Med 1985;30:168-172.
56. Li SQ, Goldstein M, Zhu J, Huber D. The no-scalpel vasectomy. J Urol 1991;145:341-344.

57. Li S, Zhu J. Ligation of vas deferens with clamping method under direct vision. Unpublished, 1984.
58. Liskin L, Benoit E, Blackburn R. Vasectomy: new opportunities. Population Reports, Series D, No. 5. Baltimore, Johns Hopkins University, Population Information Program, March 1992.
59. Liskin L, Pile JM, Quillin WF. Vasectomy—safe and simple. Popul Rep 1983;Series D(4):61-100.
60. Liskin L, Rinehart W, Blackburn R, Rutledge AH. Minilaparotomy and laparoscopy: safe, effective and widely used. Popul Rep 1985;Series C(9): 125-167.
61. Margolis A. Personal communication, to Gary K. Stewart 1992.
62. Mahgoub SE, Zeniny AE, Shourbagy ME, Tawil AE. Long-term luteal changes after tubal sterilization. Contraception 1984;30:125-134.
63. Marquette C, Koonin L, Marston-Ainley S. Vasectomies in the United States: 1991. Presented at the American Public Health Association annual meeting, November 1992.
64. Martinez-Schnell B, Wilcox LS, Peterson HB, Jamison PM, Hughes JM. Evaluating the effects of tubal sterilization on menstrual selected issues in data analysis. Stat Med 1993;12:355-363.
65. Massey FJ, Bernstein GS, O'Fallon WM, Schuman LM, Coulson AH, Crozier R, Mandel JS, Benjamin RB, Berendes HW, Chang PC. Vasectomy and health: results from a large cohort study. JAMA 1984;252:1023-1029.
66. Moss WM. Vasectomy failure after use of an open-ended technique. Fertil Steril 1985;43:667-668.
67. Nienhuis H, Goldacre M, Seagroat V, Gill L, Vessey M. Incidence of disease after vasectomy: a record linkage retrospective cohort study. Br Med J 1992;304:743.
68. Ortho Pharmaceutical Corporation. 1991 Ortho Annual Birth Control Survey. Raritan NJ.
69. Penfield AJ. Female sterilization by minilaparotomy or open laparoscopy. Baltimore MD: Urban and Schwarzenberg, 1980.
70. Peterson HB, Hulka JF, Spielman FJ, Lee S, Marchbanks PA. Local versus general anesthesia for laparoscopic sterilization: a randomized study. Obstet Gynecol 1987;70:903-908.
71. Peterson HB, DeStefano F, Rubin GL, Greenspan JR, Lee NC, Ory HW. Deaths attributed to tubal sterilization in the United States, 1977 to 1981. Am J Obstet Gynecol 1983;146:131-136.
72. Peterson HB, Xia Z, Hughes JM, Wilcox LS, Tylor LR, Trussell J. The risk of pregnancy after tubal sterilization: Findings from the U.S. Collaborative Review of Sterilization. Am J Obstet Gynecol 1996; 174:1161-1170.
73. Petitti DB. A review of epidemiologic studies of vasectomy. Biomedical Bulletin 1988;5. (Association for Voluntary Surgical Contraception, New York.)
74. Petitti DB, Klein R, Kipp H, Friedman GD. Vasectomy and the incidence of hospitalized illness. J Urol 1983;129:760-762.
75. Petitti DB, Klein R, Kipp H, Kahn W, Siegelaub AB, Friedman GD. A survey of personal habits, symptoms of illness, and histories of disease in men with and without vasectomies. Am J Public Health 1982;72:476-480.
76. Pitaktepsombati P, Janowitz B. Sterilization acceptance and regret in Thailand. Contraception 1991;44:623-637.

77. Planned Parenthood of Sacramento Valley, CA. Personal communication with Gary K. Stewart, 1993.
78. Pritchard JA, MacDonald PC Grant NF. Williams obstetrics, 17th ed. Norwalk CT: Appleton- Century-Crofts, 1985: Chapter 40.
79. Radwanska E, Headley SK, Dmowski P. Evaluation of ovarian function after tubal sterilization. J Repro Med 1982;27:376-384.
80. Radwanska E, Berger G, Hammond J. Luteal deficiency among women with normal menstrual cycles, requesting reversal of tubal sterilization. Obstet Gynecol 1979;54:189-192.
81. Ramsay IN, Russell SA. Who requests reversal of female sterilization? A retrospective study from a Scottish unit. Scott Med J 1991;36:44-46.
82. Reed TP, Erb RA. Hysteroscopic female sterilization with formed-in-place silicone rubber plugs. In: Phillips JM. Endoscopic female sterilization. Downey CA: The American Association of Gynecologic Laparoscopists, 1983.
83. Rulin MC, Davidson AR, Philliber SG, Graves WL, Cushman LF. Changes in menstrual symptoms among sterilized and comparison women: a prospective study. Obstet Gynecol 1989;74:149-154.
84. Rulin MC, Davidson AR, Philliber SG, Graves WL. Long-term effect of tubal sterilization on menstrual indices pelvic pain. Obstet Gynecol 1993;82: 118-121.
85. Schwartz DB, Wingo PA, Antarsh L, Smith JC. Female sterilizations in the United States, 1987. Fam Plann Perspect 1989;21:209-212.
86. Shain RN, Miller WB, Holden AE, Rosenthal M. Impact of tubal sterilization and vasectomy on female marital sexuality: results of a controlled longitudinal study. Am J Obstet Gynecol 1991;164:763-771.
87. Shain RN, Miller WB, Mitchell GW, Holden AEC, Rosenthal M. Menstrual pattern change one year after sterilization: results of a controlled, prospective study. Fertil Steril 1989;52:192-203.
88. Shy KK, Stergachis A, Grothaus LG, Wagner EH, Hecht J, Anderson G. Tubal sterilization and risk of subsequent hospital admission for menstrual disorders. Am J Obstet Gynecol 1992;166(6-1):1698-1706.
89. Sidney S, Queensberry CP Jr., Sadler MC et al. Vasectomy and the risk of prostate cancer in a cohort mulitphasic health check-up examinees: second report. Cancer Causes Control 1991;2:113-116.
90. Siegler AM, Hulka J, Peretz A. Reversibility of female sterilization. Fertil Steril 1985;43:499-510.
91. Soderstrom R. Clinical challenges: share warning information, court case teaches. Contra Technol Update 1981;2:8-9.
92. Soderstrom RM, Levy BS, Engel T. Reducing bipolar sterilization failures. Obstet Gynecol 1989;74:60-63.
93. Sokal DC, Zipper J, King T. Transcervical quinacrine sterilization: clinical experience. Int J Gynecol Obstet 1995;51 Supp1:S57-S69.
94. Stergachis A, Shy KK, Grothaus LC, Wagner EH, Hecht JA, Anderson G, Normand EH, Raboud J. Tubal sterilization and the long-term risk of hysterectomy. JAMA 1990;264:2893-2898.
95. Stewart FH, Guest F, Stewart GK, Hatcher RA. Understanding your body. New York: Bantam, 1987.
96. Stewart GK. Personal communication with Herbert Peterson, 1993.

97. Tietjen L, Cronin W, McIntosh N. Infection prevention for family planning service programs: a problem-solving reference manual. Durant OK: Essential Medical Information Systems, Inc., 1992.

98. Trussell J, Leveque JA, Koenig JD, London R, Borden S, Henneberry J, LaGuardia KD, Stewart F, Wilson TG, Wysocki S, Strauss M. The economic value of contraception: a comparison of 15 methods. Am J Public Health 1995;85:494-503.

99. U.S. Bureau of the Census, Statistical Abstract of the United States: 1992 (112th ed.) Washington DC, 1992.

100. Uribe-Ramirez LC, Camarena R, Hernandez F, Diaz-Garcia M. A retrospective analysis of surgical complications of four tubocclusive techniques. In: Phillips JM. Endoscopic female sterilization. Downey CA: The American Association of Gynecologic Laparoscopists, 1983.

101. Vasectomy and Prostate Cancer Conference. Department of Health and Human Services. The National Institute of Child Health and Human Development, The National Cancer Institute, The National Institute of Diabetes and Digestive and Kidney Diseases. March 2, 1993.

102. Vessey M, Huggins G, Lawless M, McPherson K, Yeates D. Tubal sterilization: findings in a large prospective study. Br J Obstet Gynaecol 1983;90: 203-209.

103. Walker AM, Jick H, Hunter JR, McEvoy J. Vasectomy and nonfatal myocardial infarction: continued observation indicates no elevation of risk. J Urol 1983;130:936-937.

104. Whong YW. Ectopic pregnancy subsequent to female sterilization. Korean Association of Voluntary Sterilization. December 1987.

105. Wilcox LS, Chu SV and Peterson HB. Characteristics of women who considered or obtained tubal reanatomosis: results from a prospective study of tubal sterilization. Obstet Gynecol 1990;75:661-665.

106. Wilcox LS, Chu SY, Eaker ED, Zeger SL, Peterson HB. Risk factors for regret after tubal sterilization: 5 years of follow-up in a prospective study. Fertil Steril 1991;55:927-933.

107. Wilcox LS, Martinez-Schnell V, Peterson HB, Ware JH, Hughes JM. Menstrual function after tubal sterilization. Am J Epidemiol 1992;135: 1368-1381.

108. Wingo PA, Huezo CM, Rubin GL, Ory HW, Peterson HB. The mortality risk associated with hysterectomy. Am J Obstet Gynecol 1985;152(7-1):803-808.

109. World Federation of Health Agencies for the Advancement of Voluntary Surgical Contraception. Safe and voluntary surgical contraception. New York: World Federation of Health Agencies, 1988.

110. World Health Organization. Mental health and female sterilization: report of a WHO collaborative prospective study. J Biosoc Sci 1984;16:1-21.

111. World Health Organization. Technical and managerial guidelines for vasectomy services. Geneva: WHO, 1988.

112. Wortman J. Vasectomy—what are the problems? Popul Rep 1975; Series D(2): 25-39.

113. Yoon IB. The Yoon Ring as compared with other sterilization methods. In: Phillips JM. Endoscopic female sterilization. Downey CA: The American Association of Gynecologic Laparoscopists, 1983.

114. Zatuchni GI, Shelton JD, Goldsmith A, Sciarra JJ (eds). Female transcervical sterilization. Philadelphia PA: Harper & Row, 1983. (PARFR Series on Fertility Regulation).

115. Zhu K, Stanford JL, Daling JR, McKnight B, Stergachis A, Brawer MK, Weiss NS. Vasectomy and prostate cancer: a case-control study in a health maintenance organization. Am J Epidemiol 1996;144:717-722.

Postpartum Contraception and Lactation

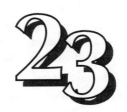

Kathy I. Kennedy, DrPH
James Trussell, PhD

- Breastmilk is the ideal source of nutrition for infants and confers immunological protection against many infections. Reproductive health care providers play an important role in promoting breastfeeding.
- The Lactational Amenorrhea Method (LAM) is a highly effective, *temporary* method of contraception. However, to *maintain* effective protection against pregnancy, another method of contraception must be used as soon as menstruation resumes, the frequency or duration of breastfeeds is reduced, bottle feeds or regular food supplements are introduced, or the baby reaches 6 months of age.
- Other good contraceptive options for lactating women are (1) barrier methods such as the male or female condom, which confer protection against sexually transmitted infections (STIs), (2) progestin-only methods, (3) the Copper T and Levonorgestrel intrauterine devices (IUDs), and (4) male or female sterilization.
- The combined pill is not a good contraceptive option for lactating women because estrogen decreases milk supply.
- Human immunodeficiency virus (HIV) can be transmitted through breastmilk. Therefore, in the United States, where safe alternatives to breastmilk are available, HIV-infected mothers are advised to avoid breastfeeding.

After childbirth, a woman soon becomes capable of becoming pregnant again since the postpartum period of infertility may be brief. Although the breastfeeding woman will have a longer period of infertility than will the nonbreastfeeding woman, her fertility usually returns during weaning, as the frequency of breastfeeds decreases. During weaning, the breastfeeding woman must use a contraceptive method to avoid an

BREASTFEEDING ESSENTIALS

Before a breastfeeding mother is discharged from the hospital after delivery, she should experience:

1. Correct positioning of the infant for breastfeeding
2. Successful latching on
3. Breaking suction

and understand:

4. The relationship between nursing frequency and milk supply
5. The let-down reflex
6. Basic breast and nipple care
7. Techniques of manual and pump expression of milk
8. Signs and symptoms of engorgement and mastitis
9. How to tell if the infant is getting enough milk[1]
10. Where to get help[2]

---

[1] See Neifiert (1996)
[2] Provide telephone numbers of lactation consultants, La Leche league or other local support group, and a clinician

Source: Modified from Bedinghaus and Melnikow (1992), with permission.

Figure 23-1 Breastfeeding essentials

unwanted pregnancy as she regains her fertility. Fortunately, most contraceptive methods are compatible with breastfeeding, and you can play an important role in promoting both contraception and breastfeeding. In addition to providing a postpartum plan for contraception, ensure that the new mother has several essential breastfeeding experiences while still in the hospital (Figure 23-1). Breastmilk is the ideal source of nutrition for infants and confers immunological protection against many infections. Health experts around the globe have declared that all women should be enabled to breastfeed exclusively for 4 to 6 months and to have access to family planning information and services that allow them to sustain breastfeeding.[87]

PHYSIOLOGIC INFERTILITY

POSTPARTUM INFERTILITY

During pregnancy, cyclic ovarian function is suspended. The corpus luteum that arises from the ovulated follicle secretes steroids, including estrogen and progesterone, that are essential in maintaining the early weeks of pregnancy. Later, steroids secreted by the placenta emerge to play a more dominant role in hormonal support of the pregnancy. Luteal and placental steroids suppress circulating levels of follicle stimulating hormone (FSH) and luteinizing hormone (LH) in the mother but more importantly disrupt their pulsatile release from her pituitary.[37] When the placenta is delivered, the inhibiting effects of estrogen and progesterone are removed, levels of FSH and LH gradually rise and pulsatile release by the pituitary of FSH and LH returns.[99]

Most nonlactating women resume menses within 4 to 6 weeks of delivery, but approximately one-third of first cycles are anovulatory, and a high proportion of first ovulatory cycles have a deficient corpus luteum that secretes sub-normal amounts of steroids. In the second and third menstrual cycles, 15% are anovulatory and a fourth of ovulatory cycles have luteal-phase defects. The first ovulation occurs on average 45 days postpartum, although few first ovulations are followed by normal luteal phases.[31]

LACTATIONAL INFERTILITY

Lactation, or breastfeeding, further extends the period of infertility and depresses ovarian function. Plasma levels of FSH return to normal follicular phase values by 4 to 8 weeks postpartum in breastfeeding women.[65] In contrast, pulsatile LH stimulation is depressed, in terms of the frequency or the amplitude of the LH pulse, in the majority of lactating women throughout most of the period of lactational amenorrhea.[18]

Nipple and areola sensitivity increases at birth.[75] Infant suckling stimulates the nerve endings in the nipple and areola. Nerve impulses are passed to the hypothalamus, stimulating the release of various hormones, including prolactin. Prolactin controls the rate of milk production but is not believed to play a major role in suppressing ovarian function.[19] Instead, suckling appears to disrupt the pulsatile release of gonadotropin releasing hormone (GnRH) by the hypothalamus,[65] perhaps by increasing hypothalamic β-endorphin production.[29] The interference with GnRH in turn averts the normal pulsatility of LH, which is required for follicle stimulation in the ovary. Small amounts of secreted estrogen are insufficient to trigger a preovulatory LH surge necessary to induce ovulation.[65,66]

Ovulation can occur even though the breastfeeding mother has not yet resumed menstruation. However, only about 60% of ovulations preceding first menses have an adequate luteal phase.[57] The probability that ovulation will precede the first menses increases with time after delivery, from 33% to 45% during the first 3 months to 64% to 71% during months 4 to 12 and 87% to 100% after 12 months.[9,57] Consequently, lactational amenorrhea becomes increasingly unreliable as an indicator of infertility beyond 6 months postpartum.

Full or nearly full (unsupplemented) breastfeeding is associated with longer periods of lactational amenorrhea and infertility than supplemented breastfeeding. Frequent stimulation of the breast by around-the-clock suckling helps maintain the cascade of neuroendocrine events producing the contraceptive effect.[47] The breastfeeding characteristics that delay the return of ovulation include a high frequency of feeds, long duration of each feed, short intervals between breastfeeds, and night feeds.[9,30] Milk production appears to be reduced far more by supplementary bottle feeds than by supplementary cup and spoon feeds.[9]

In summary:

- Full or nearly full breastfeeding (no or limited food supplements) is associated with longer periods of lactational amenorrhea and infertility than is supplemented breastfeeding.
- Breastfeeding delays the resumption of ovulation and the return of menses.
- The longer a woman breastfeeds, the more likely menstruation will return while she continues to breastfeed.
- The longer the return of menses is delayed, the more likely ovulation will precede the first menses.
- Luteal phase insufficiency is frequent in ovulatory cycles that precede first menses, particularly in the first 6 months postpartum.

CONTRACEPTIVE BENEFITS OF LACTATION

In traditional societies, and in developing countries, lactation plays a major role in prolonging birth intervals and thereby reducing fertility.[10,83,91] In developed countries, however, breastfeeding has a much smaller contraceptive impact because proportionately fewer infants are breastfed, and those who are breastfed are completely weaned at earlier ages. For example, in Indonesia, 96% of infants are breastfed, and those who are breastfed are not completely weaned until they are 2 years old on average.[86] In contrast, in the United States, only 1 in 2 infants is breastfed[49] and the mean and median time to complete weaning are only 23 weeks and 13 weeks, respectively.[94]

LACTATIONAL AMENORRHEA METHOD (LAM) OF CONTRACEPTION

Women who breastfeed could make use of breastfeeding's natural contraceptive effect. If the infant is fed only its mother's breast milk (or is given supplemental non-breastmilk feeds only to a minor extent) and the woman has not experienced her first postpartum menses, then breastfeeding provides more than 98% protection from pregnancy in the first 6 months following a birth[47,53] (Figures 23-2 and 23-3). Four prospective clinical studies of the contraceptive effect of this lactational amenorrhea method (LAM) demonstrated cumulative 6-month life-table perfect-use pregnancy rates of 0.5%, 0.6%, 1.0%, and 1.5% among women who relied solely on LAM.[43,54,72,74]

LAM requires "full or nearly full" breastfeeding because the infant who obtains nearly all nutritional requirements through breastfeeding is providing maximal suckling stimulation at the breast. As long as additional foods do not decrease this optimal amount of suckling, small amounts of supplementation should have little or no effect on the return of fertility. Thus, if LAM is to be used, supplements should be given only infrequently, in small amounts, and not by bottle (Figure 23-2). When a LAM user does give supplements, correct use of LAM can be challenged; it may be difficult to determine how much supplementation can be tolerated without affecting lactational infecundity.[53,55] (See note to Figure 23-2.) Milk expression, such as by hand pump, is not a substitute for breastfeeding in terms of its fertility-inhibiting effect.

Experience with LAM in the United States is limited. Currently, only half of new mothers initiate breastfeeding, but it is unknown whether more women would breastfeed if they appreciated the contraceptive effect of lactation (or the other benefits of breastfeeding). Some U.S.

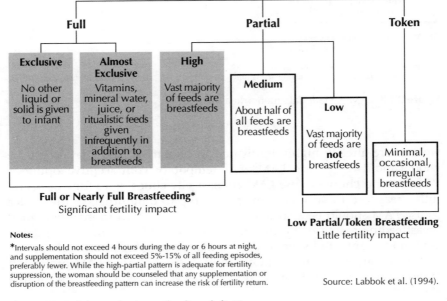

Full or Nearly Full Breastfeeding*
Significant fertility impact

Low Partial/Token Breastfeeding
Little fertility impact

Notes:

*Intervals should not exceed 4 hours during the day or 6 hours at night, and supplementation should not exceed 5%-15% of all feeding episodes, preferably fewer. While the high-partial pattern is adequate for fertility suppression, the woman should be counseled that any supplementation or disruption of the breastfeeding pattern can increase the risk of fertility return.

Source: Labbok et al. (1994).

Figure 23-2 Schema for breastfeeding definition

Ask the mother, or advise her to ask herself, these three questions:

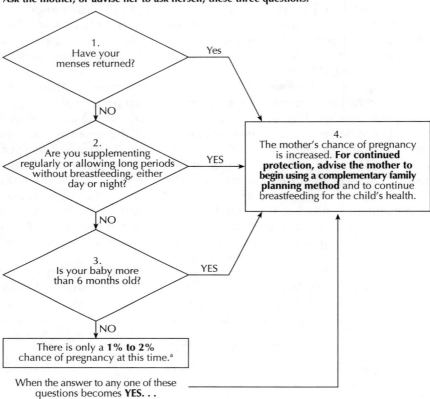

1. Have your menses returned?

Yes

NO

2. Are you supplementing regularly or allowing long periods without breastfeeding, either day or night?

YES

NO

3. Is your baby more than 6 months old?

YES

NO

4. The mother's chance of pregnancy is increased. **For continued protection, advise the mother to begin using a complementary family planning method** and to continue breastfeeding for the child's health.

There is only a **1% to 2%** chance of pregnancy at this time.[a]

When the answer to any one of these questions becomes **YES. . .**

[a] However, the mother may choose to use a complementary family planning method *at any time.*

Source: Labbok et al. (1994).

Figure 23-3 LAM: lactational amenorrhea method

women are already highly motivated to breastfeed, and they would be good candidates to use LAM as a temporary contraceptive option.[36] Women who choose to use LAM are basically choosing to fully or nearly fully breastfeed for at least some period (up to 6 months), so the choice to use LAM should be associated with the motivation to maintain good breastfeeding practices. In the United States, LAM probably is best delivered in the context of support for sound breastfeeding practices.[88]

If a woman wishes to avoid becoming pregnant after LAM protection expires, then she must begin to use another contraceptive method at that time.[45,92]

While pregnancy rates during lactational amenorrhea compare favorably with those for many other methods of contraception (Table 9-2 in

Chapter 9 on Essentials of Contraception) even greater efficacy could be achieved by both breastfeeding and using an additional method of contraception.

POSTPARTUM SEXUALITY

Most American couples resume sexual intercourse within several weeks of delivery. Among lactating women, 66% are sexually active in the first month postpartum and 88% are sexually active in the second month postpartum.[26]

Contraception is only one counseling issue for postpartum women. Women—and men—may experience reduced sexual feelings associated with bodily changes caused by pregnancy and delivery. Discussing these bodily changes may alleviate a couple's anxiety:

- Tenderness in the perineum may make intercourse painful, especially if there has been an episiotomy.
- Reduced postpartum estrogen secretion may result in diminished vaginal lubrication.
- Most women experience a heavy and bloody lochial discharge for a couple of weeks postpartum. This may interfere with a woman's sexual feeling.
- Couples may find that the exhaustion caused by the around-the-clock responsibilities of being a new parent temporarily decreases sexual drive.
- Lactation may diminish the erotic significance of the breasts. Couples need to communicate feelings about whether sucking or touching the breasts is acceptable.
- Bonding between mother and child creates skills and commitment in the mother and trust and security in the infant, but it may interfere with the mother's emotional availability to her partner.
- Conversely, a birth (especially if planned) can be an exceedingly joyous experience that can enhance sexual intimacy. To some men and women, the shape or fullness of the lactating breast is particularly arousing.

INITIATING CONTRACEPTIVE USE POSTPARTUM

Traditionally, a woman would have a postpartum follow-up consultation at 6 weeks because the uterus had involuted and healed by this time. However, a physical exam can reasonably be performed between 3 and 8 weeks postpartum. In terms of contraceptive service delivery, routinely adhering to the 6-week visit does not seem appropriate. Nearly all contraceptive methods can be used postpartum; however, the methods vary in terms of when in the postpartum period they can be initiated.[41,81,82,102] Six weeks is too late for non-breastfeeding mothers who wish to start using combined oral contraceptives, Norplant, or Depo-Provera.[34] On the other hand, 3 weeks is too soon for inserting an intrauterine device (IUD) or fitting a diaphragm. The authors therefore advocate an individual approach to timing postpartum follow-up and contraceptive initiation.

Counseling for postpartum contraception should begin in the prenatal period.[1,5,28] Many methods can be provided at the time of delivery or during the hospital stay, such as IUDs, female sterilization and, for non-breastfeeding women, Norplant or Depo-Provera. Plan in advance to provide these methods at the optimal time. Make plans during the prenatal period, so informed choice is valid and method delivery is uncomplicated, convenient, and cost-effective.

When the couple's method of choice cannot be initiated during the hospital stay after delivery, they can choose temporary methods such as LAM or condoms and make a specific action plan to initiate a longer-term method later. Schedule the first postpartum visit for the most logical time based on the couple's choice of longer-term method. For example, if a breastfeeding woman will be using progestin-only pills, her follow-up visit can be scheduled at 6 weeks postpartum, with the plan to use condoms or LAM until that time. At hospital discharge, give her a cycle of progestin-only pills (or a prescription) and a supply of lubricated condoms and instruct her when to use each to help ensure success. Most important, contact her 2 to 4 weeks after delivery to check on her postpartum recovery and to confirm and support her personal contraception plan.

If the couple has been unable to select a contraceptive method by the time of hospital discharge, the authors endorse the suggestion that a postpartum visit be scheduled for 3 weeks after delivery.[78]

Consider the following when counseling and providing contraceptives to the postpartum woman, whether or not she is breastfeeding:

- Late pregnancy is a common time for a partner's infidelity.[60] Condoms are useful in preventing STI transmission. Spermicides provide modest protection against some STIs. (See Chapter 16 on Male Condoms and Chapter 17 on Vaginal Spermicides.) Spermicides and condoms may be used safely even in the immediate postpartum period.
- Withdrawal may be a good method for couples in the postpartum period. The pregnancy rate for withdrawal is comparable with that for the diaphragm and spermicides (Table 9-2).

- Postpartum endometritis is a serious complication. The risk of introducing bacteria into the uterus is elevated before cervical closure is complete. The condom may be a particularly attractive option for some women.

- Episiotomies may still be tender. Fitting a woman for a cervical cap or diaphragm may cause discomfort.

- Avoid the diaphragm, cervical cap, and contraceptive sponge until 6 weeks after delivery. The diaphragm and cervical cap cannot be (re)fitted properly until that time. Moreover, the risk of toxic shock syndrome is increased when blood, including the postpartum lochia, is present.[24] (See Chapter 18 on Vaginal Barriers.)

- The sponge and the cervical cap (though not the diaphragm) have much higher failure rates among women who have delivered a child than among women who have not, *even during perfect use.* (See Chapter 31 on Contraceptive Efficacy.) Women need to know about this substantial decrease in efficacy for parous women.

- Postpartum abstinence, if practiced properly, is 100% effective in preventing pregnancy. It can, however, be notoriously difficult to maintain. Counsel couples about other contraceptive methods should they desire to resume intercourse.

- IUDs can be inserted postpartum, either (1) immediately after the expulsion of the placenta (postplacental insertion) or (2) during the first week postpartum (immediate postpartum insertion), though preferably within 48 hours of delivery. Expulsion rates following postpartum insertion are higher than those following interval insertion, but they are lower for postplacental than for immediate postpartum insertion.[70] Discuss this option before delivery to ensure fully informed consent. (See Chapter 21 on Intrauterine Devices.) If insertion is not performed immediately postpartum, it should be delayed. Copper T IUDs can be inserted with care at 4 to 6 weeks (but preferably 6 to 8 weeks) postpartum.[70] Some women experience mild uterine cramping when they breastfeed with an IUD in place, but the cramping does not usually interfere with lactation or with the effectiveness of the IUD. IUD insertion is less painful and removal rates for pain and bleeding are lower in the lactating mother.[12,25] Although a few case reports and a small case-control study suggested that the risk of uterine perforation is higher among breastfeeding women, other studies find no evidence of increased risk in breastfeeding women and low rates of perforation in both breastfeeding and nonbreastfeeding women.[12,25,85] Nevertheless, it seems prudent to exercise special care when inserting an IUD postpartum. An IUD can be inserted immediately after a cesarean delivery through the uterine incision.[82] Because of the risk of infection, avoid IUD insertion when a woman has had premature rupture of the membranes, prolonged labor, or fever, whether after a cesarean or a vaginal delivery.[70,85]

- Vasectomy is an appropriate postpartum choice for couples who want a permanent method. As soon as the health of the mother and infant is determined to be sound, the vasectomy can be performed. If the woman is breastfeeding, she may not need a back-up method while the vasectomy is taking effect.[18,41] As with tubal ligation, vasectomy requires counseling and reflection under non-stressful circumstances,[5] preferably before delivery.

- Tubal ligation performed during the immediate postpartum period can be a more cost-effective and simpler technique than interval sterilization.[41] Although tubal ligation is a highly effective method of contraception, a small risk of sterilization failure persists for at least a decade. However, partial salpingectomy performed postpartum carries the lowest known pregnancy risk of any female sterilization procedure.[73] Discuss immediate postpartum sterilization well before the delivery to ensure fully informed consent.[5] Take great care that the woman is confident of this choice[4] because having a tubal ligation during the postpartum period can be a risk factor for regret.[98] (See Chapter 22 on Female and Male Sterilization.) After a vaginal delivery, sterilization should be performed by minilaparotomy either within 48 hours or else delayed for 4 to 6 weeks. After 48 hours, access to the tubes is reduced and the risk of infection increased.[5] Minilaparotomy can be performed up to 6 days postpartum,[102] but the procedure will likely be more difficult and you must take precautions against infections. After a cesarean delivery, perform tubal ligation through the abdominal incision. Delay sterilization in the case of complications such as severe preeclampsia, eclampsia, premature rupture of the membranes, sepsis, fever, severe hemorrhage, or uterine rupture or perforation.[13,102]

POSTPARTUM CONTRACEPTION FOR THE NONBREASTFEEDING WOMAN

If she wishes to avoid becoming pregnant, the nonbreastfeeding woman should begin using a contraceptive method immediately postpartum or at least by the beginning of the fourth postpartum week.[34] Most nonbreastfeeding mothers have few restrictions placed on which method of contraceptive they can choose. Nonetheless, a few guidelines—in addition to those given above—are warranted:

- Combined oral contraceptives (OCs) may be prescribed immediately postpartum. However, caution women not to use them until 3 weeks after delivery.[41,82,102] The risk of postpartum thrombophlebitis and thromboembolism is greatest just after delivery.[105] Delaying combined OC use for at least 2 weeks tends to bypass the period of peak risk for postpartum thrombotic complications.[64]
- Caution women that it is difficult to practice fertility awareness before their cycles are reestablished and cyclic signs of fertility return.
- Suggest that lubricated condoms are a good option at least for the short period before the woman becomes better suited to her preferred method.
- Norplant can be inserted and Depo-Provera can be injected immediately postpartum. Discuss these options before delivery to ensure fully informed consent.

POSTPARTUM CONTRACEPTION FOR THE BREASTFEEDING WOMAN

General comments regarding contraceptive use among postpartum women are given above. In addition, the following considerations are relevant for women who are breastfeeding.

Nonhormonal Methods

Tubal ligation can be performed immediately postpartum, although it can disrupt lactation if it requires general anesthesia or separation of mother and infant. Both problems can be minimized by performing the procedure with only regional or local anesthetic.[52] Unless tubal ligation occurs on the delivery table, have the mother breastfeed her infant just before the procedure in order to reduce the transfer of the anesthetic agent to the infant. For the same reason, have her delay the next breastfeeding while the anesthesia clears from her body.[3,8]

Copper T 380A IUDs are also good choices for breastfeeding women. The copper on the Copper T does not affect the quantity or quality of breastmilk.[96] (See the following section on Hormonal Methods for information on the IUDs containing a progestin or progesterone.)

Spermicides and barrier methods have no effect on the ability to breastfeed. The lubricated condom is especially useful in the postpartum period because of increased vaginal dryness. Spermicides also may help offset dryness due to estrogen deficiency. In the United States, barrier methods are the most widely used contraceptive among lactating mothers in the first 6 months postpartum.[26] In animal studies, nonoxynol-9 is absorbed through the skin and secreted in breastmilk.[14] Questions about nonoxynol-9 secretion in breastmilk have not been completely evaluated in humans.

Lactational Amenorrhea Method (LAM) provides effective protection against pregnancy for up to 6 months postpartum. If continued protection is desired, another method of contraception must be introduced when the LAM criteria indicate a return to the risk of pregnancy. (See the detailed description of LAM earlier in this chapter.)

Fertility awareness methods can be difficult to use during the return of fertility[38] which can extend for many cycles during lactation. The couple needs to abstain for 2 weeks in order to establish a basic infertile pattern of cervical mucus (and other) symptoms. Intercourse can then occur every other night unless there is some change in the basic infertile pattern, in which case more abstinence is necessary.[71] The changing fertility symptoms after the first postpartum menses may be especially difficult for new users to identify, and may lead to an increased risk for unplanned pregnancy.[56]

Basal body temperature readings are not reliable unless a woman has at least 6 hours of uninterrupted sleep. Thus, the woman who gets up in the night to care for her infant is precluded from using the temperature symptom to help determine her fertility status.

The symptothermal method can accurately detect the onset of true fertility during breastfeeding. However, this method often requires many days of abstinence even when there is virtually no risk of pregnancy.[44] Recommend LAM to users of fertility awareness methods who are breastfeeding.[71] For up to 6 months, LAM can eliminate the requirements for abstinence with no apparent additional risk of unintended pregnancy.[46] The transition from LAM to fertility awareness methods begins with the establishment of a basic infertile pattern.[71]

Hormonal Methods

The use of hormonal contraception by a lactating woman is an area of dispute among experts.[42] All steroids pass through the breastmilk to the infant. Estrogen decreases the volume of milk.

Progestin-only contraceptives (POCs) such as Norplant, the Levonorgestrel (LNg 20) IUD, the Progestasert IUD, Depo-Provera, and minipills cause no adverse effects on lactation, and some studies suggest they may even increase milk volume. POCs do not have adverse effects on child growth or development.[27,63,82,102,103,104] These methods are good options for lactating women because they are simple to use and their contraceptive efficacy is high. (See Table 9-2 in Chapter 9 on Essentials of Contraception.)

Experts recommend that breastfeeding women delay using POC methods until 6 weeks after delivery.[41,82,102] This recommendation is based on the admittedly theoretical concern that early neonatal exposure to exogenous steroids, which have passed from the contraceptive into the milk, should be avoided if possible. The neonate's binding capacity of plasma is low, the neonatal liver is not well able to conjugate and oxidize drugs, and the immature kidneys are inefficient in excretion.[18,27] (However, the liver rapidly improves its ability to metabolize drugs, so the need to avoid exposure to exogenous steroids may be brief.[27]) Unable to be cleared from the infant's circulation, exogenous steroids or their metabolites may "compete with natural hormones for receptor sites in sex organs, brain or other tissues."[35] Experts issue their caution because animal literature has indicated long-term effects of inappropriate hormone exposure at critical postpartum periods.[35]

Although POCs would probably have no adverse effects on lactation or infant health if used soon after delivery, little research has been conducted on their immediate postpartum use, since initiation of POCs prior to 6 weeks has been discouraged. A prudent approach would be to share information about the risks and benefits of early POC use with the client, and, if the client consents, to wait until breastfeeding has been well established before starting progestin-only pills, inserting Norplant capsules, or giving the Depo-Provera injection. However, in those circumstances in which a breastfeeding woman requests Norplant insertion before leaving the hospital after delivery (especially if she plans to supplement the infant's diet relatively soon after delivery) and she has a compelling reason to start the method early, then the real long-term contraceptive benefit of using this method seems likely to exceed the theoretical risks. Because the contraceptive benefit to the lactating woman in obtaining Depo-Provera immediately postpartum is smaller and the theoretical risks might be higher (because the hormonal levels are relatively high in the immediate post-injection days), a case would be less compelling for injecting Depo-Provera before breastfeeding is well established; a woman unlikely to return for a postpartum visit may be equally unlikely to return for a repeat injection. Discuss these options before delivery to ensure fully informed consent.

Because the precipitous withdrawal of natural progesterone 2 to 3 days postpartum is the physiological trigger for lactogenesis,[15] a high dose of exogenous progestin (as with a Depo-Provera injection before the withdrawal) may interfere with the stimulus for milk synthesis. This argues for a delay in POC commencement, especially injectable formulas, until the mature milk has come in.[48] If a woman desires to use Depo-Provera immediately, encourage her to remain in the hospital until her mature milk comes in. Very early exposure to progestin-only pills is not always detrimental to lactogenesis; some studies of POCs, albeit the less potent progestin-only pills, have found no overall deleterious effect of progestin on milk volume when begun as early as the first week postpartum.[62,67] In these studies, however, the pills could have been initiated after the withdrawal of natural progesterone.

As with other progestin methods, the Progestasert IUD and the LNg 20 IUD are not recommended for use by breastfeeding women until 6 weeks postpartum.[41,81,102]

Combined oral contraceptives generally should not be used by breastfeeding mothers. A reduction in milk supply is associated with the estrogen component in combined pills, even those with low-dose preparations.[80,97] Use of combined pills may alter the composition of breastmilk, although results vary among studies; most studies report declines in mineral content. Nevertheless, the available evidence suggests that use of combined pills while nursing does not directly harm infants.[97]

Just when lactating women can begin combined pills remains a subject of disagreement. It would be ideal to avoid the use of combined oral contraceptives (OCs) entirely during breastfeeding especially since progestin-only pills are available.[33] The International Planned Parenthood Federation states that under normal circumstances, combined OCs or combined injectables should not be used by breastfeeding women at all.[41] The World Health Organization discourages the use of combined OCs until at least 6 months postpartum.[102] Other experts recommend that only after non-estrogenic methods have been rejected through informed choice can a woman begin combined OCs "after the first 8 to 12 weeks postpartum if she is still amenorrheic or whenever the service provider can be reasonably sure that the woman is not pregnant . . . ."[82]

On those occasions when a woman's informed choice is to use combined OCs during breastfeeding, it seems prudent to caution her not to use them until 2 to 3 months after delivery, and to consume the pill at the beginning of the longest interval between breastfeeds.[23] There are several reasons for this delay in initiation. First, the longer combined pill use is postponed, the better the ongoing establishment of the milk supply. Nevertheless, milk volume will still be reduced when combined OCs are started.[80] Second, the risk of postpartum thrombotic complications is highest just after delivery.[105] As a sensible health precaution, women should avoid using any method containing estrogen for at least 3 weeks. Third, the lactating woman is usually at reduced risk of becoming pregnant, especially if she is amenorrheic and fully breastfeeding. Thus, she may opt to use LAM, condoms, or other barrier methods for only a month or two, with their efficacy enhanced by lactation itself.

There is no need for breastfeeding women using progestin-only pills to switch to combined OCs during lactation. However, if it is the woman's informed choice to make this switch, it is best to do so after 6 months postpartum.[95]

Effects of Hormonal Contraception on the Breastfed Infant

Contraceptive steroids taken by the mother can be transferred to the nursing infant through breastmilk. Although the amounts are small, it is prudent to avoid exposing the neonate to exogenous steroids since they are not easily bound in plasma or conjugated by the liver or excreted, and they may compete with natural hormones for receptor sites. Also, while concern about the possible effects on the liver, sex organs, and other tissues of the neonate or premature infant is theoretical, exposure should be avoided wherever possible.

- The dose of contraceptive ethinyl estradiol (about 10 nanograms [ng] per day) reaching the infant of a mother taking combined OCs is comparable to the dose of the naturally occurring estradiol (from 6 to 12 ng per day depending on time of cycle) consumed by nursing infants of ovulatory mothers not taking combined OCs.[64]

- The quantity of progestin transferred to mother's milk varies with the type of progestin. The 17-hydroxy compounds (such as medroxyprogesterone acetate) enter the milk at approximately the same level found in the mother's blood, whereas the 19-nor compounds (such as norgestrel and norethindrone) enter the milk at only one-tenth the level in the blood.[84]

Combined OC use during lactation is not the only possible source of estrogen and progestin exposure for the infant. When a mother becomes pregnant and continues to breastfeed a prior infant, that child is exposed to estrogen and progesterone in the mother's milk. Dairy cattle may also be pregnant at the time that they are milked, so that cow's milk and infant formula made from it may have relatively high levels of estrogen and progesterone.

Although early studies of high-dose oral contraceptives did demonstrate some effect of hormones on nursing babies,[17] most of those reports were anecdotal and have not been corroborated in women using low-dose OCs. A recent study of the male offspring of women who had used depot-medroxyprogesterone acetate (DMPA) found no effect on infant hormone regulation associated with breastfeeding exposure.[93] Although the short-term effects of absorbing contraceptive steroids through breast-milk appear minimal, the long-term consequences remain unstudied.[35,42]

BREASTFEEDING: ADVANTAGES TO THE INFANT

Mother's milk has both nutritional and anti-infective advantages for the infant. The mixtures of protein, fat, carbohydrate, and trace elements change to meet the infant's evolving needs.[61] Furthermore, breastfeeding may cement the psychological bond between mother and infant. This bonding may lead to better psychological and intellectual development, though the evidence is inconclusive.[50] Finally, the infant ingests host-resistant, humoral, and allergy prophylaxis factors. These are particularly concentrated in the colostrum, the high-protein fluid secreted in the first few days postpartum.

Breastfed infants have lower risk of respiratory and gastrointestinal illness,[39,50,61] including neonatal necrotizing enterocolitis among preterm infants[58] and sudden infant death syndrome.[100] Breastfed infants are less likely to develop allergies, including eczema, cow's milk allergy, and allergic rhinitis.[61] Whether breastmilk is protective or alternative diets are allergenic cannot be determined from the available evidence.[50] Asthma may be less common and less severe among children who were breast-fed.[50] Other benefits include a decreased incidence of otitis media[50,61] and dental malocclusion and caries.[51] Preterm infants who consume mother's milk in the early weeks of life have higher IQ scores,[59] although the association may not be causal. The benefits of breastfeeding are by no means limited to infants in developing countries. All of the protective effects mentioned here have been demonstrated in children in industrialized nations.[16,39,58,100]

BREASTFEEDING AND HUMAN IMMUNODEFICIENCY VIRUS

The human immunodeficiency virus (HIV), which causes acquired immune deficiency syndrome (AIDS), can be transmitted by an infected mother to her infant in utero, during childbirth, and through breastmilk. That HIV-1 can be transmitted by breastfeeding has been conclusively demonstrated by case reports, laboratory data, and epidemiologic studies[22,77] such as prospective studies of mothers who were infected post-natally.[90] Rates of vertical transmission through all three routes combined average 25% to 30%, ranging from 13% to 43% in developing countries and from 14% to 25% in developed settings.[101] The majority of infants who are infected with HIV-1 acquire the infection in utero or during childbirth. The risk of perinatal transmission of HIV-2 is much lower than the risk of perinatal transmission of HIV-1.[2]

HIV-1 transmission via breastmilk probably is greater when the mother becomes infected postpartum than before delivery, because the maternal viral load is high during initial infection and because HIV in the milk is not yet neutralized by the anti-infective activities of the milk, such as inhibiting the binding of HIV-1 glycoproteins to CD4 molecules.[7,69,89] Although a meta-analysis attempted to quantify the risk of vertical transmission due only to breastfeeding,[20] the attributable risk of breastfeeding for HIV transmission according to time of maternal infection is not known with certainty.[77] Studies of mother to infant transmission of HIV according to breastfeeding status have produced widely varying results. The differences may be due to methodological limitations and differences among the studies, and to vast differences in the populations studied, such as women in sub-Saharan Africa versus central Europe. Confounding factors across such widely different environments and cultures are likely to differ as well.

The majority of infants who are breastfed by HIV-positive mothers do not become infected. Viral shedding into the milk is intermittent, and the persistence of HIV-specific antibodies in breastmilk confers some protection against transmission.[89] The duration of breastfeeding is not necessarily associated with HIV transmission[32] although some studies have found a substantial risk of late postnatal transmission via breastmilk.[22,77] These observations suggest the anti-HIV factors present in breastmilk do provide some protection against HIV transmission during breastfeeding.

It is clear that breastfeeding can be a route for HIV transmission. It is also clear that breastmilk is normally protective (albeit to an unknown degree) against enveloped viruses such as HIV. However, since the consequence of HIV infection through breastfeeding is virtually always fatal for the infant, it would be important to avoid even a modest risk of infection (even though the exact magnitude of the risk through breastfeeding is not yet certain). Therefore, HIV-infected mothers in the United States are advised to avoid breastfeeding.[11] In developing country settings where the risk of infant mortality from bottle feeding is high, women are advised to breastfeed regardless of their HIV status.[106]

B REASTFEEDING: EFFECTS ON THE MOTHER

Breastfeeding has a major protective effect against cancer of the ovaries (premenopausal), endometrium, and breast.[21,76,79] Breastmilk is free and always available at the right temperature, in contrast to infant formula. Breastfeeding also promotes emotional bonding between mother and infant. Finally, the breastfeeding mother experiences a rapid return of uterine tone. Oxytocin, which induces uterine contraction, is released from the posterior pituitary when the nipple is stimulated by suckling.

During lactation, the body's estrogen levels are very low, causing decreased and delayed vaginal lubrication during sexual intercourse. When cycling resumes or when the frequency of breastfeeding declines, vaginal lubrication returns to normal. Nursing mothers have added requirements for calories, protein, calcium, and iron, as well as several vitamins and other micronutrients. The increased needs for specific nutrients can be provided by a well-balanced diet. Supplements are generally unnecessary unless the diet is deficient in one or more of these nutrients.[40,107]

INSTRUCTIONS FOR AND INFORMATION ABOUT BREASTFEEDING

1. Congratulations! Enjoy your baby, rest, and keep in touch with your clinician.

2. Health experts concur that all women should be enabled to breast-feed, and to breastfeed exclusively for 4 to 6 months.

3. **If you are not breastfeeding, begin using a contraceptive method immediately.** You can become pregnant before your first menstrual period after childbirth because ovulation can begin before menstruation.

4. **If you are breastfeeding and providing bottle supplements, begin using a contraceptive method as soon as your clinician advises based on the method you have chosen.**

5. **To use the Lactational Amenorrhea Method (LAM) as a temporary method of contraception, you must feed your baby on demand, avoid any bottle feeds, and provide any minimal supplements by cup or spoon**. Begin using another method of contraception when you resume menstruation, when you reduce the frequency or duration of breastfeeds, when you introduce bottle feeds or regular food supplements, or when your baby turns 6 months old. (See Figures 23-2 and 23-3.)

6. **You can become pregnant while breastfeeding your baby,** although the risk is greatly reduced before your first menstrual period, in the first 6 months when you feed your baby on demand, avoid any bottle feeds, and provide minimal supplements by cup or spoon: your risk of pregnancy will be about 2%, equivalent to or lower than the risk associated with many other contraceptive

methods. Most U.S. women do not follow breastfeeding patterns that confer maximum protection against pregnancy. However, women who choose LAM may adopt breastfeeding behaviors that maximize both milk production and the duration of amenorrhea.

7. **Breastfeeding is a convenient, inexpensive, and nutritious way to feed your baby and it helps to protect the baby against infection, diarrhea, allergy, and sudden infant death syndrome. It also offers you protection against cancer of the breast, ovary, and uterus.**

8. **Neither intercourse nor menstruation affects the quality or quantity of your breastmilk. You do not need to stop breastfeeding because you start having intercourse again or start your period.** You can continue breastfeeding when you start using another contraceptive method.

9. **Lubricants, such as K-Y Jelly, spermicides, or saliva, may make intercourse easier after childbirth** because decreased estrogen production during breastfeeding diminishes vaginal lubrication.

10. **When you are nursing your child, your own nutrition is important.** Women can usually obtain all the calories and nutrients they need to breastfeed through their usual diet. There is no need to buy any special foods. Just eat a sensible, well-balanced diet, which is always a good idea.

11. **Avoid smoking.** Nursing women who smoke may transfer nicotine to their infant through their breastmilk. Nicotine is a poison that can harm the child. Inhaling smoke is also harmful to the baby. Smoking may also influence your ability to produce milk.

12. **Alcohol that you drink will be passed to your baby through breastmilk.** Your baby will have more difficulty metabolizing alcohol than you do, especially in the first few weeks after delivery. No good studies have been conducted to assess what level of alcohol consumption is safe. Thus it seems prudent to drink only modest amounts of alcohol.

13. **If you are using any medications while breastfeeding, be sure to tell your physician.** You can breastfeed while using virtually all common drugs. However, for some medications you may need advice concerning the best timing for ingestion to decrease infant exposure.

14. **If you are infected with HIV, the virus that causes AIDS, you could transmit the virus to your baby through breastmilk.** For this reason, most experts recommend that you not breastfeed your baby.

15. It is indeed possible to combine work and breastfeeding successfully, yet any separation of mother from infant for more than a few hours can create challenges to breastfeeding. Working women (or any breastfeeding woman!) should be sure to locate a certified lactation consultant, preferably before delivery, who can help in the event of any difficulty, from engorgement to declining milk supply. Lactation consultants are highly trained to give advice on a broad spectrum of breastfeeding issues, including the storage and transport of expressed milk, and can often help you rent an electric breast pump if you need one. The headquarters of the International Lactation Consultants Association can help you locate a certified lactation consultant near you (telephone: 919-787-5181). (See also Chapter 11 on Selected Reproductive Health Resources.)

REFERENCES

1. Acheson LS, Danner SC. Postpartum care and breast-feeding. Prim Care 1993;20:729-747.
2. Adjorlolo-Johnson G, De Cock KM, Ekpini E, Vetter KM, Sibailly T, Brattegaard K, Yavo D, Doorly R, Whitaker JP, Kestens L, Ou C-Y, George JR, Gayle HD. Prospective comparison of mother-to-child transmission of HIV-1 and HIV-2 in Abidjan, Ivory Coast. JAMA 1994;272:462-466.
3. American Academy of Pediatrics Committee on Drugs. The transfer of drugs and other chemicals into human milk. Pediatrics 1994;93:137-150.
4. American College of Obstetricians and Gynecologists. Postpartum tubal sterilization. Int J Gynaecol Obstet 1992;39:244.
5. Association for Voluntary Surgical Contraception (AVSC). Safe and voluntary surgical contraception. New York NY: AVSC International, 1995.
6. Bedinghaus JM, Melnikow J. Promoting successful breast-feeding skills. Am Fam Physician 1992;45:1309-1318.
7. Bélec L, Bouquety JC, Georges AJ, Siopathis MR, Martin PMV. Antibodies to human immunodeficiency virus in the breast milk of healthy seropositive women. Pediatrics 1990;85:1022-1026.
8. Burkman RT. Puerperium and breast-feeding. Curr Opin Obstet Gynecol 1993;5:683-687.
9. Campbell OMR, Gray RH. Characteristics and determinants of postpartum ovarian function in women in the United States. Am J Obstet Gynecol 1993;169:55-60.
10. Casterline JB, Singh S, Cleland J, Ashurst H. The proximate determinants of fertility. WFS Comparative Studies, Number 39. Voorburg, The Netherlands: International Statistical Institute, 1984.
11. Centers for Disease Control (CDC). Recommendations for assisting in the prevention of perinatal transmission of human T-lymphotropic virus type III/lymphadenopathy-associated virus and acquired immunodeficiency syndrome. MMWR 1985;34:721-726, 731-732.
12. Chi I, Potts M, Wilkens LR, Champion CB. Performance of the copper T-380A intrauterine device in breastfeeding women. Contraception 1989;39:603-618.

13. Chi IC, Thapa S. Postpartum tubal sterilization: an international perspective on some programmatic issues. J Biosoc Sci 1993;25:51-61.
14. Chvapil M, Eskelson CD, Stiffel V, Owen JA, Droegemueller W. Studies on nonoxynol-9. II. Intravaginal absorption, distribution, metabolism and excretion in rats and rabbits. Contraception 1980;22:325-339.
15. Cowie AT, Forsyth IA, Hart IC. Hormonal control of lactation. Berlin, Germany: Springer-Verlag, 1980:164-165.
16. Cunningham AS. Breastfeeding, bottlefeeding and illness: an annotated bibliography, 1986. In: Jelliffe DB, Jelliffe EFP (eds). Programmes to promote breastfeeding. Oxford, England: Oxford University Press, 1988:448-480.
17. Curtis EM. Oral-contraceptive feminization of a normal male infant. Obstet Gynecol 1964;23:295-296.
18. Díaz S, Croxatto HB. Contraception in lactating women. Curr Opin Obstet Gynecol 1993;5:815-822.
19. Diaz S, Seron-Ferre M, Croxatto HB and Veldhuis J. Neuroendocrine mechanisms of lactational infertility in women. Biol Res 1995;28:155-163.
20. Dunn DT, Newell ML, Ades AE, Peckham CS. Risk of human immunodeficiency virus type 1 transmission through breastfeeding. Lancet 1992;340:585-588.
21. Eaton SB, Pike MC, Short RV, Lee NC, Trussell J, Hatcher RA, Wood JW, Worthman CM, Blurton Jones NG, Konner MJ, Hill KR, Bailey R, Hurtado AM. Women's reproductive cancers in evolutionary context. Q Rev Biol 1994;69:353-367.
22. Ekpini ER, Wiktor SZ, Satten GA, Adjorlolo-Johnson GT, Sibailly TS, Ou CY, Karon JM, Brattegaard K, Whitaker JP, Gnaore E, De Cock KM, Greenberg AE. Late postnatal mother-to-child transmission of HIV-1 in Abidjan, Côte d'Ivoire. Lancet 1997;349:1054-1059.
23. Erwin PC. To use or not to use combined hormonal oral contraceptives during lactation. Fam Plann Perspect 1994;26:26-30, 33.
24. Faich G, Pearson K, Fleming D, Sobel S, Anello C. Toxic shock syndrome and the vaginal contraceptive sponge. JAMA 1986;255:216-218.
25. Farr G, Rivera R. Interactions between intrauterine contraceptive device use and breast-feeding status at time of intrauterine contraceptive device insertion: analysis of TCu-380A acceptors in developing countries. Am J Obstet Gynecol 1992;167:144-151.
26. Ford K, Labbok M. Contraceptive usage during lactation in the United States: an update. Am J Public Health 1987;77:79-81.
27. Fraser IS. A review of the use of progestogen-only minipills for contraception during lactation. Reprod Fertil Dev 1991;3:245-254.
28. Glasier AF, Logan J, McGlew TJ. Who gives advice about postpartum contraception? Contraception 1996;53:217-220.
29. Gordon K, Renfree MB, Short RV, Clarke IJ. Hypothalamo-pituitary portal blood concentrations of ß-endorphin during suckling in the ewe. J Reprod Fertil 1987;79:397-408.
30. Gray RH, Campbell OM, Apelo R, Eslami SS, Zacur H, Ramos RM, Gehret JC, Labbok MH. Risk of ovulation during lactation. Lancet 1990;335:25-29.
31. Gray RH, Campbell OM, Zacur H, Labbok MH, MacRae SL. Postpartum return of ovarian activity in non-breastfeeding women monitored by urinary assays. J Clin Endocrinol Metab 1987;64:645-650.

32. Guay LA, Hom DL, Mmiro F, Piwowar EM, Kabengera S, Parsons J, Ndugwa C, Marum L, Olness K, Kataaha P, Jackson JB. Detection of human immunodeficiency virus type 1 (HIV-1) DNA and p24 antigen in breast milk of HIV-1-infected Ugandan women and vertical transmission. Pediatrics 1996;98:438-444.

33. Guillebaud J. Contraception, your questions answered. New York: Churchill, 1993.

34. Guillebaud J. Postpartum contraception unnecessary before three weeks. Br Med J 1993;307:1560-1561.

35. Harlap S. Exposure to contraceptive hormones through breast milk—are there long-term health and behavioral consequences? Int J Gynaecol Obstet 1987;25(Suppl):47-55.

36. Hight-Laukaran V, Labbok MH, Peterson AE, Fletcher V, von Hertzen H, Van Look PFA. Multicenter study of the Lactational Amenorrhea Method (LAM): II. Acceptability, utility, and policy implications. Contraception 1997;55: 337-346.

37. Hodgen GD, Itskovitz J. Recognition and maintenance of pregnancy. In: Knobil E, Neill JD, Ewing LL, Greenwald GS, Markert CL, Pfaff DW (eds). The physiology of reproduction. New York NY: Raven Press, 1988: 1995-2021.

38. Howie PW. Natural regulation of fertility. Br Med Bull 1993;49:182-199.

39. Howie PW, Forsyth JS, Ogston SA, Clark A, du V Florey C. Protective effect of breast feeding against infection. Br Med J 1990;300:11-16.

40. Institute of Medicine (IOM). Nutrition during lactation. Washington DC: National Academy Press, 1991.

41. International Planned Parenthood Federation (IPPF). IMAP Statement on breast feeding, fertility and post-partum contraception. IPPF Med Bull 1996;30:1-3.

42. Johansson E, Odlind V. The passage of exogenous hormones into breast milk—possible effects. Int J Gynaecol Obstet 1987;25(Suppl):111-114.

43. Kazi A, Kennedy KI, Visness CM, Khan T. Effectiveness of the lactational amenorrhea method in Pakistan. Fertil Steril 1995;64:717-723.

44. Kennedy KI, Gross BA, Parenteau-Carreau S, Flynn AM, Brown JB, Visness CM. Breastfeeding and the symptothermal method. Stud Fam Plann 1995;26:107-115.

45. Kennedy KI, Labbok MH, Van Look PFA. Consensus statement—lactational amenorrhea method for family planning. Int J Gynaecol Obstet 1996;54: 55-57.

46. Kennedy KI, Parenteau-Carreau S, Flynn A, Gross B, Brown JB, Visness C. The natural family planning - lactational amenorrhea method interface: observations from a prospective study of breastfeeding users of natural family planning. Am J Obstet Gynecol 1991;165:2020-2026.

47. Kennedy KI, Rivera R, McNeilly AS. Consensus statement on the use of breastfeeding as a family planning method. Contraception 1989;39: 477-496.

48. Kennedy KI, Short RV, Tully MR. Premature introduction of progestin-only contraceptive methods during lactation. Contraception 1997;55:347-350.

49. Kennedy KI, Visness CM. A comparison of two U.S. surveys of infant feeding. J Hum Lact 1997;13:39-43.

50. Kovar MG, Serdula MK, Marks JS, Fraser DW. Review of the epidemiologic evidence for an association between infant feeding and infant health. Pediatrics 1984;74(4-Suppl):615-638.
51. Labbok MH. Consequences of breastfeeding for mother and child. J Biosoc Sci 1985;9(Suppl):43-54.
52. Labbok MH. Contraception during lactation: considerations in advising the individual and in formulating programme guidelines. J Biosoc Sci 1985;9(Suppl):55-66.
53. Labbok M, Cooney K, Coly S. Guidelines: breastfeeding, family planning, and the Lactational Amenorrhea Method—LAM. Washington DC: Institute for Reproductive Health, Georgetown University, 1994.
54. Labbok MH, Hight-Laukaran V, Peterson AE, Fletcher V, von Hertzen H, Van Look PFA. Multicenter study of the Lactational Amenorrhea Method (LAM): I. Efficacy, duration, and implications for clinical application. Contraception 1997;55:327-336.
55. Labbok M, Krasovec K. Toward consistency in breastfeeding definitions. Stud Fam Plann 1990;21:226-230.
56. Labbok MH, Stallings RY, Shah F, Pérez A, Klaus H, Jacobson M, Muruthi T. Ovulation method use during breastfeeding: is there increased risk of unplanned pregnancy? Am J Obstet Gynecol 1991;165:2031-2036.
57. Lewis PR, Brown JB, Renfree MB, Short RV. The resumption of ovulation and menstruation in a well-nourished population of women breastfeeding for an extended period of time. Fertil Steril 1991;55:529-536.
58. Lucas A, Cole TJ. Breast milk and neonatal necrotising enterocolitis. Lancet 1990;336:1519-1523.
59. Lucas A, Morley R, Cole TJ, Lister G, Leeson-Payne C. Breast milk and subsequent intelligence quotient in children born preterm. Lancet 1992;339:261-264.
60. Masters WH, Johnson VE. Human sexual response. Boston: Little, Brown and Company, 1966.
61. McCann MF, Liskin LS, Piotrow PT, Rinehart W, Fox G. Breastfeeding, fertility and family planning. Popul Reports 1984;12(2), Series J(24).
62. McCann MF, Moggia AV, Higgins JE, Potts M, Becker C. The effects of a progestin-only oral contraceptive (Levonorgestrel 0.03 mg) on breastfeeding. Contraception 1989;40:635-648.
63. McCann MF, Potter LS. Progestin-only oral contraception—a comprehensive review. Contraception 1994;50:S1-S198.
64. McGregor JA. Lactation and contraception. In: Neville MC, Neifert MR (eds). Lactation. Physiology, nutrition, and breast-feeding. New York: Plenum Press, 1983:405-421.
65. McNeilly AS. Suckling and the control of gonadotropin secretion. In: Knobil E, Neill JD (eds). The physiology of reproduction (Second Edition). New York: Raven Press, 1994:1179-1212.
66. McNeilly AS, Tay CCK, Glasier A. Physiological mechanisms underlying lactational amenorrhea. In: Human reproductive ecology: interactions of environment, fertility and behavior. New York NY: New York Academy of Sciences, 1994:145-155.
67. Moggia AV, Harris GS, Dunson TR, Diaz R, Moggia MS, Ferrer MA, McMullen SL. A comparative study of a progestin-only oral contraceptive

versus non-hormonal methods in lactating women in Buenos Aires, Argentina. Contraception 1991;44:31-43.

68. Neifert M. Early assessment of the breastfeeding infant. Contemp Pediatr 1996;13:142-166.

69. Newburg DS, Viscidi RP, Ruff A, Yolken RH. A human milk factor inhibits binding of human immunodeficiency virus to the CD4 receptor. Pediatr Res 1992;31:22-28.

70. O'Hanley K, Huber DH. Postpartum IUDs: keys for success. Contraception 1992;45:351-361.

71. Parenteau-Carreau S, Cooney KA. Breastfeeding, Lactational Amenorrhea Method, and natural family planning interface: teaching guide. Washington DC: Institute for Reproductive Health, Georgetown University, 1994.

72. Pérez A, Labbok MH, Queenan JT. Clinical study of the lactational amenorrhoea method for family planning. Lancet 1992;339:968-970.

73. Peterson HB, Xia Z, Hughes JM, Wilcox LS, Tylor LR, Trussell J. The risk of pregnancy after tubal sterilization: findings from the U.S. Collaborative Review of Sterilization. Am J Obstet Gynecol 1996;174:1161-1170.

74. Ramos R, Kennedy KI, Visness CM. Effectiveness of lactational amenorrhea in prevention of pregnancy in Manila, the Philippines: non-comparative prospective trial. Br Med J 1996;313:909-912.

75. Robinson JE, Short RV. Changes in breast sensitivity at puberty, during the menstrual cycle, and at parturition. Br Med J 1977;1:1188-1191.

76. Rosenblatt KA, Thomas DB. Prolonged lactation and endometrial cancer: WHO Collaborative Study of Neoplasia and Steroid Contraceptives. Int J Epidemiol 1995;24:499-503.

77. Ruff AJ. Breastmilk, breastfeeding and transmission of viruses to the neonate. Semin Perinatol 1994;18:510-516.

78. Speroff L, Darney PD. A clinical guide for contraception (Second Edition). Baltimore: Williams and Wilkins, 1996.

79. Speroff L, Glass RH, Kase NG. Clinical gynecologic endocrinology and infertility (Fifth Edition). Baltimore MD: Williams and Wilkins, 1994.

80. Tankeyoon M, Dusitsin N, Chalapati S, Koetsawang S, Saibiang S, Sas M, Gellen JJ, Ayeni O, Gray R, Pinol A, Zegers L. Effects of hormonal contraceptives on milk volume and infant growth. Contraception 1984;30:505-522.

81. Technical Guidance/Competence Working Group (TG/CWG). Recommendations for updating selected practices in contraceptive use. Volume II. Chapel Hill NC: Program for International Training in Health (INTRAH), School of Medicine, The University of North Carolina at Chapel Hill, 1997.

82. Technical Guidance Working Group (TGWG). Recommendations for updating selected practices in contraceptive use: results of a technical meeting. Volume I. Chapel Hill NC: Program for International Training in Health (INTRAH), School of Medicine, The University of North Carolina at Chapel Hill, 1994.

83. Thapa S, Short RV, Potts M. Breastfeeding, birth spacing and their effects on child survival. Nature 1988;335:679-682.

84. Toddywalla VS, Mehta S, Virkar KD, Saxena BN. Release of 19-nor-testosterone type of contraceptive steroids through different drug delivery systems into serum and breast milk of lactating women. Contraception 1980;21:217-223.

85. Treiman K, Liskin L, Kols A, Reinhart W. IUDs—an update. Popul Reports 1995;22(5). Series B(6).
86. Trussell J, Grummer-Strawn L, Rodríguez G, VanLandingham M. Trends and differentials in breastfeeding behavior: evidence from the WFS and DHS. Popul Stud 1992;46:285-307.
87. UNICEF. Innocenti Declaration on the protection, promotion and support of breastfeeding. New York NY: UNICEF, 1990.
88. Valdés V, Pérez A, Labbok M, Pugin E, Zambrano I, Catalan S. The impact of a hospital and clinic-based breastfeeding promotion programme in a middle class urban environment. J Trop Pediatr 1993;39:142-151.
89. Van de Perre P, Simonon A, Hitimana DG, Dabis F, Msellati P, Mukamabano B, Butera JB, Van Goethem C, Karita E, Lepage P. Infective and anti-infective properties of breastmilk from HIV-1-infected women. Lancet 1993;341: 914-918.
90. Van de Perre P, Simonon A, Msellati P, Hitimana DG, Vaira D, Bazubagira A, Van Goethem C, Stevens AM, Karita E, Sondag-Thull D, Dabis F, Lepage P. Postnatal transmission of human immunodeficiency virus type I from mother to infant. N Engl J Med 1991;325:593-598.
91. VanLandingham M, Trussell J, Grummer-Strawn L. Contraceptive and health benefits of breastfeeding: a review of the recent evidence. Int Fam Plann Perspect 1991;17:131-136.
92. Van Look PFA. Lactational amenorrhoea method for family planning. Br Med J 1996;313:893-894.
93. Virutamasen P, Leepipatpaiboon S, Kriengsinyot R, Vichaidith P, Muia PN, Sekadde- Kigondu CB, Mati JKG, Forest MG, Dikkeschei LD, Wolthers BG, d'Arcangues C. Pharmacodynamic effects of depot-medroxyprogesterone acetate (DMPA) administered to lactating women on their male infants. Contraception 1996;54:153-157.
94. Visness CM, Kennedy KI. Maternal employment and breast-feeding: findings from the 1988 National Maternal and Infant Health Survey. Am J Public Health 1997;87:945-950.
95. Visness CM, Rivera R. Progestin-only pill use and pill switching during breastfeeding. Contraception 1995;51:279-281.
96. Wenof M, Aubert JM, Reyniak JV. Serum prolactin levels in short-term and long-term use of inert plastic and copper intrauterine devices. Contraception 1979;19:21-27.
97. Wharton C, Blackburn R. Lower-dose pills. Popul Rep 1988;16(3), Series A(7).
98. Wilcox LS, Chu SY, Eaker ED, Zeger SL, Peterson HB. Risk factors for regret after tubal sterilization: 5 years of follow-up in a prospective study. Fertil Steril 1991;55:927-933.
99. Willson JR. The puerperium. In: Willson JR, Carrington ER, Ledger WJ, Laros RK, Mattox JH (eds). Obstetrics and gynecology. St. Louis MO: CV Mosby Company, 1987:598-607.
100. Woolridge MW, Phil D, Baum JD. Recent advances in breast feeding. Acta Paediatr Jpn 1993;35:1-12.
101. Working Group on Mother-to-Child Transmission of HIV. Rates of mother-to-child transmission of HIV-1 in Africa, America, and Europe: results from 13 perinatal studies. J Acquir Immune Defic Syndr Hum Retrovirol 1995;8:506-510.

102. World Health Organization. Improving access to quality care in family planning—medical eligibility criteria for initiating and continuing use of contraceptive methods. Geneva: Family and Reproductive Health Division, World Health Organization, 1996.

103. World Health Organization. Progestogen-only contraceptives during lactation: I. Infant growth. Contraception 1994;50:35-53.

104. World Health Organization. Progestogen-only contraceptives during lactation: II. Infant development. Contraception 1994;50:55-68.

105. World Health Organization Task Force on Oral Contraceptives. Contraception during the postpartum period and during lactation: the effects on women's health. Int J Gynaecol Obstet 1987;25(Suppl):13-26.

106. World Health Organization/UNICEF. Consensus statement from the consultation on HIV transmission and breastfeeding. J Hum Lact 1992;8:173-174.

107. Worthington-Roberts BS, Williams SR. Nutrition in pregnancy and lactation (Fifth Edition). St. Louis MO: Mosby-Year Book, Inc., 1993: 340.

Future Methods

Henry L. Gabelnick, PhD

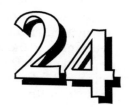

- Renewed emphasis is being placed on developing female-controlled methods that protect against both pregnancy and sexually transmitted infections (STIs).
- Researchers are investigating new delivery mechanisms for hormonal methods, with their strong record of safety and efficacy.

- New IUD designs may reduce side effects such as cramping and excess bleeding.

Concerns about product liability continue to have a major detrimental impact on development and availability of new methods. Large companies are reluctant to take risks on highly innovative approaches, and smaller companies often do not have the resources to do so. Not only have companies dropped their research programs in the face of these obstacles, but other companies have refused to supply raw materials for contraceptive products. Most new leads continue to come from public sector organizations whose budgets are severely restricted by overall government funding cutbacks. Nevertheless, a number of contraceptive leads being developed by public and private sector organizations could result in new products over the next decade. These include new barrier methods, both mechanical and chemical, new hormonal delivery systems, new intrauterine devices (IUDs), and possibly a systemic method for men. Although the search for an effective, safe immunocontraceptive also continues, none will be available for some time.

MECHANICAL BARRIER METHODS

In light of the current prevalence of infection with human immunodeficiency virus (HIV) and other sexually transmitted infections (STIs), researchers and policy makers emphasize development of methods that are more user friendly, effective, and female controlled so women may better protect themselves. Research has focused on enhancing effectiveness and minimizing annoying side effects of barrier methods, which have long provided some protection against both pregnancy and disease. Some products of this research are already on the market: the Reality Female condom and the plastic male condom.

Female condom.   Reality, the female condom now available in the United States, is a polyurethane sheath that protects all of the vaginal lining, thus providing good protection against pathogens. (See Chapter 18 on Vaginal Barriers.) Although the clinical studies of this device showed it to be about as effective as other female-controlled barrier methods such as the sponge and cervical cap, analysis of failure under perfect use (used correctly and consistently) indicate a high efficacy.[7,15] An acceptability study undertaken in New York indicated that two-thirds of the users liked the device either somewhat or very much.[8] Alternative designs and materials have been proposed but it is unlikely major investments will be made until the acceptability of a female condom is more definitively established.

Lea's Shield.   This is a one-size-fits-all diaphragm-like device with a one-way valve to allow air to escape during placement, thus creating a suction to keep the device against the cervix. The valve allows uterine and cervical fluids to escape yet is designed to prevent sperm from getting into the cervix. The results of a small clinical study conducted in the United States indicated good efficacy that compares well with other barrier methods.[12] (See Chapter 18 on Vaginal Barriers.) The device is marketed in Canada and one or two European countries. The manufacturer submitted an application to obtain approval from the Food and Drug Administration (FDA); however, the FDA review panel requested additional clinical trials.

Femcap.   This cervical cap-like barrier method has shown promise. Femcap, resembling a sailor's cap, comes in three sizes; a user's size is based on her parity.[14] A Phase II/III clinical trial has been completed. Femcap could be approved by 1998.

Silicone diaphragm.   Prototypes of an "easy-fit" silicone diaphragm are being made with the help of a group of volunteers giving feedback on device design including comfort and ease of use. This unique process could lead to a much more user-friendly device. Expanded clinical studies are planned.

Non-latex male condoms. Although very effective for fertility and disease prevention when used consistently and stored properly, the latex condom for men all too often goes unused. Some couples complain about its interference with sexual spontaneity and pleasure. Therefore, a search for better materials to improve feel and durability has been ongoing for some time. A new polyurethane condom with a traditional design was introduced in the United States in 1994. Alternative designs using polyurethane and other synthetic elastomers are also being studied for acceptability, slippage and breakage, and efficacy. (See Chapter 16 on Male Condoms.)

CHEMICAL BARRIER METHODS

New formulations of chemical barriers would ideally enhance the ease of use and increase the product's spreadability and adhesiveness on the vaginal wall to better protect against HIV and other pathogens as well as sperm. Researchers seek to reduce the amount of vaginal tissue irritation associated with heavy use of nonoxynol-9. Such irritation has been speculated to increase a woman's susceptibility to HIV infection, even though nonoxynol-9 kills HIV in the test tube. (See Chapter 17 on Vaginal Spermicides.)

Initial clinical studies have begun on new formulations similar to the currently available vaginal contraceptive film (VCF). These new versions are designed to be easier to use and may contain alternative spermicides. Gels and sponges with new active agents or additives that enhance coating of the vaginal wall are also being evaluated. One such sponge, Protectaid, now on sale in Canada, uses very low levels of active ingredients because of the theorized synergy associated with using a combination of three active ingredients. Even if the efficacy of the combination is demonstrated, it will be difficult to get FDA approval because the agency demands a higher level of proof for efficacy claims of combination products.

Scientists continue to place a priority on developing agents that will provide protection against disease without affecting sperm. Proving efficacy against pathogens, particularly HIV, while at the same time establishing safety, including lack of teratogenicity, may turn out to be a more formidable challenge than originally thought. It is doubtful any product that is a microbicide but not a spermicide will be approved in the current decade.

HORMONAL METHODS

Because hormonal methods have had a good record of safety and efficacy, particularly with the modern formulations, there would appear to be little incentive to change them drastically. However, the introduction of Norplant and Depo-Provera into the United States has spurred an increased momentum to provide improved versions or competitive products.

Drugs that have little or no activity when taken orally are being evaluated to minimize the impact of hormones on nursing babies. The prime candidates are the natural hormone progesterone and a synthetic hormone with the code name ST-1435 (now called nestorone).[11] Progesterone, which must be delivered at the rate of at least 5 mg per day, has been formulated in vaginal rings, suppositories, and injectable polymeric microspheres. The most likely candidate for approval in the next several years is the vaginal ring. Nestorone has been incorporated in skin creams, transdermal devices, vaginal rings, and subdermal implants. Although many clinical studies have been conducted, it is too early to say with any certainty which if any of the possible formulations will be available in the near future.

IMPLANTS

Implanon.   A single implant containing the progestin 3-keto-desogestrel, Implanon should remain effective for 3 to 4 years. The implant is currently undergoing large-scale clinical trials worldwide and should appear on the market soon.[6]

Norplant 2.   An improved version of Norplant containing two rods instead of six, Norplant 2 achieves similar drug levels and duration of action. FDA approval has been obtained. (See Chapter 20 on Depo-Provera, Norplant, and Minipills.)

INJECTABLES

Levonorgestrel butanoate.   A long-acting ester, levonorgestrel butanoate is an alternative to Depo-Provera. Currently being reformulated, it could be available in 5 to 7 years.

Estrogen-containing injectables.   One of the drawbacks of the implants and injectables that contain only a progestin is the disruption of normal bleeding patterns. The World Health Organization (WHO) has tested a number of monthly injectables that contain an estrogen as well as a progestin. One such combination is CycloProvera, which contains 25 mg of depo-medroxy progesterone acetate (DMPA) and 5 mg of estradiol cypionate.[10] This combination is being introduced under a licensing arrangement with WHO using the name Cyclofem. Another product called Mesigyna contains 50 mg of norethindrone enanthate and 5 mg of estradiol valerate. Both products are highly effective and minimize bleeding disruptions. WHO recently endorsed the products. It is expected that

Cyclo Provera will be registered by the Pharmacia & Upjohn Co. in the United States within the next several years.

VAGINAL RINGS

Vaginal rings provide another method of continuous delivery of progestins. The rings are being evaluated for use with a number of compounds; the most extensively tested ring contains levonorgestrel released at the rate of 20μg/day.[17] Unfortunately, problems associated with vaginal irritation have slowed commercialization. A softer, nonirritating device has been developed but commercialization has been delayed.

Also being tested are rings that contain both an estrogen and a progestin. These would be used in the same schedule as oral contraceptives: 3 weeks of drug and 1 week without to produce a withdrawal bleed. Several combinations are in various stages of development, but it is unclear when they might be available.[2]

MALE HORMONAL METHODS

Completed studies with a prototype drug, testosterone enanthate, involving more than 400 men in nine countries resulted in consistent azoospermia in 70% of the men overall and severely inhibited sperm production in almost all (98%) of the men. Overall contraceptive efficacy among the men achieving at least severe oligospermia approached 99%.[16] The major drawbacks are a long induction period requiring additional contraceptive protection and a weekly injection schedule, which is impractical.

Under study are drug delivery systems that can deliver testosterone for 2 to 3 months[3,4] and testosterone-derivative implants that are active for up to a year. Concurrently administered drugs such as peptide hormone analogs or progestins[3] are also being examined in order to improve the efficacy.

INTRAUTERINE DEVICES (IUDS)

Although not a method with universal applicability, the IUD is an excellent method for women who are not at risk for STIs.

Frameless IUD.   A frameless IUD eliminates any pressure against the uterus and thus should minimize cramping.[16] A polypropylene thread anchors the copper-releasing sleeves in the myometrium at the fundus. In another version, a biodegradable anchoring cone allows insertion immediately postpartum. Clinical trials of both devices are under way in Europe.

Levonorgestrel IUD.   The levonorgestrel IUD, which releases levonorgestrel as the active agent, is extremely effective and should provide 7 to 10 years of protection.[13] This IUD is useful for women who have a tendency to bleed excessively. Because of its effect on cervical mucus, it might have a beneficial effect on PID, although more extensive studies would be necessary. The main disadvantage is the cost, which is higher than the currently available copper devices. Although available in Europe under the name Mirena, its availability in the U.S. remains uncertain. (See Chapter 21 on Intrauterine Devices.)

IMMUNOCONTRACEPTIVES

The goal of a safe, reversible immunological approach to contraception remains elusive despite the many leads explored over the last two or three decades.

Immunocontraceptives for women.   The most advanced testing is on hCG-based approaches, either the whole molecule or fragments.[1] Both approaches, however, are abortifacients. Thus, even if efficacy, safety, reversibility, and reproducibility could be demonstrated, it is unlikely any company will pursue hCG-based vaccines. Other antigens that prevent fertilization are more promising from a political point of view but are so early in development that none will be available in this century. They include a variety of sperm and zona pellucida antigens.

Immunocontraceptives for men.   Potential vaccines for men use either luteinizing hormone releasing hormone (LHRH) or follicle stimulating hormone (FSH). Currently being tested on men with prostate cancer, a vaccine using LHRH linked to tetanus toxoid shuts down the testes to eliminate testosterone as well as sperm production. To maintain libido and potency, the user would need to supplement the vaccine with testosterone. In contrast, the FSH-based vaccine has eliminated sperm while maintaining normal testosterone levels in monkeys. Initial clinical studies on the FSH vaccine are under way in India.

THE 21ST CENTURY

Most of the methods described above are extensions and improvements of already existing methods. A recent study by the Institute of Medicine at the National Academy of Sciences[9] explored the application of modern biology and chemistry and its associated technology to the field of contraception. The panel concluded that these techniques should accelerate the progress in solving previously intractable problems. Therefore, we can look forward to future editions of *Contraceptive Technology* that will contain descriptions of truly revolutionary approaches to fertility regulation and prevention of STIs.

REFERENCES

1. Aitken RJ, Paterson M, Koothan PT. Contraceptive vaccines. Br Med Bull 1993;49:88-99.
2. Ballagh SA, Mishell DR Jr, Jackanicz TM, Lacarra M, Eggena P. Dose-finding study of a contraceptive ring releasing norethindrone acetate/ethinyl estradiol. Contraception 1994;50:535-549.
3. Bebb RA, Anawalt BD, Christensen RB, Paulsen CA, Bremner WJ, Matsumoto AM. Combined administration of levonorgestrel and testosterone induces more rapid and effective suppression of spermatogenesis than testosterone alone: a promising male contraceptive approach. J Clin Endocrin Metabol 1996; 81:757-762.
4. Behr HM, Baus S, KlieschS, Keck C, Simoni M, Nieschlag E. Potential of testosterone buciclate for male contraception: endocrine differences between responders and non-responders. J Clin Endocrin Metabol 1995;80:394-403.
5. Bhasin S, Swerdloff RS, Steiner BS, Peterson MA, Meridores T, Galmirini M, Pandian M, Goldberg R, Berman N. A biodegradable testosterone microcapsule formulation provides uniform eugonadal levels of testosterone for 10-11 weeks. JCEM 1992;74:75-83.
6. Davies GC, Li XF, Newton JR. Release characteristics, ovarian activity and menstrual bleeding pattern with a single contraceptive implant releasing 3-ketodesogestrel. Contraception 1993;47:251-261.
7. Farr G, Gabelnick H, Sturgen G, Dorflinger L. Contraceptive efficacy and acceptability of the female condom. Am J Publ Health 1994;84:1960-1964.
8. Gollub EL, Stein Z, el-Sadir W. Short-term acceptability of the female condom among staff and patients at a New York City hospital. Fam Plann Perspect 1995;27:155-158.
9. Institute of Medicine. Contraceptive research and development. Harrison PF, Rosenfield A (eds). Washington DC: National Academy Press, 1996.
10. Koetsawang S. The injectable contraceptive: present and future trends. Ann NY Acad Sci 1991;626:30-42.
11. Lahteenmaki PL, Lahteenmaki P. Concentration-dependent mechanisms of ovulation inhibition by the progestin ST-1435. Fertil Steril 1985;44: 20-24.
12. Mauck C, Glover LH, Miller E, Allen S, Archer DF, Blumenthal P, Rosensweig BA, Dominik R, Sturgen K, Cooper J, Fingerhut F, Peacock L, Gabelnick HL. Lea's Shield: a study of the safety and efficacy of a new vaginal barrier contraceptive used with and without spermicide. Contraception 1996;53:329-336.
13. Rybo G, Anderson K, Odlind V. Hormonal intrauterine devices. Ann Med 1993;25:143-147.
14. Shihata AA, Gollub E. Acceptability of a new intravaginal barrier contraceptive device (Femcap). Contraception 1992;46:511-519.
15. Trussell J, Sturgen K, Strickler J, Dominik R. Comparative contraceptive efficacy of the female condom and other barrier methods. Fam Plann Perspect 1994;26:66-72.

16. Wildemeersch D, Van der Pas H, Thiery M, Van Kets H, Parewijck W, Delbarge W. The Copper-Fix (Cu-Fix): a new concept in IUD technology. Adv Contracept 1988;4:197-205.
17. WHO Task Force on Long-Acting Systemic Agents for Fertility Regulation. Microdose intravaginal levonorgestrel contraception: a multi-centre clinical trial. I. Contraceptive efficacy and side effects. Contraception 1990;41: 105-124.
18. WHO Task Force on Methods for Regulation of Male Fertility. Contraceptive efficacy of testosterone-induced azoospermia and oligospermia in normal men. Fert Steril 1996; 65:821-829.

Preconception Care

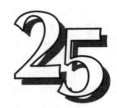

Luella Klein, MD
Felicia Stewart, MD

- Steps to assure the best possible pregnancy outcome need to begin *months* or even *years* beforehand. Reproductive tract infections acquired during pregnancy, or persisting untreated, pose multiple risks to mother, fetus, and neonate.

- Pregnancy affords an important opportunity to encourage woman to adopt healthier behaviors. For example, the 25% of women who smoke and 20% who drink alcohol can improve their chances for a healthy baby by stopping these behaviors.

Sometime during the reproductive years, most women wish to become pregnant and most men wish to become fathers. Optimal pregnancy outcomes for both mother and fetus depend on advance planning to provide the best environment for conception and pregnancy. All women and men need to know about pre-pregnancy health measures long before a pregnancy occurs. These measures include steps to protect future fertility and maintain good general health as well as steps more specifically needed when a woman contemplates pregnancy in the near future. If pregnancy occurs accidentally, the opportunity to prepare is lost; this is one of the important health reasons for avoiding unintended pregnancy. In addition, a medical visit specifically for preconception care is recommended to assure systematic review of a medical history, completion of recommended screening tests, and planning for pregnancy care.[2]

ESSENTIAL PRE-PREGNANCY INFORMATION FOR EVERYONE

Every family planning visit or routine periodic exam is an opportunity to provide preconception education and care. Ask each patient about plans for pregnancy in the future. Counsel about effective contraceptive use: how an optimal pregnancy outcome is correlated with its intendedness and the woman's ability to prepare in advance. Assess lifestyle and personal health risk factors. If appropriate, provide screening and offer preventive services. In addition to educating about the general pre-pregnancy health precautions (Table 25-1), check for diabetes in any woman with risk factors such as a family history of diabetes or obesity. Diabetes is common and, often, unsuspected. Poor control of blood sugar during the very early weeks of pregnancy is associated with a marked increase in risk for fetal abnormality.[5]

Include pre-pregnancy education and preconception planning during routine visits. Some situations pose uniquely opportune "teachable moments," when education about optimal pregnancy is likely to be directly relevant to the patient:

- A negative pregnancy test result
- Diagnosis and management of a reproductive tract infection
- Identification of possible risk of infection with the human immunodeficiency virus (HIV)
- Diagnosis of a reproductive tract abnormality
- Identification of a substance abuse problem
- Diagnosis of a significant medical problem

In each of these situations, providing information about possible consequences and planning needed for optimal future pregnancy is an essential aspect of medical management.

Negative pregnancy test visits are a common and under-exploited opportunity for intervention. As many as one-quarter of all adolescent girls who conceive have had one or more visits to learn that their pregnancy test was negative.[18] Clearly, this is a group at high risk for unintended pregnancy. In these encounters, review how to successfully use contraception and provide basic education about health precautions needed before pregnancy. If the woman intends to become pregnant in the near future, a visit specifically for structured preconception care is indicated.[2]

Table 25-1 Pre-pregnancy health precautions

Avoid toxic exposure	Tobacco, alcohol, and illicit drugs are potentially toxic to fetal development; minimizing caffeine may also be reasonable. Avoid exposure to abdominal x-ray and to potentially toxic chemicals.
Take folic acid (prenatal vitamin)	Beginning several months before pregnancy, take a vitamin that contains at least 400 micrograms (mcg) of folic acid (folate) every day to reduce the risk for neural tube defects such as spina bifida.
Make healthy diet a top priority	Dieting for weight-loss is not recommended during pregnancy. A well-balanced diet with fresh fruits and vegetables is recommended; drink 3 glasses of milk daily to ensure a total of 1500 mg of calcium, or take calcium supplements to provide this amount.
Discuss all medications with your clinician	Discuss possible pregnancy effects with your clinician before taking any medication. This includes prescription and non-prescription drugs as well as herbal or other remedies. Avoid mega-dose anything, including vitamins.
Review your immunization status	Check to be sure your immunizations are up to date, especially rubella (German measles); if not, arrange for this at least 3 months before you want to become pregnant.
Review medical and family histories for you and for the baby's father	If either of you has a family history of genetic abnormalities, counseling or testing may be helpful. If you have any serious medical problems, discuss them with your clinician before pregnancy. Make sure you do not have diabetes; if you do, careful management during early pregnancy reduces the risk of birth defects.
Avoid elevated body temperature or fever	Do what you can to avoid exposure to contagious illnesses like flu, or activities such as sauna, hot tubs, or prolonged physical exertion that might cause elevated core body temperature. Elevated temperature can increase the risk of abnormal fetal development.
Write down menstrual cycle dates	A record of the first day of each menstrual period will help your clinician determine your pregnancy due date accurately. This is especially important if tests are needed during pregnancy or if you need to have labor induced or a C-Section delivery.
Don't risk exposure to sexually transmitted infection (STI)	Avoid intercourse or use condoms carefully if there is any chance at all of STI exposure; infection such as herpes, syphilis, gonorrhea, chlamydia, or HIV/AIDS acquired during pregnancy is a very serious risk for the fetus. Get testing and treatment promptly if you have any possible STI symptoms.
Avoid toxoplasmosis and other uncommon infectious organisms	Acquiring toxoplasmosis infection during pregnancy is a serious risk for the fetus; avoid handling kitty litter (someone else should empty it every day) and wear gloves if you are handling soil outdoors. Also avoid eating raw meat or fish, or drinking unpasteurized milk.
Confirm pregnancy early	When you think you may be pregnant, have a pregnancy test and exam as soon as you can—within the first two weeks after missing your period if at all possible. If your period is abnormal or you have any pregnancy symptoms get a test right away.

THE PRECONCEPTION CARE VISIT

A preconception care visit offers the patient a battery of services to prevent problems that could affect a pregnancy. Counseling can help a woman improve her lifestyle and health habits and consider the responsibilities of carrying a pregnancy. Counseling should also be directed toward helping the patient avoid an unintended pregnancy. Risk assessment identifies the woman at risk for a poor pregnancy outcome or for whom pregnancy will endanger her health. Screening tests reveal a mother's underlying medical and genetic conditions that may require medical intervention or may require her to make a decision about how to manage a pregnancy or whether to even attempt carrying a pregnancy. Request laboratory tests to determine the patient's blood group, Rh and antibody status, blood and platelet count, and fasting blood sugar and cholesterol levels. Finally, interventions can help a woman improve her health, adopt healthier lifestyle behaviors, and arrange necessary social and family support. Table 25-2 outlines the content of a preconception care visit.

In addition to a preconception care visit, some couples need referral for more detailed evaluation and counseling by a genetics specialist or perinatologist. Arrange a referral well in advance to allow time for testing

Table 25-2 The preconception care visit

Action	Risk Reduction
Review contraceptive use	Prevent unintended pregnancy
	Decrease chance of abortion
Improve nutrition and fitness	Improve maternal health and well-being
	Decrease risk of low-birthweight infant
Advise smoking cessation (or at least a decrease in number of cigarettes smoked)	Decrease risk of pregnancy loss
	Increase birthweight
	Decrease risk of sudden infant death syndrome (SIDS)
Advise abstinence from alcohol (or at least a decrease in amount consumed)	Prevent fetal alcohol syndrome
Supplement with folic acid	Decease risk of neural tube defects
Screen for HIV infection	Decrease perinatal transmission by giving Zidovudine (AZT)
	Avoid transmission via breast milk
Screen for hepatitis B	Protect the neonate from infection by administering vaccine
Screen for other sexually transmissible infections	Protect maternal fertility
	Prevent fetal and neonatal infection
Immunize	Prevent vaccine-preventable diseases
Control diabetes	Decrease risk of congenital anomalies
Counsel about domestic violence	Prevent injuries
Screen for genetic diseases	Provide choices about pregnancy outcome
Review psychosocial status	Improve emotional support and well-being
Screen for genital infections	Decrease risk of premature delivery by treating with antibiotics

or planning for prenatal testing during the first trimester for persons with following conditions:[5]

- The woman is age 35 or older.
- Either partner has had a child with a birth defect.
- Either partner has a birth defect or genetic disorder or has a family history of birth defects or genetic disorders.
- Either partner's ethnicity indicates risk for Tay Sachs disease (Ashkenazic Jewish), sickle cell anemia (black), or thalassemia (Mediterranean ancestry) if carrier status is not already known.
- Either partner has previously experienced three or more pregnancies ending in spontaneous abortion.
- The woman has a serious medical condition, or takes medication routinely.

FAMILY AND GENETIC CONDITIONS

Explore the patient's family history and the possibility of any genetic disorders. Chronic diseases such as hypertension or diabetes in a patient's family history frequently manifest during pregnancy.[1] Genetic disorders include congenital anomalies, mental retardation, Down syndrome, cystic fibrosis, Tay Sachs disease, phenylketonuria (PKU), muscular dystrophy, bleeding disorders, and sickle cell or thalassemia or other anemias. Screening and carrier testing are available for a number of disorders. Risks for chromosomal abnormality are strongly associated with age (Table 25-3), and many couples considering childbearing in the later reproductive years are very concerned about this issue. Prenatal testing is recommended for women who are age 35 or older at the time of delivery, and may also be reasonable when the father is age 55 or older.[5]

REPRODUCTIVE AND OBSTETRIC HISTORY

Problems that occurred during the patient's past pregnancies can suggest interventions needed before or during pregnancy. Women who have had a low-birthweight infant will need focused counseling on how to improve birthweight of the next infant. Question women who have had a previous spontaneous abortion about risk factors. Women who previously delivered by cesarean section should consider a trial of labor instead of a scheduled elective cesarean delivery.

Teach the patient to record her menstrual dates, then review her pattern of menstrual cycles for evidence of ovulation. Ask whether she has ever tried to become pregnant before, and emphasize the need to use contraceptive effectively until she wants to conceive.

Table 25-3 Mother's age and rates for chromosome abnormalities

Maternal Age	Down Syndrome (per 10,000 births)	Total Chromosome Abnormalities (per 10,000 births)
15	10	22
20	5 to 7	19
25	7 to 9	21
30	9 to 12	26
35	25 to 39	56
40	85 to 137	158
45	287 to 523	537
49	758 to 1530	1,493

Source: Adapted from Cefalo et al. (1995).

REPRODUCTIVE TRACT INFECTIONS

Some reproductive tract infections (RTIs) such as chlamydia and gonor-rhea can cause a pelvic inflammatory disease (PID) that can result in tubal damage, the most common cause of preventable infertility. (See Chapter 27 on Impaired Fertility.) Untreated or inadequately treated RTIs can infect a fetus; the risk for serious consequences is especially high if the infection is acquired during pregnancy. Syphilis, chlamydia, gonor-rhea, HIV, hepatitis B, and genital herpes can lead to severe fetal, neonatal, and infant complications and fetal death. (See Table 8-3 in Chapter 8 on Reproductive Tract Infections.) Cervical and vaginal infections such as bacterial vaginosis can also affect fetal growth and infant delivery.[13]

Asymptomatic endometrial infection following vaginal, cervical, or pelvic infection may infect the amniotic sac after conception and cause preterm labor or preterm rupture of the membranes, resulting in preterm delivery.[13] Preterm delivery is the greatest cause of infant mortality, cere-bral palsy, and developmental problems. Appropriate antibiotic therapy given *before* pregnancy might prevent conditions leading to preterm delivery. However, treatment given late in the pregnancy, or after the onset of premature labor or rupture of membranes, will usually not pre-vent preterm delivery due to infection.

Counseling for HIV infection should be a part of every preconception care evaluation. Be aware of the regulations in your state regarding HIV counseling and testing. Early identification of HIV infection is especially critical in relation to pregnancy. If the mother's positive HIV status is known, Zidovudine (AZT) treatment during pregnancy can reduce the risk of maternal-infant transmission by approximately two thirds.[7,9] Because breast milk can also transmit the virus, advise HIV-infected women to avoid breastfeeding.

Women most at risk for an RTI are those who have had multiple sexual partners or a history of a prior RTI. Women under the age of 25 years have the highest incidence of sexually transmissible infections (STIs) and should be carefully screened.[4]

IMMUNIZATIONS

Evaluate the patient's immunization status for diphtheria and tetanus, measles, mumps, rubella, varicella, hepatitis B, and polio. Bring her immunizations up to date *before* she becomes pregnant. Do *not* administer attenuated live viral immunizations during pregnancy. (Measles, mumps, and rubella vaccines are the most commonly used examples of attenuated live viral immunizations.)

Certain situations pose a special risk and call for other immunizations. Patients with pulmonary disease or other chronic problems would benefit from immunization against influenza and pneumococcus. Patients exposed to young children in day care centers, schools, or neonatal intensive care units could be at risk for rubella, cytomegalovirus, or herpes simplex. Patients exposed to cats may contract toxoplasmosis and should be tested and treated before becoming pregnant. Unfortunately, many laboratories are unable to provide accurate testing on antibody levels from prior infection. Testing is of little or no value and results are difficult to interpret when one of these infections is suspected *during* pregnancy.

PSYCHOSOCIAL AND LIFESTYLE BEHAVIORS

During pregnancy, some women feel motivated to adopt healthier behaviors. Others, however, find the natural stresses that occur during pregnancy make taking on new behaviors a more challenging undertaking. Therefore, the earlier before pregnancy a woman can practice a healthy lifestyle, the better.

Smoking. About one-fourth of women age 18 and older smoke.[8] Smoking during pregnancy increases bleeding during the pregnancy and the risk of spontaneous abortion. Mothers who smoke have infants with lower birthweights, more respiratory problems, and a higher incidence of hospital admissions compared with infants of mothers who do not smoke. They are also more likely to die of sudden infant death syndrome.

Alcohol abuse. About 20% of pregnant women drink alcohol. Fetal alcohol syndrome, associated with heavy and binge drinking during pregnancy, results in mental retardation and malformations of the brain, face, and body. Because the spectrum of defects decreases as the amount of alcohol intake decreases, an effective intervention includes simply cutting back on consumption if the mother is unable to stop drinking entirely. Although an occasional single drink may not be detrimental, regular drinking, even if only light to moderate in amount, may produce lasting effects on the neonate and child.[3]

Psychological problems. Refer patients for appropriate treatment if they suffer from depression, stress, anxiety, panic disorders, or other mental illness. These conditions interfere with good health and a comfortable pregnancy. Ask the patient about domestic violence, including verbal or psychological abuse. Domestic violence occurs and may even escalate during pregnancy and the immediate postpartum interval, affecting both the woman and her offspring.[11] Help the patient assess her own risk, arrange counseling and support, and make contingency plans to protect her safety.

Financial and social support. Pregnancy care is expensive, and without adequate insurance coverage, pregnancy and delivery can be financially devastating for a family, especially if the infant is premature or has a low birthweight. Review the patient's insurance coverage and provisions for maternity leave and child care, and provide information about federal or state programs that may be able to offer help. Evaluate the patient's social and family networks and how supportive these are of a pregnancy. Encourage the patient to improve her relationships with family and friends.

NUTRITIONAL AND FITNESS STATUS

Record every patient's height and weight to identify potential problems with obesity, poor weight gain, or eating disorders such as anorexia or bulimia. Ask about the patient's general nutritional patterns. A woman who is fasting or following an unusual diet or has pica needs counseling and education. Vegetarians will need dietary vigilance to assure they obtain adequate amounts of protein, calcium, and vitamins.

Until foods are supplemented with folic acid, every patient contemplating a pregnancy should take a folic acid supplement of at least 400 micrograms (mcg). Folic acid deficiencies have been associated with an increased risk of neural tube defects.[6,16] Maintaining calcium balance during pregnancy demands a total daily intake of 1,500 mg. Additional calcium supplementation has been suggested for prevention of eclampsia, as has the administration of aspirin. The potential promise of the initial smaller studies, however, has not been confirmed in larger clinical trials.[12,15]

Exercise, physical activity, and participation in sports or hobbies help keep women fit. On the other hand, excessive exercise can decrease body weight and hormone levels necessary to maintain a healthy pregnancy. Some women who over-exercise develop amenorrhea and osteoporosis. Pregnant women should avoid activities that expose them to risk of injury. Also, balance and coordination may be altered during pregnancy, making some activities such as skiing more dangerous than they otherwise would be.

MEDICAL CONDITIONS

Treat any underlying medical conditions. A healthy woman is more likely to have a healthy pregnancy. Evaluation will be needed if the patient has autoimmune disease, epilepsy, asthma, or renal disease.

Hypertension. Chronic hypertension is associated with intrauterine growth retardation, preeclampsia, and placental abruption, any of which may be life threatening to a fetus or newborn. Blood pressure should be controlled and the patient evaluated for end-organ damage of the cardiac, vascular, and renal systems. Review her antihypertensive medications, such as ACE inhibitors, which if continued can kill the fetus, and some diuretics, which can harm the fetus.

Diabetes. Congenital anomalies are more prevalent among offspring of insulin-dependent diabetic women. When blood sugar levels are controlled for 2 to 3 months before conception, the incidence of anomalies drops to levels found in the general population. Preconception care is especially important for diabetic women because cardiac and other anomalies occur during organogenesis in the first 7 to 8 weeks of pregnancy—the time many women first become aware they are pregnant.

Medication. Many drugs and medications can be detrimental to fetal development (Table 25-4). It is reasonable to avoid treatment with any medication that is not medically indicated. A woman who takes any drug for a significant chronic medical problem should consult with her clinician to determine whether the drug or dose needs to be altered during pregnancy. Category X drugs should be avoided for all women likely to become pregnant; category D drugs should also be avoided if at all possible; if continuing treatment is necessary for the woman's health, the lowest possible dose that is therapeutically effective should be used.[5]

ENVIRONMENT AND WORK

Inquire about any hazards or exposure to teratogens, toxins, chemicals, or radiation at home or work. Also discuss work activities. If the woman's job requires prolonged standing or walking, she should plan for careful follow-up throughout pregnancy to be certain that there is no indication of fetal growth retardation or symptoms of preterm labor.[10]

Table 25-4 Common medications that may adversely affect fetal development

Isotretinoin (Accutane)	Diethylstilbestrol
Some antibiotics (including tetracycline, streptomycin, aminogylcosides)	Lindane (Kwell)
	Lithium
Some anticoagulants (dicumarol, warfarin)	Meprobamate
Some antiepileptics (including diphenylhydantoin, tridione, paramethadione, valproic acid)	Podophyllin
	Thalidomide
Benzodiazepines (including Valium, Librium)	Some thyroid drugs (propylthiouracil, iodide, methimazole)
Some cancer chemotherapeutics (including methotrexate, aminopterin)	
Chlorpropamide	Tolbutamide
Corticosteroids (including cream or ointment)	

Source: Adapted from Stewart et al. (1987).

Note: Toxic effects depend on the drug, dose and timing of exposure. These drugs (as well as others) should be avoided during pregnancy unless treatment is medically necessary and no satisfactory alternative can be substituted.

MALE PARTNER'S RISK FACTORS

Both men and women play critical roles in relation to pregnancy. Although studies of men's roles are limited, there is some evidence that paternal smoking, alcohol use, and illicit drug use may be associated with adverse pregnancy outcomes as well as impaired fertility and impaired sexual functioning.[5] The father's age is also a factor in the risk of congenital abnormalities. Men who become fathers after age 40 have a slightly higher risk of having offspring with autosomal abnormalities such as Marfan syndrome and achondroplasia, and there is some evidence that older paternal age is associated with an increased risk for Down syndrome independent of the mother's age.[5] Male exposure to toxic chemicals and drugs is associated with increased risk for infertility and pregnancy loss through spontaneous abortion.

PRENATAL CARE

One obvious advantage of preconception care is the opportunity to plan for and arrange prenatal care. Encourage the patient to register early for prenatal care so she can take advantage of early prenatal testing and, if indicated, pregnancy ultrasound. Early care will also give her time to anticipate and complete chorionic villus sampling, amniocentesis, or other recommended tests.

In addition, describe the symptoms and signs that may signal problems during early pregnancy: bleeding, spontaneous abortion, and ectopic pregnancy. (See Chapter 26 on Pregnancy Testing).

REFERENCES

1. American College of Obstetricians and Gynecologists. Genetics screening and teratology counseling. ACOG Antepartum Record. Technical bulletin 205. Washington DC: ACOG, 1994.
2. American College of Obstetricians and Gynecologists. Preconceptional care. ACOG technical bulletin 205. Washington DC: ACOG, 1995.
3. Braun S. New experiments underscore warnings on maternal drinking. Science 1996;273:738-739.
4. Cates W Jr., Holmes KK. Sexually transmitted diseases. In: Maxcey-Rosenau-Last. Preventive medicine and public health. 14th edition. In press.
5. Cefalo RC, Moos M-K. Preconceptional health care: a practical guide. 2nd ed. St Louis MO: Mosby-Year Book, Inc., 1995.
6. Centers for Disease Control and Prevention. Recommendations for the use of folic acid to reduce the number of cases of spina bifida and other neural tube defects. MMWR 1992;41:1-7.
7. Centers for Disease Control and Prevention. Zidovudine for prevention of HIV transmission from mother to infant. MMWR 1994;43:285-287.
8. Centers for Disease Control and Prevention. Cigarette smoking among adults —United States 1994. MMWR 1996;45:588-590.
9. Connor EM, Sperling RS, Gelber R, Kiselev P, Scott G, O'Sullivan MJ, VanDyke R, Bey M, Shearer W, Jacobson RL, Jimenez E, O'Neill E, Bazin B, Delfraissy J-F, Culnane M, Coombs R, Elkins M, Moye J, Stratton P, Balsley J. Reduction of maternal-infant transmission of human immunodeficiency virus type 1 with Zidovudine treatment. N Engl J Med 1994;331:1173-1180.
10. Gabbe SG, Turner LP. Reproductive hazards of the American lifestyle: work during pregnancy. Am J Obstet Gynecol 1997;176:826-832.
11. Gazmararian JA, Lazorick S, Spitz AM, Ballard TJ, Saltzman LE, Marks JS. Prevalence of violence against pregnant women: a review of the literature. JAMA 1996;275:1915-1920.
12. Levine RJ, Hauth JC, Curet LB, Sibai BM, Catalano PM, Morris CD, DerSimonian R, Esterlitz JR, Raymond EG, Bild DE, Clemens JD, Cutler JA. Trial of calcium to prevent preeclampsia. New Engl J Med 1997;337:69-76.
13. McGregor J, French JI, Parker R, Draper D, Patterson E, Jones W, Thorsgard K, McFee J. Prevention of premature birth by screening and treatment for common genital tract infections: results of a prospective controlled evaluation. Am J Obstet Gynecol 1995;173:157-167.
14. Precis V. An update in obstetrics and gynecology. Preconceptional care. Washington DC: ACOG, 1994: 64-66.
15. Roberts JM. Prevention or early treatment of preeclampsia (ed.). New Engl J Med 1997;337:124-125.
16. Schwarz RH, Johnston RB Jr. Folic acid supplementation—when and how. Obstet Gynecol 1996;88:886-887.
17. Stewart F, Guest F, Stewart G, Hatcher R. Understanding your body. New York: Bantam Books, 1987.
18. Zabin LS, Emerson MR, Ringers PA, Sedivy V. Adolescents with negative pregnancy test results. JAMA 1996;275:113-117.

Pregnancy Testing and Management of Early Pregnancy

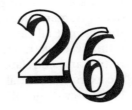

Felicia Stewart, MD

- With early pregnancy diagnosis, a woman planning to continue her pregnancy can begin prenatal precautions and medical care during the early, most vulnerable stages of fetal development.
- A woman considering abortion will have time for adequate counseling and decision making. Abortion can be performed when it is safest—early in pregnancy.

- Early pregnancy diagnosis helps ensure that ectopic pregnancy can be detected early. Early detection reduces the risk of life-threatening ectopic pregnancy complications. Early diagnosis and treatment are more likely to preserve the affected fallopian tube.

Early pregnancy diagnosis is an essential part of every family planning program. Screening very early in pregnancy can avert serious complications and provide the pregnant woman with an opportunity to learn about precautions needed during pregnancy and prenatal care resources, or about options for abortion care. Early evaluation also provides an opportunity to screen for infection with the human immunodeficiency virus (HIV). Nonjudgmental, supportive counseling and information, including accurate and specific referral options for abortion, adoption services, and prenatal care, are essential services.

Inexpensive pregnancy test kits, sensitive enough to provide accurate results as early as 1 week after fertilization, are widely available and simple to use. Thus, there is no reason to impose an arbitrary delay in pregnancy evaluation based on the date of the woman's last menstrual period. Clinical assessment and pregnancy testing should be offered as soon as the patient seeks these services.

PREGNANCY EVALUATION

Clinical evaluation for a woman who may be pregnant should include a review of pertinent history and symptoms, a laboratory test to detect human chorionic gonadotropin (hCG), and a pelvic exam. In most though not all cases, the last menstrual period date provides an accurate estimate of gestational age. A pelvic exam can confirm pregnancy test results and correlate uterine enlargement with menstrual dates. The pelvic exam is essential in identifying the possibility of abnormal pregnancy. Pregnancy diagnosis has several goals:

1. Determine whether or not the woman is pregnant.
2. Identify possible problems that require further evaluation and/or emergency intervention, such as ectopic gestation or threatened abortion.
3. Assess gestation length accurately (in weeks).
4. Help the patient make and implement her own plans for prenatal care or abortion.

History and symptoms. The most common sign that prompts a woman to seek pregnancy evaluation is an overdue menstrual period. Often the woman herself suspects pregnancy or has reason to believe that she could be pregnant. A particularly useful question to ask is simply: Do you think you are pregnant now? An unusually light or mistimed period may mean fertilization actually occurred before the last menstrual period (LMP), and for this reason, the date of the previous menstrual period (PMP) should be determined. The date when pregnancy symptoms began can help corroborate fertilization date. Breast tenderness and nipple sensitivity typically begin 1 to 2 weeks after fertilization; fatigue, nausea, and urinary frequency at about 2 weeks. Bleeding, spotting, or lower abdominal pain may signal ectopic gestation or threatened spontaneous abortion.

Physical examination. Cervical softening, blurring of the cervico-uterine angle, and uterine softening are early signs of pregnancy, appearing within the first 2 to 3 weeks after fertilization. If the uterine size does not correspond to the estimated length of gestation based on last menstrual period, consider possible reasons for the discrepancy (Table 26-1). Ultrasound evaluation often is helpful in this situation.

Table 26-1 Possible reasons for discrepancy between uterine size and menstrual dates

Uterus Smaller Than Expected	Uterus Larger Than Expected
Fertilization later than dates suggest	Fertilization earlier than dates suggest
Ectopic pregnancy	Uterine leiomyomata (fibroids)
Incomplete or missed, spontaneous abortion	Twin gestation
Error in pregnancy test	Uterine anomaly
	Hydatidiform mole

PREGNANCY TEST BIOLOGY

Pregnancy tests detect hCG in a pregnant woman's urine or serum. Correctly interpreting pregnancy test results, however, is not entirely straightforward because:

1. hCG levels change drastically over the course of pregnancy (Figure 26-1).
2. Test results, especially negative test results, must be interpreted in relation to the sensitivity, specificity, and characteristics of the particular test being used.

hCG LEVELS DURING PREGNANCY

When the blastocyst implants in the endometrium, the proliferation of trophoblastic cells initiates placental development and rapidly increasing hCG production. hCG can be detected in the woman's serum at low levels as early as 7 to 9 days after ovulation, very soon after implantation occurs. During the first 3 to 4 weeks after fertilization, the hCG level in normal pregnancy doubles approximately every 2 days so that the serum level reaches 50 to 250 mIU/ml by the time of the first missed menstrual period (Figure 26-2). hCG reaches a peak approximately 60 to 70 days after fertilization and then decreases.

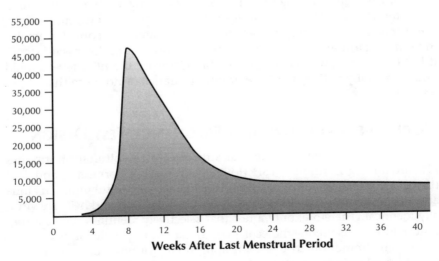

Weeks After Last Menstrual Period

Source: Braunstein et al. (1976) with permission.

Figure 26-1 hCG levels during normal pregnancy

In abnormal pregnancies, hCG levels often are abnormal. Elevated levels are normal with multiple gestation, reflecting the increased placental mass. Extremely high hCG production, with hCG levels as high as a million mIU/ml, can occur with molar pregnancy (hydatidiform mole). Such very high levels can be documented with a quantitative serum hCG test. Abnormally low hCG levels often occur before a spontaneous abortion or with an ectopic pregnancy. On the other hand, low levels may simply indicate that a normal pregnancy is earlier in gestation than menstrual dates suggest. For example, if ovulation was delayed slightly in the preceding cycle, fertilization will have actually occurred on cycle day 21 or later. Ovulation later than expected is not unusual, especially if the woman discontinued oral contraceptives in the previous menstrual cycle.

hCG Levels After Pregnancy

After a pregnancy is terminated by delivery or abortion, blood and urine hCG levels gradually decrease (Figure 26-3). The initial decrease is quite rapid, so that an hCG level after 2 weeks should be less than 1% of the level at the time the pregnancy is terminated.[4] Following full-term delivery, the level will have dropped to less than 50 mIU within 2 weeks, and hCG will be undetectable after 3 to 4 weeks. In the case of first-trimester abortion, however, initial hCG levels may be much higher. If the abortion occurs at 8 to 10 weeks of gestation when hCG may be as high as 150,000 mIU, then 2 weeks after abortion the hCG levels may still be 1,500 mIU, high enough that all pregnancy tests will still be positive. hCG may be detectable by sensitive tests for as long as 60 days after first-trimester abortion.[20] If continuing intrauterine pregnancy, retained placenta fragments, or ectopic pregnancy are possibilities, consider obtaining serial quantitative hCG levels to track an upward or downward trend. If hCG is clearing normally from the bloodstream, the hCG level should decline steadily with a half-time of disappearance of no more than 24 to 48 hours.

Hormone Structure and Pregnancy Test Design

hCG is closely related in molecular structure to the pituitary hormones LH (luteinizing hormone), FSH (follicle stimulating hormone), and TSH (thyroid stimulating hormone). Each is composed of two subunits: an alpha and a beta subunit. The alpha subunits of LH, FSH, TSH, and hCG are virtually identical. Therefore, only a test that selectively identifies the beta subunit of hCG or its unique molecular conformation is specific for hCG.

Two-site, immunometric test kits appropriate for office or home use are specific for hCG, and so is the beta subunit radioimmunoassay used for

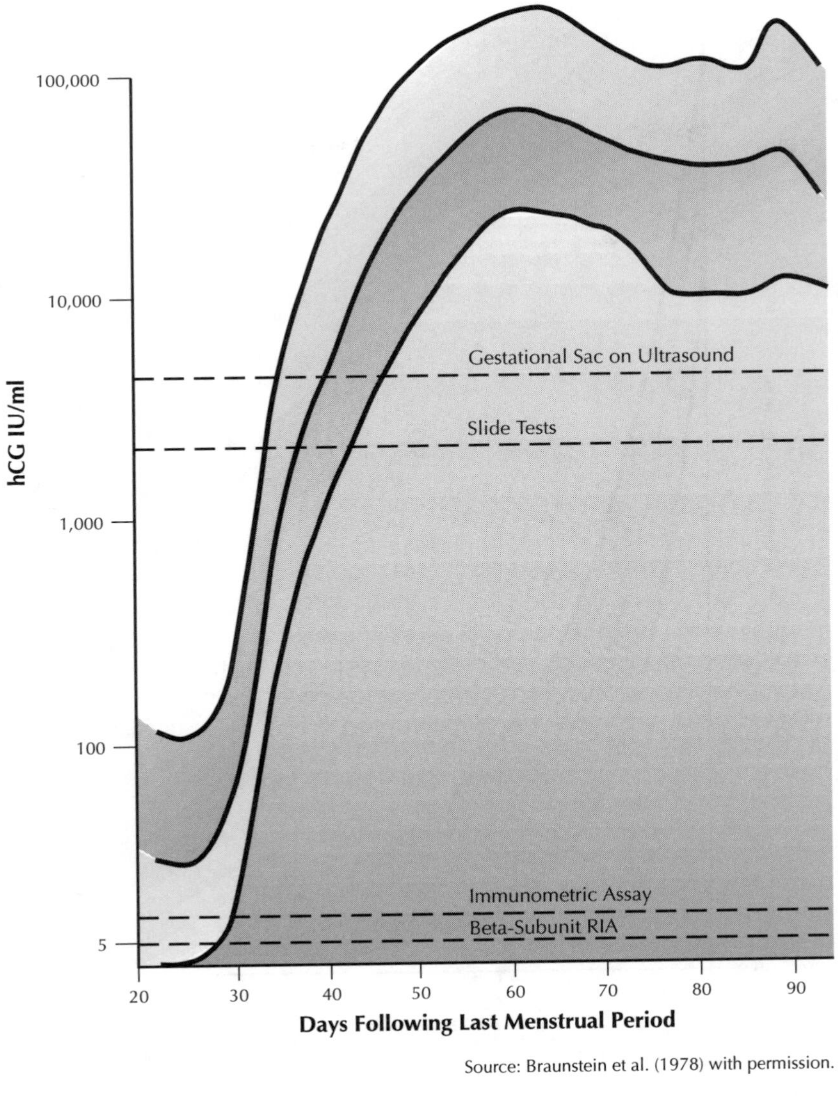
100,000
10,000
1,000
100
5
hCG IU/ml
Gestational Sac on Ultrasound
Slide Tests
Immunometric Assay
Beta-Subunit RIA
20
30
40
50
60
70
80
90
Days Following Last Menstrual Period
Source: Braunstein et al. (1978) with permission.

Figure 26-2 hCG levels in early pregnancy

quantitative serum hCG determination in the laboratory. Most agglutination inhibition slide tests, however, detect whole hCG rather than the beta subunit and therefore show at least some cross-reactivity with other hormones, especially LH. Because they are so inexpensive and simple to

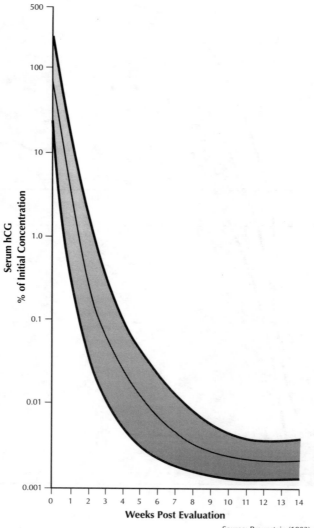

Source: Braunstein (1983) with permission.

Figure 26-3 hCG disappearance after pregnancy

use, slide tests nevertheless may be an appropriate option in certain circumstances. Other, older test methods including tube tests and radio-receptor assays are no longer needed.

PREGNANCY TEST OPTIONS

Pregnancy testing has been revolutionized with the development of monoclonal antibody techniques. Many monoclonal test kits, as well as old agglutination slide tests, are available so that the array of options is bewildering and ever-changing. Test kits suitable for use in the family planning clinic or clinician's office are shown in Table 26-2.

IMMUNOMETRIC TESTS

Immunometric tests exploit technology that has made possible the inexpensive production of pure antibody in large quantities. Immunometric tests for pregnancy are based on the ELISA (enzyme-linked immunosorbent assay) assay design; they are sometimes called "two-site" or sandwich tests and require two different antibodies. One antibody captures the beta subunit of hCG; the other antibody is conjugated to an enzyme that provides a color change. Because immunometric tests are specific for the beta subunit of hCG, cross-reaction with other hormones is not a problem. Some test kits, which may also be suitable for clinic use, are available without prescription for home use.

Specificity. Immunometric tests provide accurate qualitative (yes/no) results with hCG levels as low as 5 to 50 mIU/ml, depending on the specific test kit. With a urine test kit with a sensitivity of 25 mIU/ml, results are positive for some women as early as 3 to 4 days after implantation (10 days after fertilization); test results are positive for 98% of women within 7 days after implantation.[11]

Uses. Immunometric tests can be used to confirm pregnancy, or to "rule out" the diagnosis of pregnancy. These tests are appropriate for screening prior to procedures such as biopsy or x-ray, or prior to prescribing a drug, that would be contraindicated during pregnancy. They are also appropriate in screening for possible ectopic pregnancy. Only 1% of patients with ectopic pregnancy would be missed (falsely negative) with a urine test sensitivity of 50 mIU/ml.[4]

QUANTITATIVE BETA hCG RADIOIMMUNOASSAY

Use of an RIA "blood test" as a qualitative (yes/no) pregnancy test does not have any advantage over immunometric urine tests. Immunometric kits are equally specific for hCG and provide sensitivity that is completely satisfactory for clinical evaluation, with immediate results, and at much lower cost.

Table 26-2 Commonly used clinic and office pregnancy tests

Name (Manufacturer)	Sensitivity (mIU/ml)*	Time Required	# Steps/ Comments
Immunometric Tests: Specific for beta hCG, no LH, FSH, or TSH cross-reaction Reliably detect pregnancy 7–10 days after conception, approximately one week **before** the next period is due. Cost $0.75–$3.50**			
Acceava hCG (Biostar)	25	2–3 Min	1 Step/Urine
CARDS Q.S. hCG (Quidel)	25	3 Min	1 Step/Urine
Clinistrip 25 mIU (Clinicare Technologies)	25	3–5 Min	1 Step/Urine
Combo card (LW Scientific)	25	2–5 Min	1 Step/Urine or Serum
Double-Check (Bio-Medical Products)	25	2–5 Min	1 Step/Urine
Gravi-sticks (LW Scientific)	25	2–5 Min	1 Step/Urine
Nimbus Plus (Biomerica)	25	5 Min	1 Step/Urine
OSOM hCG (Wyntek)	25	3 Min	1 Step/Urine
Icon II hCG Hybritech (Smith-Kline Diagnostics)	20	5 Min	5 Steps/Serum
Quick Vue (Quidel)	25	3 Min	1 Step/Urine
Signify (Abbott)	25	5 Min	1 Step/Urine
SureStep hCG (Applied Biotech)	25	1 Min	1 Step/Urine
SureStep hCG Combo (Applied Biotech)	25	1 Min	1 Step/Serum or Urine
Testpack plus hCG OBC combo (Abbott)	25	5 Min	1 Step/Serum or Urine
Agglutination Inhibition Slide Tests: Test antibody reacts to whole hCG, not specific for beta hCG; cross-reaction with LH, FSH, and TSH is possible. Reliably detect pregnancy 18–21 days after conception (32–36 days after last menstrual period). All require urine specimen. Cost $1.30–$2.30**			
Wampole UCG (Wampole)	1,500–2,500	2 Min	

* Sensitivity specified as the lower limit of reliable HCG detection in product literature. Test results may be positive at lower hCG levels in some cases.
** Bulk or nonprofit agency discount purchase may reduce costs significantly.

Source: Manufacturers' product literature (1997).

Note: Slide tests that detect hCG levels of approximately 500 mIU/ml are also available, but cost as much as immunometric tests. Immunometric kits are more sensitive and easier to use.

Specificity. Because radioimmunoassay (RIA) provides accurate quantitative results with hCG levels as low as 5 mIU/ml, it can detect pregnancy reliably within 7 days after fertilization. The test may be positive a few days earlier. Because the RIA test procedure requires use of radioisotopes, it is appropriate for a laboratory associated with a hospital or large clinic.

Tests are usually performed in batches because of expense; test processing requires 1 to 2 hours.

Uses. RIA can provide a quantitative result; serial test specimens can be used to check doubling time or disappearance time when ectopic pregnancy, impending spontaneous abortion, or possible retained placental fragments are being evaluated. Very high levels can be documented to confirm the diagnosis of molar pregnancy. Be sure to specify quantitative beta hCG when ordering this test. Also, serial tests should all be ordered from the same laboratory to avoid possible confusion about assay standardization differences between laboratories.

AGGLUTINATION INHIBITION SLIDE TESTS

Inexpensive agglutination inhibition slide tests, widely used for the last 20 years, depend on binding of hCG in the patient's urine with an anti-hCG antibody in the test solution. Binding of the test antibody prevents clumping (agglutination) of latex particles in the test solution.

Specificity. Because antibodies used in most slide tests are not specific for the beta subunit of hCG, cross-reactions are possible. To minimize problems of cross-reaction with LH, FSH, or TSH, slide-test sensitivity is set so that high levels of hCG are required to give a positive test result. A cross-reaction, therefore, is unlikely to be a source of clinical confusion. However, a test specimen obtained during the brief surge of LH just before ovulation or during the perimenopausal years may cause false positive results in a slide pregnancy test because of LH cross-reaction. Cross-reactivity with TSH is unlikely because its level is normally quite low.

Uses. Slide tests are inexpensive, easy to perform, and appropriate for confirming pregnancy at and after the sixth week of gestation. hCG levels early in pregnancy (the first month after fertilization) may be below the level detected by latex agglutination slide pregnancy tests. (In rare cases, the hCG level later in pregnancy [after 16 to 20 weeks] may also decline below the sensitivity for these tests.) The slide tests are not appropriate to "rule out" pregnancy because early pregnancy, ectopic pregnancy, and impending abortion may be missed. If the initial agglutination test is negative, a more sensitive test should be used (see Immunometric Tests), or the test should be repeated a few days later.

HOME PREGNANCY TESTING

Home pregnancy test kits offer the advantages of privacy, anonymity, and convenience. Moreover, they are popular. In a national survey, approximately 33% of pregnant women reported using them.[16] In another survey, 17% of college women reported that they had used a home test at least once. Most women chose home testing because results can be obtained quickly and confidentially.[12] Because home pregnancy tests are easily accessible, a woman may identify pregnancy early and thus be more able to be an active manager of her own health care.

Specificity. Unfortunately, the accuracy of home tests in actual use may not be ideal. In one study of three commonly used home kits,[14] the predictive value was only 84% for positive home test results and 62% for negative results. Another researcher found that when test kits were used by non-technical personnel, results did not agree with standard laboratory test results in approximately 10% of 200 samples tested.[15] Test accuracy can be affected by the techniques and experience of the user, and by the user's ability to follow the test instructions precisely.[19] The most common error with home pregnancy tests is a negative result that occurs because the test was performed too early in pregnancy. An incorrect result could mislead a woman, causing her to delay in getting a clinical evaluation.

Uses. If a home test result is positive, clinical evaluation is needed to confirm the pregnancy, determine the length of gestation, and identify any possible risk for ectopic or abnormal pregnancy. If the home test result is negative, clinical evaluation also may be needed to determine the cause of menstrual delay or of the other symptoms that have prompted the test, especially if the woman does not resume normal menses soon. In either case, a second pregnancy test is likely to be indicated, so that the cost of the home kit may be an unnecessary expense. On the other hand, positive results may prompt a woman to change her lifestyle earlier than were she to wait for a clinical evaluation.

AVOIDING PREGNANCY TEST INTERPRETATION ERRORS

If pregnancy test results do not agree with other clinical signs, consider the possible reasons for the discrepancy. Plan appropriate follow-up or further evaluation to protect the patient against possible consequences of an incorrect test result:

1. Any test result can be wrong. Laboratory errors do occur, including specimen mix-up and incorrectly performed test procedures. For accurate results, instructions for the kit must be followed meticulously and timed with a stopwatch. Use control solutions to verify accuracy. Observe test-kit expiration dates.

2. Know exactly what kind of pregnancy test was performed, and what sensitivity the test has. Without this information, it is not possible to assess the clinical significance of a negative result or to evaluate the possibility of a false positive result.

3. Send all serial specimens for quantitative beta hCG assays to the same laboratory. Results of quantitative immunoassay performed by different laboratories may not be comparable because of differences between immunoassay kits and standards used by different manufacturers. Some laboratories record hCG levels in metric units; these can be roughly converted to mIU by multiplying the metric results by 5.2 (10 ng/ml = 52 mIU at the Second International Standard for hCG). Results should be multiplied by 2 for comparison to the First International Standard Preparation for hCG, which is identical to the Third International Standard. Know what standard your laboratory uses.

4. Do not base clinical management on the results of a home pregnancy test. Although home kits have excellent theoretical accuracy, their use even by trained personnel may not reliably provide the sensitivity or specificity needed for optimal clinical management.[14,15,17] Be careful about accepting the results of a pregnancy test performed in another facility, especially if critical clinical situations such as ectopic pregnancy are possible.

5. False negative results are common with agglutination inhibition tests. False negative results frequently occur because the test is performed too early or too late in pregnancy. Abnormal pregnancy, urine that is too dilute, and medication that interferes with test result may all be responsible. Use an immunometric test (Table 26-1) to "rule out" pregnancy.

6. False negative results are rare with immunometric tests but can occur if test procedures are performed incorrectly (such as excessive rinsing) or if the test reader has red-green color blindness.[3] Elevated lipids, high immunoglobulin levels, and low serum protein associated with severe kidney disease also can interfere with a test assay. If a false negative result is suspected, order a quantitative beta subunit radioimmunoassay.

7. False positive pregnancy test results are not common, but they can cause perplexing dilemmas:

- False positive results with an immunometric test are very rare, but laboratory error is always possible. If a false positive result is suspected, obtain a quantitative beta subunit radioimmunoassay.
- If an agglutination inhibition slide test is positive, but the uterus is not enlarged, perform a confirmatory immunometric test. The positive result could be caused by LH cross-reaction, in which case the immunometric test will be negative because it is specific for beta hCG.

- Slide tests also can yield false positive results because of protein or blood in the urine specimen. Consider obtaining a confirmatory immunometric test if the urine specimen shows 1+ proteinuria or more. An immunometric test is likely to give an accurate (negative) result. When a positive pregnancy test is not confirmed by the presence of a pregnancy in the uterus, do not assume the test result is false. Seriously consider the possibility of an ectopic pregnancy.

8. In very rare cases, pregnancy test results are positive even though the patient is not pregnant because hCG actually is present, originating from a source other than pregnancy. hCG levels persist after a recent pregnancy or after hCG treatment. Low levels of hCG (5–30 mIU) may be associated with tumors of the pancreas, ovaries, breast, and many others.[2] Some normal postmenopausal women also have low levels of circulating hCG-like substance, whose origin is unknown.[4]

MANAGING PROBLEMS IN EARLY PREGNANCY

Consider the possibility of spontaneous abortion or ectopic pregnancy whenever a woman in the reproductive years has symptoms such as abdominal pain, abnormal bleeding, or irregular or missed menstrual periods. The patient's history, as well as her own assessment of pregnancy risk, may be helpful. For example, in a study of women undergoing evaluation at a hospital emergency department, 63% of the women who thought they might be pregnant, were pregnant. A sensitive pregnancy test, however, is a prudent precaution to take, no matter what the woman's history indicates. In the previously cited study, 10% of women who reported a normal last menstrual period, and stated that there was no chance they could be pregnant, were nevertheless found to be pregnant.[21]

No matter what the cause or diagnosis, Rh screening is indicated for any woman with bleeding in pregnancy. The risk of Rh sensitization resulting from bleeding in early pregnancy is low, but treatment with Rh immune globulin is a wise precaution. A blood count also is indicated at the time of initial evaluation. The results may help assess the cumulative extent of bleeding and may provide an important baseline for later comparison if internal hemorrhage is suspected.

Abnormal bleeding, cramping, and abdominal pain can occur with threatened abortion, complete or incomplete spontaneous abortion, and ectopic pregnancy. However, these symptoms also can occur in an early pregnancy that subsequently progresses to a normal outcome. When these symptoms occur, perform an evaluation immediately: exclude the presence of ectopic pregnancy and arrange appropriate care for possible spontaneous abortion.

POSSIBLE ECTOPIC PREGNANCY

A woman who has clinical evidence of possible ruptured ectopic pregnancy, such as hypotension and/or postural hypotension, severe abdominal pain, guarding, or rebound tenderness requires immediate referral for emergency surgery. An ultrasensitive pregnancy test is almost certain to be positive (false negative rate is less than 1%)[4] but agglutination inhibition tests are not sensitive enough to detect the lower hCG levels associated with ectopic gestation in about 50% of cases.[1] Because intervention should not be delayed, further nonsurgical evaluation is not prudent.

More commonly, the clinician considers the possibility of ectopic pregnancy because the woman has less serious and nonspecific symptoms such as bleeding in early pregnancy, uterine enlargement that does not correlate with dates (uterus is too small), or early vacuum abortion that has failed to recover identifiable placental tissue from the uterine cavity. Often the patient is completely asymptomatic. These situations allow time for further outpatient evaluation if the patient is willing and able to monitor her own symptoms carefully. While evaluation is pending, the patient must be warned to watch for ectopic pregnancy danger signs (Table 26-3) and to return immediately for emergency care if danger signs occur. Further steps in evaluation might include the following:

1. Quantitative beta hCG assay. Although test results probably will not be available for at least 24 hours, an initial level can be compared with the beta hCG level 2 days later if diagnosis is still uncertain. A decline of 60% or more favors the diagnosis of normal hCG disappearance after spontaneous or induced abortion, or after spontaneous resolution of an ectopic pregnancy. A level of 1,000 mIU or less provides limited reassurance about the safety of outpatient management, because life-threatening intra-abdominal hemorrhage is rare with ectopic pregnancy at such an early stage of pregnancy.[18] However, clinically significant internal bleeding, while rare, has been reported even at levels below the 25 mIU/ml sensitivity of immunometric tests.

2. Pathology phone report. If an abortion has been performed, request a microscopic tissue evaluation and a report by phone. The pathologist may be able to identify placental villi and confirm intrauterine pregnancy, in which case the likelihood of simultaneous ectopic pregnancy is extremely remote.

Table 26-3 Early pregnancy danger signs

Possible Ectopic Pregnancy
Sudden intense pain, or persistent pain, or cramping in the lower abdomen, usually localized to one side or the other
Irregular bleeding or spotting with abdominal pain when period is late or after an abnormally light period
Fainting or dizziness persisting more than a few seconds. These may be signs of internal bleeding. (Internal bleeding is not necessarily associated with vaginal bleeding.)

Possible Miscarriage
Late last period and bleeding is now heavy, possibly with clots or clumps of tissue; cramping more severe than usual
Period is prolonged and heavy—5–7 days of "heaviest" days
Abdominal pain or fever

Contact your clinician immediately or go to a hospital emergency room if you develop any of these signs.

Source: Stewart et al. (1987).

3. Ultrasound evaluation. Pelvic ultrasound should be able to detect a fetus with cardiac activity inside the uterus by the 7th to 8th week of gestation dated from last menstrual period. The use of vaginal probe ultrasound moves this threshold forward by 7 to 10 days. With a vaginal probe, it is possible in some cases to detect a tiny gestational sac of 1 mm–3 mm in size in the uterus as early as 30 days after ovulation, when hCG is 900 mIU/ml or less.[8] With good abdominal ultrasound equipment and technique, a gestational sac should definitely be detected when the beta hCG is 1,800 mIU (by 5 to 6 weeks of gestation). A vaginal probe should detect a gestational sac when hCG is 1,000 mIU (by 4–5 weeks of gestation).[13]

Unfortunately, a sac-like ultrasound appearance, called a "pseudogestational sac," can occur in conjunction with ectopic pregnancy in as many as 10% of cases.[25] The other ultrasound signs of possible ectopic pregnancy, such as poorly defined adnexal mass and cul de sac fluid, are not specific enough for conclusive diagnosis. However, the diagnosis of ectopic pregnancy can be made conclusively if a gestational sac and fetal heartbeat are detected outside of the uterine cavity. The differential diagnosis usually includes intrauterine gestation earlier than menstrual dates would suggest, complete or incomplete spontaneous abortion, or pregnancy with a corpus luteum cyst. Unless intrauterine gestation can be identified with certainty or an extrauterine gestation is visible, ultrasound results do not provide a definite diagnosis.

If after completing these three diagnostic steps ectopic pregnancy cannot be excluded, arrange for surgical evaluation. Refer immediately if the patient becomes symptomatic during the process of evaluation. Laparoscopy will most likely be needed to ascertain the diagnosis.

In some cases, close observation alone may be an option: when beta hCG is low and declining, the patient remains asymptomatic, and the size of the ectopic pregnancy is small. Spontaneous abortion of an ectopic pregnancy followed by resorption occurs in as many as 83% of such cases in a reported series.[18] In this situation, the beta hCG will decline slowly to zero. Alternatively, some centers treat with methotrexate[24] or with etoposide[22] to induce dissolution of trophoblast tissue, thus causing a medical abortion. If gestation is early, it may be possible to evacuate the pregnancy through an incision in the fallopian tube wall during laparoscopic or abdominal surgery. When technically possible, this approach is preferred over salpingectomy or salpingo-oophorectomy for the patient who would like to preserve her future fertility.[1]

Early diagnosis is very important in ectopic pregnancy. Early diagnosis and intervention have helped to reduce ectopic pregnancy mortality from 35.5 deaths per 10,000 ectopic pregnancies in 1970 to 5.4/10,000 in 1988.[10] Also, early diagnosis allows more time for conservative management, which may help to preserve the woman's future fertility.

POSSIBLE SPONTANEOUS ABORTION

Approximately 15% of early pregnancies end in spontaneous abortion; the proportion is even higher if pregnancy losses are counted during the first 2 weeks of gestation, before the menstrual period is overdue and pregnancy is likely to be recognized. Missed abortion is also fairly common, but is unlikely to cause symptoms that would prompt the woman to seek care. Often the diagnosis is not suspected until prenatal exams reveal that uterine enlargement is not keeping pace with pregnancy dates, or an ultrasound evaluation fails to detect an expected fetal pole or cardiac activity at an appropriate time.

The diagnosis of spontaneous abortion may be made on the basis of a pelvic examination. If the cervix is dilated and products of conception are visible in the cervix or vagina, then abortion is inevitable. An ultrasound evaluation may help determine whether the uterine cavity is already empty. If the uterus appears to be empty and bleeding is not heavy, then uterine evacuation may not be necessary. Otherwise, vacuum aspiration can empty the uterus to resolve the woman's bleeding and cramping and to reduce the risk of infection. (See Chapter 28 on Abortion.)

Vacuum aspiration is also indicated if bleeding is so heavy that it is life-threatening or if the woman does not want to continue the pregnancy. If the pregnancy is wanted and the condition is not life-threatening, then intervention can be delayed while further evaluation is undertaken to determine whether the pregnancy may be viable. Serial quantitative beta hCG assays and an ultrasound evaluation are likely to document the diagnosis (see section on Possible Ectopic Pregnancy). When the pregnancy is desired, take time for a careful and thorough evaluation. Intervention on the basis of an initial exam or ultrasound will seem abrupt and shocking as the woman first begins to acknowledge the possibility of her loss and grief.

COUNSELING OBJECTIVES WITH PREGNANCY DIAGNOSIS

The issues surrounding personal fertility are complex, and a pregnancy diagnosis visit should provide the client an opportunity to clarify and articulate her feelings. Before beginning the physical exam and testing, find out what the woman hopes her result will be. When presenting the test results, elicit the client's reaction and allow time for her to express her feelings. Assess the woman's support system. Provide referrals if the patient feels counseling would be helpful. This is especially important if her own support system is not adequate. Emphasize that no decision based on the test results need be made that day. Encourage the woman to talk with her partner, family, or friends. Outline all the options available.

- If the client is pregnant and plans to continue her pregnancy, review precautions for optimal pregnancy (see Chapter 25 on Preconception Care) and be certain she has an appropriate resource for prenatal care. Remind her about danger signs of possible problems in pregnancy (Table 26-3).

- If the client plans to continue her pregnancy, but does not want to parent the child, refer her to a resource that can help with adoption.

- If the client is pregnant but does not plan to continue her pregnancy, refer her for abortion services. In this case, the sooner the decision is made and acted upon, the safer the procedure will be.

- If the client is not pregnant and wishes she were, counsel her about her own fertility. (See Chapter 27 on Impaired Fertility.) If appropriate, refer her for fertility evaluation and help. Remind her about precautions for optimal pregnancy and about taking a daily vitamin that includes folic acid 0.4 mg before and during pregnancy.[9]

- If the client is not pregnant, plans to continue being sexually active, and is happy with the negative test result, then birth control counseling is appropriate. A pregnancy scare can be a good bridge from risk-taking to effective, ongoing contraceptive use.

- If the client is not clear how she feels about the test result, positive or negative, consider referral for counseling. Appropriate pregnancy counseling services are likely to be available through a local abortion facility. Be sure that pregnancy counseling referral resources you recommend have been carefully evaluated. Anti-abortion groups advertise pregnancy counseling services in some communities; these agencies do not provide the nonjudgmental environment that your clients are entitled to have in making a personal decision about pregnancy. A woman who is not pregnant, but who has ambivalent feelings about pregnancy, may want to consider working with a mental health professional to clarify her feelings.

REFERENCES

1. American College of Obstetricians and Gynecologists. Ectopic pregnancy. ACOG Technical Bulletin, No. 126. March 1989.
2. Bandi ZL, Schoen I, Waters M. An algorithm for testing and reporting serum chorionic gonadotropin at clinically significant decision levels with use of 'pregnancy test' reagents. Clin Chem 1989;35:545-551.
3. Bluestein D. Monoclonal antibody pregnancy tests. Am Fam Physician 1988;38:197-204.
4. Braunstein GD. hCG testing: a clinical guide for the testing of human chorionic gonadotropin. Monograph. Abbott Park IL: Abbott Diagnostics, 1992.
5. Braunstein GD. hCG expression in trophoblastic and nontrophoblastic tumors. In: Fishman WH (ed). Oncodevelopmental markers. Academic Press, 1983:351-371.
6. Braunstein GD, Karow WG, Gentry WC, Rasor J, Wade ME. First-trimester chorionic gonadotropin measurements as an aid in the diagnosis of early pregnancy disorders. Am J Obstet Gynecol 1978;131:25-32.
7. Braunstein GD, Rasor J, Danzer H, Adler D, Wade ME. Serum human chorionic gonadotropin levels throughout normal pregnancy. Am J Obstet Gynecol 1976;126:678-681.
8. Cacciatore B, Tiitinen A, Stenman UH, Ylostalo P. Normal early pregnancy: serum hCG levels and vaginal ultrasonography findings. Br J Obstet Gynecol 1990;97:899-903.
9. Centers for Disease Control. Recommendations for the use of folic acid to reduce the number of cases of spina bifida and other neural tube defects. MMWR 1992;41(RR-14):1-7.
10. Centers for Disease Control. Ectopic pregnancy—United States, 1988-1989. MMWR 1992;41:591-594.
11. Chard T. Pregnancy tests: a review. Hum Reprod 1992;7:701-710.
12. Coons SJ, Churchill L, Brinkman ML. The use of pregnancy test kits by college students. J Am Coll Health 1990;38:171-175.
13. Deutschman M. Advances in the diagnosis of first trimester pregnancy problems. Am Fam Phys 1991;44(suppl 5):15S-30S.
14. Doshi ML. Accuracy of consumer performed in-home tests for early pregnancy detection. Am J Publ Health 1986;76:512-514.

15. Hicks JM, Iosefsohn M. Reliability of home pregnancy-test kits in the hands of lay persons. [letters to the editor]. N Engl J Med 1989;320(5):320-321.

16. Jeng LL, Moore RM, Kaczmarek RG, Placek PJ, Bright RA. How frequently are home pregnancy tests used? Results from the 1988 National Maternal and Infant Health Survey. Birth 1991;18:11-13.

17. Latman NS, Burot BC. Evaluation of home pregnancy test kits. Biomedical Instrument and Technol 1989;144-149.

18. Leach RE, Ory SJ. Modern management of ectopic pregnancy. J Repro Med 1989;34:324-338.

19. Lee C, Hart LL. Accuracy of home pregnancy tests. DICP, Ann Pharmacotherapy 1990;24:712-713.

20. Marrs RP, Kletzky OA, Howard WF. Disappearance of human chorionic gonadotropin and resumption of ovulation following abortion. Am J Obstet Gynecol 1979;135:731-736.

21. Ramoska EA, Sacchetti AD, Nepp M. Reliability of patient history in determining the possibility of pregnancy. Ann Emerg Med 1989;18:48-50.

22. Segna RA, Mitchell DR, Misas JE. Successful treatment of cervical pregnancy with oral etoposide. Obstet Gynecol 1990;76:945-947.

23. Stewart FH, Guest FJ, Stewart G, Hatcher RA. Understanding your body: every woman's guide to gynecology and health. New York: Bantam Books, 1987.

24. Stovall TG, Ling FW, Gray LA, Carson SA, Buster JE. Methotrexate treatment of unruptured ectopic pregnancy: a report of 100 cases. Obstet Gynecol 1991;77:749-753.

25. Thorsen MK, Lawson TL, Aiman EJ, Miller DP, McAsey ME, Erickson SJ, Quiroz F, Perret RS. Diagnosis of ectopic pregnancy: endovaginal vs. transabdominal sonography. AJR 1990;155:307-310.

Impaired Fertility

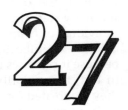

Gary K. Stewart, MD, MPH

- Maintaining a couple's ability to become pregnant until they reach their desired family size is a principal goal of reproductive health care providers.
- The first task in reproductive health care is to help individuals establish a reproductive life plan.
- The second task involves obtaining the information and skills necessary to attain such a plan.
- Basic education and fertility assessment can take place in the primary reproductive health care setting; couples who require more extensive assessment and treatment should be referred.

As a reproductive health care provider, you are entrusted with preserving an individual's fertility—to dispense and recommend only safe and effective means of contraception that will not impair fertility and to educate patients about preventing problems that may lead to impaired fertility. In addition, you can provide an initial evaluation and counsel about infertility. In some reproductive health care facilities, services may need to expand to welcome men.

The following definitions are adapted from the World Health Organization's (WHO's) definitions of infertility in a couple:

Primary infertility.   The couple has never conceived despite having unprotected intercourse for at least 12 months.

Secondary infertility.   The couple has previously conceived but is subsequently unable to conceive within 12 months despite having unprotected intercourse.

Pregnancy wastage.   The woman is able to conceive but unable to produce a live birth.

PROBABILITY OF PREGNANCY

It is estimated that 10% to 15% of couples are not able to conceive within 1 year of trying. However, this estimate represents an aggregate summary statistic and usually will be of little value when counseling an individual or couple regarding their chances of conception. The standard measure of infertility (failure to conceive in 12 months) is misleading because it confuses total inability to conceive with a delay in conception. In fact, the majority of "infertile" couples do conceive, whether or not they are treated for infertility.

If a normally fertile woman has a 20% chance of pregnancy each cycle, the cumulative pregnancy rates might be plotted as per Figure 27-1. About 95% of couples would be pregnant by the 13th cycle. On the other

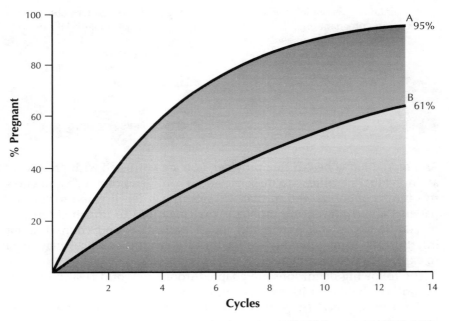

Source: Adapted from Hammond et al. (1983).

A Cumulative pregnancy curve assuming cyclic fecundability of 20%.

B Cumulative pregnancy curve assuming cyclic fecundability of 7%.

Figure 27-1 Cumulative pregnancy curves assuming two levels of fecundability

hand, if the chance of pregnancy were smaller, as for clients who are having donor insemination using frozen sperm or undergoing ovulation induction, the cumulative probabilities of pregnancy would follow a more prolonged, lower slope.[22,23,27,43] Cumulative pregnancy rates for surgically treated patients (such as those treated for endometriosis or tuboplasty) rise steeply for 12 months, then gradually stabilize until 36 months, after which pregnancies rarely occur.[21,28]

In actual populations, neither curve in Figure 27-1 is likely to be obtained. Although the probabilities of conception may remain roughly constant over time for an individual couple (assuming behavior does not change), they will decline for a group because the most fecund will become pregnant first. Of the remaining couples, only a minority (perhaps about one-fourth) will never conceive. The rest simply take a little longer to become pregnant.

REQUIREMENTS FOR FERTILITY

For a couple to produce a child unassisted by the new fertility technology, both partners must be fecund. In the United States, male infertility is principally responsible in 40% of infertile couples and female infertility in 40%. In 20% of infertile couples, the cause of infertility is either unknown or it exists in both partners.[27,49] The diagnoses of infertility are noted in Table 27-1.

Table 27-1 Male and female diagnoses of infertility in developed countries

Diagnosis	% of Couples
Female Diagnosis	
No demonstrable cause	40
Bilateral tubal occlusion	11
Acquired tubal abnormalities	12
Anovulatory regular cycle	10
Anovulatory oligomenorrhea	9
Ovulatory oligomenorrhea	7
Hyperprolactinemia	7
Male Diagnosis	
No demonstrable cause	49
Accessory gland infection	7
Idiopathic low motility	3
Primary testicular failure	10
Varicocele	11

Source: WHO (1986).

Requirements for Male Fertility

- Normal spermatogenesis and ductal system (normal count, motility, and biologic structure and function)
- Ability to transmit the spermatozoa to the female vagina, through
  - Adequate sexual drive
  - Ability to maintain an erection
  - Ability to achieve a normal ejaculation
  - Placement of ejaculate in the vaginal vault

Requirements for Female Fertility

- Adequate sexual drive and sexual function to permit coitus
- Functioning reproductive anatomy and physiology that include:
  - A vagina capable of receiving spermatozoa
  - Normal cervical mucus to allow passage of spermatozoa to the upper genital tract
  - Ovulatory cycles
  - Fallopian tubes that will function to permit the sperm and ovum to meet and allow migration of the conceptus to the uterus
  - A uterus capable of developing and sustaining the conceptus to maturity
  - Adequate hormonal status to maintain pregnancy
- Normal immunologic responses to accommodate sperm, conceptus, and fetal survival
- Adequate nutritional, chemical, and health status to maintain nutrition and oxygenation of placenta and fetus

FACTORS AFFECTING REPRODUCTIVE PERFORMANCE

Several factors affect the probability of conception (Figures 27-2 and 27-3):

Age of woman. The effects of age on fertility are moderate and do not begin to exert an effect until the late 30s (Table 27-2).[35] Older women take longer to conceive, but both clinicians and patients must carefully distinguish "waiting longer" from never being able to conceive. Women attempting pregnancy at age 40 or older have a 50% decreased fertility rate and a two-fold to three-fold increased risk of spontaneous abortion compared with younger women.[54] About 45% of older women eventually give birth. A host of other factors, including frequency of inter-

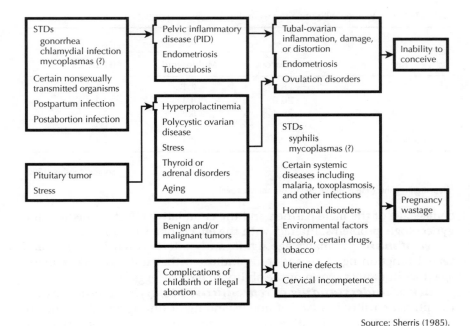

Source: Sherris (1985).

Figure 27-2 Relationships between selected direct and indirect causes of female infertility

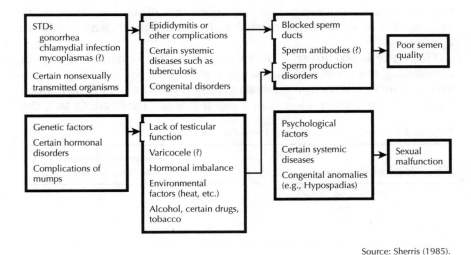

Source: Sherris (1985).

Figure 27-3 Relationships between selected direct and indirect causes of male infertility

Table 27-2 % of women with impaired fecundity, by age and parity.*

Age	Parity		
	Nulliparous	**Multiparous**	**All Parities**
15–24	8.4	7.1	7.6
25–34	20.0	8.3	10.9
35–44	36.4	8.8	11.4
15–44	20.5	8.4	10.7

Source: Mosher (1990).

*Data are from the 1988 National Survey of Family Growth.

course, age of the male partner, and the cumulative effect of medical and gynecologic problems, interact with the effects of a woman's age.[16]

Age of man. A man's age significantly affects coital frequency and sexual functioning. A recent study indicated that until age 64, a man's age does not affect sperm or the ability to fertilize eggs.[18]

Lack of understanding of reproductive biology. Another barrier to optimal fertility is a lack of understanding of timing and frequency of intercourse. Patient education is of primary importance in fertility counseling and family planning.

Coital frequency. Infrequent coitus is a common cause of infertility.[33] Coital frequency is positively correlated with pregnancy rates (Table 27-3).[30] Although the sperm count may be slightly decreased by an intercourse frequency of once per day or once every other day, the motility and number of sperm in the normal male would be sufficient to achieve a pregnancy.[39]

Timing of intercourse. Intercourse prior to ovulation is key in maximizing the chance of pregnancy (Table 27-4). Sperm cells can survive as long as 5 days in the female genital tract. The ovum has a much shorter life expectancy—less than 1 day if it is not fertilized. In fact, the

Table 27-3 Frequency of intercourse and probability of conception within 6 months

Frequency of Intercourse	% Achieving Pregnancy Within 6 Months
<1 per week	17
1 per week	32
2 per week	46
3 per week	51

Source: MacLeod (1953).

Table 27-4 Probability of conception in the absence of contraception by day of coitus with respect to estimated time of ovulation

Coital Day	Average Likelihood of Conception
−5	0.00
−4	0.11
−3	0.20
−2	0.15
−1	0.26
0 (ovulation)	0.15
1	0.09
2	0.05
3	0.00

Source: Trussell and Kost (1987).

"window of time" for fertilization is thought to last only a few hours, thus requiring sperm availability in the genital tract at or shortly before ovulation. (See Chapter 15 on Fertility Awareness Methods.)

Lubricants. Some lubricants such as Surgilube and K-Y Jelly may have some spermicidal properties. Because of their lubricating quality, some spermicidal preparations may mistakenly be used by some couples trying to conceive.

Douching. Although it is an unreliable method of contraception, douching may kill the very sperm that might have united with an egg in couples of marginal fertility. In addition, pelvic inflammatory disease (PID) and ectopic pregnancy are increased among women who douche. (See Chapter 8 on Reproductive Tract Infections.)

Multiple sexual partners. Exposure to multiple partners increases the risks for STIs, PID, cervical intraepithelial neoplasia (CIN), and other conditions that may require treatment such as freezing the cervix, laser treatment, conization and, possibly, hysterectomy. Some women develop antibodies to sperm, a condition some clinicians believe is more likely to occur in women exposed to multiple partners. Regular use of condoms (except when pregnancy is desired) may help prevent STIs, CIN, and the development of antisperm antibodies.

Sexually transmitted infections. Gonorrhea and chlamydia. In the woman, these organisms cause cervicitis and PID (associated with tubal disease and pelvic adhesions), and in the man, urethritis, epididymitis, and, possibly, accessory gland infection. PID is the major etiology of tubal infertility, although chronic cervicitis may produce subfertility in some women. Chlamydia causes severe subclinical tubal inflammation with subsequent tubal damage, despite its benign course of signs and symptoms.[20,52] Although inadequately treated chlamydial salpingitis may appear to improve, tubal damage caused by the inflammatory response will continue. PID of any etiology produces tubal scarring, resulting in bilateral intratubal adhesions that interfere with the movement of sperm and ova, either by completely occluding the tube or by damaging the delicate mucosa and cilia necessary for proper tubal functioning.[13,57] Other pelvic adhesions may limit tubal mobility, motility, or contact with the ovary, thus interfering with capture of ova. Many of the same factors that impair fertility also increase the likelihood of ectopic pregnancy, which may further damage the reproductive system.[10]

Human papilloma virus (HPV). HPV is often a precursor to cervical dysplasia. The impact upon fertility is dependent upon treatment, which may range from a required hysterectomy (should cervical cancer be diagnosed) to cryosurgery, cone biopsy, or similar treatment of the cervix for simple dysplasia. Cervical treatment may reduce fertility because of cervical transport problems subsequent to scarring or damage to the cervical mucous-producing cells, possibly leading to cervical incompetence associated with preterm deliveries and possible pregnancy loss.

Parasitic and other infectious diseases. Some parasitic and other infectious diseases can lead to infertility and fetal wastage.

Mumps, leading to orchitis (testicular inflammation), may cause secondary testicular atrophy in the small number of men infected after puberty. Bilateral orchitis occurs in perhaps 1% of adult men with mumps; most men will recover without impaired fertility.[46]

Toxoplasmosis, malaria, filariasis, schistosomiasis, leprosy (Hansen's Disease), and tuberculosis are causes of infertility not likely to be encountered in the United States.

Previous pregnancy. Child delivery associated with infection, lacerations, uterine injury, rare hemorrhagic events requiring transfusions, or hysterectomy may inhibit future successful pregnancies. Postpartum infections and postabortion infections, frequently caused by reproductive tract infections (RTIs), can be a major cause of infertility. Postabortion infections are most common where safe, legal abortions are not available.

Sickle cell disease. In men, sickle cell disease has been documented as a cause of recurring priapism with possible impotence due to tissue and nerve damage. In women, sickling crises or alterations in placental blood flow or oxygenation have been associated with an increased rate of fetal wastage.[38]

Nutrition. Women who have a body weight 10% to 15% below normal may have reduced fertility. The percentage body fat should be greater than 22% to permit regular, ovulatory cycles.[17] Women with eating disorders such as anorexia nervosa or bulimia may be at increased risk of menstrual dysfunction and may be over-represented in infertility clinics.[51] Obesity may also lead to less frequent ovulation or to less frequent intercourse, thereby contributing to fertility problems.[47]

Toxic agents. Exposure to toxic agents may emerge as one of the principle causes of infertility with no demonstrable anatomic cause. Exposure to these agents can occur from occupational hazards (e.g., farms, factories, semiconductor industry, or mines); contaminated air, water, or food supply; drug ingestion; or other exposures. Lead, toxic fumes, and exposure to pesticides are suspected contributors to infertility.[59,63] In women, lead poisoning reduces conceptions and increases the risk of fetal wastage. In men, exposure to lead can reduce both sex drive and sperm count. Pesticide exposure can also reduce sperm count.[59]

Smoking and alcohol. In men, cigarette smoking and alcohol use may cause poor sperm quality, and marijuana use has also been implicated in lower sperm motility and count. In women, both smoking and heavy alcohol use are associated with lower rates of conception[7] and increased rates of spontaneous abortion. Smoking also appears to increase slightly the risk of placenta previa. Smoking and alcohol use both negatively affect the developing fetus and may result in low birthweight babies.[49]

Medications. Narcotics, tranquilizers (such as phenothiazines), monoamine oxidase inhibitors (antidepressants), some antihypertensives, and drugs such as guanethidine and methyldopa may cause impotence. Amoebicides, antimalarial drugs, nitrofurantoin, sulfasalazine, cimetidine, certain antihypertensives, and methotrexate may affect sperm production.[9,42,44] Calcium channel blockers may inhibit sperm function. Habitual use of narcotics or barbiturates apparently decreases regularity and effectiveness of ovulation. Systemic, powerful anticancer drugs exert many tissue effects that may include testicular or ovarian failure, in some cases after only one cycle of chemotherapy. Many other prescription medications, including tetracycline, retinoic acid derivatives (Accutane), several antiseizure medications, some antidepressants, some tranquilizers, and coumadin are examples of drugs clearly associated with an increased risk of fetal defects. Many of these drugs may also be associated with fetal wastage, although they more commonly cause increased rates of malformation rather than spontaneous abortion.[49] Review current medications as part of preconception counseling.

Surgery. Sexual functioning may be reversibly or irreversibly impaired by surgery involving the penis, scrotum, prostate, and pelvis (which may cause nerve damage). Ovarian, cervical, or uterine surgery, even for benign processes, may cause subsequent difficulties with conception, ovulation, or fetal wastage. Adhesions from any pelvic or abdominal surgery may interfere with conception. Discuss surgical procedures in detail preoperatively; instruct the surgeon regarding the patient's future fertility intentions. Ask the surgeon to report on findings of the pelvic organs, and obtain a copy of the operative report for the personal files of the client.

Radiation. Exposure to radiation may be occupational, accidental, iatrogenic, or as a therapeutic component of cancer treatment. Therapeutic radiation treatments in men or women can sometimes be tailored to minimize gonadal exposure and optimize future fertility and gonadal function. In men, the testicular germinal epithelium enclosing the seminiferous tubules may be reversibly incapacitated by irradiation, and chromosomal aberrations may occur.[41] Also, testicular cancer risks may be increased by irradiation.[9] In women, irradiation may cause ovarian failure, fetal wastage, or fetal damage.[49]

Physical exertion or heat. It remains unclear whether strenuous exercise alone, particularly endurance training, can cause reproductive problems. Recent studies suggest the development of exercise-associated reproductive problems involves nutritional changes and metabolic balance to a significant degree.[14] Some highly trained women athletes such as long-distance runners and professional dancers may experience reversible amenorrhea without any apparent long-term detrimental effects on fertility.[17] Men who take frequent hot showers or whirlpool treatments and men whose occupations involve subjecting the body to high temperature (e.g., furnace workers) may subject the scrotum to temperatures high enough to reduce sperm production temporarily.[53] There is no evidence that endurance training leads to male infertility.[6]

Tight clothing. Jockey shorts and tight pants have been postulated to have the same suppressive effect on sperm production as do hot showers, because of high temperatures in the scrotal region. However, no evidence supports this hypothesis.

PREVENTING INFERTILITY

Patients may find it easier to prevent some of the problems associated with infertility if they have set goals for their future childbearing. Counseling about STIs, contraception, and sexual behaviors will be more meaningful for patients who have identified their fertility goals. You can influence patients' risk of impaired fertility in a number of ways:

- Stay current in the prevention, diagnosis, and treatment of STIs and PID.
- Be aware that contraceptive choice influences the risk of PID. Encourage sexually active young people to avoid IUDs and to use barrier methods.

- Begin or continue public health education efforts so the consequences of untreated sexual infection may be fully understood by your clients and particularly by all young people.
- Assist young persons in identifying their risk factors for STIs.
- Work within the community to ensure all individuals, including minors, have access to early and confidential diagnosis and treatment of STIs.

INTRAUTERINE DEVICES (IUDs)

The IUD is associated with an increased risk of PID.[9,15,29] However, recent studies suggest previous risk estimates may have been overestimated.[12] (See Chapter 21 on Intrauterine Devices.) Take the following actions to preserve fertility among IUD users:

- Be conservative in using IUDs for women who plan to bear children in the future. Many clinicians will not insert IUDs into nulliparous women.
- Avoid recommending the IUD to women who are at risk for STIs and PID.
- Urge further refinements in current IUDs and encourage the availability of the Levonorgestrel IUD (LNg 20), which presents a lower risk of PID.
- Screen for STIs in at-risk patients.
- Never insert an IUD into a woman with an untreated STI.
- Consider giving antibiotic prophylaxis after IUD insertion in areas where the incidence of STI is high.
- Assume that a vaginal discharge in the presence of an IUD signals an infection until proven otherwise.
- Be certain clients are aware of the danger signs of PID and know where to go and what to do if these signs occur.

ORAL CONTRACEPTIVES

Oral contraceptive users have a lower risk of symptomatic PID than do women who use the IUD or no contraceptive method,[12] probably due to decreased menstrual flow and myometrial activity, along with a less penetrable cervical mucus. Amenorrhea and temporary infertility following pill use (post-pill amenorrhea) do not appear to threaten female fertility seriously. Post-pill amenorrhea is most common among women who had irregular menses before beginning oral contraceptive therapy. (See Chapter 19 on The Pill: Oral Contraceptives.) This temporary condition is usually amenable to treatment by using standard ovulation induction drugs such as clomiphene citrate. The risk of cervical infection with chlamydia is enhanced among pill users (as compared with non-users),[12,56] although the damaging effects of inflammation may be less.[12] The question of an increased risk of CIN has not been settled. Because an increased risk of CIN occurrence among pill users may be likely, diagnose and treat the condition early. Take the following actions to preserve fertility among pill users:

- Educate patients about the positive relationship between the pill and PID.
- Urge pill users at high risk for STIs to use barrier contraception as well and to limit their number of sexual partners.
- Perform Papanicolaou smears annually.

BARRIER METHODS

Condoms and other barrier methods reduce the risk of acquiring STIs such as chlamydia and gonorrhea, both of which are associated with PID and tubal infertility. (See Chapter 16 on Male Condoms.) Because the risk of infertility increases with each episode of PID, clients who have had a previous episode of PID should be counseled about barrier methods to avoid infection. The use of condoms has been widely encouraged to reduce a woman's risk of developing immunologic reactions to sperm.[48]

STERILIZATION

A number of patients request sterilization reversal, an expensive procedure with uncertain prognosis. A number of circumstances can lead to a high degree of regret among users:[8,25,60,61] young age at the time sterilization, loss of a child, divorce or remarriage, later desire for more children, and selection of sterilization because of unhappiness with using one of the reversible methods. Take the following actions to avoid unwanted infertility of sterilization procedures:

- Emphasize the permanence of the procedure.
- Avoid using the term "tying the tubes" to describe sterilization procedures; to some patients, such reference might imply "untying the tubes" is feasible. (See Chapter 22 on Female and Male Sterilization.)
- Make sure clients have access to reversal procedures. This may require changes in laws relating to health insurance and public funding.

ABORTION

No epidemiologic evidence supports a fertility risk to women experiencing first-trimester vacuum abortions. A slightly increased risk of infertility exists when large cervical dilation is used for some dilation and curettage (D&C) abortion procedures and when the abortion is performed in the second trimester.[26] Abortions resulting in severe complications are so rare that they are not readily apparent in statistical evaluations of fertility risk. A full-term pregnancy still has a greater negative impact on long-term fertility than does safe, legal abortion. Take the following actions to preserve fertility in patients undergoing abortion:

- Advise patients of the potential for complications.
- Avoid using sharp curettes for first-trimester abortions if a vacuum aspiration may be used instead.
- Use gradual dilation with laminaria (to not more than 11 mm, if possible).
- Prescribe prophylactic antibiotics whenever interference or illegal abortion is suspected (some clinicians recommend routine antibiotic prophylaxis for all abortions).
- Vigorously treat septic abortions.
- Provide contraceptive counseling to all abortion patients.
- Screen for and treat STIs (gonorrhea and chlamydia) prior to surgery, or treat all patients with prophylactic antibiotics effective against resistant strains of disease-causing organisms.
- Follow up for early signs of infection. (See Chapter 28 on Abortion.)
- Have abortion complications treated by experienced clinicians.

FERTILITY EVALUATION

Triaging (sorting by urgency) is the important task of the first counselor to see the infertile client or couple. Discussion, investigation or referral, rather than advice to "wait and see," should be the general response to the inquiring couple who has tried unsuccessfully to conceive. Although typically the couple should try to conceive for 12 months before beginning a work-up, an evaluation may be expedited under the following conditions:

- The woman is in her late 30s. Because a steep decline in fertility occurs after age 40, women over age 35 should receive early assessment. The assessment should be concise, complete, and accomplished quickly.
- The woman reports irregular menses. This symptom could signal sporadic ovulation (which is unlikely to improve spontaneously

beyond adolescence) and may be a sign of premature ovarian senescence or failure (early menopause). Irregular or abnormal bleeding may be a symptom of PID or other gynecologic disease, making evaluation necessary.

- The medical history includes previous pelvic surgery or serious medical problems, mumps for the man, or repeated miscarriages, ectopic pregnancy, or PID for the woman. Because time is not likely to improve such problems, but rather will allow the couple's fecundity to steadily diminish, seek a diagnosis and remedy promptly.
- The woman has severe progressive dysmenorrhea or dyspareunia suggestive of endometriosis or other pelvic disease.
- The woman used an IUD in the past; had a pelvic infection; had surgery on an ovary, a tube, or uterus; or has any reason to suspect damage to her pelvic organs such as endometriosis, ovarian cyst, or fibroid. An early assessment, including a laparoscopy, may be in order, which can then lead to an early diagnosis and treatment, or to reassurance that more time is needed.
- The couple lives in an area with a high endemic incidence of STIs.
- One of the couple was exposed to DES in utero.
- Neither partner has ever produced a pregnancy, despite having had unprotected intercourse.

While funding, personnel, and laboratory resources may be limited, some basic initial services should be provided by most reproductive health care programs. The following basic services help some couples improve fertility and expedite further evaluation and treatment for others who need more. Begin with the first four items listed and, where resources and training permit, include all of the following:

- Educate the patients.
- Gather pertinent historical information.
- Provide a thorough physical exam.
- Provide a resource for reassurance, counseling, and emotional stability including referral as needed. Referral sources may be found by consulting with the American Fertility Society or the local Resolve group. (See Chapter 11 on Selected Reproductive Health Resources.)
- Systematically evaluate the possible problems:
  - Counsel couples about fertility awareness techniques and optimizing coital timing. (See Chapter 15 on Fertility Awareness Methods.)
  - Check couples for asymptomatic STI infections that could cause subfertility.

- Determine whether ovulation takes place, as indicated by basal body temperature or cervical mucus records (or urine LH test kits where available).
- Perform semen analyses.

- Make a plan and initiate treatment based upon information gathered; counsel couples with potentially serious fertility problems or undetected reasons for infertility about their options for further evaluation and treatment.
- Reassess progress at predetermined intervals.
- Refer couples to other infertility specialists or adoption agencies as needed. Explain the anticipated short-term and long-term costs and the chances for success with further treatment, and discuss the options of adoption or remaining childless.

HISTORY AND PHYSICAL ASSESSMENT

After interviewing the couple together, interview the man and woman separately to obtain confidential information. Having both partners present for the physical exams may ensure both partners understand the anatomy and related issues. This idealized scenario may not be comfortable or possible for some couples.

Before beginning the evaluation process, explain the main steps needed for diagnostic evaluation (Table 27-5). Describe the capacity of your facility. If referral becomes necessary, try to assure procedures are not duplicated unnecessarily and an orderly, agreed upon evaluation can be continued. Following a standard set of guidelines, such as the WHO flow sheet of the standardized approach to the infertile couple,[63] will enhance the effectiveness of referral prognosis.

Physical examination of the woman.   Visual evaluation of hair distribution and of body and breast development can indicate endocrinopathy or developmental deficiencies such as hypogonadism, adrenal hyperplasia, hypothyroidism, ovarian dysfunction, and hyperprolactinemia. A complete pelvic exam (palpation of uterus and adnexae, speculum exam of vagina and cervix) should reveal any uterine hypoplasia, adnexal tumors, or cervical lesions and should indicate whether dyspareunia may be a problem.

Physical exam of the man.   Again, visual inspection of sexual characteristics can identify such endocrinopathies as hypogonadism or Klinefelter's syndrome (the genetic XXY anomaly often associated with infertility). A penile exam can reveal hypospadias (displacement of the urethral opening) or phimosis (constriction of the foreskin). The testicular exam detects atrophy, tumors, epididymal cysts, cryptorchidism

Table 27-5 A fertility assessment visit schedule

The initial assessment of the couple should proceed in a systematic manner, with the objective of completing the first line of infertility evaluation within approximately 2–3 cycles. A suggested schedule for visits is as follows:

Visit 1:

> Family planning clinic visit (ideally day 5–10 of menstrual cycle)
> Ideally previous medical records obtained
> Male and female complete medical history
> Male and female physical examination
> Develop investigation plan

Between Visits:

> Male obtain physical exam if not already completed
> Male semen evaluation
> Male and female laboratory tests (although the blood tests might ideally be done later)
> Male and female be certain that all past and pertinent records are obtained
> Begin BBTs and fertility awareness record keeping

Visit 2:

> Clinic visit (pre-ovulatory day 13 of 28-day cycle or time by LH kit)
> Intercourse 12 hours prior to clinic visit
> Postcoital test

Between Visits:

> Day 22 of 28-day cycle
> Serum progesterone
> Other blood tests as indicated

Visit 3:

> Clinic visit (day 26 of 28-day cycle)
> Endometrial biopsy

Between Visits:

> Radiologist office (day 5–10 of menstrual cycle when not bleeding)
> Hysterosalpingogram

Visit 4:

> Clinic visit
> Consultation
> Review all records and information to date

Depending upon the above findings (after discussing with the patient), we would then proceed with some other investigations which might include:

- Diagnostic Laparoscopy and Hysteroscopy
- Hormonal Studies
- Immunologic Studies
- Tests of Sperm Function
- Other Tests as Indicated

(undescended testicles), vas thickening or absence, hydrocele (fluid accumulation in the testes or along the spermatic cord), or varicocele (dilation of the veins of the spermatic cord in the scrotum).

FURTHER ASSESSMENTS AND TESTS

Following the initial history, physical exam, and basic diagnostic laboratory procedures, inform the patient about the further tests that may need to be performed and about initial recommendations.[3] Trained specialists tend to rely on five traditional infertility tests: semen analysis, assessment of ovulation, postcoital test (PCT), endometrial biopsy, laparoscopy, and hysterosalpingogram (HSG).[19] This initial evaluation will identify the basic causes of infertility in about 80% of couples. The next level of evaluation is, in general, well beyond the scope of most family planning clinics, but might involve immunologic studies, test of sperm function, and other tests as indicated.

Semen evaluation. Make arrangements with the laboratory prior to bringing in a specimen for a semen evaluation (Table 27-6). If the sperm count is at least 15 to 20 million, the absolute number of sperm is probably less critical than their motility and morphology. The presence of bacteria or white blood cells, as well as semen viscosity, should also be recorded. More than one evaluation may be necessary, particularly if the results are borderline. The WHO recommends two samples taken at least 2 weeks apart (Table 27-7).[62]

Ovulation assessment. Instruct patients in recording basal body temperatures and charting mucus changes. (See Chapter 15 on Fertility Awareness Methods.) This documentation often is helpful in verifying ovulation, determining timing and frequency of intercourse, and educating the

Table 27-6 Directions for collecting semen for evaluation

1. Abstain from intercourse (no ejaculation) for at least 3 and no more than 5 days. Do not drink any alcohol or take a hot shower or hot bath immediately prior to producing the specimen.

2. Produce a semen specimen by masturbation into a small, sterile, dry, wide-mouthed jar. Be sure the entire specimen is captured in the container. We can provide the container if you wish. You may use the restroom in the office building or obtain the specimen elsewhere.

3. Take the specimen to the laboratory as soon as possible after obtaining the specimen. Note the exact time the specimen was obtained and write it and your name on the container. The specimen must arrive in the laboratory within 1 hour of collection.

4. Try to keep the specimen close to body temperature during transit.

Table 27-7 Criteria for a normal semen sample

A semen sample was considered normal if all of the following conditions were met:

Spermatozoa

Concentration	$>20 \times 10^6$/ml
Motility	>40% progressively motile
Morphology	>50% normal (ideal) forms
Viability	>60% live
Agglutination	no

Seminal Fluid

Normal Appearance
Normal Viscosity
Less Than 10^6 WBCs/ml

client about the physiology of the menstrual cycle. The timing of various tests can also be recorded and guided by this documentation.

Postcoital test. About 1 day before the woman ovulates, obtain a postcoital (Sims-Huhner) test about 12 hours after the couple has had intercourse. Draw a small amount of cervical mucus into a thin catheter from the endocervical canal. Ideally, there is an abundance of acellular, watery cervical mucus that ferns, has a spinnbarkeit of greater than 8 cm, and has greater than 10 motile sperm per high-power field. The sperm should swim with good motility and in one direction.[37]

Endometrial biopsy. Using a paracervical block, take a biopsy on cycle day 26 of a 28-day cycle (or post-ovulation day 12) to see whether the changes in the endometrium are uniform with the expected secretory effect. Occasionally, a dysynchrony can occur, producing a luteal phase problem that would require treatment with either ovulation inducers or supplemental progesterone (Clomid or progesterone suppositories). These biopsies are most useful (1) when read by an experienced histologist or pathologist who evaluates endometrial biopsies frequently enough to discriminate phases of secretory maturity and (2) when read in conjunction with patient information about the day of the menstrual cycle and serum progesterone levels.

Laparoscopy. A laparoscopy can be performed on day 26 of a 28-day cycle when an endometrial biopsy is performed. Consider this approach when you suspect pelvic pathology in a patient who has a history of PID or a long history of IUD use or who is older and just beginning her work-up. Laparoscopy is somewhat uncomfortable for the woman, but it provides considerable information about anatomical abnormalities or damage or obstruction of the tubes. It may be combined with a hysteroscopy to rule out uterine anomalies, adhesions, or submucous fibroids.

Hysterosalpingogram. HSG is typically performed early in the menstrual cycle after bleeding has stopped but prior to ovulation. Radiopaque dye inserted into the uterus and x-ray photographs document its spread through the uterus and tubes. Because HSG can cause serious recurrence of PID, prophylactic antibiotics are recommended for patients with a history of PID.

SEX SELECTION

Patients may request sex selection for various reasons. Prevention of sex-linked genetic disorders is the principal medical indication for sex selection. Many organizations have issued statements regarding the ethics of provider participation in sex selection. The American College of Obstetricians and Gynecologists (ACOG) recently published a report stating that while providers may not ethically withhold medical information from patients who request it, they are not obligated to perform an abortion, or other medical procedure, to select fetal sex. It is recommended physicians explicitly inform patients, ideally in advance, if they are unwilling to perform specific medical procedures that patients might request.[1]

There are many different techniques for sex identification and selection. Prefertilization sex selection techniques use various methods for separating X-bearing and Y-bearing sperm.[33,40] Assisted reproductive technologies, such as in-vitro fertilization and zygote intrafallopian transfer, allow for the biopsy of one or more cells from a developing preembryo at the cleavage or blastocyst stage.[25] At present, reliable techniques for selecting sex are limited to postfertilization methods.[1] After implantation of a fertilized egg, fetal cell karyotyping will provide information about fetal sex.

COSTS

Economic considerations are critical. The costs of the more technology-driven evaluations and treatment far exceed the resources of most people and most health programs. Careful consideration must be given to determine the extent of service to be covered.

B ASIC TREATMENT POSSIBILITIES

The treatment of identified problems is well outlined in general references, so it will not be described in great detail here. Instead, a highly simplified summary of the general strategies for counseling patients will be discussed. Infertility therapy, like any other medical therapy, is generally directed toward curing or improving diagnosed anatomic and physiologic problems. In addition, comprehensive infertility treatment seeks to maximize the chance of pregnancy by optimizing all conditions for conception (for example, by instructing patients about optimal timing of intercourse and by eliminating any factors that potentially diminish fertility, such as those discussed in the preceding sections of this chapter). For a significant portion of patients who have no identifiable cause of infertility, the comprehensive approach is the only therapeutic option, provided all diagnostic tests have been completed. Although specific treatments require experienced practitioners, specialized equipment, precise timing, or great expense, they are still not perfect.

Male infertility may be treated with insemination from donor sperm to overcome problems including azoospermia or impotence. Make sure donor semen does not carry any organisms that produce STIs, including HIV. Criteria for preparation, storage, and screening are set by the American Fertility Society.[2] Their current recommendation is to use sperm that has been frozen and quarantined for 6 months. If the donor is still HIV-antibody negative after 6 months, the sperm may be released. More advanced reproductive technology approaches to male infertility include intrauterine insemination, super-ovulation of the female, in-vitro fertilization (IVF), and intracytoplasmic sperm injection.[3] These techniques, however, are expensive and must be performed by highly skilled providers.

Female infertility may be treated with a wider range of approaches:

Cervical mucus problems impairing conception may be treated with insemination or uterine instillation of a small amount of specially prepared sperm.

Cervical incompetence interfering with continuing pregnancy may be treated with cerclage, bed rest, or both. Cerclage is the passage of strong suture material around the cervix, like a purse string, to prevent premature dilation.

Ovulation disorders can be treated with ovulation-inducing drugs such as clomiphene citrate, which suppresses estrogen's ovulation-suppressive effect. In women whose ovulation is suppressed by hyperprolactinemia (high blood levels of the pituitary hormone prolactin), ovulation may be induced with prolactin-suppressing drugs such as bromocriptine.

Damage to ovaries, such as torsion, surgical removal, hemorrhagic cyst, or premature menopause that has eliminated primordial follicle tissue required to produce new ova, can only be overcome by some use of high-technology fertility medicine with an ova donated from another woman.

Uterine and tubal abnormalities may be corrected by surgical procedures (in some cases microsurgery). Some congenital uterine and tubal anomalies, such as true bicornuate uterus, may not be amenable to surgical repair. In the case of tubal damage caused by endometriosis,[5] hormonal suppression of the displaced endometrial tissue may be prescribed before or instead of surgery. Tubal or pelvic scarring due to PID may be improved with microsurgery of the tube or laparotomy to allow lysis of pelvic adhesions. Currently, the delicate cilia and mucosa of the tubal lining cannot be surgically regenerated, and the variable effects of the body's capacity to repair itself produce a low rate of tubal cure. In vitro fertilization (see the following discussion) may be the only way to bypass damaged fallopian tubes.

Advanced reproductive technology, also referred to as assisted reproductive technology (ART), requires expert practitioners and procedures and results in successful pregnancies at rates near the normal fecundity rates. The following are two of the major high technology approaches:

- Gamete intrafallopian tube transfer (GIFT) involves placing a mixture of ova and sperm into the fallopian tube. It is used primarily for unexplained infertility, where the fallopian tubes appear normal. The sperm is collected, washed, incubated, and prepared prior to laparoscopic harvesting of the oocytes. At the time of laparoscopy, both the sperm and oocytes are placed into the fallopian tube. Results from the 1994 Registry of ART procedures indicates the overall live delivery rate per retrieval was 28.4%.[4]
- In vitro fertilization (IVF) involves placing mature ova (harvested either at laparoscopy or transvaginally using an ultrasound-directed needle to aspirate the oocyte) with specially prepared sperm in a laboratory tissue culture medium and incubating them to allow fertilization. Fertilized ova that have successfully attained a certain maturity (generally between two and eight cell divisions) are placed in the uterus via a transcervical catheter. National surveys indicate a pregnancy rate of 19% per treatment cycle.[34] Results from the 1994 Registry of the ART procedures indicates the overall live delivery rate per retrieval was 20.7%.[4]

GIFT and IVF frequently use ovulation stimulation drugs to increase the number of ova ready for harvest. A recent combined analysis of three epidemiologic studies found a significant association between ovarian cancer and the use of fertility drugs.[58] While other studies have presented contradictory findings and the topic remains controversial, there appears to be enough cause for concern to slightly alter the provider's approach to counseling patients. Counsel women who wish to donate eggs, particularly repeat donors, because they derive no reproductive benefit from their fertility drug exposure.[50]

A DOPTION

Many couples faced with infertility who desire children choose adoption. Licensed adoption agencies may or may not allow communication between the birth-parents and adopting parents, and they generally involve a longer wait than independent adoptions. Couples may seek the help of providers who have contact with women with unwanted pregnancies. Attorneys, clergy, friends, and independent adoption centers can also aid in matching couples with birth parents. Adopting children from other countries, older children, or children with special needs may minimize the waiting period. Present these options to infertile clients, along with referrals to adoption resources.

T HE COPING PHASE

Many couples who seek help for infertility eventually do achieve pregnancy, often in the course of preliminary investigation.[45,63] Their risk for ectopic pregnancy, miscarriage, and perinatal mortality are higher than average. Some will eventually confront the reality of childlessness.

The impact of permanent infertility, coupled with the stresses of fertility evaluation and treatment, may damage a couple's relationship or an individual's self-concept. Normal reactions to the diagnosis of infertility include processes similar to other grieving processes: surprise, denial, isolation, anger, guilt, sorrow and, finally, resolution.[36] Depression and prolonged stress can follow diagnosis and treatment. In addition, couples may experience a great strain on their relationship. (See Chapter 2 on Sexuality and Reproductive Health.) Remember how disruptive infertility diagnosis and treatment can be for couples.[31] Take an active and complementary role in helping infertile couples to cope:

- Provide information on adoption and fostering, with names and addresses of local agencies.
- Refer couples for psychological counseling if their depression appears serious.
- Refer couples to infertility networks and support groups specifically designed to help people with infertility problems. (See Chapter 11 on Selected Reproductive Health Resources.)
- Remain sensitive to the heightened vulnerability of infertility patients.

REFERENCES

1. American College of Obstetricians and Gynecologists (ACOG) Committee on Ethics. Sex selection. Committee Opinion, ACOG 1996;(177):1-4.

2. Guidelines for gamete donation: 1993. The American Fertility Society. Fertil Steril 1993;59(Suppl 1):1S-9S.
3. American Society for Reproductive Medicine. Diagnostic testing for male factor infertility. Birmingham.
4. American Society for Reproductive Medicine and the Society for Assisted Reproductive Technology Registry. Assisted reproductive technology in the United States and Canada: 1994 results generated from the ASRM/SARTR. Fertil Steril 1996;66:697-705.
5. American Society for Reproductive Medicine. Revised American Society for Reproductive Medicine classification of endometriosis: 1996. Fertil Steril 1997;67:817-821.
6. Arce JC, De Souza MJ. Exercise and male factor infertility. Sports Med 1993;15:146-169.
7. Baird DD, Wilcox AJ. Cigarette smoking associated with delayed conception. JAMA 1985;253:2979-2983.
8. Boring CC, Rochat RW, Becerra J. Sterilization regret among Puerto Rican women. Fertil Steril 1988;49:973-981.
9. Castleman M. Sperm crisis. Medical Self-Care 1980;Spring:26.
10. Cates W, Rolfs RT, Aral SO. Pathophysiology and epidemiology of sexually transmitted diseases in relation to pelvic inflammatory disease and infertility. Proceedings of the Seminar on Biomedical and Demographic Determinants of Human Reproduction. Liege, Belgium: International Union for the Scientific Study of Population, 1988.
11. Cates W, Stone KM. Family planning, sexually transmitted diseases and contraceptive choice: a literature update. Part I. Fam Plann Perspect 1992;24:75-84.
12. Cates W, Stone KM. Family planning, sexually transmitted diseases and contraceptive choice: a literature update. Part II. Fam Plann Perspect 1992;24:122-128.
13. Cates W, Wasserheit JN, Marchbanks PA. Pelvic inflammatory disease and tubal infertility: the preventable conditions. Ann New York Acad Sci 1994;709:179-195.
14. Cumming DC, Wheeler GD, Harber VJ. Physical activity, nutrition, and reproduction. Ann New York Acad Sci 1994;709:55-76.
15. Farley TM, Rosenberg MS, Rowe PJ, Chen JH, Meirik O. Intrauterine devices and pelvic inflammatory disease: an international perspective. Lancet 1992;339:785-788.
16. Frank O, Bianchi PG, Campana A. The end of fertility: age, fecundity and fecundability in women. J Biosoc Sci 1994;26:349-368.
17. Frisch RE. Fatness and fertility. Sci Am 1988;258:88-95.
18. Gallardo E, Simon C, Levy M, Guanes PP, Remohi J, Pellicer A. Effect of age on sperm fertility potential: oocyte donation as a model. Fertil Steril 1996;66:260-264.
19. Glatstein IZ, Harlow BL, Hornstein MD. Practice patterns among reproductive endocrinologists: the infertility evaluation. Fertil Steril 1997;67:443-451.
20. Gjonnaess H, Dalaker K, Anestad G, Mardh PA, Kuile G, Bergan T. Pelvic inflammatory disease: etiologic studies with emphasis on chlamydial infection. Obstet Gynecol 1982;59:550-555.
21. Guzick DS, Rock JA. Estimation of a model of cumulative pregnancy following infertility therapy. Am J Obstet Gynecol 1981:140:573-578.

22. Hammond MG, Halme JK, Talbert LM. Factors affecting the pregnancy rate in clomiphene citrate induction of ovulation. Obstet Gynecol 1983;62:196-202.
23. Hammond MG, Talbert LM. Infertility: a practical guide for the physician, 2nd ed. Oradell NJ: Medical Economics Books, 1985.
24. Hardy K, Martin KL, Leese HJ, Winston RM, Handyside AH. Human preimplantation development in vitro fertilization is not adversely affected by biopsy at the 8-cell stage. Hum Reprod 1990;5:708-714.
25. Henshaw SK, Singh S. Sterilization regret among US couples. Fam Plann Perspect 1986;18:238-240.
26. Hogue CJ, Cates W, Tietze C. Effects of induced abortion on subsequent reproduction. Epidemiol Rev 1982;4:66-94.
27. Keller DW, Strickler RC, Warren JC. Clinical infertility. Norwalk CT: Appleton-Century-Crofts, 1984.
28. Lauritsen JG, Pagel JD, Vangsted P, Starup J. Results of repeated tuboplasties. Fertil Steril 1982;37:68-72.
29. Lee NC, Rubin GL, Ory HW, Burkman RT. Type of intrauterine device and the risk of pelvic inflammatory disease. Obstet Gynecol 1983;62:1-6.
30. MacLeod J, Gold RZ. The male factor in fertility and infertility: VI. Semen quality and certain other factors in relation to ease of conception. Fertil Steril 1953;4:10-33.
31. Mahlstedt PP. The psychological component of infertility. Fertil Steril 1985;43:335-346.
32. Martin RH. Human sex pre-selection by sperm manipulation. Hum Reprod 1994;9:1790-1791.
33. Masters WH, Johnson VE. Advice for women who want to have a baby. Redbook Magazine 1975;3:70-74.
34. Medical Research International, Society for Assisted Reproductive Technology, The American Fertility Society. In vitro fertilization-embryo transfer (IVF-ET) in the United States: 1990 results from the IVF-ET Registry. Fertil Steril 1992;57:15-24.
35. Menken J, Trussell J, Larsen U. Age and infertility. Science 1986;233:1389-1394.
36. Menning BE. Counselling infertile patients. Contemp Ob/Gyn 1979; February.
37. Moghissi KS. The cervix in infertility. In: Hammond MG, Talbert LM (eds). Infertility: a practical guide for the physician. 2nd ed. Oradell NJ: Medical Economics Books, 1985:84-101.
38. Pernoll ML, Benson MC (eds). Current obstetric and gynecologic diagnosis and treatment. 6th ed. Norwalk CT: Appleton-Lange, 1987.
39. Pfeffer WH. An approach to the diagnosis and treatment of the infertile female. Med Aspects Hum Sex 1980;14:121-122.
40. Pyrzak R. Separation of X- and Y-bearing human spermatozoa using albumin gradients. Hum Reprod 1994;9:1788-1790.
41. Roland M. Infertility therapy: effects of innovations and increasing experience. J Repro Med 1980;25:41-46.
42. Schlegel PN, Chang TS, Marshall FF. Antibiotics: potential hazards to male fertility. Fertil Steril 1991;55:235-242.
43. Schwartz D, Mayaux MJ. Female fecundity as a function of age: results of artificial insemination of 2,193 nulliparous women with azoospermic husbands. N Engl J Med 1982;306:404-406.

44. Shane JM, Schiff I, Wilson EA. The infertile couple: evaluation and treatment. In: CIBA Clinical Symposia 1976;28:2-40.
45. Shane JM. Ambulatory evaluation of the infertile patient. In: Ryan GM (ed). Ambulatory care in obstetrics and gynecology. Grune & Stratton, 1980: 303-316.
46. Sherris JD, Fox G. Infertility and sexually transmitted disease: a public challenge. Popul Rep 1983 (reprinted 1985);Series L(4):113-115.
47. Shoupe D. Effect of body weight on reproductive function. In: Mishell DR, Davajan V, Lobo RA. Infertility, contraception & reproductive endocrinology, 3rd ed. Cambridge: Blackwell Scientific Publications, 1991.
48. Shushan A, Schenker JG. Immunological factors in infertility. Am J Repro Immunol 1992;28:285-287.
49. Speroff L, Glass RH, Kase NG. Clinical gynecologic endocrinology and infertility, 4th ed. Baltimore MD: Williams & Wilkins, 1989.
50. Spirtas R, Kaufman SC, Alexander NJ. Fertility drugs and ovarian cancer: red alert or red herring? Fert Steril 1993;59:291-293.
51. Stewart DE, Robinson GE, Goldbloom DS, Wright C. Infertility and eating disorders. Am J Obstet Gynecol 1990;163:1196-1199.
52. Svensson L, Westrom L, Ripa KT, Mardh PA. Differences in some clinical and laboratory parameters in acute salpingitis related to culture and serologic findings. Am J Obstet Gynecol 1980;138:1017-1021.
53. Tanagho EA, Lue TF, McClure RD. Contemporary management of impotence and infertility. Baltimore MD: Williams & Wilkins, 1988.
54. Toner JP, Flood JT. Fertility after the age of 40. Obstetrics and Gynecology Clinics of North America 1993;20:261-272.
55. Trussell J, Kost K. Contraceptive failure in the United States: a critical review of the literature. Stud Fam Plann 1987;18:237-283.
56. Washington AE, Gove S, Schachter J, Sweet RL. Oral contraceptives, Chlamydia trachomatis infection, and pelvic inflammatory disease: a word of caution about protection. JAMA 1985;253:2246-2250.
57. Westrom LV. Sexually transmitted diseases and infertility. Sexually Transmitted Diseases 1994; Mar-Apr Supp: S32-S37.
58. Whittemore AS, Harris R, Itnyre J, Halpern J, the Collaborative Ovarian Cancer Group. Characteristics relating to ovarian cancer risk: collaborative analysis of twelve US case-control studies. Am J Epidemiol 1992;136:1175-1220.
59. Whorton MD, Krauss RM, Marshall S, Milby TH. Infertility in male pesticide workers. Lancet 1977;2:1259-1261.
60. Wilcox LS, Chu SV and Peterson HB. Characteristics of women who considered or obtained tubal reanatomosis: results from a prospective study of tubal sterilization. Obstet Gynecol 1990; 75:661-665.
61. Wilcox LS, Chu SY, Eaker ED, Zeger SL, Peterson HB. Risk factors for regret after tubal sterilization: 5 years of follow-up in a prospective study. Fertil Steril 1991;55:927-933.
62. World Health Organization. WHO laboratory manual for the examination of human semen and semen-cervical mucus interactions. 2nd ed. Cambridge; New York: Published on behalf of the World Health Organization by Cambridge University Press, 1992.

63. World Health Organization Task Force on the Diagnosis and Treatment of Infertility. Workshop on the investigation of the subfertile couple. Proceedings of the 12th World Congress on Fertility and Sterility, Singapore. In: Ratman S, Teoh E, Anandakumar C (eds). Infertility in the male and female. London: Parthenon Publishing, 1986. (Advances in fertility and sterility series; vol 4).

Abortion

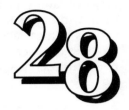

Willard Cates Jr., MD, MPH
Charlotte Ellertson, PhD, MPA

- Legally induced abortion is safer than continuing a pregnancy to term.
- Vacuum aspiration is the most commonly used abortion method, accounting for over 90% of all procedures.

- Mifepristone or methotrexate, used with misoprostol, provide alternatives to surgical methods of terminating early unwanted pregnancies.

In an ideal world, each woman would be able to plan and bear the children she wants at the time she wants. She would have available to her a variety of options to accomplish her goals. For the last few decades, women who wished to prevent pregnancy have had a number of contraceptive options. But none of these methods is perfect, even when used consistently and correctly. In addition, circumstances change, and so even women who may initially desire to become pregnant may later find themselves facing an unwanted pregnancy.

Traditionally, women wanting to end a pregnancy had few choices. Surgical techniques, although safe and effective, were essentially the only option. In recent years, however, women have gained new choices. Medical abortifacients allow a woman to terminate unwanted pregnancy earlier and without surgical intervention. Even within medical abortion, women can be offered a choice of parenteral or oral methods. During the coming decade, some of these same compounds may be developed as monthly pills for luteal use, or as menses inducers for women who do not wish to know for certain they are terminating a pregnancy.

Such technological breakthroughs demand a change in our thinking. No longer can we afford to cast contraceptives as good and abortion as a regrettable back-up. Instead, we owe it to women to provide the full range of family planning options so they can decide which is right for them without feeling judged. Several excellent review texts describe the various clinical abortion techniques in more detail.[6,16,21] This chapter provides our factual introduction to providing this important reproductive health service.

LEGAL STATUS OF ABORTION

Before 1970, legal abortion was not widely available in the United States. Beginning in 1970, however, several large states on the East and West coasts passed legislation allowing abortion under many circumstances. During the next three years, the majority of legal abortions were performed in New York and California.

On January 22, 1973, the U.S. Supreme Court decided two landmark cases—*Roe v. Wade*[38] and *Doe v. Bolton*[17]—that legalized abortion nationwide. In brief, these decisions established the "trimester framework" providing the following:

1. In the first trimester, the abortion decision and procedure must be left to the judgment of the pregnant woman and her physician. States have little scope to interfere.

2. In the second trimester, each state may choose to regulate abortion procedures in ways that are reasonably related to the pregnant woman's health.

3. In the third trimester, when a fetus is already viable, the state may choose to promote its interest in potential human life by limiting, or even prohibiting, abortion. It may not, however, impose restrictions that interfere with the life or health of the pregnant woman.

Since *Roe v. Wade*,[38] induced abortion has become one of the most commonly performed surgical procedures in the United States. Unlike in some other countries, however, abortion in America has been subject to intense debate and vigorous campaigns to limit the practice. Over the past two and a half decades, numerous and varied pieces of legislation to regulate abortion services have been introduced at the local, state, and national levels.[10] Attempts to pass a sweeping constitutional amendment overturning *Roe v. Wade* failed conclusively in 1983. Since then, abortion foes have concentrated on limiting abortion services in a piecemeal fashion[4,12] and on eliminating Medicaid funding for abortion rather than on trying to prohibit abortions outright. A landmark ruling for this approach was the 1992 Supreme Court decision in *Planned Parenthood of Southeastern Pennsylvania v. Casey*.[36] The Court ruled that states could restrict early-abortion services by enacting waiting periods, subjective counseling requirements, parental involvement provisions, and hospitalization requirements. Consequently, during the 1990s most major confrontations have occurred in state legislatures where both sides of the abortion issue are concentrating attempts to advance their agendas.

Recent legal changes, such as the Freedom of Access to Clinic Entrance (FACE) laws, promise some relief to the epidemic harassment and violence directed against abortion clinics.[23] Nearly all facilities affected by violence remain open, but the cumulative intimidation is gradually discouraging some clinicians from providing abortions. Thus the most profound threat to women's access to abortion now may be clinician supply rather than legal restrictions.[10]

CHARACTERISTICS OF WOMEN OBTAINING ABORTIONS

Data on women obtaining illegal abortions are difficult to collect and unreliable. Legal abortions, however, are reported by most state health authorities to the Centers for Disease Control and Prevention (CDC), and also form the subject of independent surveys. Between 1972 and 1990, the number of reported abortions increased substantially (Table 28-1). Most of the increase occurred between 1972 and 1980, with reported legal abortions rising from about 600,000 to 1.3 million per year.[13] During the 1980s, the number of reported legal abortions and the legal abortion rate (procedures per 1,000 women ages 15 to 44) remained remarkably stable, varying each year by less than 5%. In 1990, more than 1.4 million legal abortions, the highest number ever, were reported to CDC. Since 1990, the number of reported abortions has decreased each year by 2% to 4%; by 1994, the number of reported abortions declined to under 1.3 million.

The reported number of legal abortions is probably an underestimate. Totals provided by central health agencies are frequently lower than those obtained by direct surveys of abortion providers. Over the years, the number of legal abortions reported by CDC has been 15% lower than the number generated from independent surveys by The Alan Guttmacher Institute.[27]

Overall, women undergoing abortions tend to be young, white, and unmarried (Table 28-1). Most women have had no previous live births and are having an abortion for the first time. About half of all abortions occur before the eighth week of pregnancy, and 5 out of 6 are performed in the first trimester. Younger women tend to obtain abortions later in

Table 28-1 Characteristics of women who obtained legal abortions—United States, selected years, 1972 to 1994

	Year			
	1972	**1980**	**1990**	**1994**
Characteristics	%	%	%	%
Residence				
In-state	56.2	92.6	91.8	91.7
Out-of-state	43.8	7.4	8.2	8.3
Age (years)				
≤19	32.6	29.2	22.4	20.2
20-24	32.5	35.5	33.2	33.5
≥25	34.9	35.3	44.4	46.3
Race				
White	77.0	69.9	64.8	60.5
Black and other	23.0	30.1	35.2	39.5
Marital Status				
Married	29.7	23.1	21.7	19.9
Unmarried	70.3	76.9	78.3	80.1
Weeks of Gestation				
≤8	34.0	51.7	51.6	53.7
9–10	30.7	26.2	25.3	23.5
11–12	17.5	12.3	11.7	10.9
13–15	8.4	5.1	6.4	6.3
16–20	8.2	3.9	4.0	4.3
≥21	1.3	0.9	1.0	1.3
Total Reported Legal Abortions	**586,760**	**1,297,606**	**1,429,577**	**1,267,415**

Source: CDC (1997).

pregnancy than do older women. Finally, with the widespread availability of abortion since 1973, more than 90% of women now obtain the procedures in their states of residence.

DECIDING TO TERMINATE A PREGNANCY

The decision about how to resolve a pregnancy may begin even before a woman knows for certain she is pregnant. In fact, many women who come to the clinic seeking abortion services do not have confirmed pregnancies. Helping a woman understand she may be pregnant is an important step in assisting her make a decision about how she wants to resolve the pregnancy. Women who suspect they are pregnancy should be encouraged to come to the clinic as soon as they recognize the symptoms of pregnancy, including delayed menses. Regardless of whether a woman chooses to terminate her pregnancy or to continue it, a delay in confirming pregnancy until after the first 2 months can create problems:[9]

- Delays the start of prenatal care or the chances for early termination
- Increases the risks of complications
- Limits her options of abortion methods if the woman chooses to terminate

Clinicians and pregnancy counseling staff should provide a supportive, nonjudgmental setting in which women may explore their feelings concerning pregnancy once they find they are pregnant. If a clinic does not offer comprehensive services, women may need referrals to agencies providing services such as financial assistance, further counseling, first- and second-trimester abortions, prenatal care, and adoption. Counselors should provide each woman with an opportunity to discuss whether to continue her pregnancy. They should be empathetic, nonjudgmental and objective. The counselor should review the woman's feelings about the pregnancy, about abortion, about her partner, and about her future life plans and her ability to provide for a child at present and in the future. Some women want or need extensive discussion about these subjects; others require minimal counsel. Ambivalence is common, because for many women the decision is complicated.

In addition to providing basic factual information, the counselor should also be able to meet the counseling needs of most women and identify high-risk clients who may need more extensive education, evaluation, or counseling. Abortion providers need to follow strict criteria to ensure the woman is making an informed decision. (See Chapter 10 on Education and Counseling.)

SELECTING A METHOD OF ABORTION

Once a woman has decided to end her pregnancy, she may need assistance in selecting the best method for her. The main factor that determines which methods are possible for a specific woman is the duration of her pregnancy (Figure 28-1). For women obtaining abortions at later gestational ages, options are typically more limited. Women seeking early abortion, however, may have more than one safe and effective option. The clinician should explain to the woman the variety of abortion procedures available to her: how they are done; their discomforts, safety, success rates risks, costs, and duration; and their follow-up care. The woman should be given written information summarizing the discussion.

Surgical Methods

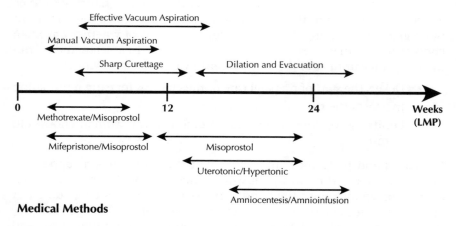

Figure 28-1 Options for terminating pregnancy, by length of pregnancy

In helping the early-abortion client decide between medical and surgical methods (Table 28-2), the important advantages to stress are that the surgical abortion is faster, more certain, and is handled for the woman by the provider, allowing the woman to remain less involved. It can also be performed under general anesthesia if the woman insists. The drawbacks of the surgical method are that many women dislike the invasiveness of the surgical procedure and the small risk of uterine perforation and infection it carries. By contrast, many women choosing medical abortion report it is more "natural" to them, as well as more private and intimate. Some women also report medical methods allow them to take a more active role in their abortions.[47]

Table 28-2 Advantages and disadvantages of early abortion methods

	Medical	Surgical
Advantages	Avoids surgery, anesthesia	Quicker
	More natural, like menses	More certain
	Less painful	Woman can be less involved
	Easier emotionally	Can be done under general
	Woman can be more in control, more involved	anesthesia
Disadvantages	Bleeding, cramping, nausea (actual or feared)	Invasive
	Waiting, uncertainty	Small risk of uterine, cervical injury, or infection
	Extra clinic visit, longer visits	

Disadvantages to medical methods are that the woman must be prepared to wait, possibly for as long as several weeks, for the abortion to occur.[24] A medical abortion is less predictable and may involve substantial cramping. Medical abortion patients will also observe more bleeding than their surgical counterparts, although the amounts are rarely clinically significant. For instance, one study of mifepristone used with a vaginal prostaglandin to treat women of 63 days or less past their last menstrual period (LMP) found the median blood loss was only about 75 milliliters (mls)[37] compared with the 50 mls typically lost during menses or nearly 500 mls typically given in a blood donation. Research from Europe and Canada suggests that over half of eligible women select medical methods.[7,8,446]

The woman may want her partner or other supportive persons to be involved in the process. Clinicians should honor the client's wishes.

PRE-ABORTION PROCEDURES

HISTORY

Take a history that covers the following information:

- Recent menstrual history
- Prior obstetric and gynecologic history, including previous surgery on the cervix or uterus, (e.g., conization of the cervix, cesarean delivery, and history of leiomyomata [fibroids]) and any complications of previous abortions
- Contraceptive history and future contraceptive desires
- Allergies or intolerance to local anesthetics, analgesics, antibiotics, anti-progestins, prostaglandins, and other drugs
- Drugs (over-the-counter, prescription, and recreational) currently being used, including anti-coagulants.
- Acute or chronic illnesses (including asthma, cardiac valvular disease, hemorrhagic disorders, or adrenal failure) that might require more evaluation, adjunctive therapy, or special care in the performance of the abortion or that might preclude one or more methods of abortion

CLINICAL EXAM

Perform a brief physical exam that includes taking vital signs, listening to the heart and lungs, and palpating the abdomen. Then perform a thorough pelvic exam. During the pelvic exam, estimate (independent of the history) the size of the pregnant uterus and check whether the cervix is anteverted or retroverted. Determine the presence of any abnormality such as uterine leiomyomata and adnexal masses that might influence the selection of a procedure. Ultrasound evaluation of the uterus may be valuable in assessing duration of pregnancy, pelvic architecture, and fetal position, as well as in diagnosing ectopic pregnancy.

LABORATORY TESTS

Recommended laboratory screening includes the following procedures:

- A urine or serum pregnancy test
- A hemoglobin or hematocrit (Offer iron supplementation to anemic women with hemoglobin <10 g/dl or hematocrit <30%.)
- An $Rh_0(D)$ determination (Women who are D-negative should be given anti-Rh_0[D] immune globulin [RhoGAM] because of the risk of isoimmunization.)
- Screening for reproductive tract infection as appropriate

S URGICAL METHODS

In the United States, surgical methods are currently the most common abortion procedures.

FIRST TRIMESTER

Vacuum aspiration is the standard first-trimester surgical method. Though used in other countries, sharp curettage is not widely available in the United States for induced abortion.

Vacuum Aspiration

Introduced to this country in 1967, vacuum aspiration is now the most widely used abortion procedure.[13,30] In 1994, 97% of abortions were performed by vacuum aspiration (suction curettage). This procedure is a safe and simple way to empty the uterus completely and quickly with minimal cervical dilation. It is most safely performed using local anesthesia, although many women request general anesthesia.

Perform a bimanual examination to determine the uterine size and angle of the cervical-uterine junction. Insert the speculum and cleanse the cervix. Using a local anesthetic such as 0.5% to 1% lidocaine amide (limiting the amount to less than 2 milligrams [mg] per pound [lb]), place a paracervical block to reduce pain. If necessary, dilate the cervix using gently sloped Pratt or Denniston dilators. Laminaria or other osmotic dilators placed up to 24 hours before the procedure can assist in dilating the cervix. (See the section on Adjunctive Techniques.) Use a tenaculum to stabilize the cervix if necessary. After inserting a vacuum cannula, introduce negative pressure to evacuate the products of conception. Most clinicians use an electrical vacuum pump to create the negative pressure, although if the woman dislikes the sound of the electric pump, manual vacuum aspiration is possible using a syringe. The cannula size generally used is 2 mm less than the number of weeks gestation (measured from LMP), although a larger size may speed the abortion procedure. When the uterus feels empty, examine the tissue to ensure the pregnancy was intrauterine rather than ectopic or a hydatidiform mole, as well as to confirm that the evacuation was complete. Tissue examination may be easier if the products of conception are suspended in saline or white vinegar and checked with backlighting.

For pregnancies less than 14 weeks gestation, vacuum aspiration can be done in a medical office, provided appropriate back-up and preparation are available for dealing with potentially adverse situations, such as allergic reactions to medication, uterine atony, uterine perforation, seizure, or cardiac arrest. Forceps are generally necessary to evacuate pregnancies later than 14 weeks gestation.

SECOND TRIMESTER

The standard surgical method used for second-trimester abortion is dilation and evacuation. A variety of adjunctive techniques make the procedure safer and more effective.

Dilation and Evacuation (D&E)

D&E allows vacuum aspiration to be performed into the second trimester.[24] D&E is especially appropriate for procedures performed between 13 and 16 weeks gestation, although some proponents use this method up through 20 or more weeks. An accurate estimate of the gestational age is crucial; intraoperative sonography may help. The cervix requires more dilation for a D&E than for a vacuum aspiration, because the products of conception in the second trimester are much larger. Osmotic dilators are often used to accommodate a gradual, less painful, and less traumatic dilation of the cervix. After administering a paracervical block or general anesthetic, remove the osmotic dilators and dilate the cervix as needed with mechanical dilators. The vacuum cannula, and other instruments as needed, can then evacuate the fetus and placenta from the uterus.

Adjunctive Techniques

Several adjunctive techniques can assist the clinician in performing second-trimester surgical abortions.

Laminaria. Dried seaweed of the genus *Laminaria* is highly hygroscopic and can, over a period of time, dilate the cervix. Laminaria are effective and relatively painless, and they decrease the risk of cervical laceration or perforation, reducing mortality by nearly 50%. Place the laminaria so they extend through the endocervical canal and dilate both the internal and external os. Usually, most of the cervical expansion occurs by 6 hours, but maximum dilation does not occur until 12 to 24 hours after placement of the laminaria.

Synthetic osmotic dilators. Two synthetic hygroscopic dilators are used in the United States. Lamicel is a magnesium sulfate-impregnated sponge. Dilapan is an expanding polymer of polyacrilonitrile. Both produce faster cervical dilation than laminaria. They have the advantages of uniform size (3 mm to 5 mm diameter), assured sterility, and easy insertion and removal. Depending on cost, these synthetic dilators may eventually replace the natural products.

Oxytocin or vasopressin. Intravenous oxytocin (TUBEX) may be used as an adjunct to vacuum aspiration to reduce the amount of bleeding. When used with second-trimester methods, oxytocin facilitates uterine contractions, hastens the abortion, and limits blood loss. Some clinicians avoid using oxytocin until the procedure is completed for fear of "trapping" the fetal skull (often the last part removed) as the uterus contracts. Other clinicians opt for vasopressin with the paracervical or intracervical block to constrict uterine vessels and decrease blood loss.

M EDICAL METHODS

In the past few years, new medical methods of early abortion have been developed.[27] In addition, some medical methods for later abortion have been refined.

FIRST TRIMESTER

Two new options for early medical abortion are available (or will be soon) in the United States. The first, mifepristone (formerly known as RU 486), together with a prostaglandin, is widely used to abort early pregnancies in several European countries[5,35,42,45] and has recently been shown to be safe and effective as well as acceptable in developing countries.[48] Clinical trials of mifepristone have been completed in the United States, and the drug has been recommended for approval by the U.S. Food and Drug Administration (FDA). Its use has recently been expanded in large-scale introductory studies. In addition, methotrexate in combination with misoprostol (both widely available) have been used successfully to terminate early pregnancies.[14,15,26,46] Women who are severely anemic should not use either method. Standard precautions for $Rh_o(D)$ isoimmunization should be used, as is the case with surgical methods.

Mifepristone and Misoprostol

Mifepristone is a 19-norsteroid with a high affinity for the progesterone receptors. The drug acts as a progesterone antagonist. The drug also binds strongly to glucocorticoid receptors, and to a lesser extent, to androgen receptors. It stimulates synthesis of prostaglandins by cells of the early decidua. Mifepristone has been investigated as an early abortifacient and as an emergency contraceptive, as well as for other indications. It is marketed for abortion in France, the United Kingdom, Sweden, and China. Supplementing mifepristone with misoprostol (Cytotec), a widely available low-dose E_1 prostaglandin analogue, increases efficacy. Mifepristone appears to be more effective the earlier in the pregnancy it is used: women with pregnancy durations of 7 weeks or less LMP experience a complete abortion about 95% of the time. Success rates decrease to about 80% in the ninth week LMP, and side effects tend to be more pronounced at this later duration of pregnancy. Large scale clinical trials of mifepristone medical abortion have not examined use beyond 9 weeks LMP.

Over 80% of women using the regimen report cramping and bleeding. In fact the drugs are intended to induce these actions to help create the abortion. Women report medical abortion is experientially similar to a miscarriage. Most pain can be managed with acetaminophen (Tylenol) or acetaminophen with codeine phosphate. It is common practice to avoid giving aspirin or ibuprofen as these analgesics are anti-prostaglandins and may counteract the effects of the misoprostol. Although bleeding may seem significant to the woman, the amount of bleeding is rarely clinically significant. Median blood loss for a similar regimen (mifepristone plus gemeprost) is less than 100 mls, although the range can extend up to several hundred mls and is significantly correlated to length of gestation.[37] Approximately 1% of women experience uterine bleeding that requires curettage; about 0.1% require transfusion. Some clinicians report treating excessive bleeding with an ergot alkaloid such as methylergonovine maleate (Methergine) before resorting to aspiration or curettage.

Mifepristone will be distributed directly to any licensed physician who is trained in abortion, pregnancy diagnosis, and gestational age assessment and can treat or refer complications to an appropriate back-up facility. Contraindications to the regimen include confirmed or suspected ectopic pregnancy or undiagnosed adnexal mass, chronic adrenal failure, concurrent long-term corticosteroid therapy, hemorrhagic disorders or concurrent anticoagulant therapy, or known allergy to mifepristone or misoprostol. Remove the IUD from IUD users before starting treatment.

The regimen involves three visits to the clinic. On the first visit, the woman takes 600 mg mifepristone. Two days later, she returns to the clinic for administration of prostaglandin. A small percentage (fewer than 5%) of women will have expelled their pregnancies before the second visit. If the woman thinks she has expelled the pregnancy between the two visits, perform a pelvic examination to assess whether the abortion has been completed. For all women who have not had complete abortions, administer two 200 µg tablets of misoprostol (400 µg total) orally. These tablets can be purchased inexpensively directly from a pharmaceutical supply house. Their shelf-life is short, however, so expiration dates of misoprostol should be checked frequently. Following administration of misoprostol, the woman should stay under observation for 4 hours or until stable. During the first 4 hours following prostaglandin, most (about two-thirds) of the abortions take place. Women should return to the clinic after about 2 weeks for a follow-up appointment to ensure their abortion is complete.

Several aspects of the mifepristone regimen remain to be refined. Preliminary research suggests a 200 mg dose of mifepristone may be as effective as a 600 mg dose.[50] Vaginal administration of the misoprostol may work as well as oral administration, or possibly even better at the later gestational ages.[19,20] Most important, the initial protocols used in the United States are based on those from Europe, where medical practice differs from the United States. As United States clinicians gain experience with the regimen, protocols may be adapted and simplified for home use.[18] For example, the misoprostol step may be administered at home by the woman herself,[41] as is the case with methotrexate abortion.

Methotrexate and Misoprostol

Methotrexate is a cytotoxic drug that has been used successfully to treat unruptured ectopic pregnancy, choriocarcinoma, psoriasis, and rheumatoid arthritis. The drug is lethal to proliferating trophoblastic tissue and causes early abortion by blocking the folic acid in fetal cells so they cannot divide. Used in combination with misoprostol, it is about 95% successful in terminating early pregnancies.[26,46]

Methotrexate regimens have been developed to terminate intrauterine pregnancies only quite recently and involve off-label use of the drug. For this reason, no single standardized protocol has been set forth. Several methotrexate-misoprostol protocols are currently used.[14,26,40] All protocols involve a minimum of two clinic visits. All require women to be of good health with no contraindications to surgical abortion and no history of chronic renal or hepatic disease, anemia, acute inflammatory bowel disease, or uncontrolled seizures. Women should discontinue using vitamins containing folate for 1 week after taking methotrexate.

Regardless of which protocol is used, on the first visit the woman receives 50 mg methotrexate per square meter of body surface, administered intramuscularly in the gluteal muscle. All protocols follow methotrexate by 800 µg misoprostol inserted vaginally. One option is to give four 200 µg tablets; advise the woman to hold the tablets in place with a tampon. In such cases, instruct women to leave the tampon in place for 12 hours or until active vaginal bleeding begins. Another option is to use vaginal suppositories (either four 200 µg suppositories or one 800 µg suppository) prepared by a local pharmacy. The optimum interval between methotrexate and misoprostol insertion has yet to be determined. In some protocols, misoprostol is administered 3 days after methotrexate, while in others, it is not administered until 5 to 7 days later.

Methotrexate protocols also vary as to whether women are required to return for misoprostol insertion or whether they can self-administer the prostaglandin at home. All protocols provide women with acetaminophen containing codeine phosphate (300 mg/30 mg). If women plan to take the misoprostol at home, instruct them to (1) use the suppository(ies) when they can rest afterwards (i.e., before bedtime); (2) drink fluids to avoid feeling dizzy when rising; (3) eat lightly because of the possibility of nausea or vomiting; (4) insert the suppository or tablets deep into the vagina with clean hands; (5) rest on their backs for at least 30 minutes; (6) expect cramping and bleeding within the next 12 hours; (7) use acetaminophen with codeine every 4 hours if needed for cramping; (8) use ibuprofen as backup only; and (9) call if they have heavy vaginal bleeding (soaking four sanitary pads within 2 hours). Some protocols provide a second dose of misoprostol to use if women have not begun bleeding within 24 hours of the initial dose.

Timing of follow-up visits varies. Some protocols require women to return to the clinic as early as 3 days after the initial misoprostol administration. Others suggest women return only after a week following misoprostol administration. If the woman has not had a complete abortion by the first follow-up visit (based on bimanual vaginal examination or vaginal ultrasound), or if her βhCG level has not declined by at least 50% at the first follow-up visit, offer an additional dose of misoprostol or a vacuum aspiration. For those accepting an additional misoprostol dose, schedule weekly follow-up appointments for up to a month, or longer if the woman opts to keep waiting for abortion to occur without surgical intervention.

SECOND TRIMESTER

Several medical agents may be used for second-trimester abortion when administered by amniocentesis and amnioinfusion. They fall into two broad groups: hypertonic solutions (e.g., saline or urea) and uterotonic drugs (e.g., prostaglandin E_2 suppositories or misoprostol). However, in 1994, these methods combined accounted for only 0.7% of all abortions in the United States.[13] They have been replaced by D&E procedures that are safer, faster, and less expensive.

Hypertonic Solutions

Two hypertonic solutions are typically used intra-amniotically.

Saline.   Saline is relatively inexpensive, readily available, and feticidal; in addition, considerable clinical experience with the procedure has been amassed. However, its disadvantages include higher rates of severe, disseminated intravascular coagulation.

Hypertonic urea.   Used to terminate second-trimester pregnancies, hypertonic urea is relatively safe with a low cost and with feticidal effects. The major disadvantage has been the high failure rate when used as a sole abortifacient. Currently prostaglandins are generally used to augment labor in urea-induced abortions.

Uterotonic Agents

Both E_1 and E_2 prostaglandins can be used for second-trimester medical abortions with or without the hypertonic agents.

Dinoprostone.   A prostaglandin E_2, Dinoprostone is marketed as PROSTIN E2, a vaginal suppository for evacuating a missed abortion. These 20 mg vaginal suppositories cause a high incidence of gastrointestinal side effects and often affect the thermoregulatory mechanism, causing a temperature elevation in some clients.

Misoprostol.   Misoprostol (Cytotec) is a synthetic E_1 prostaglandin agent approved for the prevention and treatment of gastric ulcer disease. It is used in combination with other drugs for early medical abortion, but it is also effective for second-trimester abortion. Vaginal administration of 200 µg misoprostol every 12 hours produces pregnancy termination rates comparable to prostaglandin E_2 suppositories given every 3 hours.[29] The misoprostol regimen is less expensive and entails fewer side effects than other prostaglandins.

Amniocentesis and Amnioinfusion

Amniocentesis (removal of fluid from the amniotic cavity) and amnioinfusion (infusion of medication into the amniotic cavity) are techniques central to the second-trimester instillation procedures.

Ask the woman to empty her bladder and then lie in the supine position. Cleanse the amniocentesis site with a disinfectant, and drape the site with sterile towels. No premedication is recommended. At the injection site, infiltrate the skin with a local anesthetic. Insert an 18-gauge spinal needle into the intrauterine cavity to obtain a flow of clear amniotic fluid.

Many clinicians also insert osmotic dilators in the cervix either before or at the time of the amniocentesis to expedite the procedure and decrease the incidence of cervical lacerations. Prostaglandin suppositories can help soften the cervix.

Adjunctive Techniques

Adjunctive techniques can also simplify second-trimester medical abortions, but their advantages are mixed.

Intravenous oxytocin (TUBEX) may be used with second-trimester methods to facilitate uterine contractions, hasten the abortion, and limit blood loss. When used as an adjunct to second-trimester saline abortion, oxytocin increases the risks of disseminated intravascular coagulation, cervical laceration, and water intoxication, although it decreases the risks of infection and retained products of conception.

PREVENTING ABORTION COMPLICATIONS

Compared with childbirth, as well as with other surgical procedures, legal abortion is remarkably safe.[9] In the two largest studies of legally induced abortions reported to date, the rate of major complications is less than 1 in 200 cases.[21,25] Early abortions are safer than those occurring later in pregnancy. Teenagers tend to have abortions later in gestation than do adult women, and therefore, as a group experience more complications. Adjusted for length of gestation, however, teenagers have fewer complications than do older women.[11] The abortion method influences risks of complications: dilation and evacuation, for example, is significantly safer than instillation procedures for pregnancies 13 to 20 weeks post LMP.[24]

Abortion-related problems are less likely under these conditions:

- The pregnancy is early.
- The woman is healthy.
- The woman is not ambivalent about having the abortion performed (or can cope with feelings of ambivalence).
- The woman does not have gonorrhea or chlamydia infection of the cervix.
- Osmotic dilators are used when appropriate.
- Local anesthesia is used in preference to general anesthesia.
- The uterus is carefully and completely emptied.
- The clinician carefully examines the aspirated or curetted tissue to rule out the possibility of a molar or ectopic pregnancy.
- Rh_o(D) immune globulin (RhoGAM) is given to D-negative women.

- The woman understands the warning signs for potential postabortal problems.
- Prompt follow-up care is available on a 24-hour basis.
- Prophylactic antibiotics are given to surgical patients.

Prophylactic antibiotics can reduce complications from induced abortions.[39] A common regimen is 100 mg of doxycycline, taken twice a day for 1 to 3 days. Many providers wait until after surgery to begin the antibiotics because of the problem of nausea and vomiting.

A woman's risk of dying from a legal surgical abortion has decreased greatly between 1972 and 1990, and abortion mortality is now exceedingly rare.[30] In 1972, the case fatality rate was 4.1 deaths per 100,000 legal abortions. By 1990, the rate had declined over 90% to 0.3 deaths per 100,000 procedures. Legal-abortion mortality is related to the age of the woman, the type of procedure used, and the length of gestation. Death is also associated with general health problems at the time of abortion. In recent years, a disproportionate share of deaths has been attributable to complications from general anesthesia or pulmonary embolism.[32]

Early medical abortion has been implicated in only one death, a fatal myocardial infarction linked to an injectable prostaglandin, sulprostone.[31] For this reason, sulprostone is no longer used in the abortion regimens. No deaths have been associated with other medical regimens for early abortion.

MANAGING POSTABORTION COMPLICATIONS

Legally induced abortion is, fortunately, an extremely safe procedure.[9,25] Nevertheless, any complaint of problems after an abortion procedure should be taken seriously. The recognition and management of the potential serious postabortion problems is critical.

Warning Signs After Abortion

Caution

- Fever
- Chills
- Abdominal pain, cramping, or backache
- Tenderness (to pressure) in the abdomen
- Prolonged or heavy bleeding
- Foul vaginal discharge
- Delay (6 weeks or more) in resuming menstrual periods

SHORT-TERM COMPLICATIONS

A variety of short-term complications are possible. All can be minimized by proper vigilance and prompt detection and treatment.

Infection. Postabortal infections can be minimized by screening and treating for gonorrhea, chlamydia and cervicitis before the abortion, by complete emptying of the uterus, and by administrating prophylactic antibiotics when surgical methods have been used. Infections may be heralded by cramping, fever, discharge, and pelvic discomfort. Advise women to seek help immediately if any suspicious symptoms develop after the procedure (see Warning Signs After Abortion). If retained products of conception are suspected, remove them by repeat vacuum aspiration after initiating an antibiotic. If the infection has extended beyond the uterus, hospitalize the woman and administer parenteral antibiotics.

Intrauterine blood clots. The most common problem requiring a repeat aspiration is the presence of intrauterine blood clots. These can occur either immediately or as long as 5 days after a surgical abortion; their presence is manifested by severe cramping and pain. The syndrome is diagnosed by a pelvic exam showing a large, tense, tender uterus without bleeding from the cervix. Simple vacuum aspiration remedies the problem. Ergot alkaloids (such as Methergine) used intramuscularly or orally may help prevent this problem.

Incomplete abortion. In rare cases, the abortion will be incomplete (perhaps 0.5% of surgical procedures and about 2% of medical abortions). Carefully evaluating the products of conception after the surgical procedures helps catch such failures directly, when they can most easily be remedied. A careful history and physical examination are an important part of the postabortion exam. Vacuum aspiration or curettage is the appropriate solution.

Continuing pregnancy. In rare cases, attempts to terminate the pregnancy will fail altogether (about 0.1% of surgical procedures and 0.5% to 1% of early medical abortions). A woman with a continuing pregnancy has ongoing symptoms of pregnancy, an enlarged uterus at the follow-up exam, and a persistently positive pregnancy test. Rule out an abnormal uterus (e.g., bicornuate), twin pregnancies, or an ectopic pregnancy, and then perform a surgical abortion to terminate the pregnancy. Particularly in the case of ongoing pregnancies following failed medical abortion, surgical abortion is strongly recommended because of the risk of fetal malformation.

Cervical or uterine trauma. Perforation of the uterus and laceration of the cervix are worrisome complications of surgical abortion. Depending on their severity, these complications may require attention ranging from simple observation to hysterectomy. Trauma may be prevented by using osmotic dilators for gentle cervical dilation and by applying gentle but firm and steady traction when using the tenaculum on the cervix. Advanced gestational age and previous term delivery are risk factors for uterine perforation. Using local rather than general anesthesia lowers the risk of both cervical injury and uterine perforation considerably, as does the use of osmotic dilators for late-term procedures.

Bleeding. Regardless of whether medical or surgical methods are used, bleeding during or after an abortion is common. This bleeding is not usually clinically significant. Local anesthetics, uterine-contracting agents (oxytocin administered intravenously or ergotrate administered orally or intramuscularly), vascular constricting agents (vasopressin), and uterine massage can help minimize bleeding after a pregnancy termination. After medical abortions, perhaps 1% of women require aspiration or curettage to stop the bleeding. In very rare cases, transfusion may be required (0.1 to 0.2%).

LONG-TERM COMPLICATIONS

Once pregnant, a woman can choose to terminate or continue her pregnancy. The key question involving long-term effects of this choice is whether women opting to terminate their pregnancies face greater risk of future adverse outcomes than do women who opt to continue the pregnancy. Based on this comparison, no evidence exists for long-term sequelae of the abortion option. Three areas, however, are sometimes misunderstood by the general public:

Future fertility impairments. First-trimester abortion performed by the vacuum aspiration technique has little effect on subsequent fertility or on the risk of spontaneous abortions, premature delivery, and low birthweight babies.[28]

Psychiatric sequelae. Major psychiatric sequelae associated with abortion are rare, regardless of whether medical or surgical methods have been used.[43,44] Transient feelings of stress or sadness may follow what is sometimes a difficult decision to terminate a pregnancy.[1] By contrast, feelings of relief are also common. In addition, longitudinal studies reveal no evidence of widespread long-term psychological trauma after abortion.

Breast cancer. The association between induced abortion and subsequent breast cancer has received intense scrutiny. Full-term pregnancy has an apparent dichotomous influence on breast tissue: it produces an early gestational increase in growth due to the stimulus of estrogens, but a later gestational differentiation of mammary tissue. This latter effect is apparently related to a decrease in risk of breast cancer.[34] A careful analysis of the available epidemiological studies reveals a number of biases that can cause spurious associations. Ascertainment bias is a particular hazard, because the sensitive nature of abortion can affect a woman's willingness to report a previous experience. Because of these limitations, current observational studies may not be able to resolve the important etiologic questions surrounding the relationship between induced abortion and breast cancer. However, any such association is likely to be small or non-existent.[34] Moreover, the most comprehensive analysis of induced abortion and breast cancer to date, based on the Danish population-based experience, found no association between induced abortion and breast cancer.[33]

POSTABORTION CONTRACEPTION

Fertility returns quickly following abortion. *Even within 10 days, a woman can conceive again.* For this reason it is critical that women understand their risk for subsequent pregnancy. A woman's clinic visit to terminate an unplanned pregnancy also represents a general opportunity to discuss the contraceptive options available to prevent future unintended conceptions. Make sure the woman is aware of all the options available to her and understands how to use correctly the particular contraceptive method she chooses. If the unplanned pregnancy occurred while the woman was using a barrier contraceptive (condom, spermicide, or diaphragm), review any behavioral or situational factors that may have contributed to the pregnancy. Explain the availability of emergency contraception as a back-up in case of condom breakage or of failure to use the barrier method. If the unplanned conception occurred while using hormonal methods, make sure the woman understands the recommended regimens and how to minimize chances of becoming pregnant if pills or injections are missed.

The woman may start a method of contraception as soon as she is ready to resume intercourse, or even earlier, depending on the method. Women having medical abortions do not need to abstain from intercourse and can initiate any methods except IUDs as soon as they wish. An IUD may be inserted as soon the termination of pregnancy is confirmed. In the case of women who have an uncomplicated early surgical abortion, an IUD can safely be inserted at the same time as the procedure.

REFERENCES

1. Adler NE, David HP, Major BN, Roth SH, Rosso NF, Wyatt GE. Psychological response after abortion. Science 1990;248:41-44.

2. Alan Guttmacher Institute. The limitations of U.S. statistics on abortion. New York: Alan Guttmacher Institute, 1997.
3. Alan Guttmacher Institute. Late-term abortions: Legal considerations. New York: Alan Guttmacher Institute, 1997.
4. Annas GJ. The Supreme Court, liberty, and abortion. N Engl J Med 1992;327:651-654.
5. Aubény E, Peyron R, Turpin CL, Renault M, Targosz V, Silvestre L, Ulmann A, Baulieu EE. Termination of early pregnancy (up to and after 63 days of amenorrhea) with mifepristone (RU 486) and increasing doses of misoprostol. Int J Fertil 1995;40(Supp. 2):85-91.
6. Baird DT, Grimes DA, Van Look PF (eds). Modern methods of inducing abortion. London: Blackwell Science, 1995.
7. Blayo C. L'évolution du recours à l'avortement en France depuis 1976. Population 1995;3:779-810.
8. Cameron ST, Glasier AF, Logan J, Benton L, Baird DT. Impact of the introduction of new medical methods on therapeutic abortions at the Royal Infirmary of Edinburgh. Brit J Obstet Gynecol 1996;103:1222-1229.
9. Cates W Jr. Legal abortion: The public health record. Science 1982;215: 1586-1590.
10. Cates W Jr, Grimes DA, Hogue LL. Topics for our times: Justice Blackmun and legal abortion—a besieged legacy to women's reproductive health. Am J Public Health 1995;85:1204-1206.
11. Cates W Jr, Schulz KF, Grimes DA. The risks associated with teenage abortion. N Engl J Med 1983;309:621-624.
12. Cates W Jr, Gold J, Selik RM. Regulation of abortion service: for better or worse? N Engl J Med 1979;301:720-723.
13. Centers for Disease Control and Prevention. Abortion surveillance: preliminary data—United States, 1994. MMWR 1997;45:1123-1127.
14. Creinin MD, Darney PD. Methotrexate and misoprostol for early abortion. Contraception 1993;48:339-348.
15. Creinin MD, Park M. Acceptability of medical abortion with methotrexate and misoprostol. Contraception 1995;52:41-44.
16. Darney PD, Morbuch P, Korn A. Protocols on office gynecologic surgery. London: Blackwell Science, 1996.
17. *Doe v. Bolton* 410 U.S. 179 (1973).
18. Ellertson CE, Elul B, Winikoff B. Taking the medical out of medical abortion: Can women use mifepristone/misoprostol without medical supervision? Reproductive Health Matters (forthcoming).
19. El-Refaey H, Rajasekar D, Abdalla M, Calder L, Templeton A. Induction of abortion with mifepristone (RU 486) and oral or vaginal misoprostol. N Engl J Med 1995;332:983-987.
20. El-Refaey H, Templeton A. Early induction of abortion by a combination of oral mifepristone and misoprostol administered by the vaginal route. Contraception 1994;49:111-114.
21. Grimes DA. Management of abortion. In: Rock JA, Thompson JR (eds.). TeLinde's Operative Gynecology, 8th Edition. Philadelphia: Lippincott-Raven, (in press).
22. Grimes DA. Medical abortion in early pregnancy: a review of the evidence. Obstet Gynecol 1997;89:790-796.

23. Grimes DA, Forrest JD, Kirkman AL, Radford B. An epidemic of antiabortion violence in the United States. Am J Obstet Gynecol 1991;165:1263-1268.
24. Grimes DA, Schulz KF, Cates W Jr, Tyler CW. Midtrimester abortion by dilation and evacuation. N Engl J Med 1977;296:1141-1145.
25. Hakim-Elahi E, Tovell HM, Burnhill MS. Complications of first trimester abortion: a report of 170,000 cases. Obstet Gynecol 1990;76:129-135.
26. Hausknecht RU. Methotrexate and misoprostol to terminate early pregnancy. N Engl J Med 1995;333:537-540.
27. Henshaw SK, Van Vort J. Abortion services in the United States, 1991 and 1992. Fam Plann Perspect 1994;26:100-106, 112.
28. Hogue CJ, Cates W Jr, Tietze C. Effects of induced abortion on subsequent reproduction. Epidemiol Rev 1982;4:66-94.
29. Jain JK, Mishell DR Jr. A comparison of intravaginal misoprostol with prostaglandin E$_2$ for termination of second-trimester pregnancy. N Engl J Med 1994;331:290-293.
30. Koonin LM, Smith JC, Ramick M, Green CA. Abortion surveillance—United States, 1992. MMWR 1996;45(SS-3):1-36.
31. Lancet editor. A death associated with mifepristone/sulprostone. Lancet 1991;337: 969-970.
32. Lawson H, Frye A, Atrash HA, Smith JC, Shulman HB, Ramick M. Abortion mortality, United States, 1972 through 1987. Am J Obstet Gynecol 1994;171:1365-1372.
33. Melbye M, Wohlfahrt J, Olsen JH, Frisch M, Westergaard T, Helweg-Larsen K, Andersen PK. Induced abortion and the risk of breast cancer. N Engl J Med 1997;336:81-85.
34. Michels KB, Willett WC. Does induced or spontaneous abortion affect the risk of breast cancer? Epidemiology 1996;7(5):521-528.
35. Peyron R, Aubény E, Targosz V, Silvestre L, Renault M, Elkik F, Leclerc P, Ulmann A, Baulieu EE. Early termination of pregnancy with mifepristone (RU 486) and the orally active prostaglandin misoprostol. N Engl J Med 1993;328:1509-1513.
36. *Planned Parenthood of Southeastern Pennsylvania v. Casey* 505 U.S. 833 (1992).
37. Rodger MW, Baird DT. Blood loss following induction of early abortion using mifepristone (RU 486) and a prostaglandin analogue (gemeprost). Contraception 1989;40:439-447.
38. *Roe v. Wade* 410 U.S. 113 (1973).
39. Sawaya GF, Grady D, Kerlikowske K, Grimes DA. Antibiotics at the time of induced abortion: the case for universal prophylaxis based on a meta-analysis. Obstet Gynecol 1996;87:884-890.
40. Schaff EA, Eisinger SH, Franks P, Kim SS. Combined methotrexate and misoprostol for early induced abortion. Arch Fam Med 1995;4:774-779.
41. Schaff EA, Stadalius LS, Eisinger SH, Franks P. Vaginal misoprostol administered at home after mifepristone (RU 486) for abortion. J Fam Pract 1997; 44:353-360.
42. Silvestre L, Dubois C, Renault M, Rezvani Y, Baulieu EE, Ulmann A. Voluntary interruption of pregnancy with mifepristone (RU 486) and a prostaglandin analogue. N Engl J Med 1990;322:645-648.
43. Stotland NL. The myth of the abortion trauma syndrome. JAMA 1992;268:2078-2079.

44. Urquhart DR, Templeton AA. Psychiatric morbidity and acceptability following medical and surgical methods of induced abortion. Br J Obstet Gynecol 1991;98:396-399.

45. Urquhart DR, Templeton AA, Shinewi F, Chapman M, Hawkins K, McGarry J, Rodger M, Baird DT, Bjornsson S, Macnaughton M, Lunan CB, Macrow P, Elstein M, Killick S, Hill NCW, Turnbull AC, MacKenzie IZ, Cohn M, Stewart P, Bryce F, Lilford RJ, Johnson N, Li TC, Cooke ID, Olajide F, Chard T, Lim B, Lees DAR, Subramanyan V, Grudzinskas JG, Davey A. The efficacy and tolerance of mifepristone and prostaglandin in termination of pregnancy of less than 63 days gestation: UK multicentre study—final results. Contraception 1997;55:1-5.

46. Wiebe ER. Abortion induced with methotrexate and misoprostol. Can Med Assoc J 1996;154:165-170.

47. Winikoff B. Acceptability of medical abortion in early pregnancy. Fam Plann Perspect 1995;27:142-148, 185.

48. Winikoff B, Sivin I, Coyaji K, Cabezas E, Xiao B, Gu S, Du M, Krishna U, Eschen A, Ellertson C. Safety, efficacy, and acceptability of medical abortion in China, Cuba, and India: a comparative trial of mifepristone-misoprostol versus surgical abortion. Am J Obstet Gynecol 1997;176:431-437.

49. Winikoff B, Ellertson C, Elul B, Sivin I. Acceptability of mifepristone/misoprostol abortion in the United States. (forthcoming).

50. World Health Organization Task Force on Post-ovulatory Methods of Fertility Regulation. Termination of pregnancy with reduced doses of mifepristone. Br Med J 1993;307:532-537.

Adolescent Sexual Behavior, Pregnancy, and Childbearing

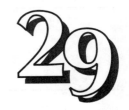

James Trussell, PhD
Josefina J. Card, PhD
Carol J. Rowland Hogue, PhD, MPH

- Each year, 1 of every 8 women aged 15 to 19 in the United States becomes pregnant. This proportion has changed little since the late 1970s.
- This overall constancy has masked two offsetting long-term trends: increasing proportions, until recently, having sexual intercourse and increasing proportions using contraception.
- Both pregnancy and birth rates among teens in the United States are very high when compared with those in other developed countries, although rates of sexual activity are similar.
- Recent research suggests the consequences of teenage childbearing are not as deleterious as has been claimed but nevertheless damage life chances for mother and child.
- While everyone agrees teenage pregnancy is a problem, no consensus about a solution exists.
- Adolescents with a negative pregnancy test are an accessible but neglected target group for intervention.

Each year, 1 in 8 women aged 15 to 19 in the United States becomes pregnant. This proportion has changed little since the late 1970s. Consequently, each year about 1.2 million pregnancies occur to those in this age group. Another 63 thousand pregnancies occur among women aged 14 and younger (Table 29-1). Each year, 1 in 17 women aged 15 to 19 gives birth. Of all births in the United States, 13% occur to women aged less than 20.[77] Each year, 1 in 40 men aged 15 to 19 fathers a child,[77] and 1 in 15 men fathers a child while he is a teenager.[47] The sheer magnitude of these statistics has generated widespread public concern. The overwhelming consensus is that adolescent pregnancy is a serious problem and public policies and programs should be implemented to reduce its incidence and ameliorate its consequences.

Table 29-1 Estimated pregnancies, births, and abortions to adolescents in 1998 (numbers in thousands), United States

Age group	Pregnancies	Births	Abortions
15–19	1,225	572	335
<20	1,288	585	349
<15	63	13	14
15–17	534	215	132
18–19	691	357	203

Note: The sum of births, induced abortions and spontaneous abortions among women age *a* will not equal pregnancies to women age *a*, because women are older when their pregnancies are resolved than when they are conceived. There are more births and induced abortions resulting from pregnancies to women under age 20 than there are births and induced abortions to women under age 20. Estimates of births, abortions and pregnancies for 1998 were obtained by assuming that 1992 rates (Henshaw 1996, 1997; Ventura et al. 1996) pertained to the projected number of women in 1998 (Day 1996).

This consensus, however, offers little guidance for formulating public policy because the reasons for concern vary widely:

- Many object to adolescents' having sex simply because they are too young.
- Others would draw an important distinction between those who are married and those who are not. Some believe sex among unmarried persons is unwise or immoral. Most pregnant adolescents (virtually all those aged 14 and younger) are unmarried at the time their pregnancy is resolved. Nearly 95% of births to women younger than 15 and 75% of births to women aged 15 to 19 occur out of wedlock.[77]
- Others would differentiate pregnancies that are intended from those that are not. More than 8 in 10 adolescent pregnancies are unintended.[19]
- Some, including many family planning clinicians, are particularly troubled by the large number of abortions obtained by adolescents: about 349 thousand each year.

Still others view a birth to an adolescent as a tragedy, reasoning that giving birth at an early age not only seriously damages the young woman's life chances and limits her options, but also creates a suboptimal environment for the child. About 585 thousand births occur to women under 20 years of age (Table 29-1). Only 1 in 3 births to women aged 15 to 19 is intended.[1] Among births to women aged 15 to 17, 1 in 5 is fathered by a male 6 or more years older.[43]

Most observers are particularly concerned about pregnancy and its consequences among the poor or the very young. Each year women younger than 15 have about 13 thousand births and 14 thousand abortions; women aged 15 to 17 have 215 thousand births and 132 thousand abortions. About three-fourths of adolescent births occur among poor women (those with family incomes ranging from below the poverty level to as much as 50% above), and about half occur among women who were both poor and unmarried.[72] Some view the problem primarily as a health issue, others as a moral issue, and yet others as an economic issue.

We have identified four categories of arguments supporting public intervention to "solve" the adolescent pregnancy problem, each suggesting different intervention strategies and target groups. These arguments may be summarized as follows:

Sex prevention. Unmarried persons, especially young persons, should not engage in sexual intercourse. Our society places far too much emphasis on sex, especially in the media, and public institutions, especially the schools, have abandoned the teaching of traditional values. The solution, therefore, is a vigorous campaign to promote chastity among the unmarried. Because other strategies to reduce adolescent pregnancy (e.g., increasing the availability of contraceptive and abortion services) have the undesirable even if unintended effect of "legitimizing" and perhaps even increasing sexual activity, they are unacceptable. The target group is very large. More than 95% of women aged 15 to 19 have never married[68] and only 52% of these are still virgins.[1] Likewise, more than 98% of men aged 15 to 19 have never married,[68] of whom only 45% are still virgins.[69]

Pregnancy prevention. Campaigns with the sole aim of promoting chastity have not proven effective. Because such large proportions of adolescents are sexually active, it is prudent to provide accurate information on reproductive biology and contraception starting at an early age. Such information is an essential component of family life education, whose primary goal should be to promote rational and informed decision-making about sexuality. Nevertheless, information will not reduce pregnancy rates unless contraceptive services are also widely available. Preventing pregnancy should reduce the incidence of adolescent childbearing and abortion. The target group here is the sexually active and those about to become sexually active.

Abortion or pregnancy support. While preventing pregnancies is an important goal, this objective will not be met in the short run. Even if high-quality sex education and contraceptive services were universally available, some adolescents would nevertheless become pregnant. Many of them do not always plan their lives carefully. Moreover, typical contraceptive failure rates even among more mature women are not low.[73]

Therefore, abortion services or programs to ameliorate the adverse consequences of adolescent childbearing must be available, particularly for the poor, who suffer the consequences to a greater extent and generate more public costs. The target group here is much smaller, consisting of abortion services for whatever fraction of the 1.3 million pregnant teenagers who do not wish to carry their pregnancy to term (at least the 3 in 10 who actually obtain abortions) and ameliorative programs for the remainder.

Societal restructuring.   Teenage childbearing is not the problem it appears to be; it is instead the symptom of the major underlying fundamental problem of poverty, an indicator of the extent to which many young people have been excluded from the American dream.[45] The target group is the poor and near-poor, and what is required is a fundamental restructuring of society so young women no longer feel they have nothing to lose by having a child at an early age. Because the problems faced by these youth are so many and so extensive, real solutions—such as better schools, safer neighborhoods, access to health care, and decent jobs for their mothers and fathers—would be very costly (and therefore very unlikely). Nevertheless, providing contraceptive and abortion services enables many poor teens to avoid childbearing.

These arguments are not mutually exclusive, and even those persons generally in agreement with one of them may not concur with all the points. Nevertheless, even this simple categorization shows the considerable discrepancies among the solutions advocated by those who view sex, those who view pregnancy, and those who view childbearing (particularly among the poor) as the main aspect of this problem and others who view teen pregnancy and childbearing not as the problem but only as a symptom. Conflict also exists (by no means limited to adolescents) about the use of abortion as a remedy for an unwanted pregnancy. We return at the end of this chapter for further discussion of intervention strategies. Before doing so, we examine trends and levels of adolescent pregnancy in the United States, contrast the U.S. experience with that in other developed countries, analyze the determinants of adolescent pregnancy, examine the incidence of sexually transmitted infections (STIs) among adolescents, and analyze the consequences of adolescent childbearing.

A BORTION, BIRTH, AND PREGNANCY RATES

Pregnancies can end in births, induced abortions, or spontaneous abortions. Data for the United States are available for only the first two outcomes; spontaneous abortions must be estimated. In 1992 (the latest year for which estimates are available), 3% of females aged 14 became pregnant. This proportion rose steadily with age (Figure 29-1) to reach 18%

of women aged 18 and 19. The fraction of pregnancies ending in an induced abortion was virtually constant with age (about 30%).

- *Birth rates* among women aged 15 to 19 declined steadily from 1970 to 1978, rose slightly until 1983 when they began to decline to a record low in 1986, rose again to peak in 1991 and declined slowly thereafter, reaching a level in 1994 about the same as that observed 2 decades earlier[77] (Figure 29-2).
- *Abortion rates* rose steadily from 1973 (the year abortion was legalized) to 1979, remained relatively constant through 1988, and declined thereafter, reaching a level in 1992 not observed since 1976.[31,32]
- *Pregnancy rates* rose slowly but steadily from 1973 to 1981, remained relatively constant through 1985, fell in 1986 and 1987, set successive record highs in 1988, 1989, and 1990, and dropped in 1992.[31]

Teenage pregnancy rates among blacks are more than twice as high as those among whites (243 per 1,000 black women versus 110 per 1,000 white women aged 15 to 19 in 1992); pregnancy rates among Hispanics (208 per 1,000 women in 1992) are nearly twice as high as those among whites and 14% lower than those among blacks.[31] Because blacks are only slightly more likely than whites to abort a pregnancy, the differential in birth rates is almost the same: 105 births per 1,000 black women versus 51 per 1,000 white women aged 15 to 19 in 1994.[77] Hispanic teenagers are much less likely to have an abortion than are blacks or whites. Consequently, the birth rate among 15- to 19-year-old Hispanics (108 per 1,000 women in 1994) is more than twice that for non-Hispanic whites (40 per 1,000) and identical to that for non-Hispanic blacks (108 per 1,000).[77] These racial and ethnic differentials are probably due in large part to differences in standards of living and in perceived life chances.

COMPARISON WITH OTHER COUNTRIES

Birth rates among women aged 15 to 19 are higher in the United States than in other developed countries[2] (Figure 29-3). Teenage birth rates in the United States are four times those in the countries of the European Union.[2] Likewise, pregnancy rates were higher in the United States than in five other countries (Canada, England and Wales, France, the Netherlands, and Sweden) examined in a cross-national comparison. Why is the experience in the United States so different? For the six-country study, the difference in pregnancy rates was not due to cross-national variations in proportions married, since the same qualitative conclusions would be

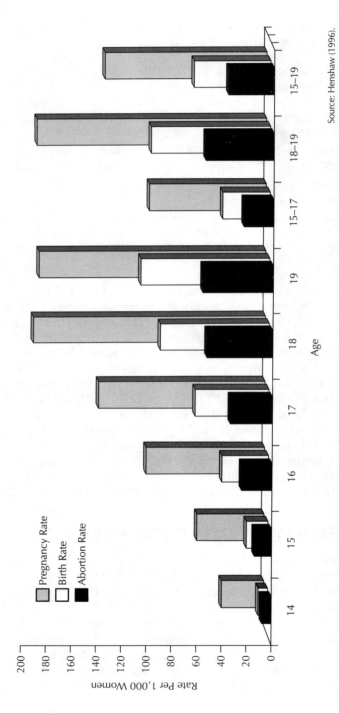

Figure 29-1 Abortions, births and pregnancies per 1,000 women aged 14–19, by age, United States, 1992

Source: Henshaw (1996).

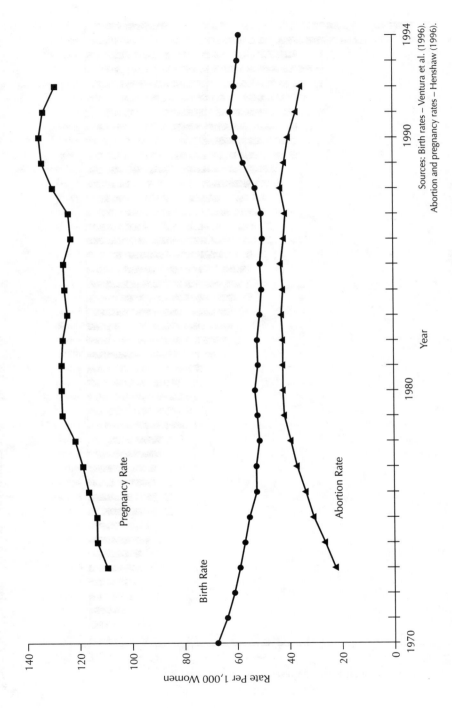

Figure 29-2 Abortions, births and pregnancies per 1,000 women aged 15–19, United States, 1970–1994

Sources: Birth rates – Ventura et al. (1996).
Abortion and pregnancy rates – Henshaw (1996).

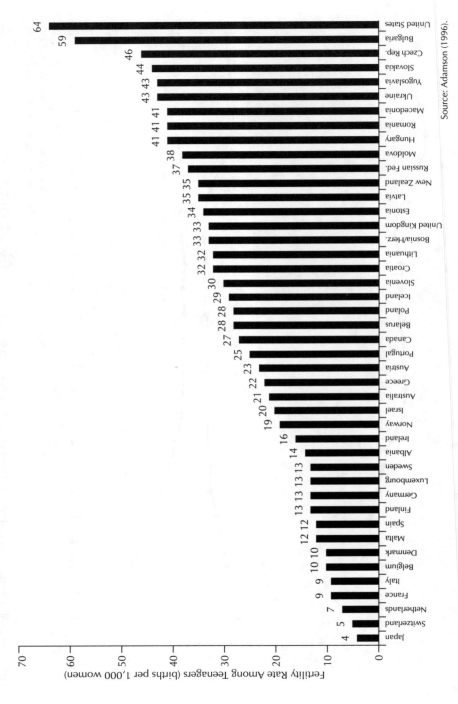

Figure 29-3 Number of births per 1,000 women aged 15–19, 1990–1995

Source: Adamson (1996).

United States 64
Bulgaria 59
Czech Rep. 46
Slovakia 44
Yugoslavia 43
Ukraine 43
Macedonia 41
Romania 41
Hungary 41
Moldova 38
Russian Fed. 37
New Zealand 35
Latvia 35
Estonia 34
United Kingdom 34
Bosnia/Herz. 33
Lithuania 33
Croatia 32
Slovenia 32
Iceland 30
Poland 29
Belarus 28
Canada 28
Portugal 27
Austria 25
Greece 23
Australia 22
Israel 21
Norway 20
Ireland 19
Albania 16
Sweden 14
Luxembourg 13
Germany 13
Finland 13
Spain 13
Malta 12
Denmark 12
Belgium 10
Italy 10
France 9
Netherlands 9
Switzerland 7
Japan 5
4

Fertility Rate Among Teenagers (births per 1,000 women)

obtained if comparisons were limited to the unmarried.[36] Part of the difference is attributable to the very high teenage pregnancy rates among U.S. blacks, but pregnancy rates for U.S. whites are still much higher than those for women in the other countries. The available evidence indicates the proportions of teenagers ever having had sexual intercourse are similar in all countries except Sweden, which has much higher proportions at each age, and Canada, where the proportions are lower but the data are less reliable. Hence, with the possible exception of Canada, higher pregnancy rates in the United States are not caused by more prevalent sexual experience. The contrast between Sweden and the United States is quite extreme: at every age greater proportions of teenagers are virgins in the United States, whereas abortion, birth, and pregnancy rates are far lower in Sweden.

The reason for higher pregnancy rates in the United States is that American teenagers are less likely to use contraceptives, or less likely to use them effectively.[36] Lower proportions of teenage women in the United States use contraceptives regularly than do teenage women in the other five countries. Among users, a smaller fraction relies on the most efficient methods, particularly the pill.

- Contraceptive supplies and services appear to be most widely available, free of charge or at low cost, to adolescents in Sweden, The Netherlands, and England and Wales.[36]
- Sex education in Sweden is compulsory and is taught in the schools at all grade levels. Information on contraception is provided, and its effectiveness is enhanced by a close link between the schools and adolescent family planning clinics. No other country approaches this level of implementation. In the Netherlands, where teenage pregnancy rates are lowest, sex education begins at an early age and is an ongoing lifelong process involving a variety of approaches and media; teen magazines and television programming are sexually explicit, focussing on real problems and feelings.[17,36]

Three factors that inhibit use of contraceptives among sexually active adolescents in the United States are largely absent in the United Kingdom, France, The Netherlands and Sweden: (1) a political culture at odds with the reality of the adolescent world,[22] (2) large pockets of deep poverty, and (3) misunderstanding about the risks and benefits of the pill.[36]

Unrealistic political culture. One segment of the population judges many types of sexual activity, particularly sexual relations among unmarried persons, to be immoral, or at best unwise, and argues that availability of contraception and abortion causes teens to have sex and should therefore be vigorously opposed. Concern about the morality of sex, while by no means absent, has far less impact on public policy in the other countries. In Sweden and The Netherlands, public policies recognize sex as a healthy and normal part of life, not only for adults but also for adolescents. At the same time, there is a strong public emphasis on personal responsibility for reproductive behavior.[17,27] In short, adolescent sex is publicly accepted as normal but adolescent pregnancy and child-bearing are not. The top public health official in these countries would never be fired, as was the Surgeon General of the United States, for suggesting that masturbation is a normal element of adolescent development and might delay the onset of intercourse. The political culture in this country hinders not only public provision of contraception but also frank public discussion about many sexual matters.[22] This political culture is all the more problematic because messages extolling sexuality are so pervasive in the mass media while messages promoting healthy and responsible sexuality, including the use of contraception, are rare. Thus, while the "Just Say No" message of the social conservatives is overwhelmed by the reality of sexual permissiveness, an effective countervailing force promoting contraceptive use is absent.

Pockets of deep poverty. The unequal distribution of income and the existence of a semi-permanent underclass in the United States guarantee many poor adolescents will perceive they are not sacrificing a bright future by having a child. In the other countries, the state redistributes income to a far greater extent. Moreover, public education, health care delivery, and other social services are more centrally controlled, thereby enabling the establishment of *national* policies far less subject to the influence of parochial interest groups.

Myths about the pill. Reliance on one of the most effective methods of pregnancy prevention, the pill, is much smaller in the United States than in the other countries, among both adolescents and older women. Despite the evidence that the pill is a good pregnancy-prevention method for sexually active adolescents (and almost all women), public perceptions in the United States are heavily influenced by myth (particularly about cancer, future fecundity, and other side effects).[42] Pills in the United States, except in selected clinics, are also much more expensive than in the other countries, where health services in general and contraceptive services in particular are heavily subsidized for all persons.

DETERMINANTS OF ADOLESCENT PREGNANCY

Although each year 1 in 8 women aged 15 to 19 becomes pregnant, 7 in 8 do not. Each year, of those who do, 3 in 10 carry the pregnancy to term. A common opinion, expressed in popular books,[16] is that many adolescents perceive (however incorrectly) having a child as an attractive alternative to their current situation. They may, for example, be bored in school or have conflicts with parents. Undoubtedly, some do believe a child is a ticket to independence or to a better life and act accordingly. Overwhelming evidence, however, shows most unmarried adolescents who become pregnant do not intend to do so.[7,19,81,82] Nevertheless, intention is seldom adequately characterized by a sharp yes-or-no dichotomy. Therefore, even though few teenagers *intend* to become pregnant out-of-wedlock, the strength of the motivation of the rest to *avoid* pregnancy varies considerably.[79] The motivation to avoid pregnancy is governed in part by a young woman's perception of the benefits of deferring parenthood. This perception is strongly influenced by both her present circumstances and her belief in her future life chances. For many disadvantaged youth, the benefits of postponed parenthood must seem remote indeed.

A common misperception is that adolescent fathers have little contact with their children. Roughly half of all adolescent fathers live with their children shortly after birth.[47] Paternal involvement persists for extended periods following the birth, even among those males who do not marry the mothers of their children.[62] Nevertheless, the frequency of contact declines markedly with time.[29]

SEXUAL BEHAVIOR

Why do unmarried adolescents become pregnant? The proximate cause is obviously vaginal sexual intercourse. In 1995, 48% of never-married women aged 15 to 19 had ever had sexual intercourse (Table 29-2). The

Table 29-2 Percentage of never-married males and females who had had sexual intercourse in 1995, United States

Sex and age	Total	Race/ethnicity		
		Non-Hispanic white	Non-Hispanic black	Hispanic
Females				
15–19	48.1	47.1	58.3	52.0
15–17	36.8	33.9	48.2	48.8
18–19	67.4	67.8	75.5	57.2
Males				
15–19	55.2	49.5	80.4	60.9
15–17	43.1	34.8	75.4	49.7
18–19	75.4	74.7	89.0	78.6

Source: Females: 1995 National Survey of Family Growth (Abma et al. 1997).
Males: 1995 National Survey of Adolescent Males (Sonenstein et al. 1997).

proportion with some sexual experience rises sharply with age at interview: 21% at age 15, 38% at age 16, 50% at age 17, 63% at age 18, and 72% at age 19. By the time they reach their 18th birthday, well over half of never-married women in the United States have had intercourse.[1] The available data suggest a reversal during the period 1988 to 1995 in the rapid secular increase in the proportion of never-married females aged 15 to 19 who had experienced sexual intercourse (27% in 1971, 36% in 1976, 42% in 1982, 50% in 1988, and 48% in 1995).[1,19,82] Not all intercourse is consensual. Among women aged 15 to 19 in 1995 who had ever had intercourse, 25% had been forced to have intercourse at least once, 51% of these before age 15.[1]

Information on adolescent males is much more limited. Data from the 1988 and 1995 National Surveys of Adolescent Males (NSAM) show that the percentage of never-married males aged 15 to 19 who had ever had intercourse declined over this time period, from 60% to 55%. There were declines in every single-year age group, with the overall decline attributable solely to a decline among whites. The data from the 1995 NSAM reveal that by their 13th birthday 4% of never-married males have become sexually active. The proportions rise to 11%, 21%, 35%, 53%, 65%, and 84% by the 14th, 15th, 16th, 17th, 18th, and 19th birthdays, respectively[69] (Table 29-2).

CONTRACEPTIVE USE

Among teenage women surveyed in 1995, 76% reported use of a contraceptive at first premarital intercourse. Of these, 83% used the condom, 5% relied on withdrawal, and only 11% used the pill.[64] Among teenage women who were currently exposed to the risk of unintended pregnancy, 19% were using no method (the same as in 1988 but substantially lower than the 30% in 1982) while 35% (down from 47% in 1988 and 44% in 1982) and 30% (up from 27% in 1988 and 15% in 1982) were relying on the pill and condom, respectively.[1,75] In addition, 8% were using the injectable and 2% the implant.

In focus group sessions, adolescents have revealed an intense desire for privacy concerning their own sexual activity and strong feelings of embarrassment when communicating about sexual matters with others: partners, friends, parents, counselors, and clinicians. Those who had not attended clinics pictured these facilities as dingy places for the poor where they would be treated impersonally and viewed as morally irresponsible.[42] Adolescents are also embarrassed to go to family physicians, who might reveal their secrets, offer unwanted moral advice, or simply not help. Their fears are not groundless: 22% of physicians in private general or family practice (but only 2% of obstetricians and gynecologists) refuse to serve minors, and 19% of general and family practitioners (18% of obstetricians and gynecologists) provide contraceptive services only with parental consent.[61] These sentiments help to explain the long delay, 23 months on average among women aged 15 to 24, between initiating sexual relations and the first family planning visit.[57]

Increasing the effective practice of contraception is difficult in part because all currently available contraceptives require the type of abstract thinking about the future that many teens have not developed. Hence, a new contraceptive that could be used to induce menses at the end of cycles during which intercourse occurred (thereby reducing the importance of planning ahead), had few side effects, was relatively inexpensive, and did not require a visit to a physician could reduce adolescent pregnancy significantly. A technological solution is unlikely, however, because (1) such a method would be considered to be an abortifacient and therefore not eligible for federal research and development support and (2) drug companies generally do not believe developing new contraceptives is profitable.[30,48] Nevertheless, more effective promotion of currently available emergency contraception could significantly reduce unintended pregnancies among teens.[74] (See Chapter 12 on Emergency Contraception.)

Another problem is that the most effective methods for preventing pregnancy do not reduce the risk of acquiring STIs. As discussed more fully below, adolescents are at especially great risk for STIs. Promoting condom use is sound public health policy. Nevertheless, some health practitioners fear it will be difficult to convince teens to use both pills and condoms. Others are concerned that if teens switch from pills to condoms, the pregnancy rate will consequently rise.

SEX EDUCATION

In a 1996 national survey, 3 in 5 teens reported that the average teen does not have enough information about how to use different methods of contraception and 45% did not think the average teen knows enough about where to obtain contraception.[37] Of those who had already had sexual intercourse, 36% reported needing to know more about how to use contraception and 30% said they need more information about where to obtain contraceptives. Three in 5 teens said the information they do receive comes too late and nearly half reported the information does not include enough detail about where to get or how to use contraceptives.

Opposition to teaching about contraceptives and where to obtain them is based on the belief that such information promotes promiscuity. The data, however, do not support this belief. Five studies based on national surveys examined whether receipt of sex education was related to initiation of intercourse. All but one of these surveys was conducted in the late 1970s or early 1980s before instruction on AIDS and skills to postpone sexual involvement was given as much emphasis as it was in the late 1980s and 1990s. Results of these studies suggest teaching of resistance skills may postpone the initiation of sexual activity while instruction about contraception may hasten the onset of sexual intercourse among young teens but not among older teens.[41] Evaluation of specific programs overcomes some of the problems that arise when interpreting results from national survey data, such as reliance on retrospective reporting (both about sex education and about initiation and frequency of intercourse), lack of information about the specific content or quality of programs (so very long-term comprehensive programs are grouped with brief superficial programs), and selection bias that would occur if sex education programs were targeted to schools with high rates of pregnancy. Evaluations of five specific programs show that none hastened the onset of sexual intercourse.[41] Two of these programs set an explicit goal of postponing sexual involvement; both succeeded even though they included instruction on contraception.

SEXUALLY TRANSMITTED INFECTIONS AMONG ADOLESCENTS

Most public attention to the consequences of teenage sexual behavior is focused on only one outcome: pregnancy. Much less attention is devoted to a second outcome: sexually transmitted infections (STIs). The incidence of STIs among adolescents increased rapidly during the 1960s and 1970s. In the 1980s and 1990s, despite the increase in awareness of STIs caused by HIV prevention messages, rates of genital infections in adolescents have stayed at high levels.[12] Two-thirds of all STI cases occur among persons under 25 years of age and one-fourth among teenagers.[14]

In the 1980s and 1990s, gonorrhea infection rates remained nearly constant among teens (with a slight rise among males offset by a decline among females) while they fell among other age groups. Nearly 175 thousand cases were reported among teens in 1995. Most clinical investigations find rates of chlamydia are at least double those of gonorrhea. The number of visits of teenage women to office-based fee-for-service practices for genital herpes infections increased from 15 thousand in 1966 to an estimated 100 thousand in 1995. The number of visits for genital warts caused by the human papillomavirus (HPV) increased from 50 thousand in 1966 to an estimated 200 thousand in 1995 among teenage women. Perhaps 10 times as many sexually active women have asymptomatic cervical HPV infection. By the end of the teenage years, about 4% of whites and 17% of blacks have been infected with herpes simplex virus type 2.[12]

By the end of 1995, 979 persons in the United States under the age of 20 with AIDS had been infected with HIV through sexual contact. Given the long latency period from infection with HIV to the development of AIDS, a considerable fraction of the 59,723 persons diagnosed with AIDS at ages 20 to 29 who had been infected through sexual contact must have been infected while still teenagers.[15]

The epidemiology of STI transmission is the same among adolescents as among adults: unprotected intercourse with multiple partners is risky. Data from the 1995 National Survey of Family Growth and 1995 National Survey of Adolescent Males show that among the 49% of unmarried females and the 50% of never-married males aged 15 to 19 who had experienced sexual intercourse in the past year, 47% of females and 50% of males had had 2 or more partners in that time period, and 25% of females and 23% of males had had 3 or more partners.[1,69] In 1995, 67% of never-married teenage males[69] and 37% of unmarried teenage females[1] reported condom use at last intercourse. This difference is also found in the CDC's Youth Risk Behavior Surveillance System. In the 1995 national survey of students in grades 9 to 12, among those who had had sexual intercourse in the 3 months preceding the survey, 61% of males but only 49% of females reported using a condom at last intercourse.[38] It is difficult to resolve the discrepancy between these two statistics. Plausible explanations are that males over-report use of condoms because they know it is the socially responsible answer or females under-report condom use when a condom is used as an adjunct to a regular method of contraception. Regardless of the answer, condom use seems to have increased among adolescents. The most plausible explanation for this increase is greater awareness of STIs, primarily HIV. Nevertheless, the disturbing fact remains that large fractions of adolescents at risk of acquiring STIs do not use condoms.

CONSEQUENCES OF ADOLESCENT CHILDBEARING

Recent research suggests the consequences of teenage childbearing are not as deleterious as has long been claimed. The reason is that most studies have compared outcomes in two groups of women: those who had a birth at an early age and those who did not. Women who give birth at an early age, however, are disadvantaged relative to those who give birth later for reasons unrelated to age at first birth. Among women who are otherwise alike, the consequences of early childbearing are not nearly so deleterious but nevertheless damage life chances for mother and child.

A considerable literature exists on the medical, social, and economic consequences of adolescent childbearing for the mother and for the child. Much of it is summarized in excellent review articles.[46,71] Unfortunately, many of the studies suffer from analytical flaws or poor experimental design, thereby rendering the conclusions suspect. Many studies report results obtained by analyzing all adolescents as one group, while the evidence suggests the experiences of younger and older adolescents may differ widely. Many studies are also based on selective samples so results are not easily generalizable.

The greatest analytical problem is determining whether the adverse conditions frequently observed among adolescent mothers are causally related to age at birth. Many studies fail to control for both maternal age and other factors correlated with age at first birth, such as socioeconomic status. Thus the adverse consequences of early childbearing per se are frequently overstated. An even more serious analytical problem arises because adolescents are able to select (or at least affect) whether or not they become pregnant or whether or not they will bear a child. Investigators can never study the consequences of adolescent childbearing by conducting a rigorous randomized trial. However, they can try to ensure adolescent mothers are compared with a control group that is as similar as possible with respect to measurable background variables at an early age, such as achievement, aptitude, motivation, and socioeconomic status. One innovative methodological approach controls for a similar family environment by comparing the experiences of pairs of sisters, one of whom gave birth as a teenager and the other of whom did not. Another compares the experiences of teenage mothers who gave birth to twins to those who gave birth to singletons; those who give birth to twins experience a truly exogenous unplanned birth.

HEALTH CONSEQUENCES

Many adverse consequences such as pregnancy-induced hypertension, anemia, toxemia, prematurity, and perinatal and maternal mortality documented in early studies were greatly overstated because the controls for socioeconomic status were inadequate or nonexistent.[35,51] The (much reduced) deleterious effects of young maternal age that are still observed when the effect of socioeconomic status is controlled may be attributable to inadequate prenatal care among adolescents.[50] Several studies have found that adolescents receiving good prenatal care exhibit pregnancy outcomes no different from, or better than, those of other women.[4] The problem, of course, is that adolescents, especially the very young, are much less likely to receive any prenatal care or, if they do, are more likely to initiate it later in the pregnancy.[77] The reasons for such behavior include not recognizing the pregnancy or desiring to conceal it, not realizing prenatal care is valuable or available, and not being able to afford it.

The relation between poor birth outcome and maternal age may, however, not be entirely attributable to the effects of prenatal care. This question was examined among white women giving birth to their first singleton child in Utah. Even in the lowest-risk group—married women whose educational attainment was appropriate for their age and who obtained adequate prenatal care—babies of mothers under 18 years of age were 1.9 times as likely to be premature, 1.7 times as likely to weigh less than 2,500 grams, and 1.3 times as likely to be small for gestational age as babies of women aged 20 to 24. Risks to babies of mothers aged 18 to 19 were lower, but still elevated.[20] These results suggest that even under optimal circumstances, young maternal age is still related to poor birth outcomes. The study design, however, only partly controls for family background.

When family background characteristics of mothers are controlled by comparing the health of children of sisters who gave birth at different ages, the effects of teen childbearing are mixed and modest.[24] For both blacks and whites, comparisons within sister-pairs (one who had a child as a teenager and one who did not) revealed less adverse effects for infants than did traditional cross-section comparisons. Generally, the differentials for whites were narrowed and for blacks were eliminated or even reversed. Compared with their sisters who first gave birth at older ages, black teen mothers were no more likely to smoke during pregnancy or to have low-birthweight babies and no less likely to breastfeed their infants or to bring them to clinics for well-baby visits. The situation was generally the opposite among whites. Further analyses that control for family-specific endowments suggest the biological effect of having a birth at younger ages is to increase birthweight marginally.[67]

One positive health consequence of teenage childbearing has been identified. The risk of breast cancer increases with the age at which a woman delivers her first full-term child. A woman who bears a child before the age of 18 faces about one-third the risk of a woman whose first birth occurs after the age of 35.[70]

Comparisons of the children of sisters have also been used to examine the effects of teenage motherhood on child development.[26] For a cross-sectional sample in which the effects of family background are not controlled, the children of women who had first births after age 19 scored consistently better on measures of child development than children of teen mothers. But in the sisters comparison, children of teen mothers did no worse than their first cousins whose mothers had first births after age 19. Other U.S. and British studies show that cognitive development of the child is influenced by the age of the mother even after the effects of background variables have been controlled. Children of young mothers fare less well, though the difference is small. In contrast, the results for the social and emotional development of the child are rather inconclusive. In all these studies, however, maternal age proved to have much less influence than did the socioeconomic variables.[4,46,54]

Socioeconomic Consequences

Evidence from the United States suggests women who have first births at an early age bear subsequent children more rapidly and have more unwanted and out-of-wedlock births, face greater marital instability, are more poorly educated, and have fewer assets and lower incomes later in life.[72] These conclusions are drawn from studies in which the effects of some important background variables, particularly childhood achievement and motivation, could not be controlled because data were not available. For example, the lower educational attainment of adolescent mothers may not be caused by their having given birth at an early age. They may have left school, even if they had not become pregnant, because they were bored or performing poorly.

One study that does address this issue directly demonstrates that although the adverse outcomes associated with early childbearing are reduced, they are not eliminated when the effects of preexisting factors are controlled.[11] This study matched each woman who bore a child before age 18 to a woman who did not, on the bases of preexisting socioeconomic status, academic achievement, aptitude, and educational expectations. The matched sample was used to study differences between groups for selected outcome variables. By age 29, only half of the women in the youngest childbearing group (under age 18) received high school diplomas, whereas nearly all those who postponed childbearing until after age 20 graduated from high school. Similar results hold for college degrees: only 2% of those who bore a child before age 18 obtained a degree before age 29 compared with 22% of those who had not given birth by age 24. Those who bore their first child at an early age also bore subsequent children more rapidly than those who postponed childbearing.

Analysis of data from three national surveys replicates findings from previous studies demonstrating that teenage childbearing leads to substantial long-term socioeconomic disadvantage when those who have births as teens are compared with all those who do not. This finding holds even when the effects of some background characteristics such as mother's and father's education and respondent upbringing in a single-parent family are controlled.[25] However, these conventional controls may not adequately make the two groups (teen mothers versus others) similar enough that the estimated effect of a teen birth can be interpreted as a causal effect. When the comparison group is confined to the sisters (who did not have births as teenagers) of the teenage mothers, a different conclusion emerges. In two of the three surveys, standard comparisons seriously overstate the costs of teenage childbearing. In the third survey, the methodology based on sister comparisons leads to the same conclusion as the conventional methodology that controls for several background characteristics.[25,34] However, even sister comparisons may overstate the deleterious consequences of teen childbearing because they may reflect differences between sisters that are unrelated to the age at first birth. For example, parents may favor, starting at an early age, the daughter they perceive to be the more able. Evidence for this concern arises from the fact that in two of three national surveys, sister comparisons show a teen birth is associated with a lower probability of graduation from high school. However, another study that carefully assessed the timing of the sequence of events (school dropout, pregnancy and birth) yielded a different conclusion. Models controlling for the effects of several background characteristics show that neither having a birth nor being pregnant (among those who carry the pregnancy to term) while in school increases the risk of subsequently dropping out. Another model reveals that having a birth after dropping out reduces the rate at which women progress to graduation.[76]

Comparisons of unmarried women who first gave birth to twins and unmarried women who first gave birth to singletons based on data from the 1970 and 1980 Censuses reveal large short-term effects of an unplanned birth on labor-force participation, poverty, and welfare receipt.[5] Consistent with the results from sister comparisons, these negative consequences are considerably smaller than those estimated in earlier studies. Most of the negative effects dissipate over time among whites but persist among blacks. Effects on poverty and welfare receipt were larger in 1980 than in 1970 and larger for blacks than whites. At the time of the 1980 Census, black but not white women who experienced an unplanned nonmarital birth were less likely to have completed high school and to be married.

Work on (primarily) black adolescents living in Baltimore who became pregnant between 1965 and 1967 has emphasized that the popular belief that early childbearing invariably leads to dropping out of school, many subsequent unwanted births, and welfare dependency is grossly oversimplified. In the period up to 5 years following the birth of their first child, these adolescent mothers did very poorly when compared with their peers who did not bear children. But a follow-up study in 1984 revealed a substantial majority finished high school, found regular employment, and eventually escaped dependence on welfare.[23] Nevertheless, the authors conclude the degree of flexibility teenage mothers have in manipulating their circumstances in later life is definitely limited and that, on average, these women did not fare as well as they would have had they been able to postpone childbearing. Their analysis of which adolescent mothers were more likely to "succeed" later in life is revealing though hardly surprising. Young mothers who had been doing well in school, who had high educational aspirations, and who had more economically secure and better-educated parents were more likely to succeed. Furthermore, those who had no more children in the 5 years following their first birth had fewer constraints in attending school and accruing job experience. The one-fourth of women who remained poor and dependent on welfare were the most likely to experience problems in later life. Hence, identifying this high-risk group is particularly important.

Given these adverse conditions associated with teenage childbearing, one would expect the children of teenage parents would be relatively disadvantaged. Indeed, such children are more likely to exhibit lower academic achievement and to show a tendency to repeat the early marriage, early childbearing, and high fertility cycle of their parents, even when the effects of other background variables are controlled.[9] The poor educational performance of the children of adolescent mothers is particularly pronounced and debilitating.[23] To what extent the adverse conditions are truly consequences of teenage childbearing as opposed to simply reflecting the preexisting poorer life chances of women who give birth as teens is still an open question. These adverse conditions are most likely to be found when the mother raises children without the support of the father or her own parents. A finding common to several studies is that those who have children at *very* young ages are less likely to leave the parental home and are therefore able to achieve a better childrearing environment.[4]

STRATEGIES TO SOLVE THE PROBLEM

Many attempts have been made to reduce the incidence of teen pregnancy in the United States and to attenuate its health, social, educational, and economic consequences for mother and child. In this section we describe the evolution of teen pregnancy prevention and care programs and examine the evidence for the effectiveness of these programs. We summarize what we know, and what we do not know, about characteristics of programs that work.

DEVELOPMENT OF INTERVENTION PROGRAMS

Largely as a result of research findings described in the previous section on the negative consequences of teen pregnancy and parenthood, "care" programs for pregnant teens, teen mothers, and their infants proliferated in the 1960s and 1970s. These programs generally provided comprehensive prenatal and postnatal health services for the young mother and her child. Many care programs also helped the teen mother stay in or return to school by providing special classes for these mothers and daycare for their children.

In the early 1980s, program planners began to look more to "prevention" as an effective way to address the problems of teen pregnancy and parenthood. New programs aimed at preventing the occurrence of early pregnancy or birth began to emerge. Many different approaches were tried, based on the research literature as well as program planners' ad hoc or ideologically based ideas about acceptable and effective means of preventing pregnancy.[52] Among the approaches tried were: *Just say no,* which teaches young people the benefits of abstinence and the skills to refuse unwanted advances; *contraceptive provision,* which facilitates access to contraception for the sexually active (e.g., by establishing school-based contraceptive clinics); *sex education,* which focuses on teaching teens about the reproductive process and about contraception; *contraceptive negotiation skills development,* which imparts skills in contraceptive discussion and negotiation with a sexual partner; and more general *life option* or *youth development* programs with broader activities such as academic remediation, job training, or adult mentoring, which are founded on the premise that the belief in a compelling personal future or goal is a strong incentive to avoid teen pregnancy. Multi-faceted programs composed of two or more of these approaches were also developed.

In the 1990s, several new developments in strategies to solve the problem emerged:

- Many programs aimed to prevent not only pregnancy among teens, but also STIs and HIV. Some of the latter programs were aimed at the general population of youth and stressed abstaining from sex, or using STI-protection when having sex. Other programs were targeted at high-risk, sexually active populations of youth such as gay and bisexual youth, runaways, and incarcerated teens. These programs focused on *safer sex,* teaching teens how to assess the riskiness of their sex-related behaviors and then lower such risk levels.

- Realizing big problems need big solutions and local input and control are essential to combating the problem, many communities embarked on *community-wide teen pregnancy prevention initiatives.* Collaboratives composed of schools, community groups, and family planning clinics were established to coordinate these efforts within the community.

- *Youth development programs* began intervening at an early point in the life of a child (e.g., junior high school, or even elementary school). These include components that go beyond teaching abstinence or contraception (e.g., academic remediation, job training) and have goals that go beyond preventing teen pregnancy (e.g., increasing rates of graduation from high school, enhancing post-graduation employment opportunities).

- The positive challenge to teach the nation's children what *healthy and responsible sex* means in the adolescent years helped to refocus the issue away from the prevailing "problem" or "disease" model.[28]

- With encouragement from President Clinton, the privately funded National Campaign to Prevent Teenage Pregnancy aims to reduce the pregnancy rate among women aged 17 and under by one-third by the year 2005.[58]

- Fiscal constraints led to a growing consensus—among funders, practitioners, and researchers alike—that program development should be guided not only by what might work (based on moral, ideological, personal, or political beliefs) but on what does work (based on *rigorous scientific evaluation*).

PROGRAM EVALUATION

The acceptance of evaluation's importance in shaping and strengthening programs was slow in coming. Although by 1990 several thousand teen pregnancy prevention programs had been developed and implemented, few good evaluations existed. A variety of reasons underlay this dearth of scientifically valid program evaluations.[8] First there were the tensions, some more real than others, between service and science. Service providers were often reluctant to direct dollars that could go toward helping those in need to scientific endeavors whose benefits were (perhaps erroneously) perceived as relatively remote. In addition, both funders and service providers were understandably wary about possible fallout from negative evaluations. Beyond these reasons, some funders felt constrained by fact or politics from providing support for approaches not in line with their mission or their legislative mandate. As the national debate grew over related issues such as abortion and the provision of contraception to minors, powerful institutions such as schools became increasingly reluctant to ally themselves with controversial issues such as school-based clinics or contraceptive education and provision.

Tensions also existed between the requirements of science and the realities of program administration. For example, scientific evaluation encouraged the random assignment of subjects to treatment and control groups; administrators often replied it was unacceptable to withhold services from those in need, especially when the funds were available to provide services to all. Scientific rigor demanded baseline and follow-up data be collected from identifiable individuals so these data could be linked; administrators often replied that, for cost and confidentiality reasons, this could not be done. Moreover, when a good evaluation was designed and implemented, it was often discovered that members of the control or comparison group had been exposed to the influence of competing similar programs, thus allowing for only a conservative test of the program's effectiveness.

Another problem was (and continues to be) the conflict between science and politics. Trends in sexual behavior cannot be monitored and programs cannot be evaluated without asking adolescents about their sexual behavior. Yet there has been an unwillingness to use public funds (or allow public authorities) to do so.

Despite these obstacles, the field made laudable progress in the 1990s. Consciousness about the importance of evaluation was raised; evaluation instrumentation advanced. Today the field is more aware of the technical challenges of program evaluation, as well as the costs and benefits associated with various research designs. Moreover, the ways in which evaluation data may serve to improve prevention programs are now better appreciated and understood.

PROGRAM PRIORITIES: PREVENTING PREGNANCY

Research described in the last section of this chapter suggests preventing adolescent pregnancy would be far more cost-effective in reducing the proportion of women who require public assistance than would increasing education or reducing subsequent fertility among adolescent mothers. Moreover, research suggests most pregnant adolescents did not intend to become pregnant. For these reasons, much greater attention has been given in recent years to the development and evaluation of teen pregnancy prevention programs and to related teen HIV prevention programs. Table 29-3 summarizes the scope and findings of eight recent reviews of existing programs and evaluations.[7,10,21,39,41,52,55,63]

Reflecting the increasingly higher standard for demonstrated program effectiveness permeating the field, these reviews of existing programs and evaluations have all used behavioral change criteria—such as delaying first sexual intercourse; reducing the number of sexual partners; reducing the frequency of intercourse; using effective protection from pregnancy or STIs at first and subsequent sexual intercourse—in judging whether a given adolescent pregnancy or HIV prevention program was effective. Such a higher standard for effectiveness evolved because the literature has consistently shown that knowledge gain in and of itself—such as an increase in knowledge about how one gets pregnant, what contraceptive options are available to the sexually active, how to protect oneself from getting an STI, where to go to obtain various contraceptive methods—does not translate automatically to behavioral change. Knowledge is a

Table 29-3 Overview of recent reviews of prevention strategies

Citation	Type[a]	Site[b]	Number	Number with ≥ one positive outcomes[c]
			Programs Reviewed	
Miller et al., 1992[d]	PP, YD	S, COM, CL	8	6
Kirby et al., 1994	PP	S	14	4
Kirby, 1995[e]	PP	S, COM, CL	22	10
	STI	S, COM, CL	10	7
	Mixture	S, COM, CL	5	2 (+1 maybe)
Moore et al., 1995[f]	PP, SP, YD	S, COM, CL	58	15 (+11 maybes)
Frost & Forrest, 1995[d]	PP	S, COM	5	5
Brown & Eisenberg, 1995	PP, SP	S, COM, CL	23	13 (+1 maybe)
Philliber & Namerow, 1995[d]	PP, YD	S, COM, CL	17	17
Card et al., 1996[e]	PP, SP	S, COM, CL	29	14
	STI	S, COM, CL	23	14
	Mixture	S, COM, CL	3	2

[a]PP = Primary Pregnancy Prevention (prevention of pregnancy before the first birth); SP = Secondary Pregnancy Prevention (prevention of pregnancy after a woman has already given birth); STI = STI/HIV/AIDS Prevention; YD = Youth Development; Mixture = equal focus on pregnancy and STI/HIV prevention.
[b]S = School-based; COM = Community-based; CL = Clinic-based.
[c]The scientific rigor of the methods used to evaluate the various programs varied greatly and these results need to be interpreted with this caution in mind.
[d]This review focused solely on programs pre-selected for their exemplary program components, evaluations, or effectiveness.
[e]Only these reviews explicitly included both pregnancy prevention and STI/HIV/AIDS prevention programs. The review by Kirby and colleagues excluded secondary prevention programs as well as STI/HIV/AIDS prevention programs aimed at special populations of high-risk youth such as homosexuals, bisexuals, drug-abusing youth, runaways, or incarcerated youth. Such programs were included in the review by Card and colleagues.
[f]This review looked at 76 programs, of which 58 utilized an experimental or quasi-experimental evaluation design.

necessary but not sufficient condition for behavior change. Behavior change is necessary if pregnancy and STIs, including HIV, are to be prevented.

Some of these recent reviews have focused only on pre-selected well-evaluated or effective programs. Others include discussions of poorly conducted evaluations or of ineffective programs. All reviews, however, include the reviewers' insights about lessons learned from the programs and evaluations that were examined. We summarize the scope, conclusions, and insights offered by each review.

The first review focused on eight adolescent pregnancy prevention programs that included rigorous evaluation designs.[52] Featured were programs seeking to influence both sexual and contraceptive risk behaviors, whether separately or in combination. The programs were eclectic in terms of type (covering both the narrowly focused pregnancy prevention programs as well as more general youth development programs) and in terms of site (some of the programs were based in schools, others in community organizations, still others in family planning clinics). Five basic principles for success emerged:

- The program goals and objectives must be clear and specific.
- The target population must be relatively young.
- The program should be intensive (i.e., the number of contacts and duration over time should be sufficient to change behavior).
- The program should be comprehensive.
- The program should leverage parent and peer support.

The second review focused on primary prevention programs based in schools.[41] Effectiveness was defined as a statistically significant positive impact on behavior, such as delayed onset of intercourse, decreased sexual activity, or increased use of contraception among the sexually active. Six distinguishing characteristics of effective programs were described. Effective programs contained the following elements:

- A narrow focus on reducing sexual risk-taking behaviors that may lead to unintended pregnancy or to STI, including HIV infection
- A foundation based upon social learning theories
- Basic information about the risks of unprotected intercourse and methods of avoiding unprotected intercourse through experiential activities designed to personalize this information
- Activities that address the social or media influences on sexual behavior
- Reinforcement of clear and appropriate values and norms against unprotected sex
- Modeling and practice in communication and negotiation skills

The third review examined 76 teen pregnancy and youth development programs to identify the range of programs under way in the United States, assess the soundness of the effort used to evaluate their effectiveness, and examine their effects on teen sexual behavior and/or knowledge.[55] Only 58 of the 76 programs had conducted experimental or quasi-experimental evaluations. The authors warned that intervention programs had generally not been informed by existing basic research studies or by theory, and existing evaluations had typically been lacking in methodological and statistical rigor. They reasoned that this deficiency accounted, in part, for the "haphazard" and "incomplete" state of knowledge about the success of teen pregnancy prevention intervention programs. Despite these caveats, they concluded that:

- Sex education programs do not increase levels of sexual activity; indeed, programs that combine education with skills development appear able to cause a moderate delay in sexual initiation.
- Initiatives that are theory-driven, have clear goals, address peer and media influences, employ small group activities, and use peer educators appear promising.
- Community-based initiatives that involve several segments of the adolescent's environment—including the school, church, and other community institutions—also appear potentially fruitful.
- Family planning services that offer approaches to reduce barriers to receiving care among adolescents appear promising.
- School-based services have only limited impact on contraceptive behavior. However, such programs combining education with counseling and access to contraceptive supplies show promise.
- There is a need to develop broader programs that focus on the factors found to predict adolescent childbearing (such as poverty, school failure, family dysfunction, and behavior problems), develop family strengths and parenting skills, and provide information about reproduction and contraceptive services.

The fourth review examined further 17 primary prevention and youth development programs among those reviewed earlier[41,55] with at least marginally credible evaluations and apparent impact on postponement of sexual intercourse, increase in contraceptive use among the sexually active, decrease in pregnancy rates, or prevention of early births.[63] Several positive strategies for combating teen pregnancy emerged:

- Strong one-on-one support from a responsible adult
- Attention to basic cognitive skills and educational achievement
- Attention to the world of work
- Attention to the specific skills necessary to avoid pregnancy
- Involvement of community members in the intervention
- Attention to the importance of peer influences
- Intervening at a young age

This review also found several strategies that do not appear to work in preventing teen pregnancy:

- Information-provision alone is not sufficient.
- Making contraceptives available is necessary but not sufficient.
- No single intervention will work for all teens or for all the teenage years.
- Abstinence programs do not appear to prevent teen pregnancy; even the most successful abstinence programs delay the onset of sexual intercourse for only a few months.
- School-based clinics do not appear to prevent teen pregnancy.

The fifth review included 49 published studies which have examined the behavioral impact of 37 educational programs designed specifically to reduce sexual risk-taking behavior among youth 18 years of age or younger.[39] Programs designed for specific high-risk groups such as homosexuals, IV drug users, or prostitutes were excluded. The criterion for effectiveness was change in sexual risk-taking behavior that was adequately demonstrated by a scientifically valid evaluation: experimental or quasi-experimental design with a suitable comparison group, measurement of outcomes over time, sufficiently large sample size (minimum of 80 in the treatment and comparison groups combined), sufficiently reliable and valid measurement of behavioral outcome variables, and proper statistical analysis. The results suggest different programs in different settings have different success outcomes. As a general rule, however, effective curricula shared similar characteristics:

- A narrow focus on reducing sexual risk-taking behaviors that may lead to STI infection or unintended pregnancy
- Social learning theories, social influence theories, or theories of reasoned action as a foundation for program development
- At least 14 hours' duration or use of small groups and small group exercises to increase the efficiency of time spent
- A variety of teaching methods designed to involve the participants and to have them personalize the information
- Basic, accurate information about the risks of unprotected intercourse and methods of avoiding unprotected intercourse
- Activities that address social pressures on sexual behaviors
- Clear and appropriate values and messages in order to strengthen individual values and group norms against unprotected sex
- Modeling and practice of communication and negotiation skills
- Training for individuals implementing the program

The sixth review focused on five rigorously evaluated teen pregnancy prevention programs that showed an ability to significantly affect at least one of the following dependent variables: delay in sexual initiation, increase in rates of contraceptive use, or decrease in proportions of teens who become pregnant.[21] Some insights into what works include:

- Among adolescents who participated in programs with role-playing exercises and interactive discussions, males were more likely than females to remain abstinent. Possibly because the support the program provided for these behaviors is seldom given to males in our society, teen boys may have benefited from such support.
- The impact on teen sexual initiation is greatest for programs aimed at younger adolescents. Among older teens, for whom delay in sexual activity is less likely, programs are more likely to affect use of contraceptives.

The authors caution that even widespread replication of these and similar programs will not eliminate teenage pregnancy in the United States. The problem and its determinants are too deeply intertwined with poverty and disadvantage to be responsive to short-term programs implemented after many teens have already become sexually active.

A seventh Institute of Medicine report reviewed 23 teen pregnancy prevention programs that had been evaluated with an experimental or quasi-experimental design measuring behavioral outcomes (e.g., sexual activity or contraceptive use).[7] The results of all evaluations had been published in peer-reviewed journals. Of the 23 programs examined, approximately one-half were found to be successful in affecting fertility-related behavior among teens. The report concludes that:

- Sexuality education programs that provide information on both abstinence and contraceptive use neither encourage the onset of sexual intercourse nor increase the frequency of intercourse among adolescents. To the contrary, programs that provide both messages appear to be effective in delaying the onset of sexual intercourse and encouraging contraceptive use, especially among younger adolescents.
- Whether abstinence-only programs have been effective in delaying initiation of first intercourse is not known.
- How to influence sexual behavior and contraceptive use by changing the surrounding socioeconomic or cultural environment is not known.

The eighth and final review employed a technique similar to the Delphi method. A panel of five experts in teen pregnancy prevention and/or teen HIV prevention research selected promising programs.[10] With the panel's assistance, four empirical criteria for assessing program effectiveness were delineated: (1) substantive relevance; (2) methodological rigor; (3) for teens at least 16 years of age, positive impact on one or more of 13 relevant fertility or STI-related behaviors (e.g., postponing or decreasing the frequency of sexual intercourse, using effective contraception); and (4) for teens 15 years of age or younger, positive impact on relevant attitudes, skills, intentions, or values. A comprehensive literature search yielded 55 candidate programs; the panel selected 30 of the 55 candidates as meeting the effectiveness criteria.

Consistent with findings of previous reviews, the selected programs varied greatly in scope, target population, and approach. The 30 programs were evenly divided between pregnancy and HIV prevention programs. Of the pregnancy prevention initiatives, 11 focused on primary prevention (averting pregnancy before the first birth) and four on secondary prevention (averting pregnancy after a woman has already given birth). The promising programs had been implemented in schools (14 programs), communities, including community-based organizations (11 programs), and clinics, both medical and family-planning (10 programs). Many are suitable for use in a variety of settings; for example, several of the school-based initiatives would work equally well in community organizations like Girls or Boys Clubs.

Several *approaches* to reducing unprotected intercourse were found in the selected programs: abstinence, behavioral skills development, community outreach, contraceptive access, contraceptive education, life option enhancement, self-efficacy/self-esteem, and sexuality or STI education. Nearly all the programs incorporate at least two of these approaches, and the typical program includes four. Similarly, the review identified eight *components*, or specific instructional methods for implementation in promising programs: adult involvement, case management, group discussion, lecture, peer counseling/instruction, public service announcements, role play, and video. Perhaps due to the large number of school-based programs in the collection, the review found group discussions, lectures, role plays, and videos are the most common instructional strategies.

The programs selected as promising were a culturally diverse lot, developed and field tested in all parts of the country, often in multiple locations, with groups of teens ranging in size from 75 to 2,500. Particular attention has been paid to the needs of high-risk youth. Thus, 10 of the 30 programs have been developed especially for teens in low-income communities with elevated rates of teen pregnancy, STIs, and HIV. Some programs are targeted toward gay, incarcerated, or runaway youth. Several programs use culturally relevant materials to appeal to particular racial or ethnic groups, especially Latinos and African-Americans.

Lessons Learned

What can we learn from the existing literature? What characteristics do effective programs share, if any? What tips concerning program development and implementation might we offer educators and practitioners working in the field? Several distinguishing characteristics of effective teen pregnancy and HIV prevention programs emerge from the literature:

1. It is important to match the duration, intensity, and content of the program to the complexity of objectives, age, culture, and level of need of the target population. Different programs will likely need to be designed for low-risk populations of teens and for high-risk populations. To be effective, programs for high-risk teens will need to be longer in duration, more intensive, and more explicit.

2. If possible, one should intervene at an early age, prior to sexual initiation. While once sexually active teens can and do revert to abstinence, effecting the reversal is a more difficult challenge than postponing sexual initiation.

3. Because the sexual-risk behaviors that teen pregnancy and HIV prevention programs are trying to change are relatively new to teens, it is important to supplement didactic conveying of information (lectures, slides, videos) with experiential learning. Most effective programs provide role-playing, modeling, and other skill-building exercises that teach teens the specific skills needed to "say no," acquire a contraceptive, or negotiate contraceptive use with a partner.

4. Teens are embedded in their families, schools, and communities. Involving parents and peers in the intervention facilitates effectiveness, in all likelihood because such involvement gives teens environmental support for the desired behavior changes.

5. At this point there is no evidence to show programs with an abstinence-only focus can delay sexual initiation for more than a few months. This finding was reinforced by a large-scale evaluation of a California-wide initiative known as ENABL (Education Now and Babies Later). ENABL was a pregnancy prevention initiative that delivered the abstinence-oriented part of a program called Postponing Sexual Involvement (PSI) to approximately 187,000 adolescents aged 12 to 14 in schools and community settings in 31 California counties. The curriculum delivered consisted of five sessions, each 45 to 60 minutes in length. The sessions focused on the risks of early sexual involvement, how to resist the social pressures that lead to early sexual involvement, how to determine limits on physically expressing affection, and how to resist pressure lines assertively.

The ENABL evaluation study[40] was published after the previous reviews, so the results are not reflected in the discussions above. The evaluation included over 7,000 teens. It was unique in that it included a follow-up data collection 17 months after the program was delivered (most evaluations of pregnancy prevention programs have had the funds to look for behavior changes at only 3, 6, and/or 12 months post-program). Consistent with previous reviews of abstinence-only programs, the ENABL evaluation found programmatically small but statistically significant effects on 8 of 18 measured mediating variables (such as beliefs and behavioral intent). Results of the 17-month follow-up analyses indicated, however, that any significant and positive effects of the program at 3 months were no longer found at 17 months post-program.

6. Because of the difficulty of delaying sexual initiation with an abstinence-only program, it is advisable to combine an encouragement of abstinence message with support for contraceptive use for sexually active teens. Effective pregnancy and HIV prevention programs typically carry a two-prong message: (1) Abstinence is a valued goal for teenagers; it is advisable to avoid having sexual intercourse while still an unmarried teenager. (2) If you and your partner do decide to have sexual intercourse, however, you should *always* protect yourselves against *both* pregnancy and STIs, including HIV.

7. At this point, caution is appropriate regarding the robustness of documented effectiveness findings. For most of the programs found effective in the above reviews, such effectiveness has been demonstrated at one site only, the site in which the program was initially developed. Whether the program will be effective at other sites—sites that could be the same or different in terms of type of culture, community, or school or in terms of the demographic and sociopsychological profile of parents and teens—still needs to be investigated.

Program Archive on Sexuality, Health & Adolescence

To facilitate the replication and re-evaluation of promising programs at new sites, a new national resource entitled Program Archive on Sexuality, Health & Adolescence (PASHA) is being developed. Bridging research and practice, PASHA is negotiating with holders of the 30 promising teen pregnancy and teen HIV prevention programs described above to obtain associated program and evaluation materials, process and document them for public use, and encourage their replication and re-evaluation across the country. To date, holders of 23 of the initial batch of 30 programs have agreed to make their programs available through PASHA.

Archiving work on all 23 of these programs has been completed and approved by the original program developer. These programs are now publicly available. The project has begun new research on the effectiveness of the PASHA programs through a comprehensive field test, replication, and re-evaluation of each program in one or more independent sites.

PROGRAM PRIORITIES: AMELIORATING THE CONSEQUENCES OF CHILDBEARING

A final strategy commanding wide public support is to ameliorate the negative consequences of adolescent childbearing. Demonstration projects have focused on three priorities for adolescent mothers:

- Ensuring a safe pregnancy and delivery
- Staying in school (particularly to increase employability)
- Avoiding additional unintended pregnancies (secondary prevention)

Health interventions are very effective. For young women in any socioeconomic category, adequate prenatal and obstetrical care greatly reduces the adverse health consequences to mother and child associated with pregnancy and childbirth at an early age.[6,46]

Some prenatal home-visitation programs for socially disadvantaged women are effective in improving women's health-related behaviors during pregnancy, reducing the incidence of preterm births and low birthweight, and reducing subsequent unintended pregnancies. The more effective programs employ nurses who visit frequently enough during pregnancy and after delivery to establish a therapeutic alliance with the family and who address the material, social, psychological, and behavioral factors associated with maternal and child health. Results of randomized trials of home-visitation programs reveal that attempts to isolate only a few important aspects of such interventions are misguided. Social support during pregnancy is ineffective at improving pregnancy outcomes unless adverse maternal health behaviors are altered. Prenatal home visits alone, without continuing comprehensive postnatal visits, are insufficient to promote well-being past delivery.[59,60]

The next priorities after ensuring a healthy delivery are to keep the mother in school and to prevent further unintended pregnancies. The results of Project Redirection—a comprehensive program whose participants (who were extremely disadvantaged when compared not only with teenagers generally but also with other teen parents) were asked to organize and frequently reorient aspects of their lives while pursuing an education, training for a job, and learning about family planning—are sobering. When compared with those not in the program who served as controls, Redirection participants were more likely to be in school or have graduated, less likely to have become pregnant, and more likely to be practicing contraception at the time of the 1-year follow-up. After 2 years, however, the differentials had vanished.[66] This finding led the investigators to conclude that the impact of the intervention lasted no longer than the participants' stay in the program. Although Project Redirection was based on a research design substantially more rigorous than is typical for teenage parent programs, the comparison group had much wider access to local social service programs than had been anticipated. Thus, comparison of Redirection participants and controls does not reveal the difference in outcomes between "no treatment" and "comprehensive treatment" groups. A supplementary analysis compared four groups: Redirection participants in the program from 1 to 2 years, Redirection participants in the program for less than 1 year, controls who were ever in a similar program, and controls who were never in any program. The results, which must be interpreted with caution since the outcomes could reflect systematic variation in uncontrolled characteristics such as motivation, suggest that the more services a mother received, the better she performed. Nevertheless, the most reasonable conclusion is that short-term assistance does not have a long-term impact on educational attainment or subsequent pregnancy.

A 5-year follow-up of Project Redirection confirmed this conclusion: the experimental and control groups had equal educational attainment and equal numbers of subsequent pregnancies, on average. The experimental group actually had a greater average number of subsequent births (but fewer abortions) than the control group. In contrast, Redirection participants, when compared with controls, worked more hours and had higher weekly earnings from employment, were less likely to be receiving welfare, and scored higher on a widely used test of parenting ability. Moreover, participants' children showed better cognitive skills and exhibited fewer behavioral problems.[65] Although these results confirm that an intensive short-term program cannot eliminate the long-term disadvantages conferred by poverty, they do provide a basis for believing the prospects for disadvantaged teenage mothers and their children can be improved by such an intervention.

Project Redirection is perhaps the best example of a comprehensive program for pregnant teenagers. Such programs have considerable appeal because they focus on the individual *after* she becomes pregnant, thereby avoiding the controversy surrounding the prevention of adolescent pregnancy and the seemingly insoluble problem of poverty. Moreover, focusing on local communities and the coordination of local programs appears to circumvent the need for additional resources. However, a review of the quality of such comprehensive programs has concluded the comprehensive model is better suited to political compromise and rhetoric than to effective problem-solving.[78] The authors argue that many comprehensive programs are based on three faulty assumptions: that the requisite services are already locally available and need only be stitched together administratively, that this goal can be accomplished without a further infusion of state and federal financial assistance, and that the adolescent pregnancy problem can be best addressed by targeting services to those already pregnant.

In summary, short-term interventions aimed at ensuring a safe pregnancy and delivery, reducing subsequent fertility, and enhancing educational attainment are expensive; only those focused on prenatal care appear to be truly effective. No Band-Aid, quick-fix, inexpensive solutions exist for ameliorating the negative outcomes associated with adolescent childbearing.

Given such outcomes—rapid subsequent fertility, low educational attainment, poor marriage prospects, high rates of marital dissolution, and out-of-wedlock childbearing—it is not surprising that a strong association between early childbearing and subsequent poverty exists.[33] Three of 4 Aid to Families of Dependent Children (AFDC) recipients under age 30 had a first birth as a teenager.[53]

PROGRAM PRIORITIES: CONCLUSIONS

A compelling question of public policy, therefore, is the relative effectiveness of fertility prevention versus ameliorative schemes for reducing poverty. Research suggests that preventing adolescent childbearing would be far more effective in reducing the proportion of young women who require public assistance than would increasing education, increasing marriage probabilities, or reducing subsequent fertility among adolescent mothers.[56] Such a finding is reassuring, because the public cost associated with teenage childbearing is substantial. In 1992, $34 billion was paid through three federal programs (AFDC, food stamps, and Medicaid) to women who first gave birth as teenagers; if all teenage births were delayed until the mother was at least 20 years old, the estimated savings would be $13 billion.[13] The cost to taxpayers of childbearing among women less than age 18 alone is $6.9 billion, consisting of $2.2 billion for welfare and food stamps, $1.5 billion in medical care expenses, $1.0 billion to construct and maintain prisons to house the criminal teen sons of adolescent mothers, $0.9 billion for foster care, and $1.3 billion in lost tax revenue from the fathers. The total annual cost to society associated with childbearing by women under age 18 together with the other disadvantages faced by adolescent mothers is $29 billion.[49]

However, those who see lifelong economic and social disadvantage as the problem, and teenage childbearing as the consequence, warn that the conventional estimates such as those presented above overstate—perhaps substantially—the costs of teenage childbearing and therefore the benefits of reducing its incidence. The subtle danger is that research and analysis based on this perspective will . . .

> . . . be used to argue that because teen pregnancy is not the linchpin that holds together myriad other social ills, it is not a problem at all. Concern about teen pregnancy has at least directed attention and resources to young, poor, and minority women. It has awakened many Americans to their diminished life chances. If measures aimed at reducing teen pregnancy are not the quick fix for much of what ails American society, there is the powerful temptation to forget these young women altogether and allow them to slip back to their traditional invisible place in American public debate. Teen pregnancy is less about young women and their sex lives than it is about restricted horizons and the boundaries of hope. It is about race and class and how those realities limit opportunities for young people. Most centrally, however, it is typically about being young, female, poor, and non-white and about how having a child seems to be one of the few avenues of satisfaction, fulfillment, and self-esteem. It would be a tragedy to stop worrying about these young women—and their partners—because their behavior is the measure rather than the cause of their blighted hopes.[44]

A sound rationale for supporting programs to reduce the incidence of adolescent pregnancy does not depend on resolving the current debate or on the accuracy of estimates about negative personal consequences or public costs. Few adolescents intentionally become pregnant. That adolescents want to avoid becoming pregnant is sufficient reason for helping them do so.

TAILORING CLINIC SERVICES FOR THE NEEDS OF TEENS

A review of more than 150 articles published since 1970 (with a focus on those published since 1980) has enriched our understanding of how clinics can best tailor their programs to meet the needs of sexually active teens.[3] Of these, 38 studies discussed aspects of adolescent behavior and sexual activity that could be related to the development of friendly and effective clinic practices, two studies on postponement of repeat teen pregnancies shed light on effective outreach and follow-up practices, and six studies reported surveys of factors associated with improved services to teenagers. Three key features of effective and friendly clinics emerged: active outreach to attract clients, comprehensive services to meet individual needs, and thorough follow-through to maintain clients in the program. This FIND, SERVE, and CARE model is an amalgam of characteristics of successful programs, presented within a theoretical context of adolescent growth and development (Table 29-4). No program was identified that contains all the aspects of outreach, clinical services, and follow-through in this model; thus, the overall impact of incorporating all programmatic aspects into one setting cannot yet be determined.

This model can be used to conduct a program audit to determine which of these "best practices" are currently in place. Program managers in charge of more than one clinic could use the audit to determine whether differences in clinic performance are related to how closely each clinic reflects the ideal for teen friendly services. In setting priorities for program improvement, the director should involve teens from the community. They might jointly develop a "wish list" of components that might hold greater promise for improved clinic services within that community. Selected components can be added sequentially, with ongoing evaluation to determine their impact on the proportion of teens being served among those in need. Additions that make an impact can be maintained, while those that do not can be replaced with other additions on the "wish list." In this systematic way, a program can be tailored to maximize its resources to meet the needs of its clientele. A related use of this model may be for the program administrator to justify additional financial support in order to add and evaluate a major new component (e.g., case management).

Adolescents with a negative pregnancy test result are an appropriate target group for contraceptive counseling and services. In one study of women aged 17 and younger seeking pregnancy tests in clinics, 62% tested negative. Many came for pregnancy tests even though they were certain they were not pregnant. Among those who had ever conceived, 1 in 4 had had a prior negative test result at a clinic. Altogether almost 3 in 5 received a negative test result in a clinic prior to becoming pregnant.[80]

Table 29-4 Quick checklist for assessing contraceptive services to teens (FIND, SERVE, CARE Model)

FIND	

Are you maximizing the value of outreach? Specifically, are you:	**By:**
Providing a *Family-oriented* service?	• Recruiting clients through their mothers (who may have been teen mothers themselves) • Recruiting clients through their sister(s), who may have been teen mothers • Knowing what the teen's family has taught about sex • Knowing whether the teen is or has been sexually abused
Providing an *Integrated* service?	• Having an active, two-way referral system with schools • Having an active, two-way referral system with community-based organizations, clubs, etc. • Maximizing community interest in the clinic through advertisements, speeches, and community-based education programs

Providing a *Needed* service targeting teens who are more likely to have early or unprotected sex?	• Knowing which teens in the community are more likely to have sex at an early age, those who
	  — Are/were sexually abused
	  — Are substance abusers
	  — Are delinquents
	  — Lack adult supervision after school
	  — Live in poverty
	  — Live with one parent
	
	• Knowing which teens in the community are more likely to have unprotected sex, those who
	  — Initiated intercourse at an early age
	  — Are teen parents
	  — Are ambivalent about parenting
	  — Had a negative pregnancy test
	
	• Knowing where those teens are in the community
	• Getting into those areas and actively recruiting

Providing a *Determined* outreach effort?	• Having a sign on the clinic that is visible • Locating the clinic in a place accessible to teenagers • Encouraging clients to tell friends about the clinic and to bring friends with them • Including active outreach activities in the base budget • Evaluating the outreach efforts

(continued)

Table 29-4 Quick checklist for assessing contraceptive services to teens (FIND, SERVE, CARE Model) *(cont.)*

SERVE	
Are you maximizing the quality of your services? Specifically, are you:	**By:**
Making the services *Safe* for teen clients?	• Including a statement of confidentiality on advertising materials • Including a statement of confidentiality on clinic forms • Explaining the confidentiality policy to teens who visit the clinic
Making the services *Elastic* to fit individuals' needs?	• Providing services in late afternoons • Providing services in the evenings • Providing services on weekends • Having few levels of hierarchy above the nursing level • Hiring female staff • Accepting governmental/state funding • Applying for external grants • Providing a mechanism to accept donations • Conducting community fund raisers • Accepting insurance coverage of services • Determining the dialects of the community • Determining literacy rates of the adolescent population • Hiring staff who speak the right languages at the right levels
Making the services *Related?*	• Working with parents in the community on ways to support teen contraceptive use • Counseling teens on ways they can involve their partners in contraceptive decision making • Encouraging teens to bring their partners and parents to clinic visits • Using peer counselors

Making the services *Varied?*	• Developing an intake screening tool that can be used to identify teens who may need additional attention which
	  — Identifies risks for early or unprotected sex (see *Needed* above)
	  — Assesses intention to use contraceptives (see *Assessed* below)
	  — Contains a sexual and contraceptive history
	
	• Hiring staff with a background in recognizing sexual abuse and in counseling teens who have been abused
	• Through course work, workshops, and/or trainings, training current staff in recognizing and addressing sexual abuse

(continued)

Table 29-4 Quick checklist for assessing contraceptive services to teens (FIND, SERVE, CARE Model) *(cont.)*

SERVE	

Making the services *Varied? (cont.)*	• Targeting materials and counseling to client's age
	• Administering medical protocols in an age-appropriate manner
	• Allowing clients to postpone the pelvic examination and blood work
	• Providing a broad range of contraceptive methods
	
	• Counseling on needed topics such as
	  — Sexual values
	  — Saying no
	  — Abstinence and alternate forms of intimacy
	  — Use, advantages, disadvantages, and effectiveness of various forms of birth control methods
	  — Signs and symptoms of STIs
	  — Family and peer relationships
	  — Decision making
	
	• Educating staff about the health and social services in the area available to teens
	• Discussing the personal goals of the client, including needs separate from family planning issues
	• Referring teen clients to health and social agencies in the area

Assuring services are *Evaluated?*	• Obtaining ongoing feedback on service quality from clients • Establishing and periodically examining goals and objectives • Measuring progress towards goals achievement • Measuring impact of new program components

CARE	
Are you maximizing client continuation? Specifically, are you:	**By:**
Establishing and maintaining *Contact*	• Getting the names and phone numbers of people the client says you may contact to help with return appointments • Getting mailing addresses that can be used • Creating a follow-up plan that does not compromise confidentiality

(continued)

Table 29-4 Quick checklist for assessing contraceptive services to teens (FIND, SERVE, CARE Model) *(cont.)*

CARE	

Developing a means to *Assess* follow-up needs	• Using a protocol to identify teens needing closer follow-up, those who
	  — Are younger
	  — Have a negative pregnancy test
	  — Are ambivalent about using contraception
	  — Are a teen parent
	  — Have experienced sexual abuse
	  — Have a lower locus of control score
	  — Have no articulated strong future goals

Assuring personal *Respect* for each client	• Developing a system to collect information on the services used by each client and the outcome of her/his visits • Having teens see the same staff from visit to visit • Having teens see few staff at a given clinic visit • Training staff to apply developmental mileposts and longitudinal plans for contraceptive continuation
Doing what is required to *Encourage* continuation	• Providing incentives for contraceptive continuation • Reviewing partner/parent involvement in ongoing contraceptive choices • Helping teens set goals and applauding their achievements?

Source: Baden and Hogue (1997).

REFERENCES

1. Abma JC, Chandra A, Mosher WD, Peterson LS, Piccinino LJ. Fertility, family planning, and women's health: new data from the 1995 National Survey of Family Growth. Vital Health Stat 1997;Series 23, Number 19.
2. Adamson P (ed). The progress of nations 1996. New York: UNICEF, 1996.
3. Baden S, Hogue CJR. Family planning services for teens: a FIND, SERVE, CARE model. Unpublished manuscript. Atlanta GA: Rollins School of Public Health, Emory University, 1997.
4. Baldwin W, Cain VS. The children of teenage parents. Fam Plann Perspect 1980;12:34-43.
5. Bronars SG, Grogger J. The economic consequences of unwed motherhood: using twin births as a natural experiment. Am Econ Rev 1994;84:1141-1156.
6. Brown SS. Can low birth weight be prevented? Fam Plann Perspect 1985;17:112-118.
7. Brown SS, Eisenberg L. The best intentions: unintended pregnancy and the well-being of children and families. Washington DC: National Academy Press, 1995.

8. Card JJ. Advances in evaluating teen pregnancy programs. TEC Networks. Number 25, June, 1990:4.
9. Card JJ. Long-term consequences for children of teenage parents. Demography 1981;18:137-156.
10. Card JJ, Niego S, Mallari A, Farrell WS. The Program Archive on Sexuality, Health & Adolescence: promising "prevention programs-in-a-box." Fam Plann Perspect 1996;28:210-220.
11. Card JJ, Wise LL. Teenage mothers and teenage fathers: the impact of early childbearing on the parents' personal and professional lives. Fam Plann Perspect 1978;10:199-205.
12. Cates W, Berman SM, Darroch JE, Berkley S. Epidemiology of sexually transmitted diseases and STD sequelae. In: Hitchcock PJ, Boruch R, Flay B, Berkeley S, Kanouse D, Whitley R, Darroch JE (eds). STDs in adolescents: challenges for the 21st century. New York NY: Oxford University Press, in press.
13. Center for Population Options. Cost of supporting teenager's babies soars 17 percent: taxpayers spend over $30 billion dollars in federal aid. Washington DC: Center for Population Options, 1994.
14. Centers for Disease Control and Prevention. Division of STD/HIV prevention annual report, 1993. Atlanta: Centers for Disease Control and Prevention, 1994.
15. Centers for Disease Control and Prevention. HIV/AIDS surveillance report: year-end edition. Atlanta: Centers for Disease Control and Prevention, 1995.
16. Dash L. When children want children: the urban crisis of teenage childbearing. New York: William Morrow, 1989. Reissued as: When children want children: an inside look at the crisis of teenage parenthood. New York: Penguin, 1990.
17. David HP, Rademakers J. Lessons from the Dutch abortion experience. Stud Fam Plann 1996;27:341-343.
18. Day JC. Population projections of the United States, by age, sex, race, and Hispanic origin: 1995 to 2050. Curr Popul Rep, Series P25-1130. Washington DC: Government Printing Office, 1996.
19. Forrest JD, Singh S. The sexual and reproductive behavior of American women, 1982-1988. Fam Plann Perspect 1990;22:206-214.
20. Fraser AM, Brockert JE, Ward RH. Association of young maternal age with adverse reproductive outcomes. N Engl J Med 1995;332:1113-1117.
21. Frost JJ, Forrest JD. Understanding the impact of effective teenage pregnancy prevention programs. Fam Plann Perspect 1995;27:188-195.
22. Furstenberg FF. When will teenage childbearing become a social problem? The implications of western experience for developing countries. Unpublished manuscript. Philadelphia PA: Population Studies Center, University of Pennsylvania, 1997.
23. Furstenberg FF, Brooks-Gunn J, Morgan SP. Adolescent mothers and their children in later life. Fam Plann Perspect 1987;19:142-151.
24. Geronimus AT, Korenman S. Maternal youth or family background? On the health disadvantages of infants with teenage mothers. Am J Epidemiol 1993;137:213-225.
25. Geronimus AT, Korenman S. The socioeconomic consequences of teen childbearing reconsidered. Q J Econ 1992;107:1187-1214.

26. Geronimus AT, Korenman S, Hillemeier MM. Does young maternal age adversely affect child development? Evidence from cousin comparisons in the United States. Popul Dev Rev 1994;20:585-609.

27. Gress-Wright J. The contraception paradox. Public Interest 1993;113:15-25.

28. Haffner DW (ed). Facing facts: sexual health for America's adolescents. New York NY: Sexuality Information and Education Council of the United States (SIECUS), 1995.

29. Hardy JB, Duggan AK, Masnyk K, Pearson C. Fathers of children born to young urban mothers. Fam Plann Perspect 1989;21:159-163, 187.

30. Harrison PF, Rosenfield A. Contraceptive research and development: looking to the future. Washington DC: National Academy Press, 1996.

31. Henshaw SK. Personal communication to James Trussell, September 19, 1996.

32. Henshaw SK. Teenage abortion and pregnancy statistics by state, 1992. Fam Plann Perspect 1997;29:115-122.

33. Hofferth SL, Moore KA. Early childbearing and later economic well-being. Am Sociol Rev 1979;44:784-815.

34. Hoffman SD, Foster EM, Furstenberg FF. Re-evaluating the costs of teenage childbearing. Demography 1993;30:1-13.

35. Hollingsworth DR, Kotchen JM, Felice ME. Impact of gynecologic age on outcome of adolescent pregnancy. In: McAnarney ER (ed). Premature adolescent pregnancy and parenthood. New York: Grune and Stratton, 1983:169-190.

36. Jones EF, Forrest JD, Goldman N, Henshaw S, Lincoln R, Rosoff JI, Westoff CF, Wulf D. Teenage pregnancy in industrialized countries. New Haven CT: Yale University Press, 1986. Summarized in Jones EF, Forrest JD, Goldman N, Henshaw S, Lincoln R, Rosoff JI, Westoff CF, Wulf D. Teenage pregnancy in developed countries: determinants and policy implications. Fam Plann Perspect 1985;17:53-63.

37. Kaiser Family Foundation. The 1996 Kaiser Family Foundation survey on teens and sex: what they say teens need to know and who they listen to. Menlo Park CA: The Henry J. Kaiser Family Foundation, June 24, 1996.

38. Kann L, Warren CW, Harris WA, Collins JL, Williams BI, Ross JG, Kolbe LJ. Youth risk behavior surveillance—United States 1995. MMWR 1996;45(SS-4).

39. Kirby D. A review of educational programs designed to reduce sexual risk-taking behaviors among school-aged youth in the United States. Springfield VA: National Technical Information Service, 1995;#PB96108519.

40. Kirby D, Korpi M, Barth RP, Cagampang HH. The impact of the Postponing Sexual Involvement curriculum among youths in California. Fam Plann Perspect 1997;29:100-108.

41. Kirby D, Short L, Collins J, Rugg D, Kolbe L, Howard M, Miller B, Sonenstein F, Zabin LS. School-based programs to reduce sexual risk behaviors: a review of effectiveness. Public Health Rep 1994;109:339-360.

42. Kisker EE. Teenagers talk about sex, pregnancy and contraception. Fam Plann Perspect 1985;17:83-90.

43. Landry DJ, Forrest JD. How old are U.S. fathers? Fam Plann Perspect 1995;27:159-161, 165.

44. Luker K. Dubious conceptions: the controversy over teen pregnancy. Am Prospect 1991;5:73-83.

45. Luker K. Dubious conceptions: the politics of teenage pregnancy. Cambridge MA: Harvard University Press, 1996.

46. Makinson C, The health consequences of teenage fertility. Fam Plann Perspect 1985;17:132-139.
47. Marsiglio W. Adolescent fathers in the United States: their initial living arrangements, marital experience and educational outcomes. Fam Plann Perspect 1987;19:240-251.
48. Mastroianni L, Donaldson PJ, Kane TT (eds). Developing new contraceptives: obstacles and opportunities. Washington DC: National Academy Press, 1990.
49. Maynard RA (ed). Kids having kids: economic costs and social consequences of teen pregnancy. Washington DC: Urban Institute Press, 1997.
50. McAnarney ER, Thiede HA. Adolescent pregnancy and childbearing: what we learned during the 1970s and what remains to be learned. In: McAnarney ER (ed). Premature adolescent pregnancy and parenthood. New York: Grune and Stratton, 1983:375-395.
51. Menken J. The health and demographic consequences of adolescent pregnancy and childbearing. In: Chilman CS (ed). Adolescent pregnancy and childbearing: findings from research. Washington DC: United States Government Printing Office, 1980:157-200.
52. Miller BC, Card JJ, Paikoff RL, Peterson, JL (eds). Preventing adolescent pregnancy: model programs and evaluations. Newbury Park CA: Sage Publications, 1992.
53. Moore KA, Burt MR. Private crisis, public cost: policy perspectives on teenage childbearing. Washington DC: The Urban Institute Press, 1982.
54. Moore KA, Snyder NO. Cognitive attainment among firstborn children of adolescent mothers. Am Sociol Rev 1991;56:612-624.
55. Moore K, Sugland BW, Blumenthal C, Glei D, Snyder N. Adolescent pregnancy prevention programs: interventions and evaluations. Washington DC: Child Trends Inc., 1995.
56. Moore KA, Wertheimer RF. Teenage childbearing and welfare: preventive and ameliorative strategies. Fam Plann Perspect 1984;16:285-289.
57. Mosher WD, Horn MC. First family planning visits by young women. Fam Plann Perspect 1988;20:33-40.
58. National Campaign to Prevent Teen Pregnancy. Prospectus for the National Campaign to Prevent Teen Pregnancy: mission, leadership, and activities. Washington DC: National Campaign to Prevent Teen Pregnancy, 1996.
59. Olds DL. Home visitation for pregnant women and parents of young children. Am J Dis Child 1992;146:704-708.
60. Olds DL, Kitzman H. Can home visitation improve the health of women and children at environmental risk? Pediatrics 1990;86:108-116.
61. Orr MT, Forrest JD. The availability of reproductive health services from U.S. private physicians. Fam Plann Perspect 1985;17:63-69.
62. Parke RD, Neville B. Teenage fatherhood. In: Hofferth SL, Hayes CD (eds). Risking the future: adolescent sexuality, pregnancy and childbearing, Volume II. Washington DC: National Academy Press, 1987:145-173.
63. Philliber S, Namerow P. Trying to maximize the odds: using what we know to prevent teen pregnancy. Prepared for a technical assistance workshop to support the CDC Teen Pregnancy Prevention Program, 1995.
64. Piccinino LJ. Personal communication to James Trussell, March 24, 1997.

65. Polit DF. Effects of a comprehensive program for teenage parents: five years after Project Redirection. Fam Plann Perspect 1989;21:164-169, 187.
66. Polit DF, Kahn JR. Project Redirection: evaluation of a comprehensive program for disadvantaged teenage mothers. Fam Plann Perspect 1985;17: 150-155.
67. Rosenzweig MR, Wolpin KI. Sisters, siblings, and mothers: the effect of teenage childbearing on birth outcomes in a dynamic family context. Econometrica 1995;63:303-326.
68. Saluter AF. Marital status and living arrangements: March 1994. Curr Popul Rep, Series P20-484. Washington DC: Government Printing Office, 1996.
69. Sonenstein FL, Pleck JH, Ku L, Lindberg LD, Turner CF. Changes in sexual behavior and contraception among adolescent males: 1988 and 1995. Unpublished manuscript. Washington DC: The Urban Institute, 1997.
70. Speroff L, Glass RH, Kase NG. Clinical gynecologic endocrinology and infertility (Fifth Edition). Baltimore MD: Williams and Wilkins, 1994.
71. Strobino DM. The health and medical consequences of adolescent sexuality and pregnancy: a review of the literature. In: Hofferth SL, Hayes CD (eds). Risking the future: adolescent sexuality, pregnancy and childbearing, Volume II. Washington DC: National Academy Press, 1987:93-122.
72. Trussell J. Teenage pregnancy in the United States. Fam Plann Perspect 1988;20:262-272.
73. Trussell J, Kost K. Contraceptive failure in the United States: a critical review of the literature. Stud Fam Plann 1987;18:237-283.
74. Trussell J, Stewart F, Guest F, Hatcher RA. Emergency contraceptive pills: a simple proposal to reduce unintended pregnancies. Fam Plann Perspect 1992;24:269-273.
75. Trussell J, Vaughan B. Selected results concerning sexual behavior and contraceptive use from the 1988 National Survey of Family Growth and the 1988 National Survey of Adolescent Males. Working Paper #91-12. Princeton NJ: Office of Population Research, Princeton University, 1991.
76. Upchurch DM, McCarthy, J. The timing of a first birth and high school completion. Am Sociol Rev 1990;55:224-234.
77. Ventura SJ, Martin JA, Matthews TJ, Clarke SC. Advance report of final natality statistics, 1994. Mon Vital Stat Rep 1996;44(11-Suppl).
78. Weatherley RA, Perlman SB, Levine MH, Klerman LV. Comprehensive programs for pregnant teenagers and teenage parents: how successful have they been? Fam Plann Perspect 1986;18:73-78.
79. Zabin LS, Astone NM, Emerson MR. Do adolescents want babies? The relationship between attitudes and behavior. J Res Adolesc 1993;3:67-86.
80. Zabin LS, Emerson MR, Ringers PA, Sedivy V. Adolescents with negative pregnancy test results: an accessible at-risk group. JAMA 1996;275:113-117.
81. Zelnik M, Kantner JF. Sexual activity, contraceptive use and pregnancy among metropolitan- area teenagers: 1971-1979. Fam Plann Perspect 1980;12:230-237.
82. Zelnik M, Kantner JF, Ford K. Sex and pregnancy in adolescence. Beverly Hills CA: Sage Publications, 1981.

Dynamics of Reproductive Behavior and Population Change

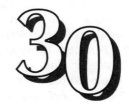

James Trussell, PhD

- Current population growth rates are very high by historical standards and cannot possibly persist indefinitely.
- Declining fertility inevitably leads to an aging of the population. Caring for an increasing proportion of elderly persons will be a significant problem in many countries.

- The impact of acquired immune deficiency syndrome (AIDS) on mortality rates and population growth could be dramatic and devastating in certain areas of the world, particularly in sub-Saharan Africa and Asia.
- Breastfeeding is an important contraceptive for a population even if an individual woman or couple cannot rely on it for very long.

In the United States, according to current experience, an average woman will bear 2 children in a lifetime that will last about 79 years. In Uganda, an average woman currently will produce 7 children; her life expectancy at birth is around 42 years. We will explore some of the reasons for these differences in the following sections. We will also examine the consequences of rapid population growth, the concepts of population momentum and population aging, and the results of governmental population policy.

Why should these issues be of concern to family planning practitioners? As firm believers in voluntary family planning, the authors of this book stress that we are dedicated to helping individuals achieve their reproductive life goals, whatever they may be. Nevertheless, individual reproductive choices do have aggregate consequences, because they determine the fertility of a population. It is only natural those involved in family planning and reproductive health would be interested in understanding how the uses of contraception and its effectiveness, the prevalence of abortion, and the duration of lactation affect the aggregate level of fertility in a population. This chapter provides a framework of analysis for answering this question.

Fertility, however, is only one of the determinants of population change. The other two components—mortality and migration—are explored below in less detail. The final section describes several methodological tools for demographic analysis. We emphasize methodology for the sake of neither rigor nor completeness. Instead, such tools are necessary to avoid common pitfalls when thinking about reproductive issues of concern to us all.

D ETERMINANTS OF FERTILITY

Why is fertility high in some populations and low in others? First, ages at menarche and menopause—which set biological limits on the start and end of childbearing—vary somewhat among populations. Second, proportions of women at each age who are sexually active and therefore exposed to the risk of pregnancy vary across populations. Third, populations vary in the spacing between initiation of sexual activity and the first live birth and in the spacing between one live birth and the next.

MENARCHE, MENOPAUSE, AND STERILITY

The average age of menarche normally varies only in a narrow range from about age 12 to about age 15.[36] The average age at menopause is much harder to measure; it is easy for a woman to know whether she has had a first period but hard to know if she has had her last. Ordinarily, menopause is assumed to have occurred if a specified period of time (e.g., 1 or 1.5 years) has passed since the last period. Menopause, too, appears to be largely confined to a rather narrow range, on average from about age 47 to age 51.[36]

The span between menarche and menopause could therefore be as short as 32 years or as long as 39 years. This difference of 7 years, all other factors being equal, could imply a difference in lifetime fertility of as much as 2 to 3 children, if, during the added 7 years, women experienced the maximum fertility rates that prevail in the primary childbearing years. For several reasons the difference is likely to be far smaller. First, as previously mentioned, it is not possible to measure directly the age at which menopause occurs, so 7 years may be an overestimate of the potential difference. Second, a difference of several years in estimated age at menopause between two populations, even if real, may mean only that in one population women have a longer period of subfecundity (reduced physiological capacity to produce a live birth) before becoming sterile. What we can observe directly is age at last birth, which seems to be near age 41 in populations not using contraception.[56] Third, differences in age at menarche are unlikely to result in differences in fertility unless entry into a sexual union is tied closely to menarche. In most populations, women do not enter sexual unions until several years after menarche. Therefore, even though differences in the childbearing span could affect lifetime fertility, in practice the effect is likely to be small, at most a difference of 1 child over a lifetime and possibly much smaller.

AGE AT MARRIAGE AND PROPORTIONS MARRIED

A major determinant of fertility differences among populations is the age at which women begin sustained sexual activity.[10] In many populations, sexual intercourse is primarily confined to marriage, so age at marriage, proportions ever marrying, and patterns of marital dissolution and remarriage are powerful determinants of fertility levels. One way to measure the impact of marriage on fertility is to compare the total fertility rates of married women with the total fertility rates of all women. Maximum fertility would be achieved if all women married at menarche and stayed married until menopause. However, this marriage pattern does not exist in any population. Estimates of the fertility-reducing effects of actual marriage patterns range from lows of 11% in Bangladesh and 14% in Senegal to highs of 40% in South Korea and 43% in Costa Rica.[19]

While proportions of older women currently married do vary across populations, this variation is too small to account for a large portion of observed differences in fertility, particularly because marital fertility rates fall with age. In contrast, there is considerable variation in the proportions of young women who are married. For example, the fraction of 15- to 19 year-old women who are married varies from lows of 1% in Japan and South Korea, 2% in Hong Kong and 4% in China to 38% in India, 48% in Bangladesh, and 58% in Sierra Leone.[60] Even if many developing countries adopted modern contraceptive practices, they are not likely to achieve growth rates lower than 1.5% per year unless age at marriage is also increased.[46] Increasing the age at marriage lowers total fertility by removing some young women from the risk of pregnancy and raises the mean age at childbearing, thereby lowering the annual population growth rate by lengthening the time between generations.[73]

Raising the age at which young women marry is almost certain to have effects other than the purely mechanically demographic. The most important is to enhance the status of women, allowing them to stay in school longer to acquire job-related skills, to work outside the home before marriage, and to enter marriage with more physical and emotional maturity and financial security. Such social changes are themselves likely to stimulate a demand for fertility control.[40] Because raising the age at which women marry so profoundly alters the social fabric, governments may be unwilling or unable to use this potential instrument of public policy. In those populations with a high prevalence of consensual unions or premarital childbearing, a change in the legal minimum age for marriage may have little effect on fertility.

BIRTH INTERVAL LENGTH

Populations also differ widely in the length of time between one birth and the next, known as the birth interval. The shorter the average interval between births, the greater the number of births that can be squeezed into the childbearing span, and vice versa. The birth interval can be divided into three parts: the period of postpartum non-susceptibility during which a woman is not at risk of conception following a birth, the waiting time to a conception leading to the next live birth once she returns to risk, and gestation period itself.[54] The last of these parts, the gestation period, does not vary from population to population. There is, however, considerable variation in the other two components.

Postpartum non-susceptibility: The period of postpartum non-susceptibility is primarily governed by the length of lactation. If women do not breastfeed, this period can be as short as 2 months. With prolonged breastfeeding, the period can be up to a year and a half on average. For example, urban women in the Philippines breastfeed for an average of 9 months and do not resume menses for an average of 4 months.[59] In rural Nigeria, women breastfeed for about 20 months and are amenorrheic about 16 months.[30] The contraceptive effect depends on the intensity (frequency and duration) of the infant's suckling, which in turn is heavily influenced by the extent of supplemental feeding, particularly by bottle.[18] (See Chapter 23 on Postpartum Contraception and Lactation.) In developing countries, particularly in sub-Saharan Africa, women may abstain from having intercourse during some or all of the period of breastfeeding.[44]

Waiting time to conceive: The length of time a sexually active woman must wait before conceiving a pregnancy that leads to a live birth is determined by the underlying fecundity (physiological capacity to produce a live birth) of the man and the woman, the frequency and timing of intercourse, the prevalence and effectiveness of use of contraception, and the frequency of abortion (both spontaneous and induced). Fetal wastage in the absence of induced abortion is certainly not constant across populations, but it is a relatively unimportant cause of differences in fertility unless there is a high prevalence of syphilis. Likewise, fecundity, which declines with age within a given population, does not seem to vary much among populations unless there is a high prevalence of pelvic inflammatory disease (PID). Of these four factors, the prevalence and effectiveness of contraceptive use and the frequency of induced abortion are the most important sources of fertility differences.

EFFECTS OF BREASTFEEDING AND CONTRACEPTION

Consider a typical developing country in which contraceptive use is low but prolonged breastfeeding is nearly universal. Postpartum non-susceptibility lasts an average of 12 months. When not using contraception or breastfeeding, young wives typically take about 6 months to become pregnant. Pregnancy lasts 9 months. Then the interval between one birth and the next (ignoring spontaneous abortions) is 12+6+9=27 months, or 2.25 years. The average fertility rate per year is therefore 1/2.25, or 444 births per 1,000 sexually active women. A common effect of modernization is to decrease breastfeeding but increase contraceptive use. However, breastfeeding often decreases before contraceptive use increases.

If breastfeeding were completely abandoned in the population described above, the period of postpartum non-susceptibility would decrease to only 2 months. Thus the typical interval between births would also decrease: 2+6+9=17 months, or 1.42 years. The average fertility rate would rise from 444 to 706 births per 1,000 sexually active women—a rise of 59%. This simple calculation demonstrates the importance of lactation as a contraceptive to a population, even though it is not dependable enough for any individual woman to rely on it for very long to prevent pregnancy. (See Chapter 23 on Postpartum Contraception and Lactation.)

As contraceptive use increases, the waiting time to conception will rise and the birth interval will lengthen accordingly. If all women use contraception that reduces the monthly risk of pregnancy by 80% (say from .1667 to .0333), then the waiting time to conception would rise to about 30 months, since the waiting time can be shown to be the reciprocal (1/p) of the monthly probability (p) of conception. This rise would more than compensate for the decrease in the postpartum non-susceptible period, since the resulting birth interval would become 2+30+9=41 months. The fertility rate would fall by 59%, from 706 to 293 per 1,000.

We ignore here and in the discussion to follow the effects of spontaneous abortion, which on average would add about 2 months to the average birth interval.

The same reasoning leads to the conclusion that breastfeeding has little effect on fertility in the United States. Suppose women use contraception that reduces the monthly probability of conception to .01. The typical birth interval would be 111 months in the absence of breastfeeding (2 months of postpartum non-susceptibility, 100 months to conceive, and 9 months of gestation). Even if breastfeeding produced an average of 8 months of postpartum non-susceptibility, then the typical birth interval would increase by only 5%; both the proportion of infants breastfed and the average duration of breastfeeding would have to increase substantially in the United States to produce even this small effect.

EFFECT OF ABORTION

Many people assume 1 abortion will prevent 1 birth. But we can easily demonstrate this assumption is false. Consider again the developing country with a birth interval among young women of 27 months (a period of postpartum non-susceptibility of 12 months, 6 months to get pregnant, and a pregnancy of 9 months). Imagine every other pregnancy is aborted. Then the waiting time to conception would consist of the following parts: 6 months to get pregnant the first time, 3 months of pregnancy until the abortion, 1 month of postpartum non-susceptibility following the abortion, and 6 more months of waiting until the next pregnancy. Thus the total waiting time goes from 6 to 16 months, a rise of 167%. But the birth interval (12+16+9 months) would increase by only 37%, from 27 to 37 months. Hence, when every other pregnancy is aborted, the fertility rate would decline by only 27%, not 50% as might initially be expected. In summary, fertility is inversely related to the length of the total birth interval. Thus, a change in any component will have a less-than-proportional impact on the total, and hence on fertility. But, one might object, an abortion certainly prevents 1 birth. However, this way of thinking ignores the fact that the next birth occurs sooner when a pregnancy is aborted than when it results in a live birth. Therefore, while an abortion prevents a particular birth, it reduces the woman's lifetime births by fewer than 1 if her reproductive behavior does not otherwise change.

In contrast, an abortion in a population practicing highly effective contraception will prevent nearly 1 birth. Suppose effective contraception reduces the monthly probability of conception to .01 and breastfeeding is minimal. The average birth interval would be 111 months, as described earlier. If every other pregnancy is aborted, then the birth interval would rise to 215 months, an increase of 94%, and the fertility rate would fall by nearly half (48%). Hence, in the United States, some abortions (those occurring to women who use contraceptives effectively) will prevent nearly 1 birth while other abortions (those occurring to women who do not use contraceptives effectively) will prevent substantially less than 1 birth.

EFFECTS OF SEXUALLY TRANSMITTED INFECTIONS

Sexually transmitted infections (STIs) substantially influence fertility in selected populations, though not in the United States.[68] Syphilis is an important cause of fetal loss among women with primary or secondary infections and may be an important factor contributing to low fertility among certain tribal groups in Burkina Faso and the Central African Republic.[36] Untreated PID caused by chlamydia and gonorrhea is a major cause of tubal infertility and sterility. The low fertility in Central Africa (a belt extending from the west coast of Cameroon and Gabon through northern Zaire into southwest Sudan) in the 1950s and 1960s[2] was attributed to a high prevalence of gonorrhea,[33] long before the additional role of chlamydia was recognized. In sub-Saharan Africa, gonorrhea and chlamydia are still common infections. Mass penicillin campaigns against gonorrhea (New Guinea), yaws (Martinique), and yaws and pinta (Cameroon, Upper Volta, Zaire, and Zambia) were followed by pronounced increases in fertility.[33,36] It is possible improved STI diagnostic and treatment services in sub-Saharan Africa as a component of prevention programs for acquired immune deficiency syndrome (AIDS) will also result in increased fertility.[15]

EFFECTS OF NUTRITION

A link between nutrition and fertility has been postulated as a relatively simple explanation for variations in marital fertility in populations that do not use contraception.[34] It is suggested the lower the nutritional status of a population, the lower its fecundity and hence fertility. If nutrition is to have a demographically important impact on fertility, it must affect the waiting time to conception or the duration of postpartum non-susceptibility. The evidence suggests chronic malnourishment may slightly increase the duration of postpartum non-susceptibility. But this effect will not amount to a difference of even 1 child in completed lifetime fertility. Nutrition does not appear to affect the waiting time to conception in chronically malnourished populations.[11,32,56] Chronic malnutrition probably does result in a delay in menarche, though, as argued above, the impact on fertility is likely to be very small. When food supplies are so short there is outright famine and starvation, fecundity and hence fertility are reduced. But when malnourishment is chronic and food intake is above starvation levels, there does not appear to be an important nutrition-fertility link.

DETERMINANTS OF MORTALITY

As living conditions in a country improve, the causes of death shift quite dramatically.[63] In developing countries, major causes of death are the infectious diseases. In developed countries such as the United States, causes of death are concentrated among degenerative diseases such as cancer and cardiovascular disease. This shift occurs primarily because infant and child mortality are much higher in developing countries. Poor nutrition makes children more susceptible to infection and less able to withstand illness that otherwise would not prove fatal. Improvement in living conditions implies better nutrition, sanitation, water supply, and access to public health measures such as vaccination against tetanus, measles, and other common diseases. With such improvements, children survive to adulthood, when degenerative diseases claim more lives.

Among Guatemalan women in 1964, for example, elimination of diarrheal, infectious, and parasitic diseases would have raised expectation of life at birth by 16.4 years, and elimination of cancer and heart disease would have added only 1.7 years. In contrast, elimination of the first three categories of diseases in the United States would have added 0.8 years and the elimination of the two degenerative causes of death 19.6 years.[65] The reason for the contrast between the United States and Guatemala is quite simple. In the United States, virtually nobody died of the diarrheal, infectious, and parasitic diseases, while in Guatemala, a smaller fraction of women lived long enough to die of cancer or heart disease. An even more interesting contrast occurs in the United States itself. As stated above, elimination of heart disease and cancer would have added 19.6 years to the expectation of life. But the contributions of the two causes were very lopsided. Cancer accounted for only 2.6 years, whereas heart disease accounted for 17.1.

REPRODUCTIVE AND SEXUAL BEHAVIORS AFFECTING MORTALITY

Reproductive and sexual behavior significantly affect mortality in three major ways. First, the total number of children women bear, the ages at which they bear children, and length of intervals between births all affect maternal and infant health. Short intervals between births are associated with higher rates of infant, child, and maternal mortality. Reducing the number of children women bear would reduce maternal morbidity and mortality, especially in populations with high fertility, poor health conditions, and high reproductive morbidity. Parents can minimize the risk of infant and child death by not bearing children at very young and very old ages, by averting high-parity births, and by lengthening the interval between births.[57] Second, breastfeeding significantly lowers the risk of infant and child death.[80] Third, unprotected sexual intercourse entails the risk of transmitting and acquiring STIs, including the human immunodeficiency virus (HIV), the virus that causes AIDS. STIs other than HIV are themselves associated with higher risks of transmitting and acquiring HIV. Pregnant women infected with HIV may transmit the infection to their infants in utero, during childbirth, or through breastmilk.

MATERNAL MORTALITY AND MORBIDITY

Each year an estimated 585,000 women worldwide die during pregnancy or childbirth. About 146,000 die from hemorrhage, 44,000 from obstructed labor, 74,000 from eclampsia (which causes convulsions and brain and kidney damage), and 87,000 from sepsis. About 20 million abortions are performed in unsafe conditions each year, resulting in the deaths of an additional 76,000 women and girls. Another 15 million women annually incur pregnancy-related or birth-related injuries, infections, or disabilities that often go untreated. As a result, about 300 million women—more than a quarter of the adult female population in developing countries—live with debilitating health problems. The most obvious and distressing is fistula, which allows leakage of urine or feces into the vagina, bypassing muscles that normally control the flow; as many as 1 million women suffer from fistula. Several million women face increased risk during childbirth each year because of the traditional practice of female genital mutilation, experienced by more than 130 million women, nearly three-quarters of whom live in Nigeria, Egypt, Ethiopia, Sudan and Kenya.[1,76]

HIV AND AIDS

During 1995, an estimated 2.7 million adults and 500,000 children were infected with HIV. By mid-1996, an estimated 27.9 million people had been infected with HIV.[3] Among those infected, more than 1 in 4 had developed AIDS; among those with AIDS, about 3 in 4 had died. In mid-1996, an estimated 21.8 million adults and children were living with HIV, 94% of whom lived in developing countries. Of the adults, 58% were men and 42% women.

Global AIDS Policy Coalition (GAPC) estimates indicate that 1993 per-capita spending on HIV prevention ranged from $0.07 to $0.44 in poor countries in sub-Saharan Africa, from $0.01 to $0.13 in poor countries in Asia, from $0.02 to $0.08 in all countries in Latin America, and from $0.25 to $2.46 in rich countries in North America and Western Europe.[49]

GAPC predicts 63 million adults will have been infected with HIV by January 1, 2001. By that time, Asia is projected to account for 52% of the cumulative number of HIV infections; sub-Saharan Africa, 38%; Latin America, 3%; North America, 2%; Western Europe, 2%; and the Caribbean, 1%. Overall, by 2001, more than 90% of all HIV infections will have occurred in developing countries.

The impact of AIDS on mortality rates and population growth could be dramatic and devastating in certain areas of the world. In several sub-Saharan African countries, AIDS has already become the leading cause of adult mortality, doubling or tripling death rates that were already eight times those in developed countries. By the year 2000, life expectancy at birth is expected to be at least 15 years lower than it would have been had HIV not appeared in Burundi, Kenya, Malawi, Rwanda, Tanzania, Uganda, Zambia, and Zimbabwe. The death rate among children from birth to age 4 will be substantially higher than it would have been in the absence of HIV in many countries, particularly in Zambia and Zimbabwe where it will be more than twice as high. In several Sub-Saharan countries, population growth rates will be at least 1 percentage point lower in the year 2000 because of HIV.[24] The prognosis is just as bleak for several countries in Asia, particularly India, Indonesia, Myanmar, and Vietnam.

DETERMINANTS OF MIGRATION

Compared with fertility and mortality, migration has received relatively less academic attention. It is also the process that is least linked to biology and most linked to economic, social, and political conditions. When assessing the determinants of migration, investigators have traditionally emphasized "push" and "pull" factors. Push factors include extraordinary events such as wars, floods, famines, political or religious persecution, and more ordinary conditions associated with depressed economic conditions: high unemployment, low wages, and little hope. Pull factors are those that attract people to a location. They are often those associated with economic opportunity: good jobs, high wages, and good public services such as education. They may also include an attractive environment, religious freedom, and proximity to family or large ethnic groups. These factors help to explain why people in the United States have been moving from the north and east to the south and west, from the frostbelt to the sunbelt. These factors also help explain rural-to-urban migration in developing and developed countries. Urban wages are typically higher, and public services are better.

The rapid growth of cities in developing countries is a matter of great concern to policymakers. However, careful examination of available data leads to several conclusions that do not support popular perceptions.[64]

First, the rate of out-migration from rural to urban areas is higher in developed than in developing countries. Second, rates of urbanization in currently developing countries are not especially high if compared with currently developed countries when they were in a similar stage of development. Third, the primary determinant of the growth of urban areas in developing countries is the rate of natural increase, which accounts for about three-fifths of the growth while net in-migration explains the remaining two-fifths. However, the rate of growth of the absolute size of the urban population, as opposed to the rate of growth of the proportion urban in the total population, is very high by historical standards—precisely because the rate of natural increase is so high. This observation suggests policies that slow the rate of natural increase, such as provision of family planning services, can have the added benefit of reducing urban growth.

U.S. IMMIGRATION POLICY[†]

The United States has one of the most generous immigration policies in the world. Prior to World War I, it took in almost all the immigrants who could make it to U.S. shores, and it still accepts about one-half of the world's immigrants each year.[51] U.S immigration policy with respect to *legal* immigration is based on three principles: family reunification, building a skilled labor force, and accepting a "fair" share of the world's refugees. The 1990 Immigration Act (IMMACT) created an annual flexible cap on immigration of 700,000 in fiscal years (FY) 1992–94, and 675,000 thereafter (not including refugees, asylees, and some other smaller categories). The annual cap can exceed 675,000 in any year to the extent family-sponsored and employment-based preference visas go unused in the previous year.[41] In addition, a pre-determined number of refugees (arrived at through negotiations between Congress and the President) is admitted annually.[47]

The number of legal immigrants admitted to the United States totaled 720,461 in FY95.[41] Of these visas, about 593,000 were subject to the overall numerical ceiling, and included 460,000 family-sponsored immigrants (divided between 238,000 family-sponsored preference migrants and 222,000 immediate relatives of U.S. citizens), 85,000 employment-based immigrants, 47,000 diversity-program migrants, and fewer than 300 dependents of formerly legalized aliens. Among the 127,000 additional legal immigrants who were not subject to the numerical cap, the largest groups consisted of refugees (107,000) and asylees (8,000).

[†]This section was prepared by Thomas J. Espenshade, Professor of Sociology and Faculty Associate, Office of Population Research, Princeton University.

Legal immigration in FY95 was 20% lower than in FY93, the largest 2-year decline in legal immigration since the early 1930s.[42‡] The number of legal immigrants may decline further as a result of policy changes legislated in the 1996 Welfare Reform Act to restrict legal immigrants' access to public benefits to which they had previously been entitled.[29]

Another principle of U.S. immigration policy is to control *illegal* or undocumented migration. In 1986, Congress passed the Immigration Reform and Control Act (IRCA). IRCA stepped up enforcement along the Mexico-U.S. border by increasing the number of Border Patrol agents and raising spending on such items as stronger fences, all-terrain vehicles, and infrared sensors. It also instituted a policy of "employer sanctions" whereby it became illegal for the first time for U.S. employers knowingly to hire undocumented migrants; previously, it had been illegal for an undocumented migrant to work in the United States but, by the terms of the "Texas proviso," not illegal for employers to hire them. Finally, IRCA contained a generous amnesty program for undocumented migrants already in the United States.**

By the end of FY95, a total of 2,680,000 aliens had been admitted for permanent U.S. residence under the IRCA provisions.[41] In addition, 142,000 dependents of legalized aliens had been granted legal permanent residence under IMMACT.[42] IRCA did not, however, achieve its major objective of slowing the flow of undocumented immigrants. In the first year IRCA reduced the gross flow of illegal immigrants entering the United States from Mexico by an estimated 44% (2.0 million versus 3.5 million). However, IRCA's effect was only two-thirds as large in the second year after enactment.[8,27] There is now general agreement that the longer-run effects of IRCA have been negligible.[7]

The most recent estimates suggest about 3.4 million undocumented migrants were U.S. residents in October 1992.[82] California led all states with 1.44 million, or 43% of the total, followed by New York with 450,000. Mexico was the leading sending country, accounting for 1.32 million undocumented migrants, or 39% of the total. El Salvador was second on the list with 327,000 illegal immigrants. Roughly half of all current undocumented migrants entered the country illegally; the remaining fraction entered on temporary nonimmigrant visas but stayed after their visas expired or violated the terms of their visas.[31]

---

‡This comparison excludes immigrants who were beneficiaries of the one-time legalization program under IRCA.

**Persons who could demonstrate they had lived continuously in the United States in illegal status since January 1, 1982 and illegal migrant farmworkers who could show they had performed at least 90 days of work in perishable crop agriculture in the 12-month period ending May 1, 1986 were entitled to apply for legal temporary residence which could later be converted to legal permanent U.S. residence.[9]

In September 1996, President Clinton signed the Illegal Immigration Reform and Immigrant Responsibility Act, whose primary purpose is to prevent the entry and employment of illegal immigrants. It doubles the number of Border Control agents, increases funding for the Immigration and Naturalization Service (INS), establishes pilot programs for employment-eligibility verification, sets federal standards for state personal-identification documents, reiterates the delegation of discretionary authority to the states to distinguish between legal immigrants, citizens, and refugees, and restricts the right of aliens to challenge INS action with class-action lawsuits or with judicial challenges of a deportation order or denial of legal resident status.[38] For family reunification, sponsors are required to have an income of at least 125% of the federal poverty level, whereas previously there were no income restrictions for sponsors. The act is also significant for what it does not contain: further restrictions on the eligibility of legal immigrants for social services, limitations on the number of legal immigrants, asylees, or refugees, the Gallegly amendment that would have denied public education to illegal immigrant children, and automatic deportation of public charges.

It is too soon to tell how effective these latest reforms will be. They do not embody dramatic changes. On the other hand, measures viewed as being extremely harsh (for example, building a fortified wall along the Mexico-U.S. border all the way from Texas to California) do not have widespread support, even when they might ultimately be more effective.[28]

POPULATION GROWTH AND AGE STRUCTURE

The age structure of a population is completely determined by its history of fertility, mortality, and migration. In Figure 30-1, we see two examples of age pyramids, one for the United States and one for Mexico. We notice immediately that the profile for the United States is more nearly vertical (or steeper). Although one might think the difference is due to mortality, it is, in fact, due almost entirely to fertility. This fact can be demonstrated by examining populations with different levels of fertility and mortality. If fertility and mortality remain constant for a long time, then the age distribution of the population will also become constant. The population itself may grow, shrink, or remain the same size, but the proportion of the population in each age group will remain the same. Such a population is known as a stable population; if its growth rate is zero, it is called stationary. The age distributions of the six stable populations resulting from combinations of three levels of fertility (total fertility rates of 2, 5, and 8 lifetime births per typical woman) and two levels of mortality (life expectations of 35

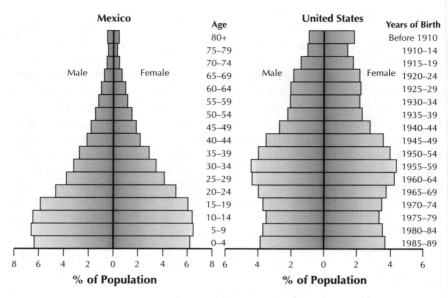

Mexico | Age | United States | Years of Birth
Male   Female | 80+ | Male   Female | Before 1910
 | 75–79 | | 1910–14
 | 70–74 | | 1915–19
 | 65–69 | | 1920–24
 | 60–64 | | 1925–29
 | 55–59 | | 1930–34
 | 50–54 | | 1935–39
 | 45–49 | | 1940–44
 | 40–44 | | 1945–49
 | 35–39 | | 1950–54
 | 30–34 | | 1955–59
 | 25–29 | | 1960–64
 | 20–24 | | 1965–69
 | 15–19 | | 1970–74
 | 10–14 | | 1975–79
 | 5–9 | | 1980–84
 | 0–4 | | 1985–89

8 6 4 2 0 2 4 6 8   6 4 2 0 2 4 6

% of Population   % of Population

Sources: INEGI (1992); United States Bureau of the Census (1992).

Figure 30-1 Age pyramids for the United States and Mexico, 1990

and 70) are shown in Figure 30-2. Mortality plays the smaller role in determining the shape of the age profile; whether women have 2 or 8 children has a far greater impact on the age profile than whether they live 35 or 70 years.

POPULATION MOMENTUM

The current age profile of a population contains momentum, just as a moving locomotive does. This momentum occurs because the number of persons already born implies much about future growth. The easiest way to understand the power of momentum is to ask how large the population would ultimately be if (1) the number of births in future years remains the same as the number this year, and (2) mortality remains constant. As is demonstrated in the last section of this chapter, a population with the same number of births each year and constant mortality will ultimately have the same age distribution as the underlying life table. Life expectancy (E) is the ratio of total person-years lived to the number of births (B). Then the total person-years lived by the population, or equivalently the total size of the stationary population, is E times B. Consider again the case of the United States and Mexico (Figure 30-1). The number of births in 1997 in Mexico was 2.6 million and the expectation of life was

72 years.[39] Hence the ultimate size of the stationary population would be 187 million or twice as large as the 1997 population. In the United States, the number of births was about 4.0 million and the life expectancy about 76 years.[39] Hence, the ultimate size would be 304 million, about 14% larger than the 1997 population. We see the Mexican population currently contains more momentum than does the U.S. population. The larger momentum results from its past high fertility, which has produced an age distribution with a very wide base (Figures 30-1 and 30-2).

These calculations are "quick and dirty" estimates. They give a precise answer to the question of what the size of the population would be if the number of births and mortality rates remained constant. But it is very unlikely the number of births in Mexico will remain the same. The age-specific fertility rates would have to fall over time for the number of births to remain constant because the number of women of childbearing age will continue to increase for many years. Therefore, the size of the Mexican population is very likely to surpass 187 million in the future. In the United States, on the other hand, the number of births would

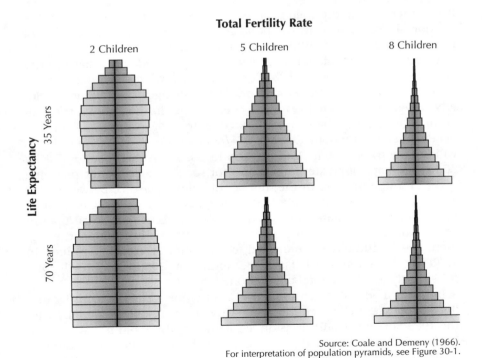

Source: Coale and Demeny (1966).
For interpretation of population pyramids, see Figure 30-1.

Figure 30-2 Age pyramids for six stable populations

decrease over time because the number of women currently of childbearing age is atypically large (the children of the baby boom). In fact, if the current age-specific mortality and fertility rates continued into the future, the size of the U.S. population (ignoring migration) would shrink to zero in the distant future since the typical woman now bears less than 1 daughter. (See the section on Gross and Net Reproduction Rates at the end of this chapter.)

SOCIETAL CONSEQUENCES OF IRREGULAR AGE DISTRIBUTIONS

Age distributions convey more than information about population momentum. Often they imply real problems for society. In the United States, the size of the population age 65 and over rose only from 17% of the size of the working age (18-64) population in 1960 to 20% in 1990. If current trends continue, however, the fraction will rise to 28% by the year 2020 and to 36% by the year 2050.[25,70] Those projections also indicate the size of the population age 85 and over will rise only from 2% of the size of the working age population in 1990 to 3% in 2020; however, it will increase rapidly thereafter, reaching 8% in 2050. This rise in the fraction of old persons in the population is mostly the consequence of the rapid decline in fertility levels, from "baby boom" to "baby bust." The increase in population over age 65 has strained the social security system, which relies on contributions of current workers to finance benefits for the current retired population. The challenge of caring for the elderly is even more severe in Japan, where changes in the age structure will occur more rapidly than in the United States. For example, the elderly dependency ratio (population age 65+/population age 15 to 64) in Japan will double from 20% in 1995 to 42% in 2020 and then rise to 57% by 2050.[78] Perhaps of greater importance for social and economic planning is the absolute increase in the number of elderly persons. Between 1990 and 2025, the size of the population age 65 and over is expected to double in the United States and Japan, triple in China, and quadruple in South Korea, Singapore, and Malaysia.[50] In the United States, the segment age 85 and older is projected to grow rapidly, from 3.0 million in 1990 to 6.5 million in 2020 and 18.2 million in 2050 when it will comprise nearly 5% of the total population.[25]

In the United States, fertility fell as a consequence of decisions by millions of couples to limit childbearing. Government policy, especially after the 1973 Supreme Court decision legalizing abortion, did not attempt to limit individual control of reproductive behavior. Two more examples reveal the potential power of government action; they also highlight the value of demographic analysis before action is taken. In 1966 the government of Romania introduced pronatalist policies, including banning virtually all abortions and discontinuing importation of oral contraceptives and intrauterine devices (IUDs). The result was as instantaneous as it was stunning.[71,72] Within 8 months the monthly birth rate doubled; within 11 months it tripled. What were the economic and social effects? Inadequate hospital care for the babies and their mothers caused infant and maternal mortality to rise sharply. As a consequence of unsafe illegal abortion, maternal mortality increased to a level 10 times that in any other European country. In the 23 years the policy was enforced, more than 10,000 women died from unsafe abortions. Many women who did not resort to unsafe abortion bore unwanted children whom they placed in institutions. Such large-scale warehousing of children overwhelmed these institutions and severely degraded the quality of care. The educational system had to digest a giant bulge of students. Other problems, such as employment and housing, also arose as the large cohorts aged. The government took action because it was worried about low levels of fertility (fertility rates in 1965 implied the typical woman who lived to age 50 would bear only 1.9 children). Its action certainly had the result of increasing fertility, but obviously the government had not thought clearly about the consequences. The ban on abortion was reversed immediately after the Ceaucescu regime was overthrown in December 1989.

Another example illustrates the problems caused by government attempts to lower fertility quickly. From 1979 through 1983, the government of China vigorously promoted the policy of 1 child per family.[††] What would be the consequences if the 1-child policy were strictly adopted? By the year 2035, about a quarter of the population would be age 65 and over, versus only about 5% today.[20] Only a tiny minority of Chinese are eligible for the state system of social security for the aged, so the state-financed system of old-age security would not be in danger of collapsing. Nevertheless, the traditional family structure would change radically in ways that would jeopardize the family's ability to care for the elderly and reduce its potential as a production unit; there would be no brothers, sisters, aunts, or uncles. The 1-child policy may have already had the unintended side-effect of inducing female infanticide or female-specific abortion due to a cultural preference for sons.[4,5,21,87] Results of demographic analysis suggest the Chinese could meet their aggregate

---

[††]Since that time, the government has pursued a more flexible policy by allowing certain categories of couples to have 2 (but never 3) children. Furthermore, clear repudiation from the central government appears to have throttled the excessive zeal with which subordinate officials implemented the policy (mandatory insertion of IUDs for women with 1 child, abortion for unauthorized pregnancies, and sterilization for couples with 2 or more children[4]).[37]

population targets by replacing the 1-child policy with a 2-child policy having a minimum age at first birth of 27 and a minimum birthspacing interval of 4 years.[13] While the 2-child policy would not avoid the adverse age distribution effect, it would offer couples greater choice (they could have 1 child any time or 2 children subject to the rules) and reduce the adverse effects on the family.

DEMOGRAPHIC TRANSITION

The populations of Western Europe tended historically to undergo first a fall in mortality and only later a fall in fertility. This observation led to a formal description of the process known as the demographic transition, which is shown in Figure 30-3. The paradigm is one of high birth

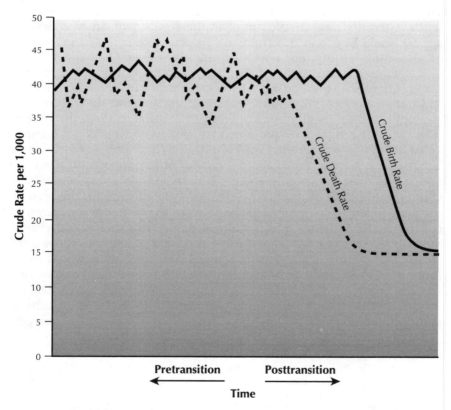

Figure 30-3 The demographic transition

and death rates in the pretransition phase. Birth and death rates were not necessarily equal in every year. Fertility was the more stable. In good years, mortality was low, but the population was subject to chronic food shortage resulting from vagaries of the weather and limited storage and transport capacities, as well as periodic epidemics. Generally, mortality fluctuated widely, and birth and death rates, on the average, balanced.

At the time of the industrial revolution, mortality fell because of improvements in living conditions such as better housing and food distribution networks and public health measures such as the provision of clean water. Lowering fertility, however, requires *individuals* to make conscious decisions about postponing marriage or controlling fertility within marriage. These personal decisions were made only after standards of living had improved considerably. Several mechanisms have been suggested. As couples realized mortality had fallen, they would need to have fewer births in order to attain the same number of surviving children. As the status of women changed, primarily through mass education, high fertility became less desirable to them.[16,17] Moreover, the economic value of children decreased: in traditional societies wealth flows upward, from the young to the old; in modern societies, wealth flows from the old to the young, as parents invest heavily in their children's education.

All developed countries have experienced a demographic transition. For some, however, the lag between the fall in mortality and the fall in fertility was short and for others, long. The strict interpretation of the classical paradigm has been shown to be incorrect. When the countries of Europe are examined on a provincial basis, the results indicate fertility sometimes fell before mortality declined and before education became general.[23] Hence, the demographic transition is a more complicated process than the simple paradigm suggests. Exhaustive analysis of the population history of England reveals it did not correspond to the prototypical high-pressure regime of high birth and death rates before the transition. Instead, mortality was, on average, moderate and fertility was kept moderate, not through control of marital fertility, but through controls on age at marriage.[86] Other pretransition societies have also been found to have moderate levels of marital fertility.[6,23]

Demographic transition theory is especially relevant if, in addition to telling us why fertility fell historically, it yields predictions about what would cause fertility to fall in currently developing countries. Appeal to the classical statement of the theory would suggest development is the best contraceptive. Indeed, this was the position taken by many at the World Population Conference in Bucharest in 1974, a conference split between those who thought family planning programs were the key to reducing fertility and hence population growth, and those who felt policy makers should concentrate on development and population would take care of itself.[26][‡‡]

A careful reading of the evidence from the historical experience of current developed countries and the recent experience of developing countries suggests that (1) declines in marital fertility occurred in a wide variety of social and economic settings, (2) deliberate attempts to limit family size were not only largely absent but also probably unknown prior to the onset of the decline in fertility, even though a substantial fraction of births may have been unwanted, (3) the decline of marital fertility and the adoption of family limitation were essentially irreversible processes once under way, (4) cultural setting had an important and independent effect on the onset and spread of fertility decline, and (5) social interaction, through which people exchange and evaluate information and ideas and exert and receive social influence, plays a central role in fertility decline.[14,45] These considerations lead one to adopt a position midway between the two extremes adopted at Bucharest. Although the empirical record confirms a loose relationship between socioeconomic modernization and fertility decline, it also reveals important innovation-diffusion and social interaction aspects of the practice of fertility control. Emphasizing the right of couples to determine the number of children they want to have and providing them with information and technical assistance to give meaning to this right, particularly when coupled with advances in the status of women and the educational power of mass media, can sharply reduce fertility.[66] Access to the broadest array of fertility-regulating technologies consistent with the principle of informed consent is essential.[62]

Considerable survey evidence suggests that large fractions of women in developing countries desire increased spacing between children or termination of childbearing.[83,84] Consequently, as three recent comprehensive reviews of and two international conferences on population and development have concluded, voluntary family planning could play an important role in aiding the development process.[35,53,58,75,85] While

---

‡‡The United States was the leader of the family planning approach in Bucharest but reversed its position at the 1984 International Conference on Population held in Mexico City due to intense political pressure from social conservatives, particularly anti-abortion groups. The U.S. position that rapid population growth does not hinder and even fosters economic development was supported only by the Vatican. Ironically, those developing countries that had been the most vocal critics of the U.S. position in Bucharest also switched sides in Mexico City. The 1994 International Conference on Population and Development held in Cairo resulted in a shift of focus away from demographic targets and toward reproductive health and the empowerment of women and sustainable development.[52]

slower population growth would benefit development in most developing countries, it would not automatically make poor countries rich and is no substitute for the elimination of market imperfections.

China illustrates an alternative to voluntary family planning that is clearly effective in reducing fertility and the rate of population growth. However, it is unlikely many other governments would have the authority to implement such compulsory policies, even if they had the desire. Human-rights issues aside, experience with mass sterilization campaigns in India suggests coercive or compulsory attempts to bring down the birth rate are more likely to bring down the government instead.

Nevertheless, it is doubtful further investments in voluntary family planning programs alone would halt rapid population growth. More than 800 million people are projected to be added to the population of developing countries in the 1990s and in each of the following two decades. The population of the developing world is estimated to grow from 4.1 billion in 1990 to 10.2 billion in 2100. Of this increase of 5.7 billion, 1.9 billion can be attributed to unwanted fertility, 1.0 billion to high desired family size and 2.8 billion to population momentum. Therefore, if such growth is to be avoided, further policy options to reduce demand for large families and to limit population momentum are needed. These include enhancing the status of women, raising the average age at childbearing by increasing age at marriage, reducing adolescent childbearing, and increasing intervals between births.[12]

MEASURING FERTILITY, MORTALITY AND POPULATION GROWTH

The population of a state, county, city, or country can change in only three ways: through births, deaths, or migration. New persons can be added by birth or in-migration; persons can exit through death or out-migration. Total world population can change in only two ways: births and deaths.

In 1997, an estimated 2.4 million people died in the United States and only 453 thousand in Uganda.[39] Does the fact that there were more than five times as many deaths in the United States as in Uganda indicate it is healthier to live in Uganda? No; there were 267.7 million people in the United States (and therefore at risk of dying) but only 20.6 million people in Uganda. If one divides the number of deaths by the population at risk, one obtains the *crude death rate* (CDR). These rates were 9 per 1,000 population (.009) in the United States and 22 per 1,000 (.022) in Uganda.

This methodological principle of controlling for population size is often overlooked. For example, in 1982 the Centers for Disease Control issued a report calling attention to its estimate that for the first time in the United States contraceptive-related deaths outnumbered pregnancy-related deaths.[67] This finding was widely (mis)interpreted by the press to mean that it is just as dangerous to prevent pregnancy as it is to become pregnant. But such reasoning ignores the fact that there are two different populations at risk in this comparison. Only women who become pregnant can die of pregnancy-related causes. A much larger number of women is at risk of death from contraception-related causes. Most of the contraceptive-related deaths were estimated to occur among women using the pill; even so, more than twice as many women used the pill as became pregnant. Hence the risk of death from prevention of pregnancy is far lower than the risk of death from pregnancy.

CRUDE RATES

Rates are defined by demographers to be the number of events divided by the average number of persons exposed to the risk of the event in a year. The denominator of a rate can also be described as the number of *person-years* lived; the concept of person-years is a natural generalization of man-hours or person-hours. Using a rate, such as the CDR, avoids the severe problems in interpretation, as illustrated above, caused by examination of the numerator alone (e.g., deaths), without reference to the population at risk (the denominator). Another example of a rate is the *crude birth rate* (CBR), the number of births in a year divided by the total mid-year population. The difference between the crude birth rate and the crude death rate is known as the *crude rate of natural increase* (CRNI). If migration is negligible, the CRNI is also the *crude growth rate* (CGR), usually referred to more simply as the growth rate; otherwise, the CGR is the sum of the crude birth rate and the crude rate of in-migration minus the sum of the crude death rate and the crude rate of out-migration.

The population of the world in mid-1997 is estimated to have been 5.840 billion. It is currently growing at a rate of 1.47% per year.[39] In 1997 about 86 million people—a number comparable to the total population of Germany, the twelfth largest country in the world—were added; this growth results in the addition of 236 thousand people every day, or nearly 10 thousand people every hour. Should this growth of 1.47% continue, in 50 years time the population would be 12 billion, and in 100 years would be 25 billion. Of course, such growth could not continue indefinitely. Indeed, the growth rate has fallen after having reached a peak of 2.04% per year in the period 1965 to 1970.[78]

DOUBLING TIME

The growth rate is a simple measure of the rapidity of population growth. It can be used to determine the length of time it would take a population to double, known as the *doubling time.* If a population is growing at a rate of r% per year, then it will double in about T=69.3/r years.*** (See Figure 30-4.)

The concept of geometric growth or doubling (1, 2, 4, 8, 16 . . .) originally led Malthus to the dismal conclusion that population would soon outstrip the food supply.[48] He reached this conclusion by arguing that if population growth continued unchecked, it would increase in a geometric sequence (1, 2, 4, 8, 16, 32, 64, 128 . . .), while food supply could grow only in an arithmetic sequence (1, 2, 3, 4, 5, 6, 7, 8 . . .). Under such conditions the ratio of food to population would diminish rapidly. Fortunately, as we all know, Malthus' prediction has thus far been incorrect. He did not foresee improvements in agricultural technology and the widespread acceptance of contraception in many societies.

Nevertheless, geometric growth is still staggering. Many students who are first introduced to the concept are surprised to learn the world population growth rate is 1.47%. After all, this number is small compared with inflation rates in excess of 10% and interest rates of 15% or more common in many countries. Still, at the current growth rate, the population of the world would double in 47 years and quadruple in 95 years. To see just how great the current growth rate is, let us compare it with the population growth rate in the past. Imagine Adam and Eve lived about 100,000 years ago. What average growth rate would result in a population of 2 growing to a population of 5.840 billion in 100,000 years? The answer is a very small number, only .0218%. Another way of looking at this issue is to determine what the population of the earth would be if it had grown at 1.47% for 100,000 years. The answer is ridiculously large: about the number 167 followed by 633 zeroes! Finally, we might work backwards from the present by asking when Adam and Eve would have lived if the population growth rate had remained constant at 1.47% ever since. A population of 2 would grow to 5.840 billion in 1,491 years; hence Adam and Eve would have lived in the Garden of Eden in the year 506 A.D., in reality just 64 years before Mohammed was born in Mecca. We see from these three calculations that the current growth rate is very large by historical standards.

PROBLEMS WITH CRUDE RATES

All the rates discussed above are called crude rates because they make no allowance for the age distribution of the population. A simple example

---

***This formula is correct for all values of r if r is the continuously compounded (exponential) rate of growth. If r is derived from the formula $r = \{P(2)/P(1) - 1.0\} \times 100$ (i.e., the population this year is r% bigger than the population last year), then the doubling time formula is a very good approximation for values of r up to 10%. The exact formula in this case, used to derive the figures in the text, is $T = \ln(2)/\ln(1 + r/100)$, where ln is the natural logarithm.

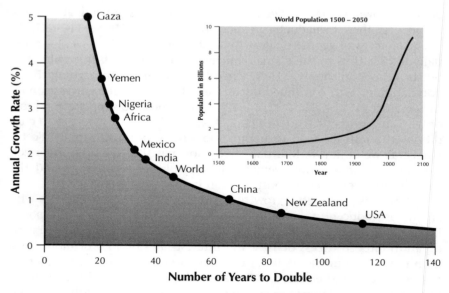

Sources: Haub and Cornelius (1997); United Nations (1995b, 1996b).

Figure 30-4 Doubling time and world population growth curve

will demonstrate they are indeed crude and more refined measurement is needed. In 1980, the CDR in Mexico was 6.2 per 1,000 population, while in the United States it was 8.8.[69] One might be tempted to conclude the United States provided a less healthy environment. In fact, however, the death rates in every age group (0 to 14, 15 to 44, 45 to 64, and 65+) were higher in Mexico. How could this anomaly arise? The answer is quite simple. The crude death rate in the United States was higher because its population was older (a much smaller fraction age 0 to 14 and a much larger fraction over age 45) than Mexico's. If the United States' age-specific death rates had prevailed in Mexico, the CDR in Mexico would have been only 3.8 instead of 6.2. Similarly, if the Mexican death rates at all ages had prevailed in the United States, the CDR would have been 11.4 instead of 8.8.

Why does the age distribution of a population affect the CDR? It does so because death rates are not the same at every age. A typical example of death rates by age is shown in Figure 30-5. Examination reveals that age-specific death rates after childhood rise with age; the probability of dying at age 60 is much higher than the probability of dying at age 40, which in turn is higher than the probability of dying at age 20. This example helps us to understand why the current CDR in the United States is

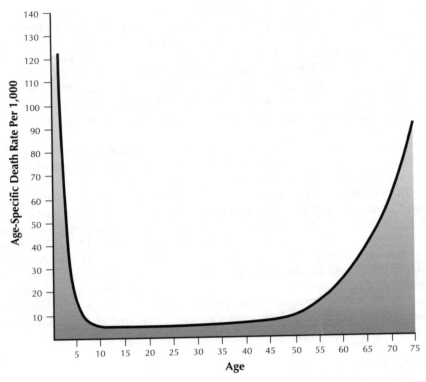

Source: Coale and Demeny (1966).

Figure 30-5 Age-specific mortality rates for a typical population with expectation of life of 50 years

higher than the CDR in Egypt, Indonesia, Iran, Libya, Malaysia, Nicaragua, Syria, Thailand, and Vietnam, although mortality, when properly measured, is higher in these countries. The crude birth rate is less problematic because childbearing, unlike death, is confined to the middle of the age distribution.

PEARL INDEX: A PROBLEMATIC CRUDE RATE

There is a parallel between problems with crude death rates and a crude technique of determining contraceptive effectiveness called the Pearl index, which is calculated as the number of unintended pregnancies divided by the number of women-years of exposure to risk of pregnancy. Each woman contributes to the denominator the number of years of exposure from the beginning of use of a method until the end of the study, until the occurrence of an unintended pregnancy, or until she stops using the method for other reasons. The problem arises because contraceptive failure rates decline with duration of use, just as in the previous mortality example death rates in adulthood rise with age. Failure rates fall with duration of use because those women most prone to fail become pregnant early after starting use, so over time the group of continuing users becomes increasingly composed of those least likely to fail. As a consequence, the longer the study runs, the more years of exposure each individual woman is allowed to contribute and the lower will be the failure rate.

Hence, two investigators using data from a survey designed to yield estimates of contraceptive failure in the United States could obtain Pearl-index pregnancy rates of 7.5 and 4.4 per 100 women-years of exposure for the condom.[74] How could the two investigators get such different rates? One (who got 4.4) allowed each woman to contribute a maximum of 5 years of exposure while the other (who got 7.5) allowed each woman to contribute only 1 year. Which investigator is incorrect? Neither. The two rates are simply not comparable. The lesson is that when comparing the effectiveness of different contraceptive methods, one must be careful to ensure that failure is measured in the same way. We suggest, in fact, that the common measure be the probabilities of failure within the first, second, third, fourth and fifth years of use, calculated by life table techniques, which are discussed below.

AGE-SPECIFIC RATES

Crude rates can often hide more than they reveal because of the influence of the age structure of the population. Therefore, demographers prefer to calculate age-specific rates. These can be one-year rates calculated for every single age, but they are more commonly 5-year rates computed for standard 5-year age groups. Age-specific death rates are computed by dividing the number of persons alive in the age group into the number of deaths to persons in that group; they may, of course, be computed for each sex separately. Age-specific birth rates are normally computed in a different way. Only women enter the denominator, since only women bear children. Births to women in each age group are divided by the number of women in that group. The problem with age-specific rates is that there are many numbers. It is inconvenient to compare fertility in the United States and Mexico by looking at 35 single-year age-specific fertility rates, or even seven 5-year rates. Hence, there is a need to combine the age-specific rates into a single fertility or mortality index free of any age-distribution effect.

TOTAL FERTILITY RATE

Suppose we simply add all the age-specific fertility rates together. If we do so in the United States, we get 2.0. What does this number mean? Recall that the fertility rate at age 20, for example, is the number of births to women age 20 divided by the number of women age 20. Thus, the age-specific fertility rate is the number of babies produced by the typical woman of that age. If we add the fertility rates at ages 20 and 21 together, we get the number of babies produced by the typical woman during the 2-year period from her 20th birthday to her 22nd birthday. Therefore, if we add all the age-specific fertility rates together, we get the number of births that the typical woman would have if she experienced the fertility rates prevailing at every age and lived through the end of the childbearing ages. Hence, at current rates, the typical woman would produce 2.0 children by age 50. This index is known as total fertility, or the *total fertility rate* (TFR).

GROSS AND NET REPRODUCTION RATES

If we count just female births (we sum the age-specific female-birth rates), the measure is known as the *gross reproduction rate* (GRR). Since there are about 105 male births for every 100 female births in all populations (except among blacks, whose sex ratio at birth is about 103 males per 100 females), the fraction of female births is about .488. Thus we have the simple relationship that the GRR = .488 × TFR. Hence, the GRR in the United States is now about .98. This number directly tells us women are not reproducing themselves; the typical female baby would by age 50 produce only 98% of a daughter. Thus, over the long run (ignoring migration), the population of the United States would shrink if these age-specific birth rates remained constant. Actually, to reach this conclusion, we must also account for the fact that each girl baby does not necessarily live through the childbearing years. If the probability of survival is also factored in, the fertility index is known as the *net reproduction rate* (NRR). It is the number of daughters that the average girl baby will subsequently produce during her lifetime. Because not all girl babies survive to age 50, the NRR is always less than the GRR; the difference increases as mortality becomes higher. If the NRR is greater than 1.0, each woman will more than replace herself so the population will in each succeeding generation grow (ignoring migration); and if the NRR is less than 1.0, it will decline. If the NRR equals 1.0, the population will ultimately neither shrink nor grow—it will become stationary, or constant.

Life Table and Expectation of Life

Since each person can die only once, it does not make sense to add the age-specific mortality rates. Instead, we use them to construct a *life table*. A life table can best be imagined as a table showing how many people are still alive at each birthday out of the total number born at a particular time. Suppose we observe 1,000 births in 1997. Then we simply record the number who have their first birthday in 1998, their second in 1999, and so forth. We can also record how many person-years were lived between birth and age 1, between age 1 and age 2, and so on. If we add up all the years lived and divide by the number who were born, we get the average number of years lived, or the expectation of life at birth. We could also find, for example, the expectation of life at age 40 by dividing the total years lived after age 40 by the number who survived to age 40. While this exercise is revealing, we usually do not want to wait the 100 or so years it would take to find the answer. It is possible, however, to take the current age-specific death rates and convert them into a life table. This life table would not, of course, represent the experience of an actual birth cohort. It tells us at what ages members of a cohort would die if current age-specific mortality rates persisted in the future. Life tables are not mere mathematical games; they affect our everyday lives, for they are used in setting insurance rates and in developing pension plans.

Life-table methodology is not restricted just to deaths. One can use the same techniques to measure contraceptive failure (where initiation of use of a method and accidental pregnancy, respectively, take the place of birth and death in the life table),[61,81] marital dissolution (marriage replacing birth and divorce or separation replacing death),[55] and other events of interest. In these other applications, the expectation of life is not always the most convenient measure; instead, one may be interested directly in the proportion failing within 6 or 12 or 24 months (e.g., contraceptive failure) or 5 years (e.g., marriage dissolution).

It is also very enlightening to realize a life table can be thought of as a stationary population. If mortality is constant, and if there is the same number of births every year, then (ignoring migration) the number of persons at each age will be the same year after year. Furthermore, the number of person-years lived in the life table between ages 6 and 7, for example, will be the same as the number of 6-year-olds in the population.

Suggested Reading

Cohen JE. How many people can the earth support? New York NY: WW Norton & Company, 1995.

Smith JP, Edmonston B (eds). The new Americans: economic, demographic, and fiscal effects of immigration. Washington DC: National Academy Press, 1997.

Tsui AO, Wasserheit J, Haaga JG (eds). Reproductive health in developing countries: expanding dimensions, building solutions. Washington DC: National Academy Press, 1997.

REFERENCES

1. Adamson P (ed). The progress of nations 1996. New York NY: UNICEF, 1996.
2. Adegbola O. New estimates of fertility and child mortality in Africa, south of the Sahara. Popul Stud 1977;31:467-486.
3. AIDS Control and Prevention (AIDSCAP) Project of Family Health International, François-Xavier Bagnoud Center for Health and Human Rights of the Harvard School of Public Health, UNAIDS. The status and trends of the global HIV/AIDS pandemic: final report. Arlington VA: AIDSCAP/FHI, 1996.
4. Aird JS. Coercion in family planning: causes, methods, and consequences. Congressional Record-Senate 1985:S7776-S7788.
5. Banister J. China's changing population. Stanford CA: Stanford University Press, 1987.
6. Barclay GW, Coale AJ, Stoto MA, Trussell TJ. A reassessment of the demography of traditional rural China. Popul Index 1976;42:606-635.
7. Bean FD, Edmonston B, Passel JS (eds). Undocumented migration to the United States: IRCA and the experience of the 1980s. Washington DC: The Urban Institute Press, 1990.
8. Bean FD, Espenshade TJ, White MJ, Dymowski RF. Post-IRCA changes in the volume and composition of undocumented migration to the United States: an assessment based on apprehensions data. In: Bean FD, Edmonston B, Passel JS (eds). Undocumented migration to the United States: IRCA and the experience of the 1980s. Washington DC: The Urban Institute Press, 1990:111-158.
9. Bean FD, Vernez G, Keely CB. Opening and closing the doors: Evaluating immigration reform and control. Washington DC: The Urban Institute Press, 1989.
10. Bongaarts J. A framework for analyzing the proximate determinants of fertility. Popul Dev Rev 1978;4:105-132.
11. Bongaarts J. Does malnutrition affect fecundity? A summary of evidence. Science 1980;208:564-569.
12. Bongaarts J. Population policy options in the developing world. Science 1994;263:771-776.
13. Bongaarts J, Greenhalgh S. An alternative to the one-child policy in China. Popul Dev Rev 1985;11:585-617.
14. Bongaarts J, Watkins SC. Social interactions and contemporary fertility transitions. Popul Dev Rev 1996;22:639-682.
15. Brunham RC, Cheang M, McMaster J, Garnett G, Anderson R. Chlamydia trachomatis, infertility and population growth in sub-Saharan Africa. Sex Transm Dis 1993;20:168-173.
16. Caldwell JC. A theory of fertility: from high plateau to destabilization. Popul Dev Rev 1978;4:553-577.

17. Caldwell JC. Mass education as a determinant of the timing of fertility decline. Popul Dev Rev 1980;6:225-255.

18. Campbell OMR, Gray RH. Characteristics and determinants of postpartum ovarian function in women in the United States. Am J Obstet Gynecol 1993;169:55-60.

19. Casterline JB, Singh S, Cleland J, Ashurst H. The proximate determinants of fertility. WFS Comparative Studies, Number 39. Voorburg, The Netherlands: International Statistical Institute, 1984.

20. Coale AJ. Population trends, population policy, and population studies in China. Popul Dev Rev 1981;7:85-97.

21. Coale AJ, Banister J. Five decades of missing females in China. Demography 1994;31:459-479.

22. Coale AJ, Demeny P. Regional model life tables and stable populations. Princeton NJ: Princeton University Press, 1966.

23. Coale AJ, Watkins SC. The decline of fertility in Europe: the revised proceedings of a conference on the Princeton European fertility project. Princeton NJ: Princeton University Press, 1986.

24. Cohen B, Trussell J. Preventing and mitigating AIDS in sub-Saharan Africa. Washington DC: National Academy Press, 1996.

25. Day JC. Population projections of the United States, by age, sex, race, and Hispanic origin: 1995 to 2050. Curr Popul Rep, Series P25-1130. Washington DC: Government Printing Office, 1996.

26. Demeny P. Bucharest, Mexico City, and beyond. Popul Dev Rev 1985;11:99-106.

27. Espenshade TJ. Undocumented migration to the United States: evidence from a repeated trials model. In: Bean FD, Edmonston B, Passel JS (eds). Undocumented migration to the United States: IRCA and the experience of the 1980s. Washington DC: The Urban Institute Press, 1990:159-181.

28. Espenshade TJ, Belanger M. U.S. public perceptions and reactions to Mexican migration. In: Bean FD, de la Garza R, Roberts BR, Weintraub S (eds). At the crossroads: Mexican migration and U.S. policy. Boulder CO: Rowman and Littlefield Publishers, 1997:227-261.

29. Espenshade TJ, Huber GA. Retrenchment in the U.S. welfare system and its effects on immigrants and refugees. Paper presented at the Conference on Immigration and the Welfare State: Germany and the United States in Comparison, Freie Universität Berlin, Germany, December 12-14, 1996.

30. Federal Office of Statistics. Nigeria Demographic and Health Survey 1990. Columbia MD: Macro International Inc, 1992.

31. Fix M, Passel JS. Immigration and immigrants: setting the record straight. Washington DC: The Urban Institute, 1994.

32. Ford K, Huffman SL, Chowdhury AKMA, Becker S, Allen H, Menken J. Birth-interval dynamics in rural Bangladesh and maternal weight. Demography 1989;26:425-437.

33. Frank O. Infertility in sub-Saharan Africa: estimates and implications. Popul Dev Rev 1983;9:137-144.

34. Frisch RE. Demographic implications of the biological determinants of female fecundity. Soc Biol 1975;22:17-22.

35. Graham-Smith F (ed). Population—the complex reality: a report of the Population Summit of the world's scientific academies. Golden CO: North American Press, 1994.

36. Gray RH. Biological factors other than nutrition and lactation which may influence natural fertility: a review. In: Leridon H, Menken J (eds). Natural fertility: patterns and determinants of natural fertility: proceedings of a seminar on natural fertility. Liege, Belgium: Ordina Editions, 1979:217-251.

37. Greenhalgh S. Shifts in China's population policy, 1984-86: views from the central, provincial, and local levels. Popul Dev Rev 1986;12:491-515.

38. Greenhouse L. How Congress curtailed the courts' jurisdiction. The New York Times, October 27, 1996:D5.

39. Haub C, Cornelius D. 1997 World population data sheet. Washington DC: Population Reference Bureau, 1997.

40. Henry A, Piotrow PT. Age at marriage and fertility. Popul Rep 1979;7, Series M(4).

41. Immigration and Naturalization Service. Immigration to the United States in Fiscal Year 1995. Washington DC: U.S. Department of Justice, 1996.

42. Immigration and Naturalization Service. Statistical yearbook of the Immigration and Naturalization Service, 1994. Washington DC: Government Printing Office, 1996.

43. INEGI (Instituto Nacional de Estadistica Geografia e Informatica. Estados unidos Mexicanos: perfil sociodemografico: XI Censo General de Poblacion y Vivienda, 1990. Aguascalientes, Mexico: INEGI, 1992.

44. Jolly CL, Gribble JN. The proximate determinants of fertility. In: Foote KA, Hill KH, Martin LG (eds). Demographic change in sub-Saharan Africa. Washington DC: National Academy Press, 1983:68-116.

45. Knodel J, van de Walle E. Lessons from the past: policy implications of historical fertility studies. Popul Dev Rev 1979;5:217-245.

46. Lesthaeghe R. Nuptiality and population growth. Popul Stud 1971;25: 415-432.

47. Levine DB, Hill K, Warren R (eds). Immigration statistics: a story of neglect. Washington DC: National Academy Press, 1985.

48. Malthus TR. An essay on the principle of population, as it affects the future improvement of society. London, England: J Johnson, 1798.

49. Mann JM, Tarantola DJM (eds). AIDS in the World II. New York NY: Oxford University Press, 1996.

50. Martin LG. Population aging policies in East Asia and the United States. Science 1991;251:527-531.

51. Martin P, Midgley E. Immigration to the United States: journey to an uncertain destination. Popul Bull 1994;49(2).

52. McIntosh CA, Finkle JL. The Cairo conference on population and development: a new paradigm? Popul Dev Rev 1995;21:223-260.

53. Menken, J (ed). World population and U.S. policy: the choices ahead. New York: WW Norton, 1986.

54. Menken J, Bongaarts J. Reproductive models in the study of nutrition-fertility interrelationships. In: Mosley WH (ed). Nutrition and human reproduction. New York: Plenum Press, 1978:261-311.

55. Menken J, Trussell J, Stempel D, Babakol O. Proportional hazards life table models: an illustrative analysis of socio-demographic influences on marriage dissolution in the United States. Demography 1981;18:181-200.

56. Menken J, Trussell J, Watkins S. The nutrition fertility link: an evaluation of the evidence. J Interdisciplinary History 1981;11:425-441.

57. National Research Council. Contraception and reproduction: health consequences for women and children in the developing world. Washington DC:
National Academy Press, 1989.

58. National Research Council. Population growth and economic development:
policy questions. Washington DC: National Academy Press, 1986.

59. National Statistics Office. Republic of the Philippines National Demographic
Survey 1993. Calverton MD: Macro International Inc, 1994.

60. Noble J, Cover J, Yanagishita M. The world's youth 1996. Washington DC:
Population Reference Bureau, 1996.

61. Potter RG. Application of life table techniques to measurement of contraceptive effectiveness. Demography 1966;3:297-304.

62. Potts M. Sex and the birth rate: human biology, demographic change, and
access to fertility-regulation methods. Popul Dev Rev 1997;23:1-39.

63. Preston SH. Mortality patterns in national populations. New York: Academic
Press, 1976.

64. Preston SH. Urban growth in developing countries: a demographic reappraisal.
Popul Dev Rev 1979;5:195-215.

65. Preston SH, Keyfitz N, Schoen R. Causes of death: life tables for national populations. New York: Seminar Press, 1972.

66. Robey B, Rutstein SO, Morris L. The fertility decline in developing countries.
Sci Am 1993;269:30-37.

67. Sachs BP, Layde PM, Rubin GL, Rochat RW. Reproductive mortality in the
United States. JAMA 1982;247:2789-2792.

68. Sherris JD, Fox G. Infertility and sexually transmitted disease: a public health
challenge. Popul Rep 1983;11, Series L(4).

69. Smith DP. Formal Demography. New York NY: Plenum Press, 1992: Table 3.3.

70. Spencer G. Projections of the population of the United States, by age, sex,
and race: 1988 to 2080. Curr Popul Rep, Series P25-1018. Washington DC:
Government Printing Office, 1989.

71. Stephenson P, Wagner M, Badea M, Serbanescu F. Commentary: the public
health consequences of restricted induced abortion—lessons from Romania.
Am J Public Health 1992;82:1328-1331.

72. Teitelbaum MS. Fertility effects of the abolition of legal abortion in Romania.
Popul Stud 1972;26:405-417.

73. Trussell J. The impact of birthspacing on fertility. Int Fam Plann Perspect
1986;12:80-82.

74. Trussell J, Menken J. Life table analysis of contraceptive failure. In: Hermalin
AI, Entwisle B (eds). The role of surveys in the analysis of family planning
programs. Liege, Belgium: Ordina Editions, 1982:537-571.

75. United Nations. Population and development: programme of action adopted
at the International Conference on Population and Development, Cairo, 5-13
September 1994. New York: United Nations, 1995a.

76. United Nations. Reproductive rights and reproductive health: a concise
report. New York: United Nations, 1996a.

77. United Nations. World population prospects: the 1994 revision. New York:
United Nations, 1995b: Table 43.

78. United Nations. World population prospects: the 1996 revision. New York:
United Nations, 1996b: Tables A.1, A.2, A.33.

79. U.S. Bureau of the Census. United States population estimates, by age and sex, based on the 1990 census: 1990 and 1991. Suitland MD: U.S. Bureau of the Census, April 16, 1992.
80. VanLandingham M, Trussell J, Grummer-Strawn L. Contraceptive and health benefits of breastfeeding: a review of the recent evidence. Int Fam Plann Perspect 1991;17:131-136.
81. Vaughan B, Trussell J, Menken J, Jones EF. Contraceptive failure among married women in the United States, 1970-1973. Fam Plann Perspect 1977;9:251-258.
82. Warren R. Estimates of the undocumented immigrant population residing in the United States, by country of origin and state of residence: October 1992. Paper presented at the annual meetings of the Population Association of America, San Francisco CA, 1995.
83. Westoff CF, Bankole A. Unmet need 1990-1994. Comparative Studies No. 16. Calverton MD: Macro International Inc, June 1995.
84. Westoff CF, Ochoa LH. Unmet need and the demand for family planning. Comparative Studies No. 5. Columbia MD: Institute for Resource Development, July, 1991.
85. World Bank. World development report, 1984. New York NY: Oxford University Press, 1984.
86. Wrigley EA, Schofield RS. The population history of England 1541-1871. Cambridge MA: Harvard University Press, 1981.
87. Yi Z, Ping T, Baochang G, Yi X, Bohua L, Yongping L. Causes and implications of the recent increase in the reported sex ratio at birth in China. Popul Dev Rev 1993;19:283-302.

Contraceptive Efficacy

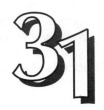

James Trussell, PhD

- Pregnancy rates during perfect use reflect how effective methods can be in preventing pregnancy when used consistently and correctly.
- Pregnancy rates during typical use reflect how effective methods are for the average person who does not always use methods correctly or consistently.

- Pregnancy rates during typical use of compliance-dependent methods generally vary widely among different groups using the same method, primarily due to differences in the propensity to use the method perfectly.
- Empirically based estimates of pregnancy rates during perfect use are sorely needed, particularly for spermicides.

A general explanation of the sources of evidence and the logic underlying the summary table on contraceptive efficacy (Table 9-2) is provided in Chapter 9 on Essentials of Contraception. This chapter more completely explains the derivation of the estimates in Table 9-2, reproduced as Table 31-1. The chapter also contains tables summarizing the efficacy literature for each method. These are arranged in the order in which they appear in summary Table 31-1. In these tables, all studies were conducted in the United States unless otherwise noted.

CHANCE

Our estimate of the percentage of women becoming pregnant among those relying on chance is based on populations in which the use of contraception is rare and on couples who report they stopped using contraceptives because they wanted to conceive. Based on this evidence, we conclude 85 of 100 sexually active couples would experience an accidental pregnancy in the first year if they used no contraception. Because this statement could be easily misinterpreted, further clarification is necessary. Available evidence in the United States suggests only about 40% of married couples who do not use contraception (but who still wish to avoid pregnancy) become pregnant within 1 year.[8] However, such couples are almost certainly selected for low fecundity or low frequency of intercourse. They do not use contraception because, in part, they are aware they are unlikely to conceive. The probability of pregnancy of 85%, therefore, is our best guess of the fraction of women now using reversible methods of contraception who would become pregnant within 1 year if they were to abandon their current method but not otherwise change their behavior. Couples who have unprotected intercourse for a year without achieving pregnancy are, by definition, infertile (but by no means are they necessarily sterile). (See Chapter 9 on Essentials of Contraception and Chapter 27 on Impaired Fertility.) Table 31-2 summarizes the efficacy studies on women who are neither using contraception nor breastfeeding.

TYPICAL USE (SPERMICIDES, PERIODIC ABSTINENCE, DIAPHRAGM, MALE CONDOM, AND PILL)

Our estimates of the probability of pregnancy during the first year of *typical* use for spermicides, periodic abstinence, the diaphragm, the male condom, and the pill are the averages of results for married women in the 1976 and 1982 National Surveys of Family Growth (NSFG) uncorrected for under-reporting of abortion[36] and for all women in the 1988 NSFG corrected for under-reporting of abortion.[12] These estimates are standardized to reflect the estimated probabilities of pregnancy that would be observed if users of each method had the same characteristics (for example, the same age distribution and the same fraction living in poverty). For alternative estimates of the efficacy of these methods during typical use, see Table 9-3 and the accompanying text. (For an explanation of how typical-use estimates of efficacy were derived for other methods, see the sections that follow.)

We reason that the correction for under-reporting of abortion produces estimates that are too high because women in abortion clinics (surveys of whom provided the information for the correction) over-report use of a contraceptive method at the time they became pregnant. Moreover, it seems likely women in personal interviews for the NSFG also tend to over-report use of a contraceptive method at the time of a conception leading to a live birth. Evidence is provided by a first-year probability of pregnancy of 6% for the IUD (a method with little scope for user error) among married women in the 1976 and 1982 NSFGs; this probability is much higher than rates observed in clinical trials of IUDs.[36] We expect over-reporting of contraceptive method use both in the NSFG and in surveys conducted in abortion clinics because the responsibility for the pregnancy is shifted from the woman (or couple) to the method. Thus, we suspect pregnancy rates based on the NSFG alone tend to be too low because induced abortions (and contraceptive failures leading to induced abortions) are under-reported but at the same time tend to be too high because contraceptive failures leading to live births are over-reported. These two sources of bias tend to cancel, whereas adjustment for under-reporting of induced abortion would make the pregnancy rates too high. However, we expect estimates based only on married women from the 1976 and 1982 NSFGs to be underestimates of the risk of pregnancy for all women, since unmarried women regularly having intercourse experience higher pregnancy rates during typical use of contraceptives than do married women.[12] We conclude the estimates based on the experience of married women in the 1976 and 1982 NSGFs uncorrected for under-reporting of abortion are likely to be too low and that those based on the experience of all women in the 1988 NSFG corrected for under-reporting of abortion are likely to be too high; our final estimate is the average of these two.

CERVICAL CAP, SPONGE, AND DIAPHRAGM

Our estimates of the probabilities of pregnancy during the first year of *perfect* use of the cervical cap and sponge correspond with results of a reanalysis of data from clinical trials in which women were randomly assigned to use the diaphragm or sponge or the diaphragm or cervical cap.[37] The results indicate that among parous women who use the sponge perfectly, 19.4% to 20.5% will experience a pregnancy within the first year. The corresponding range for nulliparous women is 9.0% to 9.5%. Among parous women who use the cervical cap perfectly, 25.7% to 27.0% will experience a pregnancy within the first year. The range for nulliparous women is 7.6% to 9.9%. In contrast, parous users of the diaphragm do not appear to have higher pregnancy rates during perfect use than do nulliparous users; 4.3% to 8.4% of all women experience an accidental pregnancy during the first year of perfect use of the diaphragm. Our revised estimates in the third column of Table 31-1 (and Table 9-2) are obtained from the midpoints of these ranges.

We next faced the problem of whether and how to revise the estimates for these methods during *typical* use (the second column). The proportions becoming pregnant during the first year of typical use for parous users of the sponge (27.4%) and cervical cap (30.3%) were about twice as high as for nulliparous users of these methods (14.0% and 15.2%, respectively). The evidence for the diaphragm is mixed. In the sponge-diaphragm trial, the proportion becoming pregnant in the first year of typical use for parous users of the diaphragm (12.4%) was marginally lower than that for nulliparous users (12.8%). In the cap-diaphragm trial, the proportion becoming pregnant among parous users (29.0%) is almost double that among nulliparous users (14.8%).[38] Faced with this information, we set the estimates for nulliparous users of the cervical cap and sponge equal to the estimate for all users of the diaphragm based on the NSFG (20%). We doubled the estimates for nulliparous users of the cervical cap and sponge to obtain the estimates for parous users.

WITHDRAWAL

Our estimate of the proportion becoming pregnant during a year of *perfect* use of withdrawal is an educated guess based on the reasoning that pregnancy resulting from pre-ejaculatory fluid is unlikely.[11,23] The estimate for *typical* use of withdrawal is the weighted average of the three life-table estimates in Table 31-8.

FEMALE CONDOM

The *typical-use* estimate for the female condom is based on the results of a 6-month clinical trial of the Reality female condom (originally classified as a vaginal pouch); 12.4% of women in the United States experienced a pregnancy during the first 6 months of use.[38] The 12-month probability of pregnancy for users of Reality in the United States was projected from the relation between the pregnancy rates in the first 6 months and the pregnancy rates in the second 6 months for users of the diaphragm, sponge, and cervical cap.[38] The probability of pregnancy during 6 months of *perfect* use of Reality by U.S. women who met the compliance criteria stipulated in the study protocol was 2.6%. Those who reported fewer than four acts of intercourse during the month prior to any follow-up visit, who did not use Reality at every act of intercourse, who ever reported not following the Reality instructions, or who used another method of contraception were censored at the beginning of the first interval where noncompliance was noted.[4] Under the assumption that the probability of pregnancy in the second 6 months of perfect use would be the same, the probability of pregnancy during a year of perfect use would be 5.1%

SPERMICIDES (PERFECT USE)

Our estimate of the proportion becoming pregnant during a year of *perfect* use of spermicides is not empirically based. We reason spermicides used alone may be less effective and certainly should be no more effective than spermicides used in conjunction with a barrier. However, six studies outside the United States,[2,3,5,6,10,25] in addition to several U.S. studies reviewed earlier,[36] have yielded very low probabilities of pregnancy during the first year of typical use of spermicides, much lower than any estimates for barriers with spermicides.

Our intuition may lead us to understate the efficacy of spermicides used alone for two reasons. First, women are instructed that a dose of spermicides used alone remains effective for only 1 hour (see Chapter 17 on Vaginal Spermicides) but the diaphragm and spermicidal cream or jelly may be inserted up to 8 hours and the cervical cap and spermicide up to 48 hours before intercourse (see Chapter 18 on Vaginal Barriers). It is possible the rules for the diaphragm and cervical cap are too lenient, thereby increasing the pregnancy rate during perfect use of these methods relative to that for spermicides used alone. On the other hand, the sponge, which may be inserted up to 24 hours before intercourse, contains 1 gram of nonoxynol-9, about 7 to 12 times the amount in an application of foam, cream, or gel and nearly 14 times the amount in each sheet of film. The sponge was designed to be used for up to 2 days (hence the name) and only concerns about toxic shock syndrome prevented labeling to that effect. Nevertheless, the sponge is no more effective during perfect use among nulliparous women than the diaphragm or cervical cap. Second, we ignore the fact that the spermicidal products used alone differ from those used in conjunction with barriers. The modern efficacy literature on spermicides is dominated by studies of suppositories, foams, and film, and high spermicide efficacy is documented only in these studies. There are few studies of creams and gels used alone, and those with the lowest pregnancy rates are more than 30 years old (Table 31-3). The biophysical properties of foams (and perhaps suppositories and film) may result in better dispersion both in the vagina and in cervical secretions. Evidence for this hypothesis can be found in an early randomized trial with a crossover design (so all subjects used each product); however, even in this study the pregnancy rates for foam are high.[17] We consider it more likely the spermicide studies suffer from flaws in analysis or design that are not apparent in the brief published descriptions. For example, an FDA advisory committee was openly skeptical of one German study:[2] "The way in which the survey was designed and the manner in which the various incentives were offered (physicians reportedly received a fee for completing survey data forms) would clearly make the data resulting from the survey unacceptable to any scientific group or regulatory agency."[18,31] Therefore, we set the pregnancy rate during perfect use of spermicides equal to the empirically based pregnancy rate during perfect use of the diaphragm.

The first clinical trial of Emko vaginal foam is also one of the few studies to compute separate pregnancy rates for cycles in which the product was used at every act of intercourse and for cycles in which unprotected intercourse occurred.[17] The design of that trial was also quite sophisticated. Women were randomly assigned to six groups. Each group used three different spermicidal products for three cycles each. The six groups represented all possible permutations of orders of use of the three products. If the pregnancy rate for three cycles of consistent use of Emko vaginal foam is extrapolated, then the implied proportion becoming pregnant in the first year of consistent use is 8.9%. (For a discussion of how *typical-use* estimates were derived, see the section on Typical Use.)

PERIODIC ABSTINENCE (PERFECT USE)

The *perfect-use* estimates for periodic abstinence are based on an empirical estimate of 3.2% for the ovulation method.[34] Common sense dictates that the newer variants of periodic abstinence should be inherently efficacious because they demand abstinence during large portions of each cycle and particularly during times near estimated peak fecundity. They are relatively ineffective in actual use because perfect use is so difficult to achieve, and the consequence of imperfect use is a high risk of pregnancy. The post-ovulation variant of periodic abstinence requires the longest periods of abstinence, followed in order by the sympto-thermal, ovulation, and calendar variants. Consequently, we have assigned probabilities of pregnancy during perfect use consistent with that ordering with the realization we can be confident only about the rate for the ovulation method. Given the dearth of evidence, higher or lower estimates for calendar rhythm would be as plausible and defensible. (For a discussion of how *typical-use* estimates were derived, see the section on Typical Use.)

MALE CONDOM (PERFECT USE)

Our estimate of the proportion becoming pregnant during a year of perfect use of the male condom is based on results from the only study of the male condom meeting modern standards of design, execution, and analysis.[40] Couples were randomly assigned to use either a latex condom or a polyurethane condom for 7 months. Adjusted for the use of emergency contraceptive pills, the six-cycle probability of pregnancy during consistent use of the latex condom was 1.2%. Assuming a constant per-cycle probability of pregnancy, the 13-cycle probability of pregnancy during consistent use would be 2.6%. This estimate is consistent with an estimate based on studies of condom breakage and slippage.[1] Under the assumption that 1.5% of condoms break or slip off the penis and that women have intercourse twice a week, then about 1.5% of women would experience condom breaks during the half-week that they are at risk of pregnancy during each cycle. The per-cycle probability of conception would be reduced by 98.5%, from 0.1358 to only 0.0020, if a condom failure results in no protection whatsoever against pregnancy, so that about 2.6% of women would become pregnant each year.[15] Unfortunately, breakage and slippage rates did not accurately predict pregnancy rates during consistent use in the clinical trial of the latex and polyurethane male condom,[40] and estimates of condom breakage and slippage during intercourse and withdrawal vary substantially across studies in developed countries,[1] from a low of 0.6% among commercial sex workers in Nevada's legal brothels[1] to a high of 7.2% among monogamous couples in North Carolina.[30] (For a discussion of how *typical-use* estimates were derived, see the section on Typical Use.)

PILL (PERFECT USE)

Although the lowest reported pregnancy rate for the combined pill during typical use is 0% (Table 31-11), recent studies indicate pregnancies do occur, albeit rarely, during perfect use. Hence we set the perfect-use estimate for the combined pill at the very low level of 0.1%. The combined pill appears to be inherently more effective than the progestin-only pill. The lowest reported proportion becoming pregnant during the first year of use of the minipill is about 1% (Table 31-10), but imperfect use in 15% to 20% of cycles probably accounts for half the pregnancies. Consequently, we set the *perfect-use* estimate for the minipill at 0.5%. (For a discussion of how *typical-use* estimates were derived, see the section on Typical Use.)

INTRAUTERINE DEVICE (IUD)

The estimates for *typical* use of the Progesterone T and the Copper T 380A IUDs are taken directly from the large study for each method shown in Table 31-12. The estimate for the LNg 20 IUD is the weighted average of the results from the two studies shown in Table 31-12. The estimate for *perfect* use of the Copper T 380A IUD was obtained by removing the pregnancies that resulted when the device was not known to be in situ,[27] on the perhaps-questionable assumption that these pregnancies should be classified as user failures and the empirically based assumption that expulsions are so uncommon that the denominator of the perfect-use pregnancy rate is virtually the same as the denominator for the typical-use rate (Table 31-12). The *perfect-use* estimates for the Progesterone T and LNg 20 IUDs were derived analogously. No differences in the *typical-use* and perfect-use estimates for LNg 20 are apparent due to the fact that only one significant digit is shown.

DEPO-PROVERA AND NORPLANT

The *typical-use* estimate for Depo-Provera is the weighted average of the seven studies of the 150 mg dose shown in Table 31-13. While imperfect use of injectables may occur if women miss a scheduled injection, each 150 mg dose probably provides more than 3 months' protection for many (perhaps most) women. For this reason, and because we have no information concerning pregnancies that may have resulted from late injections, we set the *perfect-use* estimate equal to the typical-use estimate.

The *typical-use* estimate for Norplant (6 capsules) and Norplant-2 (2 rods) is based on results from the three studies reported in Table 31-14.[27,28,29] The earlier study and one of the two arms in one of the later studies of Norplant-2 included only implants with a core made of an elastomer no longer used, and the earlier study of Norplant included both implants made with a hard tubing no longer used and implants made with the soft tubing currently used.[27,28] Because the later studies provide information on the current versions of the two implants,[28,29] their results are more relevant. Yet, although those studies recorded no pregnancies, it is highly implausible the new versions of these implants never fail. We therefore arbitrarily set the typical-use estimate at 0.05%. Because there is no scope for user error, the typical-use and *perfect-use* estimates are the same.

STERILIZATION

The weighted average of the results from the eight vasectomy studies in Table 31-16 analyzed with life-table procedures is 0.01% becoming pregnant in the year following the procedure. In these studies, pregnancies occurred after the ejaculate had been declared to be sperm-free. This perfect-use estimate of 0.01% is undoubtedly too low, because clinicians are understandably loath to publish articles describing their surgical failures, and journals would be reluctant to publish an article documenting poor surgical technique. The difference between typical-use and perfect-use pregnancy rates for vasectomy would depend on the frequency of unprotected intercourse after the procedure had been performed but before the ejaculate had been certified to be sperm-free. We arbitrarily set the *typical* and *perfect-use* estimates to 0.15% and 0.10%, respectively. For female sterilization, there is no scope for user error. The *typical-* and *perfect-use* estimates are the pooled results from the U.S. Collaborative Review of Sterilization, a prospective study of 10,685 women undergoing tubal sterilization.[20] We are less concerned about publication bias with female than with male sterilization because the largest studies of female sterilization are based on prospective, multicenter clinical trials, not retrospective reports from one investigator.

EMERGENCY CONTRACEPTION

Ten clinical trials of emergency contraceptive pills (ECPs) have compared the observed number of pregnancies among women with regular menstrual cycles with the expected number of pregnancies based on known cycle day of intercourse and published estimates of conception probabilities by cycle day.[33] These results show treatment with ECPs reduces the chance of pregnancy by at least 75%. Typically, if 100 women have unprotected intercourse once during the second or third week of their menstrual cycle, about 8 would become pregnant. If those same women used emergency contraceptive pills, only 2 would become pregnant (a 75% reduction). Postcoital administration of levonorgestrel also provides effective emergency contraception. The only randomized trial comparing the two regimens found progestin-only pills to be as effective as ECPs but result in less nausea and vomiting.[9] The World Health Organization is conducting further comparative trials. A copper-T IUD can be inserted up to 5 days after unprotected intercourse to prevent pregnancy. Copper-T IUD insertion is extremely effective, reducing the risk of pregnancy following unprotected intercourse by more than 99%.[32] Moreover, a copper-T IUD can be left in place to provide continuous effective contraception for up to 10 years.

THE LACTATIONAL AMENORRHEA METHOD (LAM)

LAM is a highly effective, *temporary* method of contraception. If the infant is being fed only on its mother's breastmilk (or is given supplemental non-breastmilk feeds only to a minor extent) and if the woman has not experienced her first postpartum menses, breastfeeding provides more than 98% protection from pregnancy in the first 6 months following a birth.[14] Four prospective clinical studies of the contraceptive effect of this Lactational Amenorrhea Method (LAM) demonstrated cumulative 6-month life-table perfect-use pregnancy rates of 0.5%, 0.6%, 1.0%, and 1.5% among women who relied solely on LAM.[13,16,19,24]

CONTRACEPTIVE CONTINUATION

Contraceptives will be effective at preventing unintended pregnancy only if women or couples continue to use them once they have initiated use. The proportions of women continuing use at the end of the first year for spermicides, periodic abstinence, the diaphragm, the male condom, and the pill were computed in two steps. In the first step, we obtained from the 1982 National Survey of Family Growth the proportions of married women continuing use if the only forms of discontinuation were (1) change of method and (2) complete termination of contraceptive use while still at risk of an unintended pregnancy.[7] Other reasons for discontinuing use of a method (such as attempting to get pregnant or not having intercourse) are not counted in the discontinuation rate because these reasons are unrelated to the method and do not apply to women seeking to avoid pregnancy and at risk of becoming pregnant. These discontinuation rates are standardized to reflect the estimated probabilities of continuation that would be observed if users of each method had the same characteristics (the same distribution by age, race, and education). In the second step, we multiplied the continuation rates excluding pregnancy (obtained in the first step) by the complement of the probability of becoming pregnant during the first year of typical use (shown in the second column of Table 31-1 and Table 9-2) to obtain the probability of continuing use among those seeking to avoid pregnancy. To obtain the estimate for the cervical cap and sponge, we substituted the probability of continuation (excluding pregnancy) for the diaphragm in the first step. To obtain the estimate for the female condom, we also substituted the probability of continuation (excluding pregnancy) for the diaphragm in the first step; the result is the same if one uses instead the probability of continuation for the male condom in the first step.

Proportions discontinuing use of Norplant, the three IUDs, and Depo-Provera for reasons related to the contraceptive are based on clinical trials. The proportion continuing use of Norplant and Norplant-2 at the end of 1 year in the randomized trial of the current versions of the implants shown in Table 31-14 was 95%.[29] This is a full 10 percentage points higher than the proportion (85%) continuing use of Norplant in the earlier trial.[27] We took as our estimate the weighted average of these two. The estimates for the Progesterone T and the Copper T 380A IUDs were taken directly from the large study for each method shown in Table 31-12. The estimate for the LNg 20 IUD is the weighted average from the two studies shown in Table 31-12. The proportion continuing use of Depo-Provera at the end of 1 year was calculated from the results of the two World Health Organization trials of the 150 mg dose injected every 90 days shown in Table 31-13; it is considerably higher than the 28.6% continuing use in a Texas study of indigent urban women in 17 clinics,[26] the 30% to 42% continuing use in a study of a hospital-based and a community-based clinic in New York City,[21] or the 23% continuing use in a study of clinics operated by Planned Parenthood of the Rocky Mountains,[39] all conducted after the drug was approved by the Food and Drug

Administration. Although results from these five studies are not strictly comparable because discontinuation for reasons such as desiring to become pregnant and no longer having intercourse was included in the Texas, New York City, and Rocky Mountain studies, the proportions continuing use would still be far lower if discontinuation for reasons unrelated to use of Depo-Provera was excluded. Note that discontinuation among users of Depo-Provera has been measured differently from discontinuation among users of other methods. A woman is considered to be a user of another method as long as she considers herself to be using that method. (See Chapter 9.) However, in studies of Depo-Provera, a woman is considered to have discontinued use if she does not return for her next shot within 14 weeks (or in some studies 15 weeks), even though contraceptive protection probably extends well beyond that period, and even if she returns thereafter and receives another injection. This convention of classifying such women as discontinuing but not pregnant at 14 (or 15) weeks leads to an overestimate of the discontinuation rate[22] and to an underestimate of the pregnancy rate if women miss an injection and become pregnant after 14 weeks but consider themselves still to be using Depo-Provera.

TEXT REFERENCES

1. Albert AE, Warner DL, Hatcher RA, Trussell J, Bennett C. Condom use among female commercial sex workers in Nevada's legal brothels. Am J Public Health 1995;85:1514-1520.
2. Brehm H, Haase W. Die alternative zur hormonalen kontrazeption? Med Welt 1975;26:1610-1617.
3. Dimpfl J, Salomon W, Schicketanz KH. Die spermizide barriere. Sexualmedizin 1984;13:95-98.
4. Farr G, Gabelnick H, Sturgen K, Dorflinger L. Contraceptive efficacy and acceptability of the female condom. Am J Public Health 1994;84:1960-1964.
5. Florence N. Das kontrazeptive vaginal-suppositorium: ergebnisse einer klinischen fünfjahresstudie. Sexualmedizin 1977;6:385-386.
6. Godts P. Klinische prüfung eines vaginalem antikonzipiens. Ars Medici 1973;2:589-593.
7. Grady WR, Hayward MD, Florey FA. Contraceptive discontinuation among married women in the United States. Stud Fam Plann 1988;19:227-235.
8. Grady WR, Hayward MD, Yagi J. Contraceptive failure in the United States: estimates from the 1982 National Survey of Family Growth. Fam Plann Perspect 1986;18:200-209.
9. Ho PC, Kwan MSW. A prospective randomized comparison of levonorgestrel with the Yuzpe regimen in post-coital contraception. Hum Reprod 1993;8:389-392.
10. Iizuka R, Kobayashi T, Kawakami S, Nakamura Y, Ikeuchi M, Chin B, Mochimaru F, Sumi K, Sato H, Yamaguchi J, Ohno T, Shiina M, Maeda N, Tokoro H, Suzuki T, Hayashi K, Takahashi T, Akatsuka M, Kasuga Y, Kurokawa H. Clinical

experience with the Vaginal Contraceptive Film containing the spermicide polyoxyethylene nonylphenyl ether (C-Film study group). Jpn J Fertil Steril 1980;25:64-68. (In Japanese; translation supplied by Apothecus Inc.)

11. Ilaria G, Jacobs JL, Polsky B, Koll B, Baron P, MacLow C, Armstrong D, Schlegel PN. Detection of HIV-1 DNA sequences in pre-ejaculatory fluid. Lancet 1992;340:1469.

12. Jones EF, Forrest JD. Contraceptive failure rates based on the 1988 NSFG. Fam Plann Perspect 1992;24:12-19.

13. Kazi A, Kennedy KI, Visness CM, Khan T. Effectiveness of the lactational amenorrhea method in Pakistan. Fertil Steril 1995;64:717-723.

14. Kennedy KI, Rivera R, McNeilly AS. Consensus statement on the use of breastfeeding as a family planning method. Contraception 1989;39:477-496.

15. Kestelman P, Trussell J. Efficacy of the simultaneous use of condoms and spermicides. Fam Plann Perspect 1991;23:226-227, 232.

16. Labbok MH, Hight-Laukaran V, Peterson AE, Fletcher V, von Hertzen H, Van Look PFA. Multicenter study of the Lactational Amenorrhea Method (LAM): I. Efficacy, duration, and implications for clinical application. Contraception 1997;55:327-336.

17. Mears E. Chemical contraceptive trial: II. J Reprod Fertil 1962;4:337-343.

18. Over-the-Counter Contraceptives and Other Vaginal Drug Products Review Panel (Elizabeth B. Connell, Chairman). Encare Oval. Memorandum to Food and Drug Administration Commissioner Donald Kennedy, February 9, 1978.

19. Pérez A, Labbok MH, Queenan JT. Clinical study of the lactational amenorrhoea method for family planning. Lancet 1992;339:968-970.

20. Peterson HB, Xia Z, Hughes JM, Wilcox LS, Tylor LR, Trussell J. The risk of pregnancy after tubal sterilization: findings from the U.S. Collaborative Review of Sterilization. Am J Obstet Gynecol 1996;174:1161-1170.

21. Polaneczky M, Guarnaccia M, Alon J, Wiley J. Early experience with the contraceptive use of depot medroxyprogesterone acetate in an inner-city clinic population. Fam Plann Perspect 1996;28:174-178.

22. Potter LS, Dalberth BT, Cañamar R, Betz M. The first cohort of DMPA users at a North Carolina family planning clinic. Unpublished manuscript. Research Triangle Park NC: Family Health International, 1997.

23. Pudney J, Oneta M, Mayer K, Seage G, Anderson D. Pre-ejaculatory fluid as potential vector for sexual transmission of HIV-1. Lancet 1992;340:1470.

24. Ramos R, Kennedy KI, Visness CM. Effectiveness of lactational amenorrhea in prevention of pregnancy in Manila, the Philippines: non-comparative prospective trial. Br Med J 1996;313:909-912.

25. Salomon W, Haase W. Intravaginale kontrazeption. Sexualmedizin 1977;6:198-202.

26. Sangi-Haghpeykar H, Poindexter AN, Bateman L, Ditmore JR. Experiences of injectable contraceptive users in an urban setting. Obstet Gynecol 1996;88:227-233.

27. Sivin I. Personal communication to James Trussell, August 13, 1992.

28. Sivin I, Lähteenmäki P, Ranta S, Darney P, Klaisle C, Wan L, Mishell DR, Lacarra M, Viegas OAC, Bilhareus P, Koetsawang S, Piya-Anant M, Diaz S, Pavez M, Alvarez F, Brache V, LaGuardia K, Nash H, Stern J. Levonorgestrel concentrations during use of levonorgestrel rod (LNG ROD) implants. Contraception 1997;55:81-85.

29. Sivin I, Viegas O, Campodonico I, Diaz S, Pavez M, Wan L, Koetsawang S, Kiriwat O, Anant MP, Holma P, el din Abdalla K, Stern J. Clinical performance of a new two-rod levonorgestrel contraceptive implant: a three-year randomized study with Norplant® implants as controls. Contraception 1997;55:73-80.

30. Steiner M, Piedrahita C, Glover L, Joanis C. Can condom users likely to experience condom failure be identified? Fam Plann Perspect 1993;25:220-223, 226.

31. Stewart FH, Stewart G, Guest FJ, Hatcher RA. My body, my health: the concerned woman's guide to gynecology. New York: John Wiley & Sons, 1979.

32. Trussell J, Ellertson C. Efficacy of emergency contraception. Fertil Control Rev 1995;4:8-11.

33. Trussell J, Ellertson C, Stewart F. The effectiveness of the Yuzpe regimen of emergency contraception. Fam Plann Perspect 1996;28:58-64, 87.

34. Trussell J, Grummer-Strawn L. Contraceptive failure of the ovulation method of periodic abstinence. Fam Plann Perspect 1990a;22:65-75.

35. Trussell J, Hatcher RA, Cates W, Stewart FH, Kost K. Contraceptive failure in the United States: an update. Stud Fam Plann 1990b;21:51-54.

36. Trussell J, Kost K. Contraceptive failure in the United States: a critical review of the literature. Stud Fam Plann 1987;18:237-283.

37. Trussell J, Strickler J, Vaughan B. Contraceptive efficacy of the diaphragm, the sponge and the cervical cap. Fam Plann Perspect 1993;25:100-105, 135.

38. Trussell J, Sturgen K, Strickler J, Dominik R. Comparative contraceptive efficacy of the female condom and other barrier methods. Fam Plann Perspect 1994;26:66-72.

39. Westfall JM, Main DS, Barnard L. Continuation rates among injectable contraceptive users. Fam Plann Perspect 1996;28:275-277.

LATE REFERENCE

40. Nelson A, Bernstein GS, Frezieres R, Walsh T, Clark V, Coulson A. Study of the efficacy, acceptability and safety of a non-latex (polyurethane) male condom: revised final report (N01-HD-1-3109). Bethesda MD: National Institute of Child Health and Human Development, September 15, 1997.

TABLE REFERENCES

Åkerlund M, Røde A, Westergaard J. Comparative profiles of reliability, cycle control and side effects of two oral contraceptive formulations containing 150 µg desogestrel and either 30 µg or 20 µg ethinyl oestradiol. Brit J Obstet Gynaecol 1993;100:832-838.

Alderman PM. The lurking sperm: a review of failures in 8879 vasectomies performed by one physician. JAMA 1988;259:3142-3144.

Apothecus Pharmaceutical Corporation. VCF®: Vaginal Contraceptive Film™. East Norwich NY: Apothecus Inc, 1992.

Archer DF, Maheux R, DelConte A, O'Brien FB, North American Levonorgestrel Study Group (NALSG). A new low-dose monophasic combination oral contraceptive (Alesse™) with levonorgestrel 100 µg and ethinyl estradiol 20 µg. Contraception 1997;55:139-144.

Ball M. A prospective field trial of the ovulation method of avoiding conception. Eur J Obstet Gynecol Reprod Biol 1976;6:63-66.

Bartzen PJ. Effectiveness of the temperature rhythm system of contraception. Fertil Steril 1967;18:694-706.

Belhadj H, Sivin I, Diaz S, Pavez M, Tejada AS, Brache V, Alvarez F, Shoupe D, Breaux H, Mishell DR, McCarthy T, Yo V. Recovery of fertility after use of the levonorgestrel 20 mcg/d or copper T 380 Ag intrauterine device. Contraception 1986;34:261-267.

Bernstein GS. Clinical effectiveness of an aerosol contraceptive foam. Contraception 1971;3:37-43.

Bernstein GS, Clark V, Coulson AH, Frezieres RG, Kilzer L, Moyer D, Nakamura RM, Walsh T. Use effectiveness study of cervical caps. Final report. Washington DC: National Institute of Child Health and Human Development, Contract No. 1-HD-1-2804, July, 1986.

Bhiwandiwala PP, Mumford SD, Feldblum PJ. A comparison of different laparoscopic sterilization occlusion techniques in 24,439 procedures. Am J Obstet Gynecol 1982;144:319-331.

Board JA. Continuous norethindrone, 0.35 mg, as an oral contraceptive agent. Am J Obstet Gynecol 1971;109:531-535.

Boehm D. The cervical cap: effectiveness as a contraceptive. J Nurse Midwifery 1983;28:3-6.

Bounds W, Guillebaud J. Randomised comparison of the use-effectiveness and patient acceptability of the Collatex (Today) contraceptive sponge and the diaphragm. Br J Fam Plann 1984;10:69-75.

Bounds W, Guillebaud J, Dominik R, Dalberth BT. The diaphragm with and without spermicide: a randomized, comparative efficacy trial. J Reprod Med 1995; 40:764-774.

Bounds W, Vessey M, Wiggins P. A randomized double-blind trial of two low dose combined oral contraceptives. Brit J Obstet Gynaecol 1979;86:325-329.

Bracher M, Santow G. Premature discontinuation of contraception in Australia. Fam Plann Perspect 1992;24:58-65.

Brehm H, Haase W. Die alternative zur hormonalen kontrazeption? Med Welt 1975;26:1610-1617.

Brigato G, Pisano G, Bergamasco A, Pasqualini M, Cutugno G, Luppari T. Vaginal topical chemical contraception with C-Film. Ginecol Clinica 1982;3:77-80. (In Italian; translation supplied by Apothecus Inc.)

Bushnell LF. Aerosol foam: a practical and effective method of contraception. Pac Med Surg 1965;73:353-355.

Cagen R. The cervical cap as a barrier contraceptive. Contraception 1986; 33:487-496.

Carpenter G, Martin JB. Clinical evaluation of a vaginal contraceptive foam. Adv Plann Parent 1970;5:170-175.

Chi IC, Laufe LE, Gardner SD, Tolbert MA. An epidemiologic study of risk factors associated with pregnancy following female sterilization. Am J Obstet Gynecol 1980;136:768-773.

Chi IC, Mumford SD, Gardner SD. Pregnancy risks following laparoscopic sterilization in nongravid and gravid women. J Reprod Med 1981;26:289-294.

Chi IC, Siemens AJ, Champion CB, Gates D, Cilenti D. Pregnancy following minilaparotomy tubal sterilization: an update of an international data set. Contraception 1987;35:171-178.

Cliquet RL, Schoenmaeckers R, Klinkenborg L. Effectiveness of contraception in Belgium: results of the second national fertility survey, 1971 (NEGO II). J Biosoc Sci 1977;9:403-416.

Corson SL. Efficacy and clinical profile of a new oral contraceptive containing norgestimate. Acta Obstet Gynecol Scand Suppl 1990;152:25-31.

Debusschere R. Effectiviteit van de anticonceptie in Vlaanderen: resultaten van het NEGO-III-onderzoek 1975-1976. Bevolking en Gezin 1980;1:5-28.

Denniston GC, Putney D. The cavity rim cervical cap. Adv Plann Parent 1981;16:77-80.

Dimpfl J, Salomon W, Schicketanz KH. Die spermizide barriere. Sexualmedizin 1984;13:95-98.

Dolack L. Study confirms values of ovulation method. Hospital Progress 1978; 59:64-66,72-73.

Dubrow H, Kuder K. Combined postpartum and family-planning clinic. Obstet Gynecol 1958;11:586-590.

Edelman DA. Nonprescription vaginal contraception. Int J Gynecol Obstet 1980;18:340-344.

Edelman DA, McIntyre SL, Harper J. A comparative trial of the Today contraceptive sponge and diaphragm. Am J Obstet Gynecol 1984; 150:869-876.

Ellis JW. Multiphasic oral contraceptives: efficacy and metabolic impact. J Reprod Med 1987;32:28-36.

Ellsworth HS. Focus on triphasil. J Reprod Med 1986;31:559-564.

Endrikat J, Jaques MA, Mayerhofer M, Pelissier C, Müller U, Düsterberg B. A twelve-month comparative clinical investigation of two low-dose oral contraceptives containing 20 µg ethinylestradiol/75 µg gestodene and 20 µg ethinylestradiol/150 µg desogestrel, with respect to efficacy, cycle control and tolerance. Contraception 1995;52:229-235.

Engel T. Laparoscopic sterilization: electrosurgery or clip application? J Reprod Med 1978;21:107-110.

Florence N. Das kontrazeptive vaginal-suppositorium: ergebnisse einer klinischen fünfjahresstudie. Sexualmedizin 1977;6:385-386.

Frank R. Clinical evaluation of a simple jelly-alone method of contraception. Fertil Steril 1962;13:458-464.

Frankman O, Raabe N, Ingemansson CA. Clinical evaluation of C-Film, a vaginal contraceptive. J Int Med Res 1975;3:292-296.

Gauthier A, Upmalis D, Dain MP. Clinical evaluation of a new triphasic oral contraceptive: norgestimate and ethinyl estradiol. Acta Obstet Gynecol Scand Suppl 1992;156:27-32.

Gibor Y, Mitchell C. Selected events following insertion of the Progestasert system. Contraception 1980;21:491-503.

Glass R, Vessey M, Wiggins P. Use-effectiveness of the condom in a selected family planning clinic population in the United Kingdom. Contraception 1974;10: 591-598.

Godts P. Klinische prüfung eines vaginalem antikonzipiens. Ars Medici 1973; 28:584-593.

Grady WR, Hayward MD, Yagi J. Contraceptive failure in the United States: estimates from the 1982 National Survey of Family Growth. Fam Plann Perspect 1986;18:200-209.

Grady WR, Hirsch MB, Keen N, Vaughan B. Contraceptive failure and continuation among married women in the United States, 1970-75. Stud Fam Plann 1983;14:9-19.

Hall RE. Continuation and pregnancy rates with four contraceptive methods. Am J Obstet Gynecol 1973;116:671-681.

Hawkins DF, Benster B. A comparative study of three low dose progestogens, chlormadinone acetate, megestrol acetate and norethisterone, as oral contraceptives. Br J Obstet Gynaecol 1977;84:708-713.

Howard G, Blair M, Chen JK, Fotherby K, Muggeridge J, Elder MG, Bye PG. A clinical trial of norethisterone oenanthate (Norigest) injected every two months. Contraception 1982;25:333-343.

Hughes I. An open assessment of a new low dose estrogen combined oral contraceptive. J Int Med Res 1978;6:41-45.

Hulka JF, Mercer JP, Fishburne JI, Kumarasamy T, Omran KF, Phillips JM, Lefler HT, Lieberman B, Lean TH, Pai DN, Koetsawang S, Castro VM. Spring clip sterilization: one-year follow-up of 1,079 cases. Am J Obstet Gynecol 1976;125:1039-1043.

Iizuka R, Kobayashi T, Kawakami S, Nakamura Y, Ikeuchi M, Chin B, Mochimaru F, Sumi K, Sato H, Yamaguchi J, Ohno T, Shiina M, Maeda N, Tokoro H, Suzuki T, Hayashi K, Takahashi T, Akatsuka M, Kasuga Y, Kurokawa H. Clinical experience with the Vaginal Contraceptive Film containing the spermicide polyoxyethylene nonylphenyl ether (C-Film study group). Jpn J Fertil Steril 1980;25:64-68. (In Japanese; translation supplied by Apothecus Inc.)

John APK. Contraception in a practice community. J R Coll Gen Pract 1973;23:665-675.

Johnston JA, Roberts DB, Spencer RB. A survey evaluation of the efficacy and efficiency of natural family planning services and methods in Australia: report of a research project. Sydney, Australia: St. Vincent's Hospital, 1978.

Jones EF, Forrest JD. Contraceptive failure rates based on the 1988 NSFG. Fam Plann Perspect 1992;24:12-19.

Jubhari S, Lane ME, Sobrero AJ. Continuous microdose (0.3 mg) quingestanol acetate as an oral contraceptive agent. Contraception 1974;9:213-219.

Kambic R, Kambic M, Brixius AM, Miller S. A thirty-month clinical experience in natural family planning. Am J Public Health 1981;71:1255-1258. Erratum. Am J Public Health 1982;72:538.

Kasabach HY. Clinical evaluation of vaginal jelly alone in the management of fertility. Clin Med 1962;69:894-897.

Kase S, Goldfarb M. Office vasectomy review of 500 cases. Urology 1973;1:60-62.

Kassell NC, McElroy MP. Emma Goldman Clinic for Women study. In: King L (ed). The cervical cap handbook for users and fitters. Iowa City IA: Emma Goldman Clinic for Women, 1981:11-19.

Keifer W. A clinical evaluation of continuous Norethindrone (0.35 mg). In: Ortho Pharmaceutical Corporation. A clinical symposium on 0.35 mg. Norethindrone: continuous regimen low-dose oral contraceptive. Proceedings of a symposium, New York City, February 22, 1971. Raritan NJ: Ortho Pharmaceutical Corporation, 1973:9-14.

Klapproth HJ, Young IS. Vasectomy, vas ligation and vas occlusion. Urology 1973;1:292-300.

Klaus H, Goebel JM, Muraski B, Egizio MT, Weitzel D, Taylor, RS, Fagan MU, Ek K, Hobday K. Use-effectiveness and client satisfaction in six centers teaching the Billings ovulation method. Contraception 1979;19:613-629.

Kleppinger RK. A vaginal contraceptive foam. Penn Med J 1965;68:31-34.

Koch JP. The Prentif contraceptive cervical cap: a contemporary study of its clinical safety and effectiveness. Contraception 1982;25:135-159.

Korba VD, Heil CG. Eight years of fertility control with norgestrel-ethinyl estradiol (Ovral): an updated clinical review. Fertil Steril 1975;26:973-981.

Korba VD, Paulson SR. Five years of fertility control with microdose norgestrel: an updated clinical review. J Reprod Med 1974;13:71-75.

Kovacs GT, Jarman H, Dunn K, Westcott M, Baker HWG. The contraceptive diaphragm: is it an acceptable method in the 1980s? Aust NZ J Obstet Gynaecol 1986;26:76-79.

Lammers P, op ten Berg M. Phase III clinical trial with a new oral contraceptive containing 150 µg desogestrel and 20 µg ethinylestradiol. Acta Obstet Gynecol Scand 1991;70:497-500.

Lane ME, Arceo R, Sobrero AJ. Successful use of the diaphragm and jelly by a young population: report of a clinical study. Fam Plann Perspect 1976;8:81-86.

Ledger WJ. Ortho 1557-O: a new oral contraceptive. Int J Fertil 1970;15:88-92.

Lehfeldt H, Sivin I. Use effectiveness of the Prentif cervical cap in private practice: a prospective study. Contraception 1984;30:331-338.

Loffer FD, Pent D. Risks of laparoscopic fulguration and transection of the fallopian tube. Obstet Gynecol 1977;49:218-222.

London RS, Chapdelaine A, Upmalis D, Olson W, Smith J. Comparative contraceptive efficacy and mechanism of action of the norgestimate-containing triphasic oral contraceptive. Acta Obstet Gynecol Scand Suppl 1992;156:9-14.

Loudon NB, Barden ME, Hepburn WB, Prescott RJ. A comparative study of the effectiveness and acceptability of the diaphragm used with spermicide in the form of C-film or a cream or jelly. Br J Fam Plann 1991;17:41-44.

Luukkainen T, Allonen H, Haukkamaa M, Holma P, Pyörälä T, Terho J, Toivonen J, Batar I, Lampe L, Andersson K, Atterfeldt P, Johansson EDB, Nilsson S, Nygren KG, Odlind V, Olsson SE, Rybo G, Sikström B, Nielsen NC, Buch A, Osler M, Steier A, Ulstein M. Effective contraception with the levonorgestrel-releasing intrauterine device: 12-month report of a European multicenter study. Contraception 1987;36:169-179.

Margaret Pyke Centre. One thousand vasectomies. Br Med J 1973;4:216-221.

Marshall J. Cervical-mucus and basal body-temperature method of regulating births: field trial. Lancet 1976;2:282-283.

Marshall S, Lyon RP. Variability of sperm disappearance from the ejaculate after vasectomy. J Urol 1972;107:815-817.

Mauck C, Glover LH, Miller E, Allen S, Archer DF, Blumenthal P, Rosenzweig BA, Dominik R, Sturgen K, Cooper J, Fingerhut F, Peacock L, Gabelnick HL. Lea's Shield®: a study of the safety and efficacy of a new vaginal barrier contraceptive used with and without spermicide. Contraception 1996;53:329-335.

McIntyre SL, Higgins JE. Parity and use-effectiveness with the contraceptive sponge. Am J Obstet Gynecol 1986;155:796-801.

McQuarrie HG, Harris JW, Ellsworth HS, Stone RA, Anderson AE. The clinical evaluation of norethindrone in cyclic and continuous regimens. Adv Plann Parent 1972;7:124-130.

Mears E. Chemical contraceptive trial: II. J Reprod Fertil 1962;4:337-343.

Mears E, Please NW. Chemical contraceptive trial. J Reprod Fertil 1962;3:138-147.

Mishell DR, El-Habashy MA, Good RG, Moyer DL. Contraception with an injectable progestin. Am J Obstet Gynecol 1968;101:1046-1053.

Morigi EM, Pasquale SA. Clinical experience with a low dose oral contraceptive containing norethisterone and ethinyl oestradiol. Curr Med Res Opin 1978;5: 655-662.

Moss WM. A comparison of open-end versus closed-end vasectomies: a report on 6220 cases. Contraception 1992;46:521-525.

Mumford SD, Bhiwandiwala PP, Chi IC. Laparoscopic and minilaparotomy female sterilisation compared in 15,167 cases. Lancet 1980;2:1066-1070.

Nelson A, Bernstein GS, Frezieres R, Walsh T, Clark V, Coulson A. Study of the efficacy, acceptability and safety of a non-latex (polyurethane) male condom: revised final report (N01-HD-1-3109). Bethesda MD: National Institute of Child Health and Human Development, September 15, 1997.

Nelson JH. The use of the mini pill in private practice. J Reprod Med 1973;10:139-143.

Peel J. The Hull family survey: II. Family planning in the first five years of marriage. J Biosoc Sci 1972;4:333-346.

Peterson HB, Xia Z, Hughes JM, Wilcox LS, Tylor LR, Trussell J. The risk of pregnancy after tubal sterilization: findings from the U.S. Collaborative Review of Sterilization. Am J Obstet Gynecol 1996;174:1161-1170.

Postlethwaite DL. Pregnancy rate of a progestogen oral contraceptive. Practitioner 1979;222:272-275.

Potts M, McDevitt J. A use-effectiveness trial of spermicidally lubricated condoms. Contraception 1975;11:701-710.

Powell MG, Mears BJ, Deber RB, Ferguson D. Contraception with the cervical cap: effectiveness, safety, continuity of use, and user satisfaction. Contraception 1986;33:215-232.

Preston SN. A report of a collaborative dose-response clinical study using decreasing doses of combination oral contraceptives. Contraception 1972;6:17-35.

Preston SN. A report of the correlation between the pregnancy rates of low estrogen formulations and pill-taking habits of females studied. J Reprod Med 1974;13:75-77.

Rice FJ, Lanctôt CA, Garcia-Devesa C. Effectiveness of the sympto-thermal method of natural family planning: an international study. Int J Fertil 1981;26:222-230.

Richwald GA, Greenland S, Gerber MM, Potik R, Kersey L, Comas MA. Effectiveness of the cavity-rim cervical cap: results of a large clinical study. Obstet Gynecol 1989;74:143-148.

Rovinsky JJ. Clinical effectiveness of a contraceptive cream. Obstet Gynecol 1964;23:125-131.

Royal College of General Practitioners. Oral contraceptives and health. New York NY: Pitman Publishing Corp., 1974.

Runnebaum B, Grunwald K, Rabe T. The efficacy and tolerability of norgestimate/ ethinyl estradiol (250 µg of norgestimate/35 µg of ethinyl estradiol): results of an open, multicenter study of 59,701 women. Am J Obstet Gynecol 1992;166: 1963-1968.

Salomon W, Haase W. Intravaginale kontrazeption. Sexualmedizin 1977;6:198-202.

Sangi-Haghpeykar H, Poindexter AN, Bateman L, Ditmore JR. Experiences of injectable contraceptive users in an urban setting. Obstet Gynecol 1996;88:227-233.

Schirm AL, Trussell J, Menken J, Grady WR. Contraceptive failure in the United States: the impact of social, economic, and demographic factors. Fam Plann Perspect 1982;14:68-75.

Schmidt SS. Vasectomy. JAMA 1988;259:3176.

Schwallie PC, Assenzo JR. Contraceptive use-efficacy study utilizing Depo-Provera administered as an injection once every six months. Contraception 1972;6:315-327.

Schwallie PC, Assenzo JR. Contraceptive use-efficacy study utilizing medroxyprogesterone acetate administered as an intramuscular injection once every 90 days. Fertil Steril 1973;24:331-339.

Scutchfield FD, Long WN, Corey B, Tyler CW. Medroxyprogesterone acetate as an injectable female contraceptive. Contraception 1971;3:21-35.

Sheps MC. An analysis of reproductive patterns in an American isolate. Popul Stud 1965;19:65-80.

Sheth A, Jain U, Sharma S, Adatia A, Patankar S, Andolsek L, Pretnar-Darovec A, Belsey MA, Hall PE, Parker RA, Ayeni S, Pinol A, Foo CLH. A randomized, double-blind study of two combined and two progestogen-only oral contraceptives. Contraception 1982;25:243-252.

Shihata AA, Trussell J. New female intravaginal barrier contraceptive device: preliminary clinical trial. Contraception 1991;44:11-19.

Shroff NE, Pearce MY, Stratford ME, Wilkinson PD. Clinical experience with ethynodiol diacetate 0.5 mg daily as an oral contraceptive. Contraception 1987;35:121-134.

Sivin I. Personal communication to James Trussell, August 13, 1992.

Sivin I, El Mahgoub S, McCarthy T, Mishell DR, Shoupe D, Alvarez F, Brache V, Jimenez E, Diaz J, Faundes A, Diaz MM, Coutinho E, Mattos CER, Diaz S, Pavez M, Stern J. Long-term contraception with the Levonorgestrel 20 mcg/day (LNg 20) and the Copper T 380Ag intrauterine devices: a five-year randomized study. Contraception 1990;42:361-378.

Sivin I, Lähteenmäki P, Ranta S, Darney P, Klaisle C, Wan L, Mishell DR, Lacarra M, Viegas OAC, Bilhareus P, Koetsawang S, Piya-Anant M, Diaz S, Pavez M, Alvarez F, Brache V, LaGuardia K, Nash H, Stern J. Levonorgestrel concentrations during use of levonorgestrel rod (LNG ROD) implants. Contraception 1997a;55:81-85.

Sivin I, Shaaban M, Odlind V, Olsson SE, Diaz S, Pavez M, Alvarez F, Brache V, Diaz J. A randomized trial of the Gyne T 380 and Gyne T 380 Slimline intrauterine copper devices. Contraception 1990;42:379-389.

Sivin I, Stern J. Long-acting, more effective copper T IUDs: a summary of U.S. experience, 1970-1975. Stud Fam Plann 1979;10:263-281.

Sivin I, Viegas O, Campodonico I, Diaz S, Pavez M, Wan L, Koetsawang S, Kiriwat O, Anant MP, Holma P, el din Abdalla K, Stern J. Clinical performance of a new two-rod levonorgestrel contraceptive implant: a three-year randomized study with Norplant® implants as controls. Contraception 1997b;55:73-80.

Smith C, Farr G, Feldblum PJ, Spence A. Effectiveness of the non-spermicidal fit-free diaphragm. Contraception 1995;51:289-291.

Smith GG, Lee RJ. The use of cervical caps at the University of California, Berkeley: a survey. Contraception 1984;30:115-123.

Smith M, Vessey MP, Bounds W, Warren J. C-Film as a contraceptive. Br Med J 1974;4:291.

Squire JJ, Berger GS, Keith L. A retrospective clinical study of a vaginal contraceptive suppository. J Reprod Med 1979;22:319-323.

Stim EM. The nonspermicidal fit-free diaphragm: a new contraceptive method. Adv Plann Parenthood 1980;15:88-98.

Tatum HJ. Comparative experience with newer models of the copper T in the United States. In: Hefnawi F, Segal SJ (eds). Analysis of intrauterine contraception. Amsterdam, The Netherlands: North Holland, 1975:155-163.

Tietze C, Lewit S. Comparison of three contraceptive methods: diaphragm with jelly or cream, vaginal foam, and jelly/cream alone. J Sex Res 1967;3:295-311.

Tietze C, Lewit S. Evaluation of intrauterine devices: ninth progress report of the cooperative statistical program. Stud Fam Plann 1970;1:1-40.

Tietze C, Poliakoff SR, Rock J. The clinical effectiveness of the rhythm method of contraception. Fertil Steril 1951;2:444-450.

Trussell J, Grummer-Strawn L. Contraceptive failure of the ovulation method of periodic abstinence. Fam Plann Perspect 1990;22:65-75.

Trussell J, Hatcher RA, Cates W, Stewart FH, Kost K. Contraceptive failure in the United States: an update. Stud Fam Plann 1990;21:51-54.

Trussell J, Kost K. Contraceptive failure in the United States: a critical review of the literature. Stud Fam Plann 1987;18:237-283.

Tyler ET. Current developments in systemic contraception. Pac Med Surg 1965;93:79-85.

Valle RF, Battifora HA. A new approach to tubal sterilization by laparoscopy. Fertil Steril 1978;30:415-422.

Vaughan B, Trussell J, Menken J, Jones EF. Contraceptive failure among married women in the United States, 1970-1973. Fam Plann Perspect 1977;9:251-258.

Vessey M, Huggins G, Lawless M, McPherson K, Yeates D. Tubal sterilization: findings in a large prospective study. Br J Obstet Gynaecol 1983;90:203-209.

Vessey M, Lawless M, Yeates D. Efficacy of different contraceptive methods. Lancet 1982;1:841-842.

Vessey MP, Lawless M, Yeates D, McPherson K. Progestogen-only oral contraception. Findings in a large prospective study with special reference to effectiveness. Br J Fam Plann 1985;10:117-121.

Vessey MP, Villard-Mackintosh L, McPherson K, Yeates D. Factors influencing use-effectiveness of the condom. Br J Fam Plann 1988;14:40-43.

Vessey M, Wiggins P. Use-effectiveness of the diaphragm in a selected family planning clinic population in the United Kingdom. Contraception 1974;9:15-21.

Vessey MP, Wright NH, McPherson K, Wiggins P. Fertility after stopping different methods of contraception. Br Med J 1978;1:265-267.

Wade ME, McCarthy P, Braunstein GD, Abernathy JR, Suchindran CM, Harris GS, Danzer HC, Uricchio WA. A randomized prospective study of the use-effectiveness of two methods of natural family planning. Am J Obstet Gynecol 1981;141:368-376.

Westoff CF, Potter RG, Sagi PC, Mishler EG. Family growth in metropolitan America. Princeton NJ: Princeton University Press, 1961.

Wolf L, Olson HJ, Tyler ET. Observations on the clinical use of cream-alone and gel-alone methods of contraception. Obstet Gynecol 1957;10:316-321.

World Health Organization. A multicentered phase III comparative clinical trial of depot-medroxyprogesterone acetate given three-monthly at doses of 100 mg or 150 mg: I. Contraceptive efficacy and side effects. Contraception 1986;34:223-235.

World Health Organization. A multicentered phase III comparative study of two hormonal contraceptive preparations given once-a-month by intramuscular injection: I. Contraceptive efficacy and side effects. Contraception 1988;37:1-20.

World Health Organization. A prospective multicentre trial of the ovulation method of natural family planning. II. The effectiveness phase. Fertil Steril 1981;36:591-598.

World Health Organization. Multinational comparative clinical evaluation of two long-acting injectable contraceptive steroids: norethisterone oenanthate and medroxyprogesterone acetate. Contraception 1977;15:513-533.

World Health Organization. Multinational comparative clinical trial of long-acting injectable contraceptives: norethisterone enanthate given in two dosage regimens and depot-medroxyprogesterone acetate. Final report. Contraception 1983;28:1-20.

Woutersz TB. A low-dose combination oral contraceptive: experience with 1,700 women treated for 22,489 cycles. J Reprod Med 1981;26:615-620.

Woutersz TB. A new ultra-low-dose combination oral contraceptive. J Reprod Med 1983;28:81-84.

Wyeth Laboratories. NORPLANT® SYSTEM Prescribing Information. Philadelphia PA: Wyeth Laboratories, December 10, 1990.

Yoon IB, King TM, Parmley TH. A two-year experience with the Falope ring sterilization procedure. Am J Obstet Gynecol 1977;127:109-112.

Table 31-1 Percentage of women experiencing an unintended pregnancy during the first year of typical use and the first year of perfect use of contraception and the percentage continuing use at the end of the first year: United States

Method (1)	% of Women Experiencing an Unintended Pregnancy within the First Year of Use		% of Women Continuing Use at One Year[3] (4)
	Typical Use[1] (2)	Perfect Use[2] (3)	
Chance[4]	85	85	
Spermicides[5]	26	6	40
Periodic Abstinence	25		63
Calendar		9	
Ovulation method		3	
Sympto-thermal[6]		2	
Post-ovulation		1	
Cap[7]			
Parous women	40	26	42
Nulliparous women	20	9	56
Sponge			
Parous Women	40	20	42
Nulliparous Women	20	9	56
Diaphragm[7]	20	6	56
Withdrawal	19	4	
Condom[8]			
Female (Reality)	21	5	56
Male	14	3	61
Pill	5		71
Progestin only		0.5	
Combined		0.1	
IUD			
Progesterone T	2.0	1.5	81
Copper T 380A	0.8	0.6	78
LNg 20	0.1	0.1	81
Depo-Provera	0.3	0.3	70
Norplant and Norplant-2	0.05	0.05	88
Female Sterilization	0.5	0.5	100
Male Sterilization	0.15	0.10	100

Emergency Contraceptive Pills: Treatment initiated within 72 hours after unprotected intercourse reduces the risk of pregnancy by at least 75%.[9]
Lactational Amenorrhea Method: LAM is a highly effective, *temporary* method of contraception.[10]

(continued)

Table 31-1 Percentage of women experiencing an unintended pregnancy during the first year of typical use and the first year of perfect use of contraception and the percentage continuing use at the end of the first year: United States

Source: Updated from Trussell and Kost (1987) and Trussell et al. (1990b). See text.

[1]Among *typical* couples who initiate use of a method (not necessarily for the first time), the percentage who experience an accidental pregnancy during the first year if they do not stop use for any other reason.

[2]Among couples who initiate use of a method (not necessarily for the first time) and who use it *perfectly* (both consistently and correctly), the percentage who experience an accidental pregnancy during the first year if they do not stop use for any other reason.

[3]Among couples attempting to avoid pregnancy, the percentage who continue to use a method for one year.

[4]The percentages becoming pregnant in columns (2) and (3) are based on data from populations where contraception is not used and from women who cease using contraception in order to become pregnant. Among such populations, about 89% become pregnant within one year. This estimate was lowered slightly (to 85%) to represent the percentage who would become pregnant within one year among women now relying on reversible methods of contraception if they abandoned contraception altogether.

[5]Foams, creams, gels, vaginal suppositories, and vaginal film.

[6]Cervical mucus (ovulation) method supplemented by calendar in the pre-ovulatory and basal body temperature in the post-ovulatory phases.

[7]With spermicidal cream or jelly.

[8]Without spermicides.

[9]The treatment schedule is one dose within 72 hours after unprotected intercourse, and a second dose 12 hours after the first dose. The Food and Drug Administration has declared the following brands of oral contraceptives to be safe and effective for emergency contraception: Ovral (1 dose is 2 white pills), Alesse (1 dose is 5 pink pills), Nordette or Levlen (1 dose is 4 light-orange pills), Lo/Ovral (1 dose is 4 white pills), Triphasil or Tri-Levlen (1 dose is 4 yellow pills).

[10]However, to maintain effective protection against pregnancy, another method of contraception must be used as soon as menstruation resumes, the frequency or duration of breastfeeds is reduced, bottle feeds are introduced, or the baby reaches 6 months of age.

Table 31-2 Summary of studies of pregnancy rates among women neither contracepting nor breastfeeding[a]

Reference	N for Analysis	Life Table 12-Month % Pregnant	Characteristics of the Sample	LFU (%)[g]	Comments
Grady et al., 1986	1,028	43.1	All married	20.6[f]	1982 NSFG; estimate far too low; see text
Sivin and Stern, 1979	420	78.1	48% nulliparous	?	Following removal of copper-medicated IUD for planned pregnancy
Vessey et al., 1978	779	82	All nulligravid	?	Britain; Oxford/FPA study following cessation of method use for planned pregnancy; conceptions leading to a live birth
Tatum, 1975	553	84.6		17.2	Following removal of copper-medicated IUD for planned pregnancy
Sivin, 1987	96	87	All parous	?	Chile, Dominican Republic, Finland, Sweden, United States; following removal of Norplant for planned pregnancy
Tietze and Lewit, 1970	378	88.2	89% aged 15–29	19.0	Following removal of nonmedicated IUD for planned pregnancy
Sheps, 1965	397	88.8	All married Hutterites	?	Conceptions leading to the first live birth following marriage among women reporting no fetal losses before the first conception
Vessey et al., 1978	1,343	89	All parous	?	Britain; Oxford/FPA study following cessation of method use for planned pregnancy; conceptions leading to a live birth
Belhadj et al., 1986	110	94.0[c]	All parous; aged 18–36	9.1	Brazil, Chile, Dominican Republic, Singapore, United States; following removal of medicated IUD for planned pregnancy

Notes:

[a] Updated from Trussell and Kost (1987), Table 1.

[c] Calculated by James Trussell from data in the article.

[g] Most of these studies incorrectly report the loss to follow-up probability as the number of women lost at any time during the study divided by the total number of women entering the study. Thus, these are the probabilities presented in the table. However, the correct measure of LFU would be a gross life-table probability. When available, gross 12-month probabilities are denoted by the letter "g."

[f] Nonresponse rate for entire survey.

For table references, see reference section.

Table 31-3 Summary of studies of contraceptive failure: spermicides[a]

Reference	Method Brand	N for Analysis	Risk of Pregnancy					Characteristics of the Sample	LFU (%)[g]	Comments
			Life-Table 12-Month % Pregnant	Pearl Index Pregnancy Rate						
				Index	Total Exposure	Maximum Exposure				
Edelman, 1980	S'positive	200		0.0	2,682 Mo.	?			?	Study conducted by Jordan-Simner, Inc., as reported by Edelman
Squire et al., 1979	Semicid Suppository	326	0.3					69% aged 20–34; 55% married; "well educated"; "highly motivated"; 24% prior use of oral contraceptives	0.0[c]	89% reported exclusive use of foam
Soloman and Haase, 1977	Patentex (Encare) Oval	1,652		0.3[c]	34,506 Cy.	54 Mo.		13% aged 15–20, 48% aged 21–30, 33% aged 31–40, 6% aged 41–45, 42% nulliparous	?	Subjects who used for less than one year excluded? Germany
Iizuka et al., 1980	Vaginal Contraceptive Film (C-Film)	168		0.6	2,161 Mo.	?		All women had been pregnant before; 20% aged <25, 64% aged 25–34, 17% aged 35+	?	Japan
Brehm and Haase, 1975	Patentex (Encare) Oval	10,017		0.9[c]	63,759 Cy.	?		18% aged <21, 20% aged >35; 46% parity 0	?	Germany; FDA rejected this study because of flawed design (see text)
Florence, 1977	a-gen 53	103		1.2[c]	2,255 Cy.	61 Mo.		17% aged 17–20, 51% aged 21–30, 20% aged 31–40, 12% aged 41+	?	Belgium
Dimpfl et al., 1984	Patentex (Encare) Oval	482	1.5					22% aged <21, 25% aged >31; 44% parity 0; 60% married	?	Denmark, Germany, Poland, Switzerland

(continued)

Table 31-3 Summary of studies of contraceptive failure: spermicides[a] *(cont.)*

Reference	Method Brand	N for Analysis	Life-Table 12-Month % Pregnant	Pearl Index Index	Pearl Index Total Exposure	Pearl Index Maximum Exposure	Characteristics of the Sample	LFU (%)[g]	Comments
Bushnell, 1965	Emko Vaginal Foam	130		1.8	2,737 Mo.	57 Mo.	Aged 17–51; 76% aged 20–35	?	
Godts, 1973	a-gen 53	56		1.9[c]	1,344 Cy.	32 Mo.	21% aged 18–20, 46% aged 21–30, 18% aged 31–40, 14% aged 41+; all gravid	?	
Carpenter and Martin, 1970	Emko Pre-fil Vaginal Foam	1,778		3.4[c]	17,200 Cy.	18 Cy.	69% aged 21–35; 24% ≥12 years education; 44% no previous contraceptive experience	14.2[c]	All women agreed to exclusive use of foam
Brigato et al., 1982	Vaginal Contraceptive Film (C-Film)	37		3.9[c]	924 Mo.	?		?	Italy
Wolf et al., 1957	Preceptin Vaginal Gel	112		4.2[c]	1,145 Mo.	29 Mo.	All aged 13–40; mean age = 25[i]; all married	8.9[c]	
Bernstein, 1971	Emko Pre-fil Vaginal Foam	2,932		4.3[c]	28,332 Cy.	20 Cy.	70% aged 21–35; 39% ≥12 years education	16.1[c]	All women agreed to exclusive use of foam
Tyler, 1965	Delfen Vaginal Foam	672		6.0	9,486 Cy.	>16 Mo.	Rates for full applicator doses and half doses combined	?	
Apothecus, 1992	Vaginal Contraceptive Film (C-Film)	761		6.5	6,501 Mo.	?			Belgium, Netherlands, Britain, Germany, Switzerland, Denmark, Sweden, Israel, Egypt; results never published; quality of study unknown

(continued)

Table 31-3 Summary of studies of contraceptive failure: spermicides[a] *(cont.)*

Reference	Method Brand	N for Analysis	Life-Table 12-Month % Pregnant	Pearl Index	Total Exposure	Maximum Exposure	Characteristics of the Sample	LFU (%)[g]	Comments
			Risk of Pregnancy						
				Pearl Index Pregnancy Rate					
Kleppinger, 1965	Delfen Vaginal Foam	138		7.5	1,116 Mo.	19 Mo.	53% aged 21–30; 27% postpartum	0.0[c,g]	
Dubrow and Kuder, 1958	Delfen Vaginal Cream	338		7.6	633 Mo.	12 Mo.	Mean age = 25; 93% ≤12 years education; 39% black; 45% Puerto Rican[i]	59.5[c]	
Dubrow and Kuder, 1958	Preceptin Vaginal Gel	835		8.1	3,728 Mo.	23 Mo.	Mean age = 25; 93% ≤12 years education; 39% black; 45% Puerto Rican[i]	45.1[c]	
Wolf et al., 1957	Delfen Vaginal Cream	875		8.9[c]	5,232 Mo.	30 Mo.	All aged 13–40; mean age = 25[t]; all married	13.0[c]	
Frankman et al., 1975	Vaginal Contraceptive Film (C-Film)	237		9.0	1,866 Mo.	23 Mo.		?	Sweden; data included in Apothecus (1992)
Rovinsky, 1964	Delfen Vaginal Cream	251		9.1	2,915 Mo.	67 Mo.	70% aged 20–34; 55% Puerto Rican; 10% ≥13 years education	28.0[c]	
Vessey et al., 1982		?		11.9	303 Yr.	?	All white; at recruitment aged 25–39 and married; at enrollment, all women had been using the diaphragm, IUD, or pill successfully for at least 5 months	0.3[t,v]	Britain; Oxford/FPA study

(continued)

Table 31-3 Summary of studies of contraceptive failure: spermicides[a] *(cont.)*

Reference	Method Brand	N for Analysis	Risk of Pregnancy					Characteristics of the Sample	LFU (%)[g]	Comments
			Life-Table 12-Month % Pregnant	Pearl Index Pregnancy Rate						
				Index	Total Exposure	Maximum Exposure				
Jones and Forrest, 1992		267	13.4					Aged 15–44[t]	21[r]	NSFG 1988; probability when standardized and corrected for estimated underreporting of abortion = 30.2[s]
Vaughan et al., 1977		596	14.9[s]					Aged 15–44; all married[t]	19.0[r]	NSFG 1973
Grady et al., 1983		1,106	17.5[s,c]					Aged 15–44; all married[t]	18.2[r]	NSFG 1973 and 1976
Schirm et al., 1982		1,106	17.9[s]					Aged 15–44; all married[t]	18.2[r]	NSFG 1973 and 1976
Mears, 1962	Emko Aerosol Foam (nonoxynol 10-11)	425		18.0[c]	722 Cy.	3 Cy.		Pearl index of 9.3 among consistent and 48.4 among inconsistent users	>20[c,t]	Britain; postal trial; random assignment to foam, foaming tablet, or pessary with crossover design
Kasabach, 1962	Koromex A Jelly	242		21.0[c]	2,058 Mo.	24 Mo.		36% aged 25–35; all married; 68% "had a high school education"; all parous	19.3[c]	
Bracher and Santow, 1992		89	21.5					27% aged <20, 56% aged 20–29, 17% aged 30+; 49% parity 0; 87% married or cohabiting	25[r]	Australian Family Survey; first use of method

(continued)

Table 31-3 Summary of studies of contraceptive failure: spermicides[a] *(cont.)*

			Risk of Pregnancy						
			Life-Table 12-Month % Pregnant	Pearl Index Pregnancy Rate					
Reference	Method Brand	N for Analysis		Index	Total Exposure	Maximum Exposure	Characteristics of the Sample	LFU (%)[g]	Comments
Grady et al., 1986		284	21.8[s]				Aged 15–44; all married[t]	20.6[r]	NSFG 1982
Frank, 1962	Koromex A Jelly	824		24.8[c]	5,767 Mo.	12 Mo.	72% aged 21–35	17.0[c]	
Dingle and Tietze, 1963	Lactikol	170		23.5	1,789 Mo.	36 Mo.	Median age = 24.5	3.2[t]	
Tietze and Lewit, 1967	Emko Vaginal Foam	779	28.3				86% < age 30; all married; 47% ≥ high school completion; 75% nonwhite	6.9[g]	
Dingle and Tietze, 1963	Durafoam	421		28.5	2,985 Mo.	36 Mo.	Median age = 26.1	3.2[t]	
Mears, 1962	Genexol Pessary (nonoxynol 10-11)	425		30.3	730 Cy.	3 Cy.		>20[c,t]	Britain; postal trial; random assignment to foam, foaming tablets, or pessary with crossover design
Tietze and Lewit, 1967	Cooper Creme and Creme Jel, Koromex A, Lactikol Creme and Jelly, Lanesta Gel	806	36.8				79% < age 30; all married; 53% ≥ high school completion; 75% nonwhite	3.4[g]	
Mears, 1962	Volpar Foaming Tablets (phenyl mercuric acetate)	425		48.2[c]	728 Cy.	3 Cy.	Pearl index of 44.4 among consistent and 64.1 among inconsistent users	>20[c,t]	Britain; postal trial; random assignment to foam, foaming tablet, or pessary with crossover design

(continued)

Table 31-3 Summary of studies of contraceptive failure: spermicides[a] *(cont.)*

Reference	Method Brand	N for Analysis	Life-Table 12-Month % Pregnant	Pearl Index Pregnancy Rate Index	Total Exposure	Maximum Exposure	Characteristics of the Sample	LFU (%)[g]	Comments
				Risk of Pregnancy					
Mears and Please, 1962	Staycept Cream (hexyl resorcinol)	678		49.6[c]	707 Cy.	3 Cy.	Pearl index of 31.4 among consistent and 132.0 among inconsistent users	>41[c,t]	Britain; postal trial; random assignment to cream, foaming tablet, or pessary with crossover design
Mears and Please, 1962	Genexol Pessary (quinine)	678		52.2	647 Cy.	3 Cy.		>41[c,t]	Britain; postal trial; random assignment to cream, foaming tablet, or pessary with crossover design
Smith et al., 1974	Vaginal Contraceptive Film (C-Film)	63[c]		55.7[c]	194[c] Mo.	<15[c] Mo.	Aged 16–35	9.5[c]	Britain; trial terminated for ethical reasons

(continued)

| | | | Risk of Pregnancy | | | | | | |
| | | | Pearl Index Pregnancy Rate | | | | | | |
Reference	Method Brand	N for Analysis	Life-Table 12-Month % Pregnant	Index	Total Exposure	Maximum Exposure	Characteristics of the Sample	LFU (%)[g]	Comments
Mears and Please, 1962	Volpar Foaming Tablets (phenyl mercuric acetate)	678		59.0[c]	705 Cy.	3 Cy.	Pearl index of 47.8 among consistent and 106.7 among inconsistent users	>41[c,t]	Britain; postal trial; random assignment to cream, foaming tablet, or pessary with crossover design

Notes:

[a] Updated from Trussell and Kost (1987), Table 2.

[c] Calculated by James Trussell from data in the article.

[g] Most of these studies incorrectly report the loss to follow-up probability (LFU) as the number of women lost at any time during the study divided by the total number of women entering the study. Thus, these are the probabilities presented in the table. However, the correct measure of LFU would be a gross life-table probability. When available, gross 12-month probabilities are denoted by the letter "g."

[i] Nonresponse rate for entire survey.

[s] Standardized: Vaughan et al., (1977) (1973 NSFG)—intention (the average of probabilities for preventers and delayers); Grady et al., (1983) (1973 and 1976 NSFG)—intention. Our calculation (the average of probabilities for preventers and delayers); Schirm et al., (1982) (1973 and 1976 NSFG)—intention, age, and income; Grady et al., (1986) (1982 NSFG)—intention, age, poverty status, and parity; Jones and Forrest (1992) (1988 NSFG)—duration, age, marital status, and poverty status.

[t] Total for all methods in the study.

[v] The authors report that LFU for "relevant reasons (withdrawal of cooperation or loss of contact)" was 0.3% per year in the 1982 study. In the 1982 study, women had been followed for 9.5 years on average; if 0.3% are LFU per year, then 2.8% would be LFU in 9.5 years. LFU including death and emigration is about twice as high as LFU for "relevant reasons."

For table references, see reference section.

Table 31-4 Summary of studies of contraceptive failure: periodic abstinence[a]

Reference	Method	N for Analysis	Life-Table 12-Month % Pregnant	Risk of Pregnancy / Pearl Index Pregnancy Rate — Index	Total Exposure	Maximum Exposure	Characteristics of the Sample	LFU (%)[g]	Comments
Trussell and Grummer-Strawn, 1990	Ovulation	725	3.2				Mean age = 30; proven fertility; agreed to use OM alone; cohabiting; 765 of 869 learned OM to satisfaction of teachers; 725 entered effectiveness study	?	Reanalysis of W.H.O. (1981) trial; probability based on 13 cycles of *perfect* use
Rice et al., 1981	Calendar + BBT	723	8.2				Aged 19–44; 9% aged 19–24, 54% aged 25–34, 37% aged 35–44; all parity 1+	3.4[c]	United States, France, Colombia, Canada, Mauritius
Dolack, 1978	Ovulation	329		10.5[c]	3,354 Cy.	?	Aged 19–48; mean age = 28; 40% had used oral contraceptives prior to study	18.0[c]	
Johnston et al., 1978	Cervical Mucus + BBT + Other Signs	268	13.3[c]				73% aged 22–32; all married or de facto married; 48% ≥12 years education (n = 460)	33.9[c,f]	Australia; probability based on 13 cycles
Wade et al., 1981	Cervical Mucus + BBT + Calendar	239	13.9[c]				Aged 20–39; 78% married	11.4[c,g]	Random assignment to OM or CM + BBT + Cal
Johnston et al., 1978	Calendar + BBT + Other Signs	192	14.3				73% aged 22–32; all married or de facto married; 48% ≥12 years education (n = 460)	33.9[c,f]	Australia; probability based on 13 cycles
Tietze et al., 1951	Calendar	409		14.4	7,267 Mo.	>60 Mo.	57% aged 25–34	13.4[c,f]	

(continued)

Table 31-4 Summary of studies of contraceptive failure: periodic abstinence[a] (cont.)

			Risk of Pregnancy					
				Pearl Index Pregnancy Rate				
			Life-Table 12-Month % Pregnant		Total Exposure	Maximum Exposure		
Reference	Method	N for Analysis		Index			Characteristics of the Sample	LFU (%)[g]	Comments
Vessey et al., 1982	Rhythm	?		15.5	161 Yr.	?	All white; at recruitment aged 25–39 and married; at enrollment, all women had been using the diaphragm, IUD, or pill successfully for at least 5 months	0.3[t,v]	Britain; Oxford/FPA study
Klaus et al., 1979	Ovulation	?	15.8[n]				67% aged 18–34; 52% ≥13 years education; some use of concurrent methods	2.9[n]	Probability based on only 12 cycles
Johnston et al., 1978	Cervical Mucus + BBT + Other Signs + Other Methods	94	16.0				78% aged 22–32; all married or de facto married; 53% ≥12 years education ("other" not limited to rhythm)	33.9[c,t]	Australia; probability based on 13 cycles
Grady et al., 1986	Rhythm	167	16.1[s]				Aged 15–44; all married[t]	20.6[r]	NSFG 1982
Ball, 1976	Ovulation	124		16.8[c]	1,626 Cy.	22 Cy.	Aged 20–39	1.6[c]	Australia
Bracher and Santow, 1992	Rhythm	137	17.9				14% aged <20, 75% aged 20–29, 11% aged 30+; 46% parity 0; 92% married or cohabiting	25[r]	Australian Family Survey; first use of method
Kambic et al., 1981, 1982	Ovulation or Cervical Mucus + BBT	235	18.2[n]				81% aged 20–34; 83% married; approx. 30% used barrier methods concurrently[t]	6.5[n]	
Grady et al., 1983	Rhythm	412	18.3[s,c]				Aged 15–44; all married[t]	18.2[r]	NSFG 1973 and 1976

(continued)

Table 31-4

Table 31-4 Summary of studies of contraceptive failure: periodic abstinence[a] (cont.)

Reference	Method	N for Analysis	Risk of Pregnancy				Characteristics of the Sample	LFU (%)[g]	Comments
			Life-Table 12-Month % Pregnant	Pearl Index Pregnancy Rate					
				Index	Total Exposure	Maximum Exposure			
Johnston et al., 1978	Ovulation + Other Methods	71	18.8				80% aged 22–32; all married or de facto married; 49% ≥12 years education ("other" not limited to rhythm)	33.9[c,t]	Australia; probability based on 13 cycles
Vaughan et al., 1977	Rhythm	220	19.1[s]				Aged 15–44; all married[l]	19.0[r]	NSFG 1973
W.H.O., 1981	Ovulation	725	19.6				Mean age about 30; proven fertility; agreed to use OM alone; 54% desired no more children; 765 of 869 learned OM to satisfaction of teachers; 725 entered effectiveness study	?	New Zealand, India, Ireland, Philippines, El Salvador; probability based on 13 cycles
Jones and Forrest, 1992	Rhythm	289	20.9				Aged 15–44[t]	21[r]	NSFG 1988; probability when standardized and corrected for estimated underreporting of abortion = 31.4[s]
Bartzen, 1967	BBT	335		21.3[c]	4,824 Cy.	58 Mo.	Aged 19–45; mean age = 28	11.6[c]	
Schirm et al., 1982	Rhythm	412	23.7[s]				Aged 15–44; all married[l]	18.2[r]	NSFG 1973 and 1976
Marshall, 1976	Ovulation + BBT	84		23.9[c]	1,195 Cy.	32 Mo.	67% aged 20–34	1.2[c]	Britain
Johnston et al., 1978	Ovulation	586	26.4				69% aged 22–32; all married or de facto married; 44% ≥12 years education	33.9[c,t]	Australia; probability based on 13 cycles

(continued)

Table 31-4 Summary of studies of contraceptive failure: periodic abstinence[a] (cont.)

Reference	Method	N for Analysis	Risk of Pregnancy					Characteristics of the Sample	LFU (%)[g]	Comments
			Life-Table 12-Month % Pregnant	Pearl Index Pregnancy Rate						
				Index	Total Exposure	Maximum Exposure				
Wade et al., 1981	Ovulation	191	37.2[c]					Aged 20–39; 74% married	13.8[c-g]	Random assignment to OM or CM + BBT + Cal

Notes:

[a] Updated from Trussell and Kost (1987), Table 3.

[c] Calculated by James Trussell from data in the article.

[g] Most of these studies incorrectly report the loss to follow-up probability (LFU) as the number of women lost at any time during the study divided by the total number of women entering the study. Thus, these are the probabilities presented in the table. However, the correct measure of LFU would be a gross life-table probability. When available, gross 12-month probabilities are denoted by the letter "g."

[h] Only net probabilities available for this study.

[i] Nonresponse rate for entire survey.

[s] Standardized: Vaughan et al., (1977) (1973 NSFG)—intention (the average of probabilities for preventers and delayers); Grady et al., (1983) (1973 and 1976 NSFG)—intention. Our calculation (the average of probabilities for preventers and delayers); Schirm et al., (1982) (1973 and 1976 NSFG)—intention, age, and income; Grady et al., (1986) (1982 NSFG)—intention, age, poverty status, and parity; Jones and Forrest (1992) (1988 NSFG)—duration, age, marital status, and poverty status.

[t] Total for all methods in the study.

[v] The authors report that LFU for "relevant reasons (withdrawal of cooperation or loss of contact)" was 0.3% per year in the 1982 study. In the 1982 study, women had been followed for 9.5 years on average; if 0.3% are LFU per year, then 2.8% would be LFU in 9.5 years. LFU including death and emigration is about twice as high as LFU for "relevant reasons."

For table references, see reference section.

Table 31-5 Summary of studies of contraceptive failure: cervical cap and other female barrier methods with spermicide[a]

Reference	Method Brand	N for Analysis	Life-Table 12-Month % Pregnant	Pearl Index Pregnancy Rate — Index	Pearl Index Pregnancy Rate — Total Exposure	Pearl Index Pregnancy Rate — Maximum Exposure	Characteristics of the Sample	LFU (%)[g]	Comments
Shihata and Trussell, 1991	Fem Cap	106	4.8					0.0[g]	Probability based on 13 cycles
Denniston and Putney, 1981	Prentif Cavity-rim	110	8.0[b,n]				98% aged 20–35; 70% nulliparous	20.9[c]	
Cagen, 1986	Prentif Cavity-rim	620	8.1[n]				87% aged 20–34; 80% always used spermicide and 14% never did	38.5[c]	LFU = "no response"
Koch, 1982	Prentif Cavity-rim	372	8.4				76% aged 20–29; 65% college graduates	8.0[c]	Women advised also to use condom for the first several cap uses
Mauck et al., 1996	Lea's Shield	79	8.7[b]				Mean age = 29.6; mean education = 14.2 years; 19% nulliparous	6.4[b,g]	
Richwald et al., 1989	Prentif Cavity-rim	3,433	11.3				Mean age 29.0; 91% white non-Hispanic; 80% unmarried; almost 60% college graduates; 64% one or more previous pregnancies; 6.1% failure rate among perfect users, 11.9% among imperfect users	18[g]	Women advised to use extra spermicide or use condoms during first 2 months of use; 15 sites; 14 in Los Angeles, 1 in Santa Fe

(continued)

Table 31-5 Summary of studies of contraceptive failure: cervical cap and other female barrier methods with spermicide[a] *(cont.)*

			Risk of Pregnancy						
			Life-Table 12-Month	**Pearl Index Pregnancy Rate**					
Reference	**Method Brand**	**N for Analysis**	**% Pregnant**	**Index**	**Total Exposure**	**Maximum Exposure**	**Characteristics of the Sample**	**LFU (%)[g]**	**Comments**
Powell et al., 1986	Prentif Cavity-rim and Vimule	477	16.6				67% aged 25–34 "about half" unmarried; 97% high school graduates; 17% using the pill when fitted for cap	43.8[c]	Canada; back-up methods encouraged (including the emergency contraceptive pills used by 23 women in cases of cap dislodgement)
Bernstein et al., 1986	Prentif Cavity-rim	687[c]	17.4				95% aged ≤35, 16% married, 96% ≥ high school completion	26.3[c,g]	Random assignment to the diaphragm or cervical cap
Kassell and McElroy, 1981	Prentif Cavity-rim	90		18.1[c]	731 Mo.	12 Mo.	Mean age = 23.6; mean education = 14.7 years	10.0[c]	
Boehm, 1983	Prentif Cavity-rim	47		18.1[c]	397 Mo.	12 Mo.		31.6	All women reported exclusive use of cap
Lehfeldt and Sivin, 1984	Prentif Cavity-rim	130	19.1				37% aged 16–25; 72% college graduates; 91% nulliparous	7.2[c]	All women agreed to exclusive use of cap

(continued)

Table 31-5 Summary of studies of contraceptive failure: cervical cap and other female barrier methods with spermicide[a] *(cont.)*

Reference	Method Brand	N for Analysis	Risk of Pregnancy				Characteristics of the Sample	LFU (%)[g]	Comments
			Life-Table 12-Month % Pregnant	Pearl Index Pregnancy Rate					
				Index	Total Exposure	Maximum Exposure			
Smith and Lee, 1984	Prentif Cavity-rim and Vimule	33	27.0				80% aged 20–29; clients at university student health service	1.5–4.6[c]	Regular users for whom the cap (with spermicide) was the sole method used "during the fertile portion of the cycle"

Notes:
[a]Updated from Trussell and Kost (1987), Table 4.
[b]6-month net probability; 12-month probability not available.
[c]Calculated by James Trussell from data in the article.
[g]Most of these studies incorrectly report the loss to follow-up (LFU) probability as the number of women lost at any time during the study divided by the total number of women entering the study. Thus, these are the probabilities presented in the table. However, the correct measure of LFU would be a gross life-table probability. When available, gross 12-month probabilities are denoted by the letter "g."
[n]Only net probabilities available for this study.
For table references, see reference section.

Table 31-6 Summary of studies of contraceptive failure: sponge[a]

Reference	N for Analysis	Life-Table 12-Month % Pregnant	Characteristics of the Sample	LFU (%)[g]	Comments
Jones and Forrest, 1992	227	14.5	Aged 15–44[t]	21[t]	NSFG 1988
Edelman et al., 1984	722	17.0	89% aged 20–34, 28% married; 77% ≥13 years education; 94% white, 49% never-married; 38% used oral contraceptives prior to entering study	33.2[c,g]	Random assignment to the diaphragm or sponge
McIntyre and Higgins, 1986	723	17.4	89% aged 20–34, 28% married; 77% ≥13 years education; 94% white, 49% never-married; 38% used oral contraceptives prior to entering study	33.2[c,g]	A reanalysis of data used by Edelman et al. (1984); random assignment to the diaphragm or sponge; much higher probability for parous women
Bounds and Guillebaud, 1984	126	24.5	92% aged 20–34; all married/consensual union; "most" ≥13 years education; 99% white	1.7[g]	Britain; random assignment to the diaphragm or sponge

Notes:

[a] Updated from Trussell and Kost (1987), Table 4.

[c] Calculated by James Trussell from data in the article.

[g] Most of these studies incorrectly report the loss to follow-up (LFU) probability as the number of women lost at any time during the study divided by the total number of women entering the study. Thus, these are the probabilities presented in the table. However, the correct measure of LFU would be a gross life-table probability. When available, gross 12-month probabilities are denoted by the letter "g."

[r] Nonresponse rate for entire survey.

[t] Total for all methods in the study.

For table references, see reference section.

Table 31-7 Summary of studies of contraceptive failure: diaphragm with spermicide[a]

Reference	N for Analysis	Risk of Pregnancy				Characteristics of the Sample	LFU (%)[g]	Comments
		Life-Table 12-Month % Pregnant	Pearl Index Pregnancy Rate					
			Index	Total Exposure	Maximum Exposure			
Stim, 1980	1,238		1.1[c]	911 Yr.	4 Yr.	Median age = 24	19.5	Fit-free diaphragm without spermicides; continuous wearing with brief daily removal for cleaning but not within 6 hours after intercourse; 1,238 women given device, with follow-up of 997
Lane et al., 1976	2,168	2.1[c]				61% aged 21–34; 71% unmarried; 92% white	1.2[c-g]	Probability downward biased due to improper exposure allocated to women LFU
Vessey and Wiggins, 1974	4,052		2.4	5,909 Mo.	>60 Mo.	All white; at recruitment aged 25–39 and married; all had been using the diaphragm for at least 5 months at enrollment; no previous pill use	1.0[v]	Britain; Oxford/FPA study
Vessey et al., 1982	?		5.5	2,582 Yr.	24 Mo.	All white and aged 25–34; all married at recruitment; at enrollment, all women had been using the diaphragm, IUD, or pill successfully for at least 5 months	0.3[l,v]	Britain; Oxford/FPA study
Loudon et al., 1991	269		8.7	2,350 Mo.	12 Mo.	Mean age = 28.6; 57% gravidity 0; 68% married or cohabiting; 54% already using the diaphragm at start of trial	>3.7	Britain; random assignment of spermicide: either C-Film or jelly

(continued)

Table 31-7 Summary of studies of contraceptive failure: diaphragm with spermicide[a] (cont.)

Reference	N for Analysis	Risk of Pregnancy				Characteristics of the Sample	LFU (%)[g]	Comments
		Life-Table 12-Month % Pregnant	Pearl Index Pregnancy Rate					
			Index	Total Exposure	Maximum Exposure			
Dubrow and Kuder, 1958	873		9.3	5,814 Mo.	48 Mo.	Mean age = 25; 39% black; 45% Puerto Rican; 93% ≤12 years education[f]	38.0[c]	
Jones and Forrest, 1992	472	10.4				Aged 15–44[f]	21[f]	NSFG 1988; probability when standardized and corrected for estimated under-reporting of abortion = 22.0[s]
Hall, 1973	347	10.6				Approximately 75% aged 20–24; 47% black; 38% Hispanic; all postpartum	16.0	
Bounds and Guillebaud, 1984	123	10.9				90% aged 20–34; all married/consensual union; "most" ≥13 years education; 96% white	0.0	Britain; random assignment to the diaphragm or sponge
Edelman et al., 1984	717	12.5				88% aged 20–34; 55% never married; 76% ≥13 years education; 94% white; 39% used oral contraceptives prior to entering study	37.8[c-g]	Random assignment to the diaphragm or sponge
McIntyre and Higgins, 1986	717	12.9				88% aged 20–34; 55% never married; 76% ≥13 years education; 94% white; 39% used oral contraceptives prior to entering study	37.8[c-g]	A reanalysis of data used by Edelman et al. (1984); random assignment to the diaphragm or sponge
Vaughan et al., 1977	166	13.1[s]				Aged 15–44; all married[f]	19.0[f]	NSFG 1973

(continued)

Table 31-7 **819**

Table 31-7 Summary of studies of contraceptive failure: diaphragm with spermicide[a] (cont.)

Reference	N for Analysis	Risk of Pregnancy				Characteristics of the Sample	LFU (%)[g]	Comments
		Life-Table 12-Month % Pregnant	Pearl Index Pregnancy Rate					
			Index	Total Exposure	Maximum Exposure			
Dingle and Tietze, 1963	189		14.3	2,012 Mo.	36 Mo.	Median age = 22.8	3.2[t]	
Grady et al., 1983	349	14.3[c,s]				Aged 15–44; all married[t]	18.2[t]	NSFG 1973 and 1976
Bernstein et al., 1986	707[c]	16.7				96% aged ≤35; 17% married; 97% ≥ high school completion	33.5[c,g]	Random assignment to the diaphragm or cervical cap
Grady et al., 1986	257	17.0[s]				Aged 15–44; all married[t]	20.6[t]	NSFG 1982
Tietze and Lewit, 1967	1,197	17.9				86% aged <30; all married; 60% ≥ high school completion; 50% white	7.2[g]	
Schirm et al., 1982	349	18.6[s]				Aged 15–44; all married[t]	18.2[t]	NSFG 1973 and 1976
Kovacs et al., 1986	324	20.9[t]				28% aged 24–26	52.2	Australia
Bracher and Santow, 1992	219	21.0				12% aged <20; 77% aged 20–29, 11% aged 30+; 56% parity 0; 87% married or cohabiting	25[t]	Australian Family Survey; first use of method
Bounds et al., 1995	80	21.2				Mean age = 29.6; 60% nulliparous	1.3	Britain; probability during consistent use = 12.3; random assignment to diaphragm with spermicide or diaphragm only
Smith et al., 1995	110	24.1				Mean age = 28.8	26.0	Britain; fit-free diaphragm without spermicide; continuous wearing with brief daily removal for cleaning but not within 6 hours after intercourse

(continued)

Table 31-7 Summary of studies of contraceptive failure: diaphragm with spermicide[a] *(cont.)*

| | | Risk of Pregnancy | | | | | | |
| | | Life-Table | Pearl Index Pregnancy Rate | | | | | |
Reference	N for Analysis	12-Month % Pregnant	Index	Total Exposure	Maximum Exposure	Characteristics of the Sample	LFU (%)[g]	Comments
Bounds et al., 1995	84	28.6				Mean age = 29.5; 55% nulliparous	0.0[g]	Britain; diaphragm without spermicide; probability during consistent use = 19.3; random assignment to diaphragm only or diaphragm with spermicide

Notes:

[a]Updated from Trussell and Kost (1987), Table 5.

[c]Calculated by James Trussell from data in the article.

[g]Most of these studies incorrectly report the loss to follow-up (LFU) probability as the number of women lost at any time during the study divided by the total number of women entering the study. Thus, these are the probabilities presented in the table. However, the correct measure of LFU would be a gross life-table probability. When available, gross 12-month probabilities are denoted by the letter "g."

[i]Nonresponse rate for entire survey.

[s]Standardized: Vaughan et al., (1977) (1973 NSFG)—intention (the average of probabilities for preventers and delayers); Grady et al., (1983) (1973 and 1976 NSFG)—intention. Our calculation (the average of probabilities for preventers and delayers); Schirm et al., (1982) (1973 and 1976 NSFG)—intention, age, and income; Grady et al., (1986) (1982 NSFG)—intention, age, poverty status, and parity; Jones and Forrest (1992) (1988 NSFG)—duration, age, marital status, and poverty status.

[t]Total for all methods in the study.

[v]The authors report that LFU for "relevant reasons (withdrawal of cooperation or loss of contact)" was 0.3% per year in the 1982 study and "about 10 per 1,000" per year in the 1974 study. In the 1982 study, women had been followed for 9.5 years on average; if 0.3% are LFU per year, then 2.8% would be LFU in 9.5 years. LFU including death and emigration is about twice as high as LFU for "relevant reasons."

For table references, see reference section.

Table 31-8 Summary of studies of contraceptive failure: withdrawal

Reference	N for Analysis	Life-Table 12-Month % Pregnant	Pearl Index Pregnancy Rate			Characteristics of the Sample[w]	LFU (%)[g]	Comments
			Index	Total Exposure	Maximum Exposure			
Vessey et al., 1982	?		6.7	674 Yr.	?	All white; at recruitment aged 25–39 and married; at enrollment, all women had been using the diaphragm, IUD, or pill successfully for at least 5 months	0.3[t,v]	Britain; Oxford/FPA study
Bracher and Santow, 1992	94	14.2				25% aged <20, 66% aged 20–29, 9% aged 30+; 57% parity 0; 92% married or cohabiting	25[t]	Australian Family Survey; first use of method
Westoff et al., 1961	~74		16.7	1,287 Mo.	?	All married; all white	5.7[t]	FGMA study
Cliquet et al., 1977	2,316	17.3				All aged 30–34 living in Belgium; 93% living as married[t]	22[t]	Belgium; 1971 National Survey on Family Development (NEGO II)
Debusschere, 1980	3,561	20.8				Aged 16–44 living in Flanders; 85% married[t]	40[t]	Belgium; 1975–1976 National Survey on Family Development (NEGO III)
Peel, 1972	62		21.9	1,640 Mo.	60 Mo.	All married	2.9[t]	Britain; Hull Family Survey

Notes:
[a] Updated from Trussell and Kost (1987), Table 1.
[c] Calculated by James Trussell from data in the article.
[g] Most of these studies incorrectly report the loss to follow-up probability (LFU) as the number of women lost at any time during the study divided by the total number of women entering the study. Thus, these are the probabilities presented in the table. However, the correct measure of LFU would be a gross life-table probability. When available, gross 12-month probabilities are denoted by the letter "g."
[r] Nonresponse rate for entire survey.
[t] Total for all methods in the study.
[v] The authors report that LFU for "relevant reasons (withdrawal of cooperation or loss of contact)" was 0.3% per year in the 1982 study. In the 1982 study, women had been followed for 9.5 years on average; if 0.3% are LFU per year, then 2.8% would be LFU in 9.5 years. LFU including death and emigration is about twice as high as LFU for "relevant reasons."
[w] Unless otherwise noted, characteristics refer to females.
For table references, see reference section.

Table 31-9 Summary of studies of contraceptive failure: condom[a]

Reference	N for Analysis	Life-Table 12-Month % Pregnant	Pearl Index Pregnancy Rate			Characteristics of the Sample[w]	LFU (%)[g]	Comments
			Index	Total Exposure	Maximum Exposure			
Potts and McDevitt, 1975	397	2.1[b]				77% males ≥ age 40; all married	4.8[c]	Britain; postal trial of spermicidally lubricated condom
Peel, 1972	96		3.9	3,689 Mo.	60 Mo.	All married	2.9[t]	Britain; Hull Family Survey
Glass et al., 1974	2,057	4.2				All white; at recruitment aged 25–39 and married; at enrollment, all women had been using the diaphragm, IUD, or pill successfully for at least 5 months	<1.0[v]	Britain; Oxford/FPA study
Vessey et al., 1988	?		4.4	10,000[c] Yr.	24 Mo.	All white; at recruitment aged 25–39 and married; at enrollment, all women had been using the diaphragm, IUD, or pill successfully for at least 5 months	?	Britain; Oxford/FPA study
Nelson et al., 1997	383	5.0[d]				14% aged <21, 77% aged 21-34, 8% aged 35+; 69% living with partner; 44% nulligravid[t]	4.6[c,d,g]	Avanti plastic condom; random assignment to Avanti plastic or Ramses latex condom
John, 1973	85		5.7[c]	261 Yr.	>7 Yr.	?	?	Britain; retrospective study
Vessey et al., 1982	?		6.0	4,317 Yr.	24 Mo.	All white and aged 25–34; all married at recruitment all women were using the diaphragm, IUD, or pill successfully for at least 5 months	0.3[t,v]	Britain; Oxford/FPA study
Nelson et al., 1997	384	6.4[d]				14% aged <21, 77% aged 21-34, 8% aged 35+; 69% living with partner; 44% nulligravid[t]	4.7[c,d,g]	Ramses latex condom; random assignment to Ramses latex or Avanti plastic condom

(continued)

Table 31-9 Summary of studies of contraceptive failure: condom[a] *(cont.)*

Reference	N for Analysis	Risk of Pregnancy				Characteristics of the Sample[w]	LFU (%)[g]	Comments
		Life-Table 12-Month % Pregnant	Pearl Index Pregnancy Rate					
			Index	Total Exposure	Maximum Exposure			
Jones and Forrest, 1992	1,728	7.2				Aged 15–44[t]	21[r]	NSFG 1988; probability when standardized and corrected for estimated under-reporting of abortion = 15.8[b]
Bracher and Santow, 1992	262	8.1				16% aged <20, 65% aged 20–29, 19% aged 30+; 48% parity 0; 83% married or cohabiting	25[r]	Australian Family Survey; first use of method
Schirm et al., 1982	1,223	9.6[s]				Aged 15–44; all married[t]	18.2[r]	NSFG 1973 and 1976
Grady et al., 1983	1,223	9.7[s,c]				Aged 15–44; all married[t]	18.2[r]	NSFG 1973 and 1976
Vaughan et al., 1977	696	10.1[s]				Aged 15–44; all married[t]	19.0[r]	NSFG 1973
Grady et al., 1986	526	13.8[s]				Aged 15–44; all married[t]	20.6[r]	NSFG 1982
Westoff et al., 1961	~212		13.8[c]	10,062 Mo.	?	All married	5.7[r]	FGMA study

Notes:

[a] Updated from Trussell and Kost (1987), Table 6.

[b] 24-month probability; 12-month probability not published.

[c] Calculated by James Trussell from data in the article.

[d] 6-month probability; 12 month probability not available.

[e] Most of these studies incorrectly report the loss to follow-up probability (LFU) as the number of women lost at any time during the study divided by the total number of women entering the study. Thus, these are the probabilities presented in the table. However, the correct measure of LFU would be a gross life-table probability. When available, gross 12-month probabilities are denoted by the letter "g."

[f] Nonresponse rate for entire survey.

[g] Standardized: Vaughan et al., (1977) (1973 NSFG)—intention (the average of probabilities for preventers and delayers); Grady et al., (1983) (1973 and 1976 NSFG)—intention. Our calculation (the average of probabilities for preventers and delayers); Schirm et al., (1982) (1973 and 1976 NSFG)—intention, age, and income; Grady et al., (1986) (1982 NSFG)—intention, age, poverty status, and parity; Jones and Forrest (1992) (1988 NSFG)—duration, age, marital status, and poverty status.

[t] Total for all methods in the study.

[v] The authors report that LFU for "relevant reasons" (withdrawal of cooperation or loss of contact)" was 0.3% per year in the 1982 study. In the 1982 study, women had been followed for 9.5 years on average; if 0.3% are LFU per year, then 2.8% would be LFU in 9.5 years. LFU including death and emigration is about twice as high as LFU for "relevant reasons."

[w] Unless otherwise noted, characteristics refer to females.

For table references, see reference section.

Table 31-10 Summary of studies of contraceptive failure: minipill[a]

Reference	Method Brand	N for Analysis	Life-Table 12-Month % Pregnant	Pearl Index Pregnancy Rate			Characteristics of the Sample	LFU (%)[g]	Comments
				Index	Total Exposure	Maximum Exposure			
Postlethwaite, 1979	Femulen (Ethynodiol diacetate 0.5 mg)	309	1.1[c]				Aged 17–48	21.0[c]	Britain
Shroff et al., 1987	Femulen (Ethynodiol diacetate 0.5 mg)	425	1.1[n]				72% aged 16–34; 25% nulligravid	12.7[c]	Britain; authors employed by manufacturer
Board, 1971	Micronor (Norethindrone 0.35 mg)	154		1.3	1,882 Mo.	19 Mo.		?	
Keifer, 1973	Micronor (Norethindrone 0.35 mg)	151		1.68	2,141 Mo.	26 Mo.	Aged 18–45; 84% aged 21–35; 74% previous oral contraceptive users; at least 32% current users at start	4.6[c]	
Vessey et al., 1985		?		1.98[c]	404 Yr.	12 Mo.	All white and aged 25–34; all married at recruitment; at enrollment, all women had been using the diaphragm, IUD, or pill successfully for at least 5 months	0.3[tv]	Britain; Oxford/FPA study
Korba and Paulson, 1974	Ovrette (Norgestrel 0.075 mg)	2,202		2.19[c]	29,006 Mo.	67 Mo.		?	Authors employed by manufacturer
McQuarrie et al., 1972	Micronor (Norethindrone 0.35 mg)	318		2.64[c]	3,453 Cy.	27 Mo.	Aged 16–42; mean age = 26; all white	2.2[c]	

(continued)

Table 31-10 Summary of studies of contraceptive failure: minipill[a] (cont.)

Reference	Method Brand	N for Analysis	Risk of Pregnancy					Characteristics of the Sample	LFU (%)[g]	Comments
			Life-Table 12-Month % Pregnant	Pearl Index Pregnancy Rate						
				Index	Total Exposure	Maximum Exposure				
Nelson, 1973	Megestrol acetate (0.5 mg)	342		2.7	3,552 Mo.	41 Mo.		14.6[c]	
Jubhari et al., 1974	Quingestanol acetate (0.3 mg)	382	2.9[n]				Mean age = 23; "predominantly white, single and nulliparous"	14.0	
Hawkins and Benster, 1977	Norethisterone (0.35 mg)	200	6.8				Mean age = 25; postpartum women, 71% within 3 months of delivery[t]	5.2[c]	Britain
Hawkins and Benster, 1977	Megestrol acetate (0.5 mg)	174	8.7				Mean age = 25; postpartum women, 71% within 3 months of delivery[t]	8.4[c]	Britain
Sheth et al., 1982	Levonorgestrel (0.30 mg)	128	9.5[n]				Mean age = 25.7	2.1[t]	Yugoslavia, India
Hawkins and Benster, 1977	Chlormadinone acetate (0.5 mg)	182	9.6				Mean age = 26; postpartum women, 71% within 3 months of delivery[t]	3.3[c]	Britain
Sheth et al., 1982	Norethisterone (0.35 mg)	130	13.2[n]				Mean age = 25.6	2.1[t]	Yugoslavia, India

Notes:

[a]Updated from Trussell and Kost (1987), Table 8.

[c]Calculated by James Trussell from data in the article.

[g]Most of these studies incorrectly report the loss to follow-up (LFU) probability as the number of women lost at any time during the study divided by the total number of women entering the study. Thus, these are the probabilities presented in the table. However, the correct measure of LFU would be a gross life-table probability. When available, gross 12-month probabilities are denoted by the letter "g."

[n]Only net probabilities available for this study.

[t]Total for all methods in the study.

[t]The authors report that LFU for "relevant reasons (withdrawal of cooperation or loss of contact)" was 0.3% per year in the 1982 study. In the 1985 study, women had probably been followed for 12.5 years on average; if 0.3% are LFU per year, then 3.7% would be LFU in 12.5 years. LFU including death and emigration is about twice as high as LFU for "relevant reasons." For table references, see reference section.

Table 31-11 Summary of studies of contraceptive failure: combined oral contraceptives[a]

Reference	Method Brand	N for Analysis	Risk of Pregnancy				Characteristics of the Sample	LFU (%)[g]	Comments
			Life-Table 12-Month % Pregnant	Pearl Index Pregnancy Rate					
				Index	Total Exposure	Maximum Exposure			
Preston, 1972	Norlestrin 2.5 (80%)	378	0.0[c]				Aged 15–46; 46% aged 25–34; 36% white; 64% on pill at start	9.5	Author employed by manufacturer; pill not marketed
Ledger, 1970	Ortho-Novum 1/80	144	0.0[c]				All aged 14–43; mean age = 24; mostly graduate students or wives of students	14.0[c]	
Woutersz, 1981	Lo/Ovral	1,700		0.12	22,489 Cy.	53 Cy.	65% aged 20–29; 55% on pill at start	23.8	Author employed by manufacturer
Korba and Heil, 1975	Ovral	6,806		0.19	127,872 Cy.	110 Cy.	Mean age = 25; 26% white; approximately 80% had not used other contraceptives within 3 months	?	Mexico, Puerto Rico, United States; author employed by manufacturer
Lammers and op ten Berg, 1991	Mercilon	1,684		0.20	25,970 Cy.	36 Cy.	23% aged <20, 51% aged 20–29, 14% aged 30–34; 12% aged 35+	?	Authors employed by manufacturer; Belgium, Denmark, Finland, France, Hungary, Netherlands, Norway, Poland, Sweden, Switzerland, West Germany, Yugoslavia
Ellis, 1987	Ortho-Novum 7/7/7	619		0.22	909[c] Yr.	?	Mean age = 24.5; 40.5% nulligravid	?	United States, Canada, France

(continued)

Table 31-11 Summary of studies of contraceptive failure: combined oral contraceptives[a] (cont.)

			Risk of Pregnancy						
			Life-Table 12-Month % Pregnant	Pearl Index Pregnancy Rate					
Reference	Method Brand	N for Analysis		Index	Total Exposure	Maximum Exposure	Characteristics of the Sample	LFU (%)[g]	Comments
Morigi and Pasquale, 1978	Modicon	1,168		0.24[c]	16,345 Cy.	53 Cy.	Aged 13–54; 85% aged 19–36; 61% previous use of oral contraceptives	?	Mexico, Puerto Rico, Canada, United States; author employed by manufacturer
Hughes, 1978	Ovamin	453	0.24[c]				Aged 16–40; % new users not stated	11.9[c]	Britain
Vessey et al., 1982	50 µg estrogen	?		0.25	10,400 Yr.	24 Mo.	All white and aged 25–34; all married at recruitment; at enrollment, all women had been using the diaphragm, IUD, or pill successfully for at least 5 months	0.3[v]	Britain; Oxford/FPA study
Runnebaum et al., 1992	Ortho-Cyclen	59,701		0.27[c]	342,348 Cy.	6 Cy.	Mean age = 24.0; 32% parous	?	Germany
Royal College, 1974		23,611		0.34	?	48 Mo.	75% aged 20–34; all married/living as married; 62% on pill at start (20% new users)	32.0[c]	Britain
Woutersz, 1983	Nordette	1,130		0.35	11,064 Cy.	31 Cy.	71% aged 20–30; 48% no use of hormones and not pregnant within 60 days of start	8.1[c]	Author employed by manufacturer

(continued)

Table 31-11 Summary of studies of contraceptive failure: combined oral contraceptives[a] (cont.)

Reference	Method Brand	N for Analysis	Life-Table 12-Month % Pregnant	Pearl Index Pregnancy Rate			Characteristics of the Sample	LFU (%)[g]	Comments
				Index	Total Exposure	Maximum Exposure			
Vessey et al., 1982	<50 µg estrogen	?		0.38	3,158 Yr.	24 Mo.	All white and aged 25–34; all married at recruitment; at enrollment, all women had been using the diaphragm, IUD, or pill successfully for at least 5 months	0.3[t,v]	Britain; Oxford/FPA study
Gauthier et al., 1992	Ortho Tri-Cyclen	661	0.57[b]				Mean age = 27.9; 24% nulligravid	?	France; 2 authors employed by manufacturer
Åkerlund et al., 1993	Mercilon	485		0.57[c]	4,543 Cy.	12 Mo.	Mean age = 23.8	?	Denmark, Norway, Sweden; random assignment to Mercilon or Marvelon; cycles excluded if the pill-taking period was less than 18 or more than 33 days or if the pill-free period was less than 5 or more than 9 days
Preston, 1974 and 1972	Norlestrin 2.5 (60%)	1,192		0.63[c]	14,536 Cy.	>18 Cy.	Aged 14–47; 35% aged 25–34; 47% white; 56% on pill at start	13.7	Author employed by manufacturer; pill not marketed
London et al., 1992	Triphasil (Tri-Levlen)	2,124		0.80	11,306 Cy.	6 Cy.	Mean age = 25.5	?	Random assignment to Triphasil or Ortho Tri-Cyclen

(continued)

Table 31-11 Summary of studies of contraceptive failure: combined oral contraceptives[a] *(cont.)*

Reference	Method Brand	N for Analysis	Life-Table 12-Month % Pregnant	Pearl Index Pregnancy Rate — Index	Pearl Index Pregnancy Rate — Total Exposure	Pearl Index Pregnancy Rate — Maximum Exposure	Characteristics of the Sample	LFU (%)[g]	Comments
Åkerlund et al., 1993	Marvelon (Ortho-Cept, Desogen)	497		0.83[c]	4,688 Cy.	12 Mo.	Mean age = 23.1	?	Denmark, Norway, Sweden; random assignment to Marvelon or Mercilon; cycles excluded if the pill-taking period was less than 18 or more than 33 days or if the pill-free period was less than 5 or more than 9 days
Corson, 1990	Lo/Ovral	737		0.94[c]	9,727 Cy.	24 Cy.	Mean age = 24.3	?	Random assignment to Lo/Ovral or Ortho-Cyclen
London et al., 1992	Ortho Tri-Cyclen	2,110		0.94	11,006 Cy.	6 Cy.	Mean age = 25.6	?	Random assignment to Ortho Tri-Cyclen or Triphasil
Preston, 1974 and 1972	Norlestrin 2.5 (40%)	1,393		0.94[c]	15,265 Cy.	>18 Cy.	Aged 13–42; 27% aged 25–34; 39% white; 49% on pill at start	16.3	Author employed by manufacturer; pill not marketed
Endrikat et al., 1995	Mercilon	219		1.04[c]	2,496 Cy.	12 Cy.	Mean age = 25.0	?	Austria, France; random assignment to Mercilon or Meliane; cycles excluded if more than two pills were missed or pill-taking was irregular

(continued)

Table 31-11

Table 31-11 Summary of studies of contraceptive failure: combined oral contraceptives[a] (cont.)

Reference	Method Brand	N for Analysis	Life-Table 12-Month % Pregnant	Pearl Index Pregnancy Rate			Characteristics of the Sample	LFU (%)[g]	Comments
				Index	Total Exposure	Maximum Exposure			
Ellsworth, 1986	Triphasil	1,264		1.09	8,349 Cy.	34 Cy.	All < age 38	?	17 U.S. centers
Archer et al., 1997	Alesse	1,477	1.1[b]				Mean age = 27.0; 47% nulliparous	4.7	Cycles in which 3 or more consecutive active pills were missed and all subsequent cycles from that subject excluded from analysis
Corson, 1990	Ortho-Cyclen	736		1.11[c]	9,351 Cy.	24 Cy.	Mean age = 24.6	?	Random assignment to Ortho-Cyclen or Lo/Ovral
Preston, 1974 and 1972	Norlestrin 1.0 (60%)	1,872		1.47[c]	20,341 Cy.	>18 Cy.	Aged 14–44; 30% aged 25–34; 42% white; 55% on pill at start	13.1	Author employed by manufacturer; pill not marketed
Preston, 1974	Norlestrin 1.0 (20%)	276		1.59[c]	2,449 Cy.	?		?	Author employed by manufacturer; pill not marketed
Vaughan et al., 1977		2,434	2.0[s]				Aged 15–44; all married[t]	19.0[r]	NSFG 1973
Bracher and Santow, 1992		1,830	2.2				42% aged <20, 49% aged 20–29, 9% aged 30+; 67% parity 0; 45% married or cohabiting	25[t]	Australian Family Survey, first use of method

(continued)

Table 31-11 Summary of studies of contraceptive failure: combined oral contraceptives[a] (cont.)

Reference	Method Brand	N for Analysis	Life-Table 12-Month % Pregnant	Pearl Index Pregnancy Rate			Characteristics of the Sample	LFU (%)[g]	Comments
				Index	Total Exposure	Maximum Exposure			
Schirm et al., 1982		4,487	2.4[s]				Aged 15–44; all married[t]	18.2[r]	NSFG 1973 and 1976
Grady et al., 1983		4,487	2.5[c,s]				Aged 15–44; all married[t]	18.2[r]	NSFG 1973 and 1976
Bounds et al., 1979	Microgynon-30	55	2.6[c]				Aged 16–39; mean age = 26; 62% used oral contraceptives as last contraceptive before study	5.5[c]	Britain; probability based on only 12 cycles
Grady et al., 1986		856	2.9[s]				Aged 15–44; all married[t]	20.6[r]	NSFG 1982
Jones and Forrest, 1992		3,041	5.1				Aged 15–44; all married[t]	21[r]	NSFG 1988; probability when standardized and corrected for estimated under-reporting of abortion = 7.3[s]
Preston, 1974	Norlestrin 1.0 (40%)	313		5.80[c]	1,570 Cy.	?		?	Author employed by manufacturer; pill not marketed
Bounds et al., 1979	Loestrin-20	55	5.9[c]				Aged 16–39; mean age = 26; 65% used oral contraceptives as last contraceptive before study	5.5[c]	Britain; probability based on only 12 cycles

(continued)

Table 31-11 Summary of studies of contraceptive failure: combined oral contraceptives[a] *(cont.)*

Reference	Method Brand	N for Analysis	Risk of Pregnancy				Characteristics of the Sample	LFU (%)[g]	Comments
			Life-Table 12-Month % Pregnant	Pearl Index Pregnancy Rate					
				Index	Total Exposure	Maximum Exposure			
Preston, 1974	Norlestrin 2.5 (20%)	178		10.45[c]	871 Cy.	?		?	Author employed by manufacturer; pill not marketed

Notes:

[a] Updated from Trussell and Kost (1987), Table 8.

[b] 12-cycle probability; 12-month probability not available.

[c] Calculated by James Trussell from data in the article.

[d] Most of these studies incorrectly report the loss to follow-up (LFU) probability as the number of women lost at any time during the study divided by the total number of women entering the study. Thus, these are the probabilities presented in the table. However, the correct measure of LFU would be a gross life-table probability. When available, gross 12-month probabilities are denoted by the letter "g."

[e] Nonresponse rate for entire survey.

[f] Standardized: Vaughan et al., (1977) (1973 NSFG)—intention (the average of probabilities for preventers and delayers); Grady et al., (1983) (1973 and 1976 NSFG)—intention. Our calculation (the average of probabilities for preventers and delayers); Schirm et al., (1982) (1973 and 1976 NSFG)—intention, age, and income; Grady et al., (1986) (1982 NSFG)—intention, age, poverty status, and parity; Jones and Forrest (1992) (1988 NSFG)—duration, age, marital status, and poverty status.

[g] Total for all methods in the study.

[h] The authors report that LFU for "relevant reasons (withdrawal of cooperation or loss of contact)" was 0.3% per year in the 1982 study. In the 1982 study, women had probably been followed for 9.5 years on average; if 0.3% are LFU per year, then 2.8% would be LFU in 9.5 years. LFU including death and emigration is about twice as high as LFU for "relevant reasons."

For table references, see reference section.

Table 31-12 Summary of studies of contraceptive failure: IUD[a]

Reference	Method Brand	N for Analysis	Life-Table 12-Month % Pregnant	Characteristics of the Sample	LFU (%)[g]	Comments
Luukkainen et al., 1987	LNg20	1,821	0.1	15% aged 17–25, 60% aged 26–35, 25% aged 36–40; 7% parity 0, 27% parity 1, 50% parity 2, 16% parity 3+	5.7[c]	Denmark, Finland, Hungary, Norway, Sweden
Sivin et al., 1990	LNg20	1,124	0.2	Mean age = 26.6; mean parity = 2.4	5.7[g,x]	Brazil, Chile, Dominican Republic, Egypt, Singapore, United States
Sivin et al., 1990	TCu380A Slimline	698	0.3	Mean age = 28.5; mean parity = 2.7; 47.4% prior IUD use	6.0	Randomized trial of TCu380A and TCu380A Slimline. Egypt, Chile, Sweden, Dominican Republic, Brazil
Sivin et al., 1990	TCu380A	298	0.4	Mean age = 28.1; mean parity = 2.6; 49.0% prior IUD use	9.7	Randomized trial of TCu380A and TCu380A Slimline. Egypt, Chile, Sweden, Dominican Republic, Brazil
Sivin and Stern, 1979	TCu380A	3,536	0.8	72% age 20–29; 64% nulliparous	18.3[n]	
Gibor and Mitchell, 1980	Progestasert	6,261	2.0[n]		?	Authors employed by manufacturer; United States (51%), Canada (5%), and at least 11 other countries
Bracher and Santow, 1992		408	3.9	10% aged <20, 68% aged 20–29, 22% aged 30+; 25% parity 0; 87% married or cohabiting	25[t]	Australian Family Survey, first use of method
Vaughan et al., 1977		576	4.2[s]	Aged 15–44; all married[t]	19.0[r]	NSFG 1973

(continued)

Table 31-12 Summary of studies of contraceptive failure: IUD[a] *(cont.)*

Reference	Method Brand	N for Analysis	Life-Table 12-Month % Pregnant	Characteristics of the Sample	LFU (%)[g]	Comments
Schirm et al., 1982		1,070	4.6[s]	Aged 15–44; all married[t]	18.2[r]	NSFG 1973 and 1976
Grady et al., 1983		1,070	4.8[r,s]	Aged 15–44; all married[t]	18.2[r]	NSFG 1973 and 1976
Grady et al., 1986		235	5.9[s]	Aged 15–44; all married[t]	20.6[r]	NSFG 1982

Notes:

[a]Updated from Trussell and Kost (1987), Table 7.

[c]Calculated by James Trussell from data in the article.

[g]Most of these studies incorrectly report the loss to follow-up (LFU) probability as the number of women lost at any time during the study divided by the total number of women entering the study. Thus, these are the probabilities presented in the table. However, the correct measure of LFU would be a gross life-table probability. When available, gross 12-month probabilities are denoted by the letter "g."

[n]Only net probabilities available for this study.

[r]Nonresponse rate for entire survey.

[s]Standardized: Vaughan et al., (1977) (1973 NSFG)—intention (the average of probabilities for preventers and delayers); Grady et al., (1983) (1973 and 1976 NSFG)—intention. Our calculation (the average of probabilities for preventers and delayers); Schirm et al., (1982) (1973 and 1976 NSFG)—intention, age, and income; Grady et al., (1986) (1982 NSFG)—intention, age, poverty status, and parity.

[t]Total for all methods in the study.

[x]Irving Sivin, personal communication to James Trussell, August 13, 1992.

For table references, see reference section.

Table 31-13 Summary of studies of contraceptive failure: injectables[a]

Reference	Method Brand	N for Analysis	Life-Table 12-Month % Pregnant	Characteristics of the Sample	LFU (%)[g]	Comments
W.H.O., 1988	Depo-Provera 25 mg + Estradiol Cypionate 5 mg (30-Day)	1,168	0.0	Aged 18–35; mean age = 26; proven fertility	11.4[g]	Egypt, Thailand, Mexico, Guatemala, Cuba, Indonesia, Pakistan, U.S.S.R., Philippines, Italy, Hungary, Chile
W.H.O., 1986	Depo-Provera 150 mg (90-Day)	607	0.0	Mean age = 27.7[l]	8.6[g]	7 developing countries
Mishell et al., 1968	Depo-Provera 150 mg (90-Day)	100	0.0[c]	59% aged 21–30	24.0[c]	Injection immediately postpartum
Howard et al., 1982	Norigest 200 mg (56-Day)	383	0.0[c]		6.5[n]	Britain
W.H.O., 1983	Depo-Provera 150 mg (90-Day)	1,587	0.1	Mean age = 27.4[l]	8.1	87% of women from 9 developing countries
W.H.O., 1988	Norigest 50 mg + Estradiol Valerate 5 mg (30-Day)	1,152	0.18	Aged 18–35; mean age = 26.7; proven fertility	10.5[g]	Egypt, Thailand, Mexico, Guatemala, Cuba, Indonesia, Pakistan, U.S.S.R., Philippines, Italy, Hungary, Chile
Sangi-Haghpeykar et al., 1996	Depo-Provera 150 mg (3-Month)	536	0.2	25% nulligravid; mean age = 24.4; primarily low income	5.4[c]	
Scutchfield et al., 1971	Depo-Provera 150 mg (90-Day)	650	0.2[c]	66% aged 20–34; 50% married	6.8[n]	
Schwallie and Assenzo, 1973	Depo-Provera 150 mg (90-Day)	3,857	0.3	86% aged 20–39	18.6	Primarily United States; also Chile, Jamaica, Mexico; authors employed by manufacturer
W.H.O., 1983	Norigest 200 mg (60-Day)	789	0.4	Mean age = 27.4[l]	7.1	87% of women from 9 developing countries
W.H.O., 1986	Depo-Provera 100 mg (90-Day)	609	0.4	Mean age = 27.7[l]	8.2[g]	7 developing countries

(continued)

Table 31-13 Summary of studies of contraceptive failure: injectables[a] *(cont.)*

Reference	Method Brand	N for Analysis	Life-Table 12-Month % Pregnant	Characteristics of the Sample	LFU (%)[g]	Comments
W.H.O., 1983	Norigest 200 mg (84-Day)	796	0.6	Mean age = 27.4[l]	7.4	87% of women from 9 developing countries
W.H.O., 1977	Depo-Provera 150 mg (84-Day)	846	0.7	87% aged 20–34	6.2	10 developing countries
Schwallie and Assenzo, 1972	Depo-Provera 300 mg (180-Day)	991	2.3[n]	88% aged 20–39	28.9	United States, Chile; authors employed by manufacturer
W.H.O., 1977	Norigest 200 mg (84-Day)	832	3.6	84% aged 20–34	5.8	10 developing countries

Notes:

[a]Updated from Trussell and Kost (1987), Table 9.

[c]Calculated by James Trussell from data in the article.

[g]Most of these studies incorrectly report the loss to follow-up (LFU) probability as the number of women lost at any time during the study divided by the total number of women entering the study. Thus, these are the probabilities presented in the table. However, the correct measure of LFU would be a gross life-table probability. When available, gross 12-month probabilities are denoted by the letter "g."

[n]Only net probabilities available for this study.

[l]Total for all methods in the study.

For table references, see reference section.

Table 31-14 Summary of studies of contraceptive failure: Norplant[a]

Reference	Method Brand	N for Analysis	Life-Table 12-Month % Pregnant	LFU (%)[g]	Comments
Sivin et al., 1997a	Norplant-2 (2 Rods)	199	0.0[x]	2.0	Chile, Dominican Republic, Singapore, Thailand, United States; current version with core of rods made of new elastomer; random assignment to new or old version of Norplant-2
Sivin et al., 1997b	Norplant-2 (2 Rods)	600	0.0[x]	0.5	Chile, Egypt, Finland, Singapore, Thailand, United States; current version with core of rods made of new elastomer; random assignment to Norplant-2 or Norplant
Sivin et al., 1997a	Norplant-2 (2 Rods)	199	0.0[x]	0.5	Chile, Dominican Republic, Singapore, Thailand, United States; old version with core of rods made of an elastomer no longer used; random assignment to old or new version of Norplant-2
Sivin et al., 1997b	Norplant (6 Capsules)	598	0.0[y]	0.2	Chile, Egypt, Finland, Singapore, Thailand, United States; current version of capsules made of soft tubing; random assignment to Norplant or Norplant-2
Sivin, 1992	Norplant-2 (2 Rods)	1,389	0.09[y]	1.1[g]	Chile, Dominican Republic, Finland, Sweden, United States; old version with core of rods made of an elastomer no longer used
Sivin, 1992	Norplant (6 Capsules)	2,470	0.09[z]	2.1[g]	Brazil, Chile, Denmark, Dominican Republic, Finland, Jamaica, Sweden, United States; data include both capsules made of hard tubing no longer used and capsules made of soft tubing currently used

Notes:
[a]Updated from Trussell and Kost (1987), Table 9.
[c]Calculated by James Trussell from data provided by Sivin (1992).
[g]Proportion LFU in the first year (number of women LFU in the first year divided by the number entering the study); gross 12-month life-table probabilities denoted by the letter "g."
[x]Proportions becoming pregnant in the second and third years are 0.0% and 0.0%, respectively.
[y]Proportions becoming pregnant in the second and third years are 0.37% and 0.35%, respectively.
[z]Three pregnancies removed because conception preceded implant; if these are included, proportion becoming pregnant is 0.21%. Proportions becoming pregnant in the second, third, fourth, and fifth years are 0.5%, 1.2%, 1.6%, and 0.4%, respectively (Wyeth Laboratories 1990).
For table references, see reference section.

Table 31-15 Summary of studies of contraceptive failure: female sterilization[a]

Reference	Procedure	N for Analysis	Life-Table 12-Month Percent Pregnant	Pearl Index Pregnancy Rate — Index	Pearl Index Pregnancy Rate — Total Exposure	Pearl Index Pregnancy Rate — Maximum Exposure	Characteristics of the Sample	LFU (%)[g]	Comments
Engel, 1978	Laparoscopy	182	0.0[c]				"No failures" presumably some women followed for at least 12 months	?	
Valle and Battifora, 1978	Laparoscopy	165	0.0[c]				"Failure rate after 2 years follow-up is zero" all aged 22–38; 80% had at least 12 months follow-up	?	
Vessey et al., 1983	Procedures other than laparotomy and laparoscopy	345		0.0	331 Yr.	12 Mo.	All white; at recruitment aged 25–39 and married; at enrollment, all women had been using the diaphragm, IUD, or pill successfully for at least 5 months	0.3[v]	Britain; Oxford/FPA study
Chi et al., 1980	Culdoscopy: Pomeroy	392	0.0				Mean age = 32[t]	?	IFRP (19 countries)
Loffer and Pent, 1977	Laparoscopy	1,717		0.0[c]		≥6 Mo.	Duration of follow-up not reported	?	
Chi et al., 1987	Minilaparotomy: Pomeroy	445	0.0[c]				Median age = 32	31.6	IFRP (19 countries)
Peterson et al., 1996	Postpartum partial salpingectomy	1,637	0.06				43% aged 18–27, 38% aged 28–33, 18% aged 34+	8.8	U.S. Collaborative Review of Sterilization
Peterson et al., 1996	Unipolar coagulation	1,432	0.07				20% aged 18–27, 39% aged 28–33, 42% aged 34+	5.0	U.S. Collaborative Review of Sterilization
Bhiwandiwala et al., 1982	Rocket Clip	630	0.18[u]					42.1[c,t]	IFRP (27 countries)

(continued)

Table 31-15 Summary of studies of contraceptive failure: female sterilization[a] (cont.)

Reference	Procedure	N for Analysis	Life-Table 12-Month % Pregnant	Risk of Pregnancy Pearl Index Pregnancy Rate			Characteristics of the Sample	LFU (%)[g]	Comments
				Index	Total Exposure	Maximum Exposure			
Peterson et al., 1996	Bipolar coagulation	2,267	0.23				31% aged 18–27, 35% aged 28–33, 35% aged 34+	10.5	U.S. Collaborative Review of Sterilization
Chi et al., 1980	Minilaparotomy	3,988	0.24				Mean age = 32[t]	?	IFRP (19 countries)
Bhiwandiwala et al., 1982	Electrocoagulation	6,542	0.26[u]					42.1[c,t]	IFRP (27 countries)
Vessey et al., 1983	Laparotomy: all procedures	743		0.28	716 Yr.	12 Mo.	All white; at recruitment aged 25–39 and married; at enrollment, all women had been using the diaphragm, IUD, or pill successfully for at least 5 months	0.3[t,v]	Britain; Oxford/FPA study
Mumford et al., 1980	Minilaparoscopy: Pomeroy	2,022	0.3[u]					?	IFRP (23 countries)
Chi et al., 1980	Electrocoagulation	3,594	0.32[c]					?	IFRP (19 countries)
Bhiwandiwala et al., 1982	Tubal Ring	5,046	0.47[u]					42.1[c,t]	IFRP (27 countries)
Mumford et al., 1980	Minilaparoscopy: Ring	1,324	0.51[u]					?	IFRP (23 countries)
Vessey et al., 1983	Laparoscopy: Tubal Diathermy	776		0.53	755 Yr.	12 Mo.	All white; at recruitment aged 25–39 and married; at enrollment, all women had been using the diaphragm, IUD, or pill successfully for at least 5 months	0.3[t,v]	Britain; Oxford/FPA study

(continued)

Table 31-15 Summary of studies of contraceptive failure: female sterilization[a] *(cont.)*

Reference	Procedure	N for Analysis	Risk of Pregnancy Life-Table 12-Month % Pregnant	Pearl Index Pregnancy Rate Index	Pearl Index Pregnancy Rate Total Exposure	Pearl Index Pregnancy Rate Maximum Exposure	Characteristics of the Sample	LFU (%)[g]	Comments
Chi et al., 1981	Tubal Ring	4,106	0.54[c]					?	IFRP (19 countries)
Peterson et al., 1996	All methods combined	10,685	0.55				33% aged 18–27, 35% aged 28–33, 32% aged 34+	10.8	U.S. Collaborative Review of Sterilization
Chi et al., 1980	Laparoscopy: Rocket Clip	457	0.59				Mean age = 32[t]	?	IFRP (19 countries)
Peterson et al., 1996	Rubber band	3,329	0.59				30% aged 18–27, 36% aged 28–33, 34% aged 34+	12.1	U.S. Collaborative Review of Sterilization
Mumford et al., 1980	Laparoscopy: Rings	4,262	0.60[u]					?	IFRP (23 countries)
Vessey et al., 1983	Laparoscopy: Rings, Clips, etc.	379		0.60	334 Yr.	12 Mo.	All white; at recruitment aged 25–39 and married; at enrollment, all women had been using the diaphragm, IUD, or pill successfully for at least 5 months	0.3[t,v]	Britain; Oxford/FPA study
Peterson et al., 1996	Interval partial salpingectomy	425	0.73				28% aged 18–27, 32% aged 28–33, 40% aged 34+	7.3	U.S. Collaborative Review of Sterilization
Chi et al., 1987	Minilaparotomy: Rings and Clips	1,416		0.79	1,143 Yr.	12 Mo.	Median age = 32 years	13.5	IFRP (19 countries)
Yoon et al., 1977	Falope Ring	902		1.33[c]	3,617[c] Mo.	12 Mo.		21.0[c]	

(continued)

Table 31-15 Summary of studies of contraceptive failure: female sterilization[a] (cont.)

Reference	Procedure	N for Analysis	Life-Table 12-Month % Pregnant	Pearl Index Pregnancy Rate Index	Total Exposure	Maximum Exposure	Characteristics of the Sample	LFU (%)[g]	Comments
Peterson et al., 1996	Spring Clip	1,595	1.82				44% aged 18–27, 30% aged 28–33, 26% aged 34+	16.4	U.S. Collaborative Review of Sterilization
Hulka et al., 1976	Spring Clip	1,079	2.3[c]					9.5[c]	United States, UK, Jamaica, Thailand, Singapore, El Salvador (defective clips)
Chi et al., 1981	Spring Clip	1,699	4.19[c]					?	IFRP (19 countries) (defective clips)
Chi et al., 1980	Culdoscopy; Tantalum Clip	498	8.19				Mean age = 32[f]	?	IFRP (19 countries)

Notes:

[a]Updated from Trussell and Kost (1987), Table 10.

[c]Calculated by James Trussell from data in the article.

[g]Most of these studies incorrectly report the loss to follow-up (LFU) probability as the number of women lost at any time during the study divided by the total number of women entering the study. Thus, these are the probabilities presented in the table. However, the correct measure of LFU would be a gross life-table probability. When available, gross 12-month probabilities are denoted by the letter "g."

[f]Total for all methods in the study.

[i]Study did not report whether the cumulative life-table probability was net or gross.

[v]The authors report that LFU for "relevant reasons (withdrawal of cooperation or loss of contact)" was 0.3% per year in the 1983 study. In the 1983 study, women had probably been followed for 10 years on average; if 0.3% are LFU per year, then 3.0% would be LFU in 10 years. LFU including death and emigration is about twice as high as LFU for "relevant reasons."

For table references, see reference section.

Table 31-16 Summary of studies of contraceptive failure: vasectomy[a]

Reference	N for Analysis	Life-Table 12-Month % Pregnant	Pearl Index Pregnancy Rate			Characteristics of the Sample	LFU (%)[g]	Comments
			Index	Total Exposure	Maximum Exposure			
Moss, 1992	6,220	0.0c					?	1 pregnancy 10 years after vasectomy
Schmidt, 1988	5,000	0.0c					?	Presumably 0 pregnancies
Alderman, 1988	5,331	0.0c				5,331 of 8,879 had at least 2 post-op semen tests	?	Canada; 4 pregnancies, 4.5–8.6 years after vasectomy
Philip et al., 1984	16,039	0.0c				16,039 of 16,796 requested post-op semen samples	?	Britain; 6 pregnancies, 1.3–3 years after vasectomy; 3 pregnancies in first year among 757 men who did not supply post-op semen samples
Kase and Goldfarb, 1973	500	0.0c				2% ≥ age 41	?	1 pregnancy 15 months after vasectomy
Vessey et al., 1982	?		0.08	2,500 Yr.	24 Mo.	Females all white; females at recruitment aged 25-39 and married; at enrollment, all women had been using the diaphragm, IUD, or pill successfully for at least 5 months	0.3[LV]	Britain; Oxford/FPA study
Margaret Pyke Center, 1973	1,000	0.1c				24% ≥ age 41	?	Britain; 1 pregnancy in first year
Klapproth and Young, 1973	1,000	0.2c				35% ≥ age 41	10.0?	2 pregnancies, 3 and 4 months after vasectomy

(continued)

Table 31-16   843

Table 31-16 Summary of studies of contraceptive failure: vasectomy[a] *(cont.)*

Reference	N for Analysis	Risk of Pregnancy					Characteristics of the Sample	LFU (%)[g]	Comments
		Life-Table 12-Month % Pregnant	Pearl Index Pregnancy Rate						
			Index	Total Exposure	Maximum Exposure				
Marshall and Lyon, 1972	200	0.5[c]					Age 25–60; "majority" aged 35–39	?	1 pregnancy 3 months after vasectomy

Notes:

[a]Updated from Trussell and Kost (1987), Table 10.

[c]Calculated by James Trussell from data in the article.

[g]Most of these studies incorrectly report the loss to follow-up (LFU) probability as the number of women lost at any time during the study divided by the total number of women entering the study. Thus, these are the probabilities presented in the table. However, the correct measure of LFU would be a gross life-table probability. When available, gross 12-month probabilities are denoted by the letter "g."

[i]Total for all methods in the study.

[l]The authors report that LFU for "relevant reasons (withdrawal of cooperation or loss of contact)" was 0.3% per year in the 1982 study. In the 1982 study, women had probably been followed for 9.5 years on average; if 0.3% are LFU per year, then 2.8% would be LFU in 9.5 years. LFU including death and emigration is about twice as high as LFU for "relevant reasons."

For table references, see reference section.

Index

pelvic mass, 126-129
premenstrual tension syndrome (PMS), 114-120
vulvar lesions, 120-124
Mestranol, 406
Methotrexate and misoprostol, 690-691
and see Abortion
Mifepristone and misoprostol, 689-690
and see Abortion
Minilaparotomy *see* Sterilization
Minipills, 472-479, 483-484, 496, 503-506; 825 *see also* Progestin-only contraceptives
advantages and disadvantages, 473-479
effectiveness, 472; 825(t)
instructions, 503-506
and lactation, 483-484
and menstrual changes, 496
missed pills, 504-505
precautions, 479
warning signs, 506
Molluscum contagiosum, 122, 202
Mucopurulent cervicitis, 202-203

National Opinion Research Center (NORC), 15, 17-19
National Survey of Family Growth (NSFG), 212-214
Natural family planning, 309
Net reproduction rate, 771
Nongonococcal urethritis, 203-204
Nonoxynol-9, 358; products, 358(t)
Nonvoluntary sexual activity, 20
Norplant, 471-479, 483-484, 488-494, 501-505; 786- 838(t) *see also* Progestin-only contraceptives
advantages and disadvantages, 473-479
effectiveness, 471; 786, 838(t)
insertion, 488-492
instructions, 501-503
and lactation, 483-484
and menstrual changes, 494
missed pills, 504-505
precautions, 479
removal, 492-494
warning signs, 503
No-scalpel vasectomy technique, 567 *see also* Sterilization, Vasectomy

Oligomenorrhea, 105-107
Oral contraceptives, 27, 149; 405-466; 663-664; 787, 827(t)
advantages and disadvantages, 409-418
amenorrhea, 437
brand names, 430(t);

breakthrough bleeding, 439-440
breast tenderness, 441
and cancer, 410, 417-418, 458-459
and cardiovascular disease, 414-416, 425
deep vein thrombosis (DVT), 424-425
depression, 442
drug interactions, 449-450, 456-457; effects of hormones in, 419(t)
effectiveness, 408-409; 780-781, 785, 827(t)
fertility return, 409; 663-664
glucose tolerance effects, 416, 430
headaches, 444-445
influence on sexual behavior, 27
instructions, 450-459
and lactation, 429, 440-441; 602-603
lipids, 411, 416, 437
and menstrual changes, 410; 413, 454-455
missed pills, 452-453
nausea, 446-447
and pelvic inflammatory disease, 425-426
precautions, 420(t)
and pregnancy, 426, 447, 455-456
problems associated with, 437-450
providing, 426-437
and sexually transmitted infection, 413-414
warning signals, 457
weight gain, 447-448
Orgasmic disorders, 38-39
Ovarian cancer screening, 59-61

Pap smear, 44-45
abnormal results, 52-59
reporting systems, 50-52
screening intervals, 51(t)
Pearl index, 769-770
Pelvic inflammatory disease, 204-206; 425-426; 516; 538
and IUDs, 515-538
and oral contraceptives, 425-426
Pelvic mass, 126-129
adenomyosis, 129
benign uterine tumors, 128-129
cysts, 127-128
infection, 127
ovarian cancer, 129
postmenopausal masses, 129
pregnancy-related, 126-127
Periodic health examination guidelines, 3-5(t)

Network

Organizations involved in family planning, reproductive health, and population activities

Advocates for Youth
1025 Vermont Avenue NW, Suite 200
Washington, DC 20005
202-347-5700
202-347-2263 FAX
email: info@advocatesforyouth
http://www.advocatesforyouth.org

AIDS Clinical Trials Information Service (ACTIS)
P.O. Box 6421
Rockville, MD 20849
800-874-2572
301-519-5671 FAX
email: actis@cdcnac.org
http://www.actis.org

Alan Guttmacher Institute (AGI)
120 Wall Street
New York, NY 10005
212-248-1111
212-248-1951 FAX
email: info@agi-usa.org
http://www.agi-usa.org/

American Association of Sex Educators, Counselors, and Therapists
P.O. Box 238
Mount Vernon, IA 52314
319-895-8407
319-895-6203 FAX
email: info@aasect.org
http://www.aasect.org

American College Health Association
P.O. Box 28937
Baltimore, MD 21240
410-859-1500
410-859-1510 FAX
email: acha@acess.digex.net
http://www.acha.org

American College of Obstetricians and Gynecologists (ACOG)
P.O. Box 96920
Washington, DC 20090
202-863-2518
202-484-5107 FAX
http://www.acog.org

American Public Health Association (APHA)
1015 15th Street NW, Suite 300
Washington, DC 20005
202-789-5600
202-789-5661 FAX
email: comments@msmail.apha.org
http://www.apha.org

American Social Health Association (ASHA)
P.O. Box 13827
Research Triangle Park, NC 27709
919-361-8400
919-361-8425 FAX
email: shabro@ashastd.org
http://www.ashastd.org

American Society for Reproductive Medicine (ASRM)
1209 Montgomery Highway
Birmingham, AL 35216
205-978-5000
205-978-5005 FAX
email: asrm@asrm.com
http://www.asrm.com

Association of Reproductive Health Professionals (ARHP)
2401 Pennsylvania Avenue NW, Suite 350
Washington, DC 20037
202-466-3825
202-466-3826 FAX
email: arhp@aol.com
http://www.arhp.org

AVSC International
79 Madison Avenue
New York, NY 10016
212-561-8000
212-779-9439 FAX
email: info@avsc.org
http://www.avsc.org

California Family Planning Council
3600 Wilshire Boulevard, Suite 600
Los Angeles, CA 90010
213-386-5614
213-368-4410 FAX
email: mis2@larfpc.org
http://family.hampshire.edu/fpca/
  larfhome.html

Catholics for a Free Choice
1436 U Street NW, Suite 301
Washington, DC 20009
202-986-6093
202-332-7995 FAX
email: cffc@igc.apc.org
http://www.cath4choice.org

CDC National AIDS Clearinghouse (CDC NAC)
P.O. Box 6003
Rockville, MD 20849
800-458-5231
301-519-6616 FAX
email: aidsinfo@cdcnac.org
http://www.cdcnac.org

Columbia University
Center for Population and Family Health
60 Haven Avenue, B-3
New York, NY 10032
212-304-5261
212-305-7024 FAX
http://cpmcnet.columbia.edu/dept/sph/popfam

Centers for Disease Control and Prevention (CDC)
1600 Clifton Road NE
Atlanta, GA 30333
(Call for mailstop)
404-639-3311
404-639-7394 FAX
email: netinfo@cdc.gov
http://www.cdc.gov

Centre for Development and Population Activities (CEDPA)
1717 Massachusetts Avenue NW, Suite 200
Washington, DC 20036
202-667-1142
202-332-4496 FAX
email: cmail@cedpa.org
http://www.cedpa.org

Committee on Population, National Academy of Science
2101 Constitution Avenue NW, HA-172
Washington, DC 20418
202-334-3167
202-334-3768 FAX
email: cpop@nas.edu
http://www2.nas.edu/cpop/index.html

Contraceptive Research and Development Program (CONRAD)
1611 North Kent Street, Suite 806
Arlington, VA 22209
703-524-4744
703-524-4770 FAX
email: info@conrad.org
http://www.conrad.org

East-West Center Program on Population
1601 East-West Road
Honolulu, HI 96848
808-944-7444
808-944-7490 FAX
email: pop@ewc.hawaii.edu
http://www.ewc.hawaii.edu

Education Program Associates (EPA)
1 West Campbell Avenue
Room 40
Campbell, CA 95008
408-374-3720
408-374-7385 FAX
email: vwoll@epa.org

Emory University Family Planning Program
Department of Gynecology and Obstetrics
69 Butler Street SE
Atlanta, GA 30303
404-616-3709
404-521-3589 FAX
http://www.emory.edu/WHSC/MED/
    FAMPLAN/choices.html

Education and Training Resource Associates (ETR)
P.O. Box 1830
Santa Cruz, CA 95061
408-438-4060
408-438-3618 FAX
http://www.etr.org

Family Health International (FHI)
P.O. Box 13950
Research Triangle Park, NC 27709
919-544-7040
919-544-7261 FAX
http://www.fhi.org

Ford Foundation
320 East 43rd Street
New York, NY 10017
212-573-5000
212-599-4584 FAX
http://www.fordfound.org

Johns Hopkins University
Center for Communication Programs
111 Market Place, Suite 310
Baltimore, MD 21202
410-659-6300
410-659-6266 FAX
email: webadmin@jhuccp.org
http://www.jhuccp.org

Hewlett Foundation
525 Middlefield Road, Suite 200
Menlo Park, CA 94025
650-329-1070
650-329-9342 FAX
http://www.hewlett.org

International Planned Parenthood Federation (IPPF)
120 Wall Street, 9th Floor
New York, NY 10005
212-248-6400
212-248-4221 FAX
email: info@ippfwhr.org
http://www.ippfwhr.org

IPAS
P.O. Box 999
Carrboro, NC 27514
919-967-7052
919-929-0258 FAX
email: ipas@ipas.org

International Union for the Scientific Study of Population (IUSSP)
34, rue des Augustins
B-4000 Liège, Belgium
32-4-222-4080
32-4-222-3847 FAX
email: fdevpop1@vm1.ulg.ac.be

John Snow, Inc.
44 Farnsworth Street
Boston, MA 02111
617-482-9485
617-482-0617 FAX
email: jsinfo@jsi.com
http://www.jsi.com

Kaiser Family Foundation
2400 Sand Hill Road
Menlo Park, CA 94025
650-854-9400
650-854-8037 FAX
email: meic@kff.org
http://www.kff.org

National Abortion Federation (NAF)
1755 Massachussetts Ave., NW
Washington, DC 20036
202-667-5881
202-667-5890 FAX
email: naf@prochoice.org
http://www.prochoice.org

National Abortion and Reproductive Rights Action League (NARAL)
1156 15th Street NW, Suite 700
Washington, DC 20005
202-973-3000
202-973-3096 FAX
email: NARAL@NARAL.org
http://www.naral.org

National Association of Nurse Practitioners in Reproductive Health (NANPRH)
1090 Vermont Avenue NW, Suite 800
Washington, DC 20005
202-408-7025
202-408-0902 FAX
email: nanprh@aol.com
http://www.nurse.org/nanprh

National Family Planning and Reproductive Health Association (NFPRHA)
122 C Street NW, Suite 380
Washington, DC 20001
202-628-3535
202-737-2690 FAX
email: info@nfprha.org
http://www.nfprha.org

National Institute of Child Health and Human Development (NICHD)
Center for Population Research
6100 Executive Blvd, Room 8B07-NIH
Bethesda, MD 20892
301-496-1101
301-496-0962 FAX

Pathfinder International
9 Galen Street, Suite 217
Watertown, MA 02172
617-924-7200
617-924-3833 FAX
email: information@pathfind.org
http://www.pathfind.org

Planned Parenthood Federation of America (PPFA)
810 Seventh Avenue
New York, NY 10019
212-541-7800
800-230-PLAN
212-245-1845 FAX
email: communications@ppfa.org
http://www.plannedparenthood.org

Population Action International (PAI)
1120 19th Street NW, Suite 550
Washington, DC 20036
202-659-1833
202-293-1795 FAX
email: pai@popact.org
http://www.populationaction.org

Population Association of America (PAA)
721 Ellsworth Drive, Suite 303
Silver Spring, MD 20910
301-565-6710
301-565-7850 FAX
email: info@popassoc.org
http://www.popassoc.org

Population Communication Services
Johns Hopkins University
111 Market Street, Suite 310
Baltimore, MD 21202
410-659-6300
410-659-6266 FAX
http://www.jhuccp.org.com

Population Council
1 Dag Hammarskjold Plaza
New York, NY 10017
212-339-0500
212-755-6052 FAX
email: pubinfo@popcouncil.org
http://www.popcouncil.org

Population Institute
107 2nd Street NE
Washington, DC 20002
202-544-3300
202-544-0068 FAX
email: web@populationinstitute.org
http://www.populationinstitute.org

Population Reference Bureau (PRB)
1875 Connecticut Avenue NW, Suite 520
Washington, DC 20009
202-483-1100
202-328-3937 FAX
email: popref@prb.org
http://www.prb.org

Princeton University
Office of Population Research
21 Prospect Avenue
Princeton, NJ 08544
609-258-4870
609-258-1039 FAX
email: opr@opr.princeton.edu
http://opr.princeton.edu/

Program for International Training and Health (INTRAH)
University of North Carolina
208 North Columbia St.
CB #8100
Chapel Hill, NC 27514
919-966-5636
919-966-6816 FAX
email: intrah@med.unc.edu
http://www.med.unc.edu/intrah/

Program for Appropriate Technology in Health (PATH)
4 Nickerson Street
Seattle, WA 98109
206-285-3500
206-285-6619 FAX
email: hgeorges@path.org
http://www.path.org

Reproductive Health Technologies Project (RHTP)
1818 N Street NW, Suite 450
Washington, DC 20036
202-530-2900
202-530-2901 FAX
email:rhtp@basshowes.com

Rockefeller Foundation
420 Fifth Avenue
New York, NY 10018
212-869-8500
212-852-8441 FAX
http://www.rockfound.org

Sexuality Information and Education Council of the United States (SIECUS)
130 West 42nd Street, Suite 350
New York, NY 10036
212-819-9770
212-819-9776 FAX
email: siecus@siecus.org
http://www.siecus.org

United Nations Population Division
Department of Economics and Social Affairs
2 United Nations Plaza
DC 2-1950
New York, NY 10017
212-963-2147 FAX
email: popin@undp.org
http://www.undp.org/popin

United Nations Population Fund (UNFPA)
220 East 42nd Street
New York, NY 10017
212-297-5211
212-297-4915 FAX
email: ryanw@unfpa.org
http://www.unfpa.org/

University of Michigan
Population Studies Center
1225 South University Avenue
Ann Arbor, MI 48109
313-998-7275
313-998-7415 FAX
http://www.psc.lsa.umich.edu/

University of North Carolina
Carolina Population Center
123 West Franklin Street
Chapel Hill, NC 27516
919-966-2157
919-966-6638 FAX
email: cpcnews@unc.edu
http://www.cpc.unc.edu

U.S. Agency for International Development (USAID)
Office of Population
Bureau for Research and Development
G/PHN/POP
Washington, DC 20523
202-712-0869
202-216-3404 FAX
email: jshelton@usaid.gov
http://www.info.usaid.gov/

World Bank
Health, Nutrition and Population Department
1818 H Street NW
Washington, DC 20433
202-473-0632
202-522-3234 FAX
http://www.worldbank.org

World Health Organization
Special Programme of Research, Development, and Research Training in Human Reproduction
1211 Geneva 27
Switzerland
41-22-791-2111
41-22-791-0746 FAX
http://www.who.ch/programmes/hrp/

ARDENT MEDIA, INC.

AN INVITATION TO YOU FROM ARDENT MEDIA

Ardent Media seeks to expand its offerings in the health field, including mental and psychological health. As our name implies, we are open to publishing and distributing information in electronic form as well as print.

We are seeking material in formats such as internet web sites, video, audio and CD-ROM in addition to book and booklet material.

If you or your organization has produced material and is seeking distribution, or is planning to write or produce such material, please contact us.

We prefer that you fax or write us a description of your material prior to sending it. Please write us at Box 286, Cooper Station P.O. New York, N.Y., 10276-0286 or Fax us at (212) 861-0998. Thank you.

Contraceptive Technology
Reader Survey

The authors of *Contraceptive Technology (CT)* ask that you take a few minutes to fill out this survey so they can better meet your needs in providing reproductive health care. Whether you are a new reader or one who has read several editions, we would greatly appreciate your insights.

1. What edition of CT are you looking at as you fill out this questionnaire?

    _____

2. How often do you refer to CT? (Circle answer.)

    First time reader   **Less than once a week**   **Once a week**

    2-3 times a week   **4-5 times a week**

3. How many people usually read your copy of CT?

    One (only you)   **Two 3-5   6-20**

4. What do you find most helpful about the book?

    _____
    _____
    _____
    _____
    _____

5. Which sections do you refer to the most?

    a. _____
    b. _____
    c. _____

6. What aspect or section of the book do you feel is in greatest need of improvement?

    _____
    _____
    _____
    _____
    _____

7. What sections do you refer to the least?

    a. _____
    b. _____
    c. _____

8. What could we do to improve the book to make it more useful to you?

_____

_____

_____

_____

_____

ABOUT YOU

1. Residence (City, State or Province, Country) _____

2. Age: Educational degree:

3. Describe your current position: _____

4. Circle your most important site of work:

   Managed care organization Private practice health department

   Family planning clinic   Hospital   Other _____

5. Circle the number of women you have provided personal contraceptive or STI services in the past year:

   None   1-10   11-100   101-500   501-5000   More than 5000

6. Circle the number of years you have worked part-time or full-time in family planning on reproductive health:

   Less than 1 year   1-2 years   3-5 years   6-10 years   11-20 years

   More than 20 years

7. How many editions of *Contraceptive Technology* (now in its 17th edition) have you owned?

8. Have you attended any of the annual *Contraceptive Technology* conferences

   Yes   No

9. Would you like more information about our conferences?

   No   Yes (fill out address below)

10. Name and address: (optional)

    Name _____

    Address _____

    _____

    City _____ State _____ Zip _____

    Fax _____ email _____

Thank you for taking the time to help us serve you better!
The Authors

Please photocopy or clip out this page and mail to:
Ardent Media
Box 286 Cooper Station P.O.
New York, New York 10276-0286
or Fax to 1-212-861-0998
You may mail or fax it along with your order.

Contraceptive Technology
New Media Survey

As our thank you for completing the new media survey and the ABOUT YOU survey on adjoining page, you will receive a special prepublication discount on any new media published by us.

In addition, the most helpful surveys will receive free access to any web site updates of the book for one year, or a free CD-ROM when published and a free copy of *Safely Sexual* upon publication.

1. Do you use the internet or other new media for any reason?
   ❏ **No** ❏ **Yes** (circle **Internet**   **CD-ROM**)

2. Do you use the internet or other new media to find medical information?
   ❏ **No** ❏ **Yes** (circle **Internet**   **CD-ROM**)

3. Would you be interested in having access to an electronic version of *Safely Sexual or Contraceptive Technology* if it were offered on the Internet or on a CD-ROM?
   ❏ **CT** ❏ **Safely Sexual** ❏ **Both**

4. Would you be interested in receiving electronic updates of *Contraceptive Technology* and/or *Safely Sexual?*
   ❏ **CT** ❏ **Safely Sexual** ❏ **Both**

5. How often would you like to receive electronic updates?
   ❏ Every 3 months   ❏ Every 6 months   ❏ Other

6. Would you be interested primarily in receiving electronic updates of specific chapters of *CT*? If yes, please specify your top 5 choices in order of preference by chapter number. 1____ 2____ 3____ 4____ 5____

7. What would you consider a fair price for an update of a chapter or the entire *CT* book?   chapter _____   book _____

8. Please let us know if you are interested in our plans for a *CT* and *Safely Sexual* CD-ROM. Please indicate below in the right margin what you would consider a fair price for each option.

   ❏ I am interested in a CD-ROM linked to a web site.
   ❏ I am interested in a CD-ROM only.
   ❏ I am interested in a CD-ROM packaged with a copy of the books.
   ❏ I am interested in a CD-ROM with text and illustrations of *CT* or *Safely Sexual* only.
   ❏ I am interested in an enhanced CD-ROM with additional information. such as ❏ audio ❏ video
      ❏ selected readings or source material ❏ color graphics
   ❏ I am interested in approx. _____copies.

9. Please specify any specific subject material you would like to see on a CD-ROM or web site that is not included in *Contraceptive Technology*.
   Please use additional sheet re: above question.

Thank you
Please photocopy or clip out this page and mail to:
Ardent Media
Box 286 Cooper Station P.O.
New York, New York 10276-0286
or Fax to 1-212-861-0998
You may mail or fax it along with your order.

Order Form

Name _____

Address _____

_____

City _____ State _____ Zip _____

Telephone _____

Fax _____ email _____

Method of Payment: ☐ Check ☐ Money Order
☐ Purchase Order (institutions Only) ☐ MasterCard ☐

Credit Card #: _____

Expiration Date _____

Signature _____

Prices are subject to change without notice. All sales final.
No returns. Our standard returns policy applies for bookstores.

Contact Ardent Media for discount information on quantity orders (25 copies or more) at our fax (212) 861-0998 or write to the address in New York on this page.

Description		Unit Price	Quantity	Total
Contraceptive Technology New 17th Edition Emergency Contraception and STI Guidelines	paper	$39.95		
	cloth	$59.50		
Contraceptive Technology 16th Edition AIDS and Abnormal Pap Smears	paper	$14.00		
Alive and Well: A Path for Living in a Time of HIV	paper	$11.95		
The World of Human Sexuality Behaviors, Customs and Beliefs	cloth	$49.95		
Lovemaps	cloth	$19.95		
Helping Women Keep Well	cloth	$16.95		
Safely Sexual* Forthcoming 1999	paper	$16.95		
	cloth	$29.95		
Family Planning at your Fingertips	paper	$19.95		
Emergency Contraception The Nation's Best-Kept Secret	paper	$12.95		

Subtotal

10% Postage and handling (minimum $4.75)

NY residents add sales tax (NYC 8.25%)

TOTAL DUE (US funds only)

*For **Safely Sexual**, order by MasterCard, Visa, or Purchase Order only.

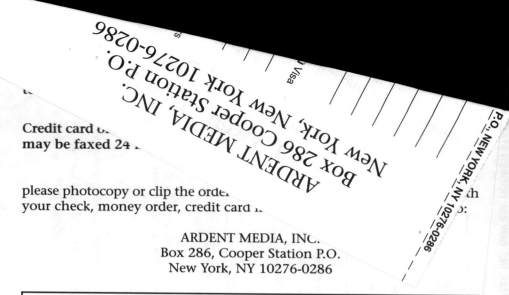

Credit card o...
may be faxed 24 ...

please photocopy or clip the orde...
your check, money order, credit card ...

ARDENT MEDIA, INC.
Box 286, Cooper Station P.O.
New York, NY 10276-0286

This 17th edition of Contraceptive Technology is current until publication of the 18th edition, which is scheduled for release in Fall 2000. Please write or fax ARDENT MEDIA in New York to be notified of the publication of the 18th edition and receive a prepublication discount offer. Please state if you are a nonprofit organization and the number of copies you are interested in purchasing.

Bulk Purchase Discounts: For discounts on orders of 25 copies or more of any book listed on the order form, please fax (212) 861-0998 or write the address above. Please state if you are a nonprofit organization and the number of copies you are interested in purchasing. Bulk discount orders are nonreturnable.

Note to Book Sellers:
All book returns require written permission and label from the publisher. Write to the address above or fax to the number above for permission.

Special Notice to Internet Users:
Contraceptive Technology will soon have its own website. If you would like to be notified, please fax or write us and include your e-mail address, regular mailing address and fax number if available. A chat room is planned for you to communicate with the authors and other readers.

ARDENT MEDIA, INC.
Box 286 Cooper Station P.O.
New York, New York 10276-0286

Order Form

Description		Unit Price	Quantity	Total
Contraceptive Technology New 17th Edition	paper	$39.95		
Emergency Contraception and STI Guidelines	cloth	$59.50		
Contraceptive Technology 16th Edition AIDS and Abnormal Pap Smears	paper	$14.00		
Alive and Well: A Path for Living in a Time of HIV	paper	$11.95		
The World of Human Sexuality Behaviors, Customs and Beliefs	cloth	$49.95		
Lovemaps	cloth	$19.95		
Helping Women Keep Well	cloth	$16.95		
Safely Sexual* Forthcoming 1999	paper cloth	$16.95 $29.95		
Family Planning at your Fingertips	paper	$19.95		
Emergency Contraception The Nation's Best-Kept Secret	paper	$12.95		

*For **Safely Sexual**, order by MasterCard, Visa, or Purchase Order only.

Name _____

Address _____

City _____ State ____ Zip ____

Telephone _____

Fax _____ email _____

Method of Payment: ❑ Check ❑ Money Order
❑ Purchase Order (institutions Only) ❑ MasterCard ❑ Visa

Credit Card #: _____

Expiration Date _____

Signature _____

Prices are subject to change without notice. All sales final.
No returns. Our standard returns policy applies for bookstores.

Contact Ardent Media for discount information on quantity orders (25 copies or more) at our fax (212) 861-0998 or write to the address in New York on this page.

Subtotal	
10% Postage and handling (minimum $4.75)	
NY residents add sales tax (NYC 8.25%)	
TOTAL DUE (US funds only)	

ARDENT MEDIA, INC.
Ordering Information

1-800-218-1535

Credit card orders (VISA or MasterCard) or institutional purchase orders may be placed toll-free 9 A.M. – 5 P.M. EST weekdays at the above telephone number.

Credit card orders (VISA or MasterCard) or institutional purchase orders may be faxed 24 hours to 1-212-861-0998

or

please photocopy or clip the order form on the opposite side and mail with your check, money order, credit card information, or purchase order to:

ARDENT MEDIA, INC.
Box 286, Cooper Station P.O.
New York, NY 10276-0286

This 17th edition of Contraceptive Technology is current until publication of the 18th edition, which is scheduled for release in Fall 2000. Please write or fax ARDENT MEDIA in New York to be notified of the publication of the 18th edition and receive a prepublication discount offer. Please state if you are a nonprofit organization and the number of copies you are interested in purchasing.

Bulk Purchase Discounts: For discounts on orders of 25 copies or more of any book listed on the order form, please fax (212) 861-0998 or write the address above. Please state if you are a nonprofit organization and the number of copies you are interested in purchasing. Bulk discount orders are nonreturnable.

Note to Book Sellers:
All book returns require written permission and label from the publisher. Write to the address above or fax to the number above for permission.

Special Notice to Internet Users:
Contraceptive Technology will soon have its own website. If you would like to be notified, please fax or write us and include your e-mail address, regular mailing address and fax number if available. A chat room is planned for you to communicate with the authors and other readers.